Textbook of Fetal Abnormalities

To my parents, without whose help and support I would not have entered medicine. To Beky, my wife, who means so much to me, and to Gabriella, who has given me so much happiness. *P. T.*

To my family, Dick, Katie, Marianne and David, for all their help and support. *J. M. McH.*

Dedicated to my wife Jean, and children Elizabeth, Rachel and Richard, for their understanding and encouragement. *D. W. P.*

For Churchill Livingstone

Commissioning Editor: Michael J. Houston
Design Direction: Ian Dick

Textbook of
Fetal Abnormalities

Peter Twining FRCR BSc BS MB
Consultant Radiologist, Directorate of Radiology, University Hospital, Queen's Medical Centre, Nottingham, UK

Josephine M. McHugo FRCPCH FRCR FRCP
Consultant Radiologist, Ultrasound Department, Birmingham Women's Hospital, Queen Elizabeth Medical Centre, Birmingham, UK

David W. Pilling FRCPCH FRCR DMRD DCH ChB MB
Consultant Radiologist, The Fetal Centre, Liverpool Women's Hospital, Liverpool, UK

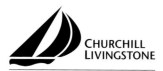

CHURCHILL
LIVINGSTONE

LONDON EDINBURGH NEW YORK PHILADELPHIA ST LOUIS SYDNEY TORONTO 2000

CHURCHILL LIVINGSTONE
An imprint of Harcourt Publishers Limited

© Harcourt Publishers Limited 2000

🌊 is a registered trade mark of Harcourt Publishers
Limited 2000

First published 2000

ISBN 0 443 053294

British Library Cataloguing in Publication Data
A catalogue record for this book is available from the
British Library.

Library of Congress Cataloging in Publication Data
A catalog record for this book is available from the
Library of Congress.

Note
Medical knowledge is constantly changing. As new
information becomes available, changes in treatment,
procedures, equipment and the use of drugs become
necessary. The editors, contributors and the publishers
have, as far as it is possible, taken care to ensure that the
information given in this text is accurate and up to date.
However, readers are strongly advised to confirm that the
information, especially with regard to drug usage,
complies with latest legislation and standards of practice.

The
publisher's
policy is to use
**paper manufactured
from sustainable forests**

Printed in China

Contents

List of contributors

Lenore Abramsky
Senior Research Officer, Department of Medical and Community Genetics, Imperial College School of Medicine, London, UK

R. Bryan Beattie MRCOG MD
Consultant in Fetal Medicine, University Hospital of Wales, Cardiff, UK

Frances A. Bu'Lock MRCP MD
Consultant in Paediatric Cardiology, Glenfield Hospital, Leicester, UK

Lyn S. Chitty MRCOG PhD BSc
Consultant and Senior Lecturer in Genetics and Fetal Medicine, Institute of Child Health, London; Fetal Medicine Unit, Obstetric Hospital, London, UK

Peter A. Farndon
Professor, Clinical Genetics Unit, Birmingham Women's Hospital, Birmingham, UK

Anne S. Garden FRCOG MBChB
Senior Lecturer in Obstetrics and Gynaecology, Honorary Consultant Obstetrician Gynaecologist, Liverpool Women's Hospital, Liverpool, UK

Gail ter Haar PhD MSc DSc(Oxon) MA(Oxon)
Head, Therapeutic Ultrasound, Royal Marsden Hospital, Sutton, UK

David James DCH FRCOG MA MD
Professor of Feto-Maternal Medicine, School of Human Development, University Hospital, Queen's Medical Centre, Nottingham, UK

Mark Kilby MRCOG MD BS MB
Senior Lecturer and Consultant in Fetal Medicine, Division of Reproductive and Child Health, Birmingham Women's Hospital, Birmingham, UK

Josephine M. McHugo FRCPCH FRCR FRCP MB
Consultant Radiologist, Ultrasound Department, Birmingham Women's Hospital; Head of Specialty, Honorary Senior Lecturer, Birmingham University, Birmingham, UK

John J. Morrison MRCOG BSc DCH BAO MD BCh MB
Professor of Obstetrics and Gynaecology, Clinical Science Institute, University College Hospital Galway, Galway, Ireland

David W. Pilling FRCPCH FRCR DMRD DCH ChB MB
Consultant Radiologist, Liverpool Women's Hospital, Liverpool, UK

Sarah A. Russell FRCR ChB MB
Consultant Radiologist, St Mary's Hospital; Honorary Lecturer, University of Manchester, Manchester, UK

Gurleen Sharland FRCP MD BSc
Senior Lecturer and Honorary Consultant, Department of Fetal Cardiology, Guy's Hospital, London, UK

A. Pat M. Smith DRCOG MD MBChB
Honorary Lecturer in Obstetrics and Gynaecology, Aberdeen Maternity Hospital, Aberdeen, UK

Peter Twining FRCR BSc BS MB
Consultant Radiologist, Directorate of Radiology, University Hospital, Queen's Medical Centre, Nottingham, UK

Srinivas Vindla MRCOG BSc MB
Research Fellow, Department of Obstetrics, Derby City General Hospital, Derby, UK

Stephen A. Walkinshaw MRCOG MD BSc(Hons)
Consultant in Fetal and Maternal Medicine, Liverpool Women's Hospital, Liverpool, UK

Michael J. Weston FRCR MRCP ChB MB
Consultant Radiologist, St James's University
Hospital; Honorary Senior Clinical Lecturer,
University of Leeds, Leeds, UK

Martin Whittle FRCP(Glas) FRCOG MD ChB MB
Professor of Fetal Medicine and Academic Head of
Division of Reproductive and Child Health,
Birmingham Women's Hospital, Birmingham, UK

Preface

The field of obstetric ultrasound and in particular, the detection of fetal abnormalities is a rapidly evolving subject. It seemed evident therefore that given the many advances that had occurred in the last few years there was a need for an up-to-date textbook written by recognised experts in the field. It is now over two years since the first editorial meeting took place and the idea of compiling a comprehensive textbook of fetal abnormalities has become a reality.

The textbook is illustrated with state-of-the-art images in order to improve the demonstration of a particular abnormality, backed up with pathological images where appropriate. An accurate pathological diagnosis is essential in terms of auditing the quality of obstetric ultrasound and also to improve the understanding of the various abnormalities concerned. Each chapter is extensively referenced with seminal articles and the most up-to-date papers, so that the references not only support the text, but also can act as a starting point for researching an individual topic in depth.

The editors hope that this textbook will be a standard reference work and will be used in the daily activities of most busy obstetric departments. It is hoped that the book will be of interest to obstetricians, sonographers and radiologists who work in busy departments of obstetrics and obstetric ultrasound. It should also be of interest to clinical geneticists, paediatricians, paediatric surgeons, paediatric pathologists and any other specialist involved in the counselling or management of a mother carrying a fetus with an abnormality.

Finally, the editors would like to thank all the contributors for their excellent chapters. We hope that the textbook will help to answer some of the questions and problems that are encountered in the diagnosis and management of fetal abnormalities.

1999

Peter Twining
Josephine M. McHugo
David W. Pilling

CHAPTER 1

Introduction

Peter Twining

For hundreds of thousands of years the fetus has been an inaccessible patient, surrounded by warm amniotic fluid and protected by the uterine and anterior abdominal walls.

In ancient times congenital abnormalities were only apparent at birth and were probably a cause of wonderment and may even have been considered to have a magical or symbolic importance. Indeed many abnormalities have been incorporated into mythology and legend such as the mermaid based on sirenomelia and the cyclops derived from cyclopia associated with holoprosencephaly.

In the early 20th century major abnormalities such as severe hydrocephalus could be suspected from clinical examination and confirmed by plain radiology. However, it was not until the advent of obstetric ultrasound that the full range of fetal disease could be diagnosed and this ushered in the concept of the fetus as a patient.

The early ultrasound scanners were a far cry from the modern compact ultrasound machines. Static scanning probes attached to heavy gantry assemblies controlled by a myriad of knobs and switches made ultrasound scanning a difficult and time-consuming affair. With the introduction of real time imaging the fetus could at last be visualized with relative ease and images obtained in spite of fetal somersaults and evasive movements.

Over the last 20 years obstetric ultrasound has revolutionized the clinician's approach to the fetus and we have learnt an enormous amount about fetal physiology and also the natural history of fetal malformations and fetal disease.

Each new development of ultrasound has added a little more information to our understanding of the fetus. High resolution images have meant that we can now see finer and finer detail within the fetus (Figs 1.1 and 1.2). In this way fetal structural abnormalities may be better defined and the extent and severity of an anatomical defect clearly outlined (Figs 1.3 and 1.4). Using this information an accurate prenatal diagnosis can be made and this diagnosis together with the likely prognosis can be conveyed to the parents.

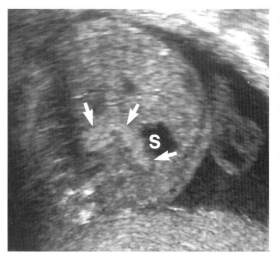

Fig. 1.1 Fetal pancreas. Transverse section through fetal abdomen at 20 weeks' gestation, showing the fetal pancreas (arrows). S, stomach.

This improvement in resolution, however, has also created a number of problems as more and more minor anomalies and normal variants are being detected (Figs 1.5 and 1.6) for which the true significance is not completely established. This does create difficulties when counselling patients and can produce significant maternal anxiety.

Another important development is colour flow Doppler and power colour flow imaging where flow within the arteries and veins can be demonstrated (Figs 1.7 and 1.8). This has contributed significantly to our understanding of the fetal circulation and fetal physiology and is particularly important in the assessment of cardiac disease (Fig. 1.9).

The other major advance is the application of 3D ultrasound to obstetrics and there is no doubt that this will provide a further new insight into fetal disease not only for the parent who will for the first time truly 'see' their baby's abnormality but also for the clinician who will be able to provide more accurate counselling following examination of the 3D images (Fig. 1.10).

It is hoped that this textbook will provide the information to help in the diagnosis of fetal abnormalities and give a concise account of the likely outcome for fetuses once an accurate diagnosis is made.

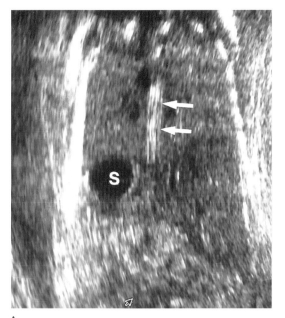 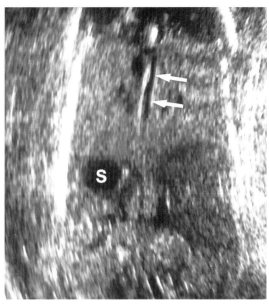

A B

Fig. 1.2 Fetal oesophagus. Coronal section through fetal thorax at 20 weeks' gestation showing fetal oesophagus (arrows). S, stomach. (A) Oesophagus collapsed. (B) Oesophagus during swallowing.

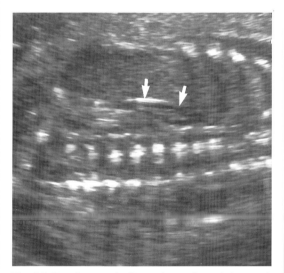 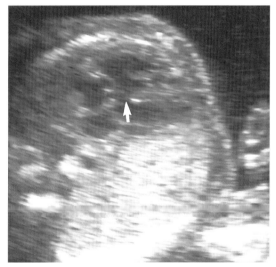

Fig. 1.3 Renal agenesis. Coronal scan through the renal fossa, showing absent kidney and adrenal gland within renal fossa (arrows).

Fig. 1.4 Cystic adenomatoid lung (type III) associated with a ventricular septal defect. Transverse section through fetal thorax, showing displacement of the heart by the dense cystic adenomatoid lung and a ventricular septal defect (arrow).

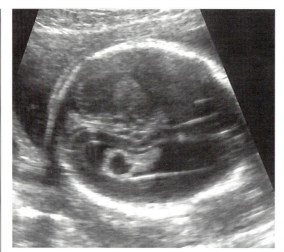

Fig. 1.5 Choroid plexus cyst.

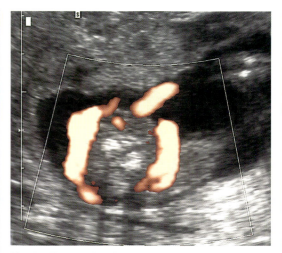

Fig. 1.8 Power colour flow image of neck, showing a nuchal cord.

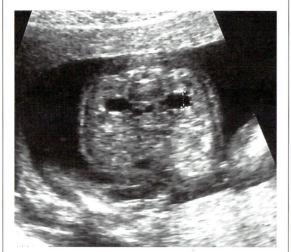

Fig. 1.6 Mild renal pelvic dilatation.

For the parents the diagnosis of a fetal abnormality is usually an unexpected and shattering experience and the approach to the parents is now truly multidisciplinary involving many different clinicians including obstetricians, radiologists, paediatricians, paediatric surgeons and clinical geneticists. In this way each expert in his or her field can help to give the parents as much information as possible. In view of this in addition to

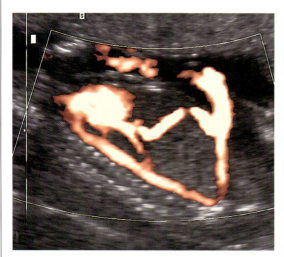

Fig. 1.7 Power colour flow of fetal circulation. Sagittal scan of 20-week fetus, showing fetal circulation.

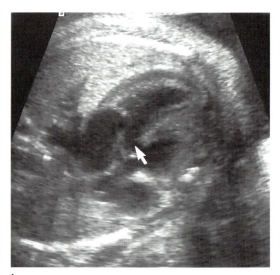

A

Fig. 1.9 Large ventricular septal defect. (A) B-mode image, showing large ventricular septal defect (arrow).

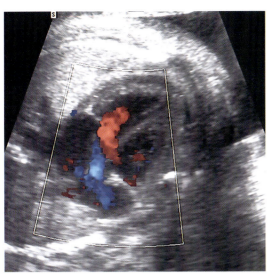

B

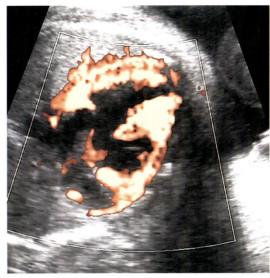

C

Fig. 1.9 Large ventricular septal defect. (B) Colour flow image, showing flow across the defect. (C) Myocardial motion image, highlighting the cardiac wall and enhancing visualization of the defect.

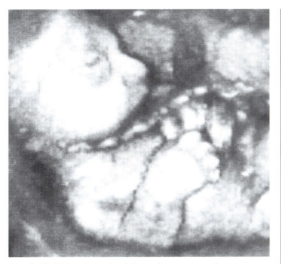

Fig. 1.10 3D picture of a fetus with micrognathia

chapters covering the various types of fetal malformation that may be detected, there are also sections on the geneticists' approach to fetal abnormalities and a section on patient counselling. Also included is a chapter on fetal therapy as some fetal disease is now amenable to treatment. In this respect the ultimate aim has been achieved: once we have the fetal patient it is inevitable there should be fetal therapy.

It is clear therefore that obstetric ultrasound has come a long way from the early days of static scanners and has revealed that long hidden world of the fetus and in so doing has greatly improved our understanding of fetal disease. It has also introduced the possibility of fetal therapy.

CHAPTER 2

Safety of ultrasound

Gail ter Haar

Introduction

It is generally accepted that B-mode ultrasound imaging is a risk-free procedure. The energy levels employed are sufficiently low that there are no significant thermal effects, and it is improbable that any biologically harmful non-thermal effects will occur for this mode. The other commonly used diagnostic mode, Doppler, carries with it the possibility for tissue heating, which, under some circumstances, may be biologically significant. This factor should be taken into account when potentially sensitive targets are exposed to Doppler ultrasound. While the hazard from this technique stems from the ultrasonic field, the risk to the patient arises from the way in which the procedure is carried out. It is therefore essential that those performing ultrasound scans are properly trained, and well versed in the way in which ultrasound interacts with the tissues through which it passes.

This chapter introduces the two mechanisms of heat and cavitation which are thought to be those with the greatest potential for causing tissue damage in an ultrasonic beam. Reported biological effects that have relevance to diagnostic, obstetric ultrasound are then discussed, and existing epidemiological evidence for the safety of ultrasound is reviewed. In conclusion, statements on the safety of ultrasound in clinical use issued by various international bodies are presented, and general recommendations for its safe use are made.

Ultrasonic fields

While it has been demonstrated that Doppler ultrasound can lead to an increase in temperature when it is incident on bone (see p. 11), this is only of biological significance at the highest power levels available. There is, however, evidence that there is an upward trend for output levels of ultrasound machines.

Ultrasonic fields may be described by a number of different parameters. The frequency range used for medical diagnostic transducers is 2 to 20 MHz (1 MHz is 10^6 cycles.s^{-1}). The choice of transducer frequency for any one investigation is determined by the depth of the tissues of interest, the lowest frequencies being used for the deepest sites. The choice of frequency has some bearing on the biophysical effects produced in tissue. At high frequencies, the attenuation (and thus the absorption) is largest, and so thermal effects may be expected to be greatest, whereas at low frequencies, it is cavitation that may be of most concern.

An ultrasound wave may be described as a pressure wave, the local pressure at any point in the beam oscillating between two values, one (positive pressure amplitude, p^+) being greater, and the other (negative pressure amplitude, p^-) being less than ambient pressure. The ultrasonic field is often described in terms of the peak positive and negative pressures found in the beam. Typically, these are in the range 1 to 5 MPa (1 MPa is 10 bar).

Another descriptor of the ultrasonic field is its total energy. This is the total energy emitted from the transducer, and is typically between 100 and 300 mW for a diagnostic probe. The heating potential of a beam can be characterized by the total power. The ultrasound field is bounded in space, and may be emitted in short pulses. For B-mode imaging the pulses are typically 1 μs long, whereas for pulsed Doppler the pulses are longer, typically of 10 μs lengths. The number of pulses emitted per second (pulse repetition frequency) varies from 1 kHz for B-mode applications to 10 kHz for Doppler devices. Intensity is defined as the energy crossing unit area in unit time, and this is the parameter often used to characterize an ultrasound beam. It has the units of Watt.cm^{-2}. Since the ultrasound pressure distribution varies both in time and in space, a number of different intensity parameters may be defined. The most commonly quoted are both averages over time. These are the spatial peak, temporal average intensity (I_{SPTA}) and the spatial average, temporal

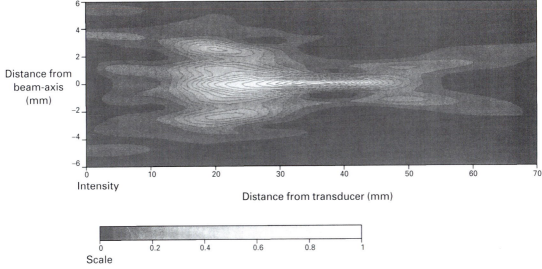

Distance from beam-axis (mm)

Intensity

Distance from transducer (mm)

Scale

Fig. 2.1 Spatial distribution of the time-averaged intensity from a typical diagnostic ultrasound transducer. It can be seen that the peak intensity is about 35 mm from the transducer face. (Courtesy of the National Physical Laboratory.)

average intensity (I_{SATA}). Figure 2.1 shows the distribution of the time-averaged intensity in space for a diagnostic transducer. The spatial peak intensity (I_{SPTA}) lies around 35 mm from the transducer face. I_{SPTA} reflects the highest energy to be found in the beam, whereas I_{SATA} represents the average energy over the area of interest. I_{SPTA} is thus higher than I_{SATA}. In these intensities, the time interval over which the average is taken is 1 s. An alternative time interval is the duration of a pulse, which gives us pulse-averaged intensities.

Henderson et al[1] surveyed the outputs of a number of common diagnostic scanners. They compared their results with those obtained 4 years earlier by Duck & Martin.[2] The results are summarized in Figures 2.2 to 2.5, which show the ranges of values obtained, and the mean value, for M-mode, B-mode, pulsed Doppler and colour Doppler modes.

There appears not to have been any significant change in the peak negative pressure over the 4 years between the two surveys (1991–1995) (Fig. 2.2). The mean and maximum values of I_{SPTA} increased for all modes of operation, with the scanned modes showing greatest increase (Fig. 2.3). The mean I_{SPTA} in B-mode increased six-fold, while that for colour Doppler more than

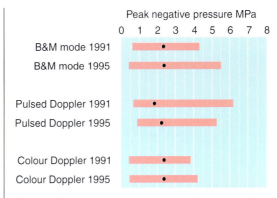

Fig. 2.2 Bar chart showing the range of peak negative pressure measured in different modes in two surveys, 4 years apart.[1,2] The average value is shown [●].

doubled. Where the data were available, a similar result was found for intracavitary probes (Fig. 2.4) (Duck & Martin did not give values for pulsed Doppler for these probes). The mean I_{SPTA} in B-mode had increased by nearly a factor of five.

A study of the change in total acoustic power over the 4 years between the two surveys shows that, while the total power for M-mode has remained more or less constant, that in B-mode is generally higher, and for pulsed Doppler, the maximum and mean powers are approximately doubled (Fig. 2.5).

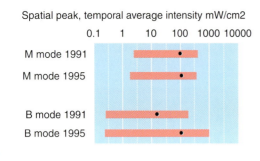

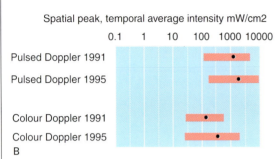

A

B

Fig. 2.3 Bar charts showing the change in spatial peak, temporal average intensity (I_{SPTA}) in two surveys, 4 years apart.[1,2] The range of values measured, and the mean [●] are shown. (A) M- and B-modes. (B) Pulsed Doppler and colour Doppler modes.

These results emphasize the importance of keeping a vigilant eye on the safety of diagnostic ultrasound. If acoustic outputs continue to increase, then applications that may once have been thought to be hazard-free may become so no longer. This is especially important, of course, in obstetrics, where the target of interest, the developing embryo or fetus, represents probably the most biologically sensitive tissue ever exposed to diagnostic ultrasound.

Thermal effects

As an ultrasonic wave travels through tissue, its energy content is reduced. This attenuation of the beam's energy is due to the two processes of scattering and absorption. Energy that is scattered back from the forward beam direction is used to form an ultrasound image or to give the required Doppler information. The energy absorbed from the beam gives rise to tissue heating.

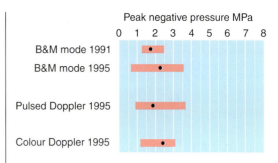

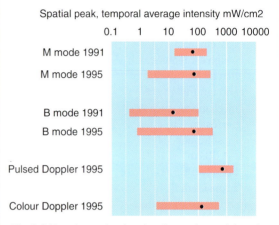

Fig. 2.4 Bar charts showing the change in spatial peak, temporal average intensity (I_{SPTA}) and in peak negative pressure for intracavitary probes, in two surveys, 4 years apart.[1,2] The range of values measured, and the mean [●] are shown.

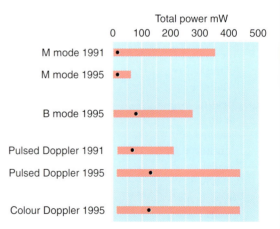

Fig. 2.5 Bar chart showing the change in total power, obtained in two surveys, 4 years apart.[1,2] The range of values measured, and the mean [●] are shown.

Roughly, an ultrasonic beam that has intensity I_0 at the transducer has a reduced intensity I_x after it has travelled a distance x from the transducer, where $I_x = I_0 e^{-\mu x}$. Here μ is the intensity attenuation coefficient for the medium through which the beam has travelled. The energy lost from the beam is given by μI, of which 60 to 90% is absorbed.[3] If we consider a tissue for which the attenuation coefficient is 2.6 dB.cm^{-1} and the density is 1 g.cm^{-3} (such as, for example, liver at 3 MHz), we can calculate that the temperature rise induced by an intensity of 1 W.cm^{-2} is 0.14°C.s^{-1} (8.64°C.min^{-1}). This rough estimate of temperature rise assumes that all the attenuated energy is absorbed, and ignores any tissue cooling from mechanisms such as conduction or perfusion. The attenuation coefficients for most human soft tissues are very similar[4] (~1 dB.cm^{-1} at 1 MHz), although skin has a higher value (~4 dB.cm^{-1} at 1 MHz). Bone has a considerably higher attenuation than the soft tissues (~10 dB.cm^{-1} at 1 MHz). This coefficient is frequency (f) dependent, varying as $f^{1.1}$ for the soft tissues, and as f^2 for bone.[5] Thus, as the frequency is increased, the amount of tissue heating for a given intensity may also be expected to increase.

As a general 'rule of thumb', the amount of heating obtained will be increased by a factor three on moving from one imaging mode to the next in the order: simple imaging (lowest), M-mode, colour Doppler imaging, and pulsed Doppler (highest).[6]

Assessment of the hazard arising from a given temperature rise draws largely on the thermal teratology literature. The limitation of this data base is that it deals mainly with whole body and large volume heating. Heating as a result of a diagnostic ultrasound beam will be limited to the (relatively small) scanned volume. Despite this, useful conclusions may be drawn from the data available.

When pregnant animals are exposed to hyperthermia, a number of effects ranging from abortion and stillbirth to small or malformed offspring may result. The severity of the reaction depends, amongst other factors, on the stage of pregnancy and the nature of the heat exposure. If the hyperthermia is experienced during the pre-implantation stage, it is likely that the embryo will either die, or survive to develop normally. Developmental defects occur when there is a hyperthermic insult at the relevant susceptible stage of gestation, the early stages of organogenesis being the most sensitive. Non-proliferative tissues are the least sensitive to thermal damage. Neural tube defects, microphthalmia and microcephaly have all been induced by heat in experimental animals.[7] There is considerable debate as to whether it is the absolute temperature or the temperature rise above the normal that is important in predicting effects.

Experimental measurement of the temperature rise induced by ultrasonic beams has concentrated mainly on the interface between bone and soft tissue because of the high energy absorption in bone. Bosward et al[8] studied the temperature rises induced in fetal guinea pig brains, both in the mid-cerebral region, and next to the occipital and parietal bones. They found that temperature rises were greatest next to bone, and that these increased with increasing mineralization (gestational age). While the mid-brain temperatures never exceeded 1°C in the live animal for 260 mW incident power at 3.2 MHz, the temperature at the bone surface rose by 5.2°C for the oldest fetuses studied. Drewniak et al,[9] in a study using fetal femurs, also demonstrated an increase in temperature rise with advancing gestational age. Duggan et al[10] have measured the rise in temperature due to 3.5 MHz pulsed Doppler exposures of the brain of the fetal sheep in utero (124 days' gestation, where term is 147 days). In these studies, the thermocouple probe was placed within the first millimetre of depth subdurally, in the cerebral cortex. The transducers were operated at 600 mW (I_{SPPA} 8.9 W.cm^{-2}, I_{SPTA} 0.3 W.cm^{-2}) and 2 W (I_{SPPA} 27.3 W.cm^{-2}, I_{SPTA} 1.7 W.cm^{-2}). The maximum temperature rises recorded for these two powers were 3°C (600 mW) and 12.5°C (2 W) in the dead fetus, and 1.7°C (600 mW) and 8.8°C (2 W) in the live, perfused, fetus. Exposure times were 120 s.

In the perfused animals, the temperature reached after 80 s was 1.5°C for the lower power and about 10.5°C for the higher power. Equilibrium was being approached by 120 s. It can be seen in Figure 2.5 that machines do not currently have maximum power levels as high as 600 mW, the peak in 1995 reaching 440 mW with a mean of 124 mW.[1] In 1995, the USA Food and Drug Administration (FDA) limited the in situ I_{SPTA} to 720 mW.cm^{-2} for machines that have an output display (see p. 15), and to 94 mW.cm^{-2} for those that do not. It is very unlikely that the lower output devices would lead to significant brain heating in the human fetus, but Duggan et al's results[9] would indicate that this possibility exists for the higher powered machines. This emphasizes the importance for operators to be aware of the heating potential of Doppler beams. Clearly there is the need for considerably more research into this topic. An interesting approach, that allows rapid comparison of bone heating from different ultrasound devices, is that of O'Neill et al[11] who have demonstrated comparable temperature rises in a tissue–bone phantom. It is also clear that, in the absence of bone, the temperature rises induced, even by the highest power clinical machines, are likely to be biologically insignificant.[12]

Duggan & McCowan[13] found, for pulsed Doppler ultrasound examination of the carotid artery for singleton pregnancies between 18 and 38 weeks of gestation, that the median scan time was 31 s. It is probable that this is typical of the time that Doppler probes are held stationary during any examination. There is a well-established relationship between thermal exposure time and the severity of a hyperthermic effect.[14] Miller & Ziskin[15] conducted a literature review of thermal bio-effects and showed that a temperature of 43°C can be maintained without hazard for 1 min, 44°C for 30 s. It is therefore clear that, where high temperatures may be expected, care should be taken not to hold the probe stationary for longer than necessary to get the required diagnostic information.

The World Federation for Ultrasound in Medicine and Biology (WFUMB)[16] surveyed the existing literature in 1992 and issued the following statements:

1. *Based solely on a thermal criterion, a diagnostic exposure that produces a maximum temperature rise of 1.5°C above normal physiological levels (37°C) may be used without reservation in clinical examinations.*
2. *An in situ temperature rise to, or above, 41°C (4°C above normal temperature) for 15 minutes should be considered hazardous in embryonic and fetal exposures; the longer this temperature is maintained, the greater is the likelihood for damage to occur.*

An additional statement designed to cover the possibility of abnormal maternal physiological states which may enhance sensitivity to heat-induced damage was added:

3. *The possible influence of potentiating factors should also be considered. This indicates that Doppler ultrasound in a febrile patient might present an additional embryonic and fetal risk.*

While these statements are useful from a biological standpoint, it remains difficult for the clinical ultrasound user to judge the temperature rise being induced in a scanned tissue volume while an examination is being conducted. The thermal index (see p. 15) has been introduced to help with this assessment.

Cavitation

Acoustic cavitation, a term used to describe the behaviour of gas bubbles in an acoustic field, has had a number of definitions.[17] In the context of ultrasound safety the definition: 'the formation and activity of gas- or vapour-filled cavities (bubbles) in a medium exposed to an ultrasonic field'[17] seems the most useful. This definition encompasses both the formation and subsequent activity of micron-sized resonant bubbles and the action of ultrasound on larger, stabilized gas spaces, such as occur in the lung.

Two types of cavitation have been identified, namely non-inertial (stable) and inertial (collapse or transient). Stable cavities oscillate in response to an applied ultrasonic pressure field. The bubble's diameter varies about an equilibrium value and the bubble can exist for a large number of cycles. Acoustic streaming (motion of fluids) and high shear stresses may be associated with stable cavitation. Inertial cavitation (previously termed collapse or transient cavitation) occurs when a gas-filled cavity expands during part of the acoustic cycle and then collapses very rapidly to a tiny fraction of its original volume. At the point of collapse, very high temperatures and pressures may be produced, and associated with these may be light emission, the formation of reactive chemical species and tissue destruction. Where inertial cavitation has taken place, vacuoles can be seen under histological examination. The shear stresses associated with bubble oscillation result in damage such as membrane disruption.[18] The potential for cavitation damage does not depend strongly on the imaging mode being used, since average pulse amplitudes are much the same for each mode.[6]

Experimental evidence, from work carried out in liquids, gels and mammalian tissues, indicates that acoustic cavitation associated with the activity of microbubbles is unlikely to be an important source of hazard when clinical diagnostic ultrasound examinations take place. However, evidence has come to light that suggests that damage can occur, under some experimental circumstances, when low ultrasound exposure levels are incident on pre-existing stabilized gas bodies such as the alveoli in the lung. Following the demonstration that extracorporeal shock wave lithotripsy (ESWL) could cause haemorrhage in canine lungs,[19] a flurry of experiments using pulsed ultrasound exposures was published. Lung haemorrhage has been induced in mouse lungs following exposures to ultrasound pulses with amplitudes around 1 MPa.[20–24]

Tarantal & Canfield[25] have seen evidence for haemorrhage in monkey lungs, and both Harrison et al[26] and Zachary et al[24] have reported some damage in the lungs of minipigs. The effect appears to be more marked in young animals than in adults, and does not occur in animals exposed in utero, where the lungs are fluid filled. The mechanism by which this damage is caused is not understood, and neither is the physiological significance. However, it appears that the presence of stabilized gas bodies results in damage from lower ultrasound exposures than those required to cause damage in the absence of gas.

Haemorrhage has also been demonstrated in the mouse intestine. Miller & Thomas[27] implicated thermal mechanisms in the production of intestinal haemorrhage by 1 MHz continuous wave ultrasound, whereas Dalecki et al[28] found haemorrhage in the absence of significant heating. As with the lung haemorrhage, stabilized gas bodies are necessary for the induction of this effect at diagnostic exposure levels.

Dalecki et al[29] have used ESWL to demonstrate haemorrhage induced in fetal tissues following exposure of late-term, pregnant mice. The haemorrhage was always seen in tissues near developing bone or cartilaginous structures such as the head, limbs or ribs. The investigators hypothesize that this effect is due to relative motion of the soft tissue and the partially ossified bones, leading to tearing of fragile blood vessels. The pressure threshold quoted is similar to that for lung haemorrhage.

Epidemiological evidence

While laboratory studies give important insight into the mechanisms by which ultrasound may constitute a hazard to the developing fetus, problems of scaling and species differences mean that it is important to consider the results from epidemiological surveys when assessing the safety of diagnostic ultrasound usage in humans.

We can be reasonably certain that diagnostic ultrasound does not cause damage on a large scale since this would already have become obvious. Epidemiological surveys have therefore concentrated on possible subtle effects, including those indicated by laboratory studies.

The clearest answer to the various questions addressed by epidemiology has come from two studies concerned with the possibility that there could be a relationship between ultrasound received in utero (B-mode and continuous wave Doppler), and childhood malignancies.[30,31] Neither of these two large case control surveys could find an association between ultrasound exposures in utero and the incidence of childhood cancer. This correlates well with the findings of laboratory experiments designed to study ultrasonically induced genetic effects, which give no indication that medical ultrasound is capable of inducing mutations in mammalian tissues in vivo. This finding is true for exposures for which inertial cavitation does not occur.[32]

A number of experimental studies has indicated that there might be a connection between ultrasound and reduction in birthweight, although this has not been a consistently reproducible finding.[33–35] Similarly, epidemiological studies of birthweight have yielded contradictory results, although the balance of evidence indicates that there is no correlation with ultrasound exposure. Early surveys[36–38] involved B-mode examination of the mother, and while two[36,37] showed no difference in birthweight between the experimental and control groups, a third[38] showed an increase in weight in the scanned group. A more recent survey[39] of mothers, who were offered five Doppler ultrasound examinations in the third trimester, showed a statistically significant increase in the number of babies with birthweight below the 10th centile, with a non-significant decrease in mean birthweight of 25 g. Unfortunately, since decreased birthweight was not a prior hypothesis of this study, there are methodological concerns with this report. However, the finding indicates that further investigation may be warranted. Whatever the result of future studies, it should be remembered that the exposure pattern used in this last survey[39] was atypical of common obstetric management. It is interesting that apparently, on the one hand, B-mode ultrasound can lead to an increase in birthweight,[38] while, on the other, Doppler exposures can lead to a decrease.[39]

Two studies have explored the possible relationship between in utero ultrasound exposures and delayed speech in children. In a Canadian survey[40] 72 children were matched with 144 controls. It was found that children exposed to ultrasound at least once in utero had a higher probability of exhibiting speech delay than those who were not. In contrast, a Norwegian randomized, follow-up study[41] demonstrated that ultrasonically exposed children were less likely to be referred to a speech therapist than their unexposed counterparts. Neither study is perfect. The Canadian study was not assessed blind, and so may have laid itself open to mis-classification, while speech delay was not a prior hypothesis of the otherwise well-designed Norwegian study, and so the finding may have been a result of chance. This subject is therefore still open, and a properly designed prospective study is indicated.

A number of neurological developmental end points have been studied. Scheidt et al[42] looked at 123 variables at birth and at 1 year. There was no difference between exposed and unexposed children for 121 of these variables, although there was a statistically significant higher proportion of children with abnormal grasp or tonic neck reflex in the experimental group. The biological importance of this is uncertain, and the result may be due to the influence of chance in multiple hypothesis testing. Stark et al[43] looked at 16 outcomes including hearing, visual acuity, colour vision, cognitive function, behaviour and a complete neurological examination. They could find no association between ultrasound and these outcomes. They did, however, find that a significantly greater proportion of ultrasound exposed children were dyslexic.

While there were some questions about the statistical methods used in this study, it is clear that further work was necessary on this topic. Salvesen et al[44,45] undertook a survey of various aspects of childhood development. The ultrasound exposures were 'routine' and were carried out during weeks 19 and 32 of pregnancy. There was no increased prevalence of dyslexia,[44] or adverse effect on visual acuity or hearing.[45] However, a possible association between ultrasound in utero and non-right-handedness was highlighted.[46] While this was a weak association, it is important that this study should be repeated, and if the results were to be replicated, then it would be essential to identify the biological mechanism causing the effect.

Output display

In this chapter, mention has been made of thermal and cavitational effects. However, it can be difficult to predict the extent of these effects during any one diagnostic ultrasound examination. In order to help the user, the USA has introduced an Output Display Standard (ODS).[47] This standard was, in part, drawn up in response to the FDA's regulations.[48] The FDA set application-specific, maximum, intensity levels in 1985. For fetal, abdominal, intra-operative, small organ, neonatal and adult cephalic imaging, the maximum permitted I_{SPTA} level was 94 mW.cm^{-2}, for peripheral vascular applications it was 720 mW.cm^{-2} and for cardiac applications 430 mW.cm^{-2}. Manufacturers may still opt to restrict outputs to these maxima (Track 1 declaration), but many feel that this is unduly restrictive. They can instead now apply a maximum I_{SPTA} of 720 mW.cm^{-2} to all applications, provided that they provide the facility to display the indices defined within the ODS (Track 3). This standard defines two biophysical indices: the thermal index and the mechanical index. If these indices are displayed in real time, the educated operator has information available which helps in making decisions about the risk:benefit ratio of the investigation underway. The thermal index, TI, is defined by the equation:

$$TI = W_0/W_{DEG}$$

where W_0 is the source power of the transducer and W_{DEG} is the source power required to increase the tissue temperature by 1°C. The ODS describes the theoretical algorithms drawn up to calculate W_{DEG} for a large number of different tissue models and transducer configurations. The calculations are designed to be reasonably conservative, while taking perfusion into account. Three different thermal indices are identified: the soft tissue thermal index (TIS), the bone thermal index (TIB), and the cranial bone thermal index (TIC). These three indices reflect the areas for concern on thermal grounds. The two bone indices differ in that TIC is meant to cover situations in which bone lies at the surface, whereas TIB is designed for use when bone lies at the ultrasound beam's focus. An example of the application of TIB is in second and third trimester fetal imaging. TIC would be used, for example, in adult cephalic imaging.

The mechanical index, MI, is intended to provide information about the non-thermal biophysical processes in the beam. It is defined by:

$$MI = p_r/\sqrt{f}$$

where p_r is the peak rarefactional pressure in MPa, reduced (derated) to take into account tissue attenuation in the beam path, and f is the ultrasonic frequency (MHz). An attenuation of 0.3 dB.cm^{-1}.MHz^{-1} is assumed. The basis for this formula is largely empirical.

The ODS requires that these indices should be displayed if the equipment has sufficiently high output that TI or MI may reach a value greater than unity. If this possibility exists, then the index must be displayed from a value of 0.4. This allows the operator to know when the system is approaching critical values of the indices and to make appropriate clinical decisions. The International Electrotechnical Commission (IEC) has a different approach to this topic, namely to classify ultrasonic fields in terms of those that can be used without any concern for hazard, and those for which a hazard may exist. One way in which this may be achieved is by defining suitable threshold values for the thermal and mechanical indices and to use these for allocating fields to the different classes; another is to define thresholds for temperature rise and pressure amplitude, values above which may constitute some hazard to the patient.

Clinical safety statements

The European Federation of Societies for Ultrasound in Medicine and Biology issued a clinical safety statement in 1998[49] which reads:

> Diagnostic ultrasound has been widely used in clinical medicine for many years with no proven deleterious effects. However, as the use of ultrasound increases, with the introduction of new techniques, with a broadening of the medical indications for ultrasound examinations, and with increased exposure continuous vigilance is essential to ensure its continued safe use.
>
> A broad range of ultrasound exposure is used in the different diagnostic modalities currently available. Doppler imaging and measurement techniques may require higher exposure than those used in B- and M-modes, with pulsed Doppler techniques having the potential for the highest levels.
>
> Modern equipment is subject to output regulation. The recommendations contained in this statement assume that the ultrasound equipment being used is designed to international or national safety requirements and that it is used by competent and trained personnel.

B- and M-modes
Based on scientific evidence of ultrasonically induced biological effects to date, there is no reason to withhold B- or M-mode scanning for any clinical application, including the routine clinical scanning of every woman during pregnancy.

Doppler for fetal heart monitoring (CTG)
The power levels used for fetal heart monitoring (CTG) are sufficiently low that the use of this modality is not contra-indicated, on safety grounds, even when it is to be used for extended periods.

Doppler mode (Colour flow imaging, power Doppler & pulsed Doppler)
Exposure used in Doppler modes are higher than for B- and M-modes. There is considerable overlap between the ranges of exposure which may be used for colour flow imaging and power Doppler, and for pulsed Doppler techniques. The clinical user should be aware that pulsed Doppler at maximum machine outputs and colour flow imaging with small colour boxes have the greatest potential for biological effects.

In general, the informed use of Doppler ultrasound is not contra-indicated. However, at the maximum machine output settings, significant thermal effects at bone surfaces cannot be excluded. The user is advised to make use of any exposure information provided by the manufacturer (for example in the form of displayed safety indices) to gain awareness of the highest output conditions, and to act prudently to limit exposure of critical structures, including bone and regions including gas. Where on-line display is not available, particular care should be taken to minimize exposure times.

Ultrasound exposure during pregnancy
The embryonic period is known to be particularly sensitive to any external influences. Until further scientific information is available, investigations using pulsed or Doppler ultrasound should be carried out with careful control of output levels and exposure times.

With increasing mineralization of the fetal bone as the fetus develops the possibility of heating fetal bone increases. The user should prudently limit exposure of critical structures such as the fetal skull or spine during Doppler studies.

The American Institute of Ultrasound in Medicine (AIUM) issued a statement on non-human mammalian in vivo biological effects in 1992.[50] This statement refers to the thermal and mechanical indices referred to earlier on page 12:

> Information from experiments utilizing laboratory mammals has contributed significantly to our understanding of ultrasonically induced biological effects and the mechanisms that are most likely responsible. The following statement summarizes observations relative to specific ultrasound parameters and indices. The history and rationale for this statement are provided in 'Bio-effects and safety of Diagnostic Ultrasound'.[50]

In the low MHz frequency range there have been no independently confirmed adverse biological effects in non-human mammalian tissues exposed in vivo under experimental ultrasound conditions, as follows:

a. When a thermal mechanism is involved, these conditions are unfocused beam intensities* below 100 mW.cm,[-2] focused[+] beam intensities below 1 W.cm,[-2] or thermal index values less than 2. Furthermore, such effects have not been reported for higher values of thermal index when it is less than

$$6 - \frac{\log_{10}t}{0.6}$$

where t is the exposure time in minutes, including off time for pulsed exposures.

b. When a nonthermal mechanism is involved,[#] in tissues that contain well-defined gas bodies, these conditions are in situ peak rarefactional pressures below approximately 0.3 MPa or mechanical index values less than approximately 0.3. Furthermore, for other tissues no such effects have been reported.

In addition, the AIUM has issued a statement (1995) based on the available epidemiological data base:

---

*Free field spatial peak, temporal average (SPTA) for continuous wave and pulsed exposures.

[+]Quarter power (–6 dB) beam width smaller than four wavelengths or 4 mm, whichever is less at the exposure frequency.

[#]For diagnostically relevant ultrasound exposures.

> Based on epidemiological evidence to date and on current knowledge of interactive mechanisms, there is insufficient justification to warrant a conclusion that there is a causal relationship between diagnostic ultrasound and adverse effects.

Summary

There is currently no evidence that there is any hazard presented to the patient by B-mode scanning. Considerable effort has been put into basic mechanistic studies, biological effects' investigations and epidemiological research, and no cause for concern has been highlighted. However, it has been demonstrated in laboratory studies that the acoustic power levels involved in Doppler examinations may be sufficient to cause biologically significant temperature rises in the vicinity of bone. It has therefore been advised by international bodies[49,51] that care should be exercised when extended examinations are necessary over calcified bone. It appears that acoustic cavitation is unlikely to be a hazard in obstetric uses of ultrasound.

In order to minimize any possible biological effects of diagnostic ultrasound (and to maximize the benefits), it is important that ultrasound users are properly trained, and that they understand the functions of the different controls available to them on their ultrasound equipment. For example, it is clear that altering the receiver controls (receiver gain, grey scale processing and M-mode time base) will have no effect on potential hazard as these control only the returning signal, but changing other settings, i.e. those associated with the output pulse, will have some effect on the beam's potential to produce heat or cavitation. It is not always easy to predict whether setting changes will increase or decrease any possible hazard, but the introduction of the display of thermal and mechanical indices is designed to aid the user in assessment of this. In addition, it must be remembered that, as well as consideration of the acoustic output characteristics, thought must be given to the biological sensitivity to heat or cavitation of the target volume. High intensities in the uterine wall may present less of a hazard than a lower intensity in the developing embryo or fetus. Advice on safety aspects of Doppler and transvaginal ultrasound for the clinical user is available in the literature.[51,52]

With appropriate use, diagnostic ultrasound can continue to be thought of as a modality with a very low risk:benefit ratio, especially in the hands of a trained operator.

References

1. Henderson J, Willson K, Jago JR, Whittingham TA. A survey of the acoustic outputs of diagnostic ultrasound equipment in current clinical use. Ultrasound Med Biol 1995; 21:699–705.
2. Duck FA, Martin K. Trends in diagnostic ultrasound exposure. Ultrasound Med Biol 1991; 36:1423–1432.
3. ter Haar GR. Ultrasonic biophysics: thermal mechanisms. In: Hill CR, ed. Physical principles of medical ultrasound. Chichester: Ellis Horwood 1986; 379–388.
4. Duck FA. Physical properties of tissue. A comprehensive reference book. London: Academic Press; 1990.
5. Bamber JB. Attenuation and absorption. In: Hill CR, ed. Physical principles of medical ultrasound. Chichester: Ellis Horwood; 1986:4.
6. European Committee for Ultrasound Radiation Safety. What happens when you alter the settings on your diagnostic ultrasound machine? Safety considerations. Eur J Ultrasound 1995; 2:329–330.
7. Edwards MJ. Hyperthermia as a teratogen: a review of experimental studies and their clinical significance. Teratogenesis Carcinog Mutagen 1986; 6:563–582.
8. Bosward K, Barnett SB, Wood AFK, Edwards MJ, Kossoff G. Heating of guinea pig fetal brain during exposure to pulsed ultrasound. Ultrasound Med Biol 1993; 19:415–424.
9. Drewniak JL, Carnes KI, Dunn F. In vitro ultrasonic heating of fetal bone. J Acoust Soc Am 1989; 86:1254–1258.
10. Duggan PM, Liggans GC, Barnett SB. Ultrasonic heating of the brain of the fetal sheep in utero. Ultrasound Med Biol 1995; 21:553–560.
11. O'Neill TP, Winkler AJ, Wu J. Ultrasound heating in a tissue-bone phantom. Ultrasound Med Biol 1994; 20:579–588.
12. ter Haar GR, Duck FA, Starritt HC, Daniels S. Biophysical characterisation of diagnostic equipment – preliminary results. Phys Med Biol 1989; 34:1533–1542.
13. Duggan PM, McCowan LME. Reference ranges and ultrasound exposure conditions for pulsed Doppler studies of the fetal carotid artery. J Ultrasound Med 1993; 12:719–722.
14. Sapareto SA, Dewey WC. Thermal dose determination in cancer therapy. J Radiat Oncol Biol Phys 1984; 10:787–800.
15. Miller MW, Ziskin MC. Biological consequences of hyperthermia. Ultrasound Med Biol 1989; 15:707–722.
16. WFUMB World Federation for Ultrasound in Medicine in Biology Symposium on Safety and Standardisation in Medical Ultrasound: Issues and recommendations regarding thermal mechanisms for biological effects of ultrasound. Ultrasound Med Biol 1992; 18: no. 9.
17. ter Haar GR. Ultrasonic biophysics: cavitation. In: Hill CR, ed. Physical principles of medical ultrasound. Chichester: Ellis Horwood 1986:388–408.
18. Leighton TG. The acoustic bubble. London: Academic Press; 1995; 5 (Effects and mechanisms).
19. Delius M, Enders G, Heine G, Stark J, Remberger K, Brendel W. Biological effects of shock waves; lung haemorrhage by shock waves in dogs – pressure dependence. Ultrasound Med Biol 1987; 16:61–67.
20. Child SZ, Hartman CL, Schery LA, Carstensen EL. Lung damage from exposure to ultrasound. Ultrasound Med Biol 1990; 16:817–825.
21. Raeman CH, Child SZ, Carstensen EL. Timing of exposures in ultrasonic haemorrhage of murine lung. Ultrasound Med Biol 1993; 19:507–512.
22. Frizzell LA, Chen E, Lee C. Effects of pulsed ultrasound on the mouse neonate: hind limb paralysis and lung haemorrhage. Ultrasound Med Biol 1994; 20:53–63.
23. Holland CK, Deng CX, Apfel RE, Alderman JL, Fernandez LA, Taylor KJW. Direct evidence of cavitation in vivo from diagnostic ultrasound. Ultrasound Med Biol 1996; 22:917–925.
24. Zachary JF, O'Brien WD. Lung haemorrhage induced by continuous and pulsed wave (diagnostic) ultrasound in mice, rabbits and pigs. Vet Pathol 1995; 32:43–54.
25. Tarantal A, Canfield DR. Ultrasound induced lung damage in the monkey. Ultrasound Med Biol 1994; 20:53–63.
26. Harrison GH, Eddy HA, Wang J-P, Liberman FZ. Ultrasound Med Biol 1995; 21:981–983.
27. Miller DL, Thomas RM. Ultrasound contrast agents nucleate inertial cavitation in vitro. Ultrasound Med Biol 1995; 21:1059–1065.
28. Dalecki D, Raeman CH, Child SZ, Carstensen EL. Intestinal haemorrhage from exposure to pulsed ultrasound. Ultrasound Med Biol 1995; 21:1067–1072.
29. Dalecki D, Child SZ, Raeman CH, Penney DP, Mayer R, Cox C, Carstensen EL. Thresholds for fetal hemorrhages produced by a piezoelectric lithotripter. Ultrasound Med Biol 1997; 23:287–297.
30. Kinnier Wilson LM, Waterhouse JAH. Obstetric ultrasound and childhood malignancies. Lancet 1984; ii:997–999.
31. Cartwright RA, McKinney PA, Hopton PA et al. Ultrasound examination in pregnancy and childhood cancer. Lancet 1984; ii:999–1000.

32. European Committee for Ultrasound Radiation Safety. Diagnostic ultrasound: genetic aspects. Eur J Ultrasound 1994; 1:91–92.

33. O'Brien WD. Dose-dependent effect of ultrasound on fetal weight in mice. J Ultrasound Med 1983; 2:1–8.

34. Child SZ, Hoffman D, Strasser D, Carstensen EL, Gates AH, Cox C, Miller MW. A test of I^2t as a dose parameter for fetal weight reduction from exposure to ultrasound. Ultrasound Med Biol 1989; 15:39–44.

35. Barnett SB, Williams AR. Identification of mechanisms responsible for fetal weight reduction in mice following ultrasound exposure. Ultrasonics 1990; 28:159–165.

36. Lyons EA, Dyke C, Toms M, Cheang M. In utero exposure to diagnostic ultrasound: a 6 year follow up. Radiology 1988; 166:687–690.

37. Salvesen KA, Jacobsen G, Vatten LJ, Eik-Nes SH, Bakketeig LS. Routine ultrasonography in utero and subsequent growth during childhood. Ultrasound Obstet Gynecol 1993; 3:6–10.

38. Waldenström U, Axelsson O, Nilsson S, Eklund G, Fall O, Lindeberg S, Sjödin Y. Effects of one-stage ultrasound screening in pregnancy: a randomised controlled trial. Lancet 1988; ii:585–588.

39. Newnham JP, Evans SF, Michael CA, Stanley FJ, Landau LI. Effects of frequent ultrasound during pregnancy: a randomised controlled trial. Lancet 1993; 342:887–891.

40. Campbell JD, Elford RW, Brant RF. Case control study of prenatal ultrasonography exposure in children with delayed speech. Can Med Assoc J 1993; 149:1435–1440.

41. Salvesen KA, Vatten LJ, Bakketeig LS, Eik-Nes SH. Ultrasound Obstet Gynecol 1994; 4:101–103.

42. Scheidt PC, Stanley F, Bryla DA. One year follow-up of infants exposed to ultrasound in utero. Am J Obstet Gynecol 1978; 131:743–748.

43. Stark CR, Orleans M, Haverkamp AD, Murphy J. Short- and long-term risks after exposure to diagnostic ultrasound in utero. Obstet Gynecol 1984; 63:194–200.

44. Salvesen KA, Bakketeig LS, Eik-Nes SH, Undheim JO, Økland O. Routine ultrasonography in utero and school performance at age 8–9 years. Lancet 1992; 339:85–89.

45. Salvesen KA, Vatten LJ, Jacobsen G, Eik-Nes SH, Økland O, Molne K, Bakketeig LS. Routine ultrasonography in utero and subsequent vision and hearing at primary school age. Ultrasound Obstet Gynecol 1992; 2:243–247.

46. Salvesen KA, Vatten LJ, Eik-Nes SH, Hugdahl K, Bakketeig LS. Routine ultrasonography in utero and subsequent handedness and neurological development. BMJ 1993; 307:159–164.

47. AIUM/NEMA. Standard for real-time display of thermal and mechanical indices on diagnostic ultrasound equipment. AIUM Publications; 1992. Available from American Institute of Ultrasound in Medicine, 14750 Sweitzer Lane, Suite 100, Laurel, MD 20707.

48. FDA. 510(k) Guide for measuring and reporting acoustic output of diagnostic ultrasound medical devices, December 1985. Available from Center for Devices and Radiological Health, US Food and Drug Administration, Rockville, MD.

49. European Federation of Societies for Ultrasound in Medicine and Biology (EFSUMB). Clinical safety statement for diagnostic ultrasound. Tours, 1998.

50. Bioeffects and safety of diagnostic ultrasound. American Institute of Ultrasound in Medicine: 1993.

51. European Committee for Ultrasound Radiation Safety. Guidelines for safe use of Doppler ultrasound for clinical applications. Eur J Ultrasound 1995; 2:167–168.

52. European Committee for Ultrasound Radiation Safety. Transvaginal ultrasonography – safety aspects. Eur J Ultrasound 1994; 1:355–357.

CHAPTER 3

The routine fetal anomaly scan

John J. Morrison
Lyn S. Chitty

Introduction

Routine fetal anomaly scanning in the mid-trimester is widely performed throughout Europe. The effectiveness of ultrasound screening in this way has been a source of great debate in recent years. It is imperative that such screening in an unselected population of pregnant women should be sensitive and specific and should have a high predictive value even when the prevalence of the condition is low. In epidemiological terms, such a screening test must also be safe and cost effective, and should ideally lead to some intervention for which benefit can be measured. Routine ultrasound is perceived as being of value in accurate determination of gestational age, diagnosis of multiple gestation, localization of placental site and assessment of fetal wellbeing[1–5] but these advantages have not been demonstrated to result in clear benefit in outcome.[6,7] Major structural malformations occur in 2 to 3% of fetuses and account for 20 to 30% of perinatal mortality in developed countries.[8–10] The vast majority of such malformations occur in pregnancies of low-risk women, i.e. they are sporadic and cannot be anticipated.[11] It is for these reasons that routine ultrasonography, as distinct from that which is indication based, has been advocated for detection of fetal anomalies.[5,12,13] It was felt that such a policy would contribute to optimal obstetric and neonatal care and might improve the chances of survival by assuring appropriate place and timing of delivery. In some cases prenatal treatment might be possible. In addition, for lethal malformations or those associated with severe handicap, early detection at routine fetal anomaly scan would allow couples to consider the option of termination of pregnancy. This review will concentrate on the benefits and pitfalls of ultrasonography in pregnancy in relation to detection of fetal malformations.

Sensitivity and specificity

There is great variation in the sensitivity of ultrasonography in detection of fetal anomalies from the numerous studies reported. This variation is due to the selection criteria of subjects (i.e. screening ultrasonography or indication based), the expertise of operators (tertiary level centres or otherwise), differences in the severity of abnormalities, gestational age at scanning, variation in ascertainment of abnormalities postnatally and the type of equipment available. A review of the randomized clinical trials of routine ultrasonography reported before 1985 found no improvement in pregnancy outcome, concluding that malformations were not identified in sufficient quantities to influence outcome statistics or that they were identified and not aborted.[14] However, significant technological advances have taken place since then and these early results may not be representative of the current situation. In 1989, Lys et al[15] reported results from routine ultrasound scans on 8316 pregnancies and identified only 14% of malformations while at the same time others reported detection rates of 34.4%[16] and 58.1% (39.4% before 24 weeks) were reported.[17] The Helsinki Ultrasound Trial in 1990[5] reported a detection rate of 36% for one centre, and 76.9% for another centre where more time was allocated to the screening examination, for ultrasonography performed between 16 and 20 weeks' gestation. Chitty et al in 1991 analyzed the findings for 8432 pregnancies that underwent routine ultrasonography between 18 and 20 weeks' gestation in a UK district general hospital and found a sensitivity of 74.4% (95% confidence interval 66.7% to 82.1%) for detection of fetal abnormalities (excluding chromosomal abnormality where there was no sonographic marker).[18] In 1992, Luck[19] reported an overall sensitivity of 85% but this study excluded facial clefts and minor degrees of talipes and did not give adequate details regarding postnatal confirmation of abnormalities. Shirley et al[20] reported a sensitivity of 60.7% in a similar setting for routine scans at 19 weeks' gestation.

In 1993, publication of the results of the Routine Antenatal Diagnostic Imaging with Ultrasound (RADIUS) trial[21] carried out in the USA concluded that routine ultrasonography, compared with selective use of ultrasonography, did not improve perinatal outcome. This was a highly publicized study and its most controversial result was the poor sensitivity achieved in detection of fetal anomalies with routine ultrasound (34.8% overall and 16.6% before 24 weeks' gestation). The reasons for this low detection rate were not clear and no information was given concerning the type of anomalies missed. This result stimulated much discussion concerning the efficacy and cost-effectiveness of a screening test for identification of malformed fetuses in a low-risk population.[22,23] A subsequent report from the participants in the RADIUS trial attempted to analyze the anomalies missed and the reasons that perinatal outcome were similar in the screened and non-screened groups.[24] They concluded that the low detection rate in the RADIUS trial, in comparison with other studies,[5,18,19,20] may have been due to poor training of sonographers in some centres, differing criteria for defining major malformations, the fact that the prevalence of some malformations may vary in different geographical areas and, finally, differences in the detection and documentation of congenital malformations in the neonatal period from one centre to the next. Other reports since the RADIUS trial have yielded equally variable results. In Austria, screening-based ultrasonography detected 50% of malformations during the years 1990–1991 with a sensitivity of 18% before 24 weeks' gestation.[25] The sensitivity in a Spanish study was 78.3% overall and 59.4% before 22 weeks' gestation.[26] The Belgian Multicentric Study reported sensitivities of 51.1% in total and 41% before 23 weeks' gestation for the period 1990–92.[27] In Italy, the sensitivity varied from 19% in one region to 30.1% in another which led the authors to question the value of routine screening for fetal anomalies.[28]

In contrast to sensitivity, the specificity of routine ultrasonography for detecting fetal malformations is very good and appears to be consistently greater than 99%.[16,17,18,19,20,27]

The only caution concerning this figure is that not all abnormalities are immediately evident on physical examination in the neonatal period and most studies do not include long-term follow-up in childhood. However, it seems that ultrasound screening for fetal malformations is a useful tool in confirming the presence of a normal fetus but its success in detecting the malformed fetus is variable.

Alternative screening policies

Indication-based sonography

Indication-based sonography, also known as selective or targeted sonography, refers to ultrasound scans performed on the basis of previous clinical details, the results of serum biochemical screening (e.g. alphafetoprotein and human chorionic gonadotrophin) or suspicion of fetal anomaly on ultrasound. Using this policy, early studies have reported sensitivities of 96%[29] and 99%.[30] Bernaschek et al[25] compared screening-based and indication-based sonography in Vienna. While the detection rate for abnormalities was generally poor in this study they found that more malformations were diagnosed by means of screening-based than indication-based scanning (18% versus 5% before 24 weeks). The most important advantage of sonographic screening, they concluded, was early diagnosis to allow for possible intra-uterine treatment or safe termination of pregnancy. In Edinburgh, the screening policy is based on a routine scan between 8 and 14 weeks followed by measurement of maternal serum alphafetoprotein at 16 weeks' gestation.[31] Any further ultrasound is performed on clinical indication only. Using these criteria, Chambers et al[31] analyzed the results from a teaching hospital between 1988–91 and reported that 130 (51%) anomalies were detected of which 64% were diagnosed before 24 weeks. In addition 11 chromosomal anomalies were diagnosed by amniocentesis, resulting in a final sensitivity of 37% before 24 weeks' gestation. The authors comment that this is comparable to some earlier reports of routine screening and conclude that until there is clear evidence of improved, obstetric decision-making, a reduction in childhood handicap and less parental suffering, the case has not yet been made for a policy of routine mid-trimester sonographic screening. However, the weaknesses in this approach are that the majority of congenital malformations occur in women with no identifiable risk factors,[11] that alterations in alphafetoprotein levels are associated with some malformations only, and that routine ultrasound detection rates of 60 to 85% have been reported for UK district general hospitals.[18–20]

First trimester ultrasound screening

Advances in the development of transvaginal probes have made it possible to examine the fetal anatomy in the first trimester.[32,33] Although there are many reports looking at high-risk populations or specific abnormalities, there are relatively few reports of routine, first trimester, anomaly scanning.[34,35] Achiron & Tadmor[36] compared transabdominal and transvaginal sonography in the first trimester. They found an improved detection rate using transvaginal sonography, but also reported a significant proportion of abnormalities which were not seen when scanned before 13 weeks but which were clearly visualized at a routine 18- to 20-week scan. As with second trimester screening, there may be difficulties in interpretation of findings, for example the spontaneous resolution of cystic hygroma detected in the first trimester has been reported[32] and an understanding of normal embryological development is essential before a diagnosis is made. In addition, Bronshtein et al[34] reported that a significant number of anomalies are transient at this time. Economides et al[35] reported high incidences of choroid plexus cysts (3.6%) and hydronephrosis (3.2%) in fetuses scanned at 12 to 13 weeks and the natural history of abnormalities needs to be more accurately defined before this technique can be considered for widespread application to the low-risk population. The relatively high, false-negative rates reported make it unlikely that first trimester anomaly scanning will ever replace the routine, second trimester scan.

Perinatal mortality and morbidity

Ultrasound screening in pregnancy for evaluation of gestational age, multiple pregnancy diagnosis, placental localization and assessment of fetal wellbeing has in some studies been shown to decrease the number of induced labours in post-term pregnancies[1,37] but without significant effect on perinatal outcome. It appears that routine, fetal anomaly scanning can improve detection of fetal malformations but translation of this into measurable perinatal benefit is more complex. Whilst perinatal mortality has been dramatically reduced in developed countries since 1950, the relative contribution of congenital malformations has increased substantially during this time owing to progress in managing other causes of fetal and neonatal deaths.[11] Congenital malformations now account for 20 to 30% of all perinatal deaths.[8–10] It would therefore seem likely that if routine fetal anomaly scanning were to allow for the interventions previously mentioned, a reduction in perinatal mortality should be observed. Most of the reports cited in earlier paragraphs do not include perinatal mortality as an outcome measure. Furthermore, it is not a good yardstick of perinatal care at any period of gestation.[38,39] Perinatal morbidity and long-term handicap in childhood are better outcome measures and these have not been adequately assessed in relation to the use of routine ultrasonography for detection of fetal malformations.

The only data available on the effects of fetal anomaly scanning on perinatal outcome are the results of randomized controlled trials comparing the effects of routine versus selective ultrasonography. The Helsinki

Ultrasound Trial was the first to report a clear reduction in perinatal mortality which was reduced by 47% in singleton and 58% in twin pregnancies.[5] Nearly half of this reduction was due to induced abortions as a result of the detection of malformations, an effect which some have referred to as a 'statistical artefact'.[6] The RADIUS trial,[21] which also assessed all potential benefits of ultrasound screening in pregnancy, including diagnosis of fetal malformations, had in its design outcome measures of perinatal mortality and both moderate and severe neonatal morbidity. The conclusion from this study was that screening ultrasonography did not improve perinatal outcome as compared with the selective use of ultrasonography on the basis of clinical indications. The outcome measures of preterm delivery, birthweight and outcome for multiple pregnancies, post-term pregnancies and small-for-gestational-age infants were similar in both groups. The detection of major anomalies by ultrasound did not alter outcome. However, fewer women terminated pregnancies complicated by fetal anomalies in the RADIUS study than the Helsinki study (33% versus 61%). As any potential effect on perinatal mortality is likely to be termination of pregnancy for lethal abnormalities this may explain some of this difference. Finally, Bucher & Schmidt[7] in their meta-analysis of four randomized clinical trials of routine ultrasonography versus selective ultrasonography reported that there was no difference in pregnancy outcome in terms of the live birth rate, the miscarriage rate or low Apgar scores (the last as a measure of perinatal morbidity). The perinatal mortality rate was, however, significantly lower in the routinely screened group but this effect was attributable to the results of the Helsinki Ultrasound Trial as discussed above. The authors concluded that routine ultrasound scanning may be useful in screening for fetal malformations in that it reduces perinatal deaths but does so without improving the number of live births. However, some of these studies were carried out in the early 1980s when the level of knowledge and the standard of equipment

were much less advanced. Other criticisms of this meta-analysis include the fact that all four studies had relatively small numbers with different objectives and screening policies and only one had the detection of fetal malformations as a specific aim.[5]

Parents' views

The offer of an ultrasound scan seems to be popular among parents but the full implications of such an offer, and the fact that it can be readily declined, are not always understood.[40,41] To compound this situation, observational studies of midwives and obstetricians suggest that the information they provide to parents concerning prenatal diagnostic tests can frequently be insufficient or inaccurate.[42,43] In 1995 Smith & Marteau reported their findings from six UK hospitals in relation to consultations with prospective mothers by midwives and obstetricians about prenatal diagnostic investigations.[44] They found that fetal anomaly scans were discussed in only 65% of such consultations (in comparison to 79% for biochemical screening) and were presented as being optional to just 11% of women. The objectives of the fetal anomaly scan were mentioned in only 37% of consultations. The implications of an abnormal finding were explained in 15% of consultations and only 1% of women were told what a negative scan result would mean. The possibility of false-positive or false-negative scan results was never mentioned in the consultations studied. The authors concluded that lack of knowledge of fetal anomaly scanning of midwives and consultants, the non-invasive nature of the test and the additional information (i.e. dates, placental site and multiple pregnancy) provided by the test, together with the perceived positive experience of the scan, may account for the lack of information women received to enable them to make an informed choice.

A Swedish study has recently investigated the choice of women who are well informed concerning all prenatal diagnostic tests.[41] All women in the study were given standard written and verbal information by 10 weeks' gestation outlining their choices. The midwives involved were given a course of lectures in genetics and fetal malformations prior to the study so that they could give uniform information to the parents. A group of women having standard antenatal care was used as controls. In the study group (1004 women) no woman declined the offer of an ultrasound examination and only 1% chose the option of a scan at 9 to 11 weeks' gestation only, i.e. for dating and detection of twins. These women had all been informed that they could decline the test and that it was a form of prenatal diagnosis. No woman in the control group (1408 women) declined the offer of an ultrasound scan either. It appears that well informed or not, and irrespective of maternal age, expectant mothers in this population welcomed the option of a routine fetal anomaly scan. Parents must be made aware of the implications of an anomaly scan. Once the abnormality has been detected, it is too late to decide that they would rather not have had that information.

Safety of ultrasound

Safety is a prime concern for an investigative tool that is widely used for screening purposes in the population. It is known that ultrasound at high intensity results in a rise in temperature with subsequent damage to tissues.[45] However, the upper limits of diagnostic ultrasound intensities are much lower than levels at which tissue hyperthermia and cavitation damage may be expected.[46] Studies in which pregnant monkeys have been exposed to ultrasound at diagnostic intensities for prolonged periods of time in the first trimester have shown no increase in the rate of congenital malformations, stillbirths or abortions.[47] However, in recent years there has been some concern over safety.

Two randomized, controlled trials of ultrasonographic screening in pregnancy were carried out in Trondheim and Alesund, Norway in 1979–81.[1,2] Of the subjects recruited for these studies, 1244 children, who had undergone routine ultrasonographic screening in utero at 19 and 32 weeks' gestation, and 1184 controls, where ultrasound had been performed only if clinically indicated (19% had a scan), were available for long-term, cohort studies. At ages 4 and 7, there was no demonstrable difference between the study group and controls in vision or hearing[48] and at ages 8 to 9, there was no statistically significant difference in oral reading, reading comprehension, spelling, arithmetic, dyslexia or overall school performance.[49] In addition, at ages 8 to 9, the groups were assessed with regard to attention, motor control, perception, neurological development and handedness during the first year of life.[50] The only difference found was an increased incidence of left-handedness in the screened group. The implications of such an association are that early brain damage to the left hemisphere, however subtle, would cause a shift in hand preference in otherwise genotypic right-handers. However, the authors did point out that this may be a possible chance finding among a number of non-significant findings.

An Australian study,[51] which received much attention at the time of its publication, set out to investigate whether intensive routine ultrasound monitoring during pregnancy (18, 24, 28, 34 and 38 weeks) had any bearing on outcome in comparison to the use of a single scan at 18 weeks' gestation in a control group. A total of 2834 pregnant women were randomly allocated to the study and control groups. The monitoring included continuous-wave Doppler flow studies. There was no difference between the groups in Apgar scores, umbilical artery blood gases, frequency and type of neonatal resuscitation, proportion and duration of admissions to the neonatal intensive care unit, requirements for ventilation and oxygen or the proportions with hyaline membrane disease, intraventricular haemorrhage, seizures and bronchopulmonary dysplasia. The gestational age at birth and the proportions and types of congenital malformations were similar in the two groups. However, the proportion of liveborn infants with birthweights less than the 10th centile was greater in the group who were intensively monitored (relative risk 1.35; 95% confidence intervals 1.09 to 1.67; $p = 0.006$) as was birthweight less than the 3rd centile (relative risk 1.65; 95% confidence intervals 1.09 to 2.49; $p = 0.020$). These results were accompanied by a trend towards reduction in mean birthweight in the study group of approximately 25 g which was not statistically significant. In the correspondence that followed this report the authors provided the absolute figures that had led to this result (35 of 1368 infants [2.56%] in the control group and 58 of 1375 infants [4.22%] in the study group were less than the 3rd centile).[52] This finding had not been a planned outcome measure from the study and hence could have occurred as a result of chance, as was pointed out in the report. These findings are at variance with reports which have shown that prolonged exposure to real time ultrasound (up to 20 hours before 20 weeks' gestation) had no effect on fetal growth.[53] Interestingly, by 1 year of age there was no measurable difference in growth between the screened and control groups in the Australian study.[54] The possibility of an adverse effect on fetal growth by ultrasound remains as yet unanswered and there is a considerable need for further data. Furthermore, the intensity of scanning in this study was far higher than would be practised in a routine ultrasound screening programme for anomalies.

Transvaginal ultrasound in the first trimester uses probes that are closer to the fetus and which may therefore result in increased fetal exposure. In comparison with grey scale imaging, the intensity of the beam with colour Doppler is increased ten-fold and with pulsed Doppler 100-fold. Increased gain can also be employed with power Doppler.[55] It is important that sonographers are aware of the potential for increased risk with these advances and that their safety limitations have not yet been assessed.

In conclusion there are no reproducible adverse biological effects of fetal exposure to diagnostic ultrasound. In the UK, the Chief Medical Officer has stated that 'there is no unequivocal evidence of damage from diagnostic ultrasound exposure in man, woman or fetus' and that 'exposures should be justified and limited to the minimum necessary for the diagnostic purpose'.[56] In the USA for the last 20 years, ultrasound machines have been subject to restrictions in maximum acoustical output by regulation of the Food and Drug Administration.[57] The principle of keeping exposures as low as reasonably achievable for the diagnostic objective has been promoted on both sides of the Atlantic. It must also be remembered that another key element in the safety of fetal ultrasound is the user. The knowledge and skill of the user are central to the potential for ultrasound to confer benefit or undue harm. Inappropriate indications, poor technique and misinterpretation of ultrasonography pose a greater threat to the safety of the fetus than the possibility of bioeffects from the exposure.

Topographic detection of fetal abnormalities

The general detection of fetal abnormalities with ultrasound has been discussed above. In this section the detection of fetal abnormalities will be discussed in relation to the different anatomical compartments. In Tables 3.1, 3.2 and 3.3 some of the results of ultrasound screening from five of the studies previously discussed[18,19,20,21,59] are shown.

Central nervous system abnormalities

The incidence of abnormalities of the fetal central nervous system has been estimated at approximately 5.3 to 6.2 per thousand[58,59] and they account for approximately 12 to 31% of all fetal malformations in series reported.[18,25,26,27,28,59] The most commonly diagnosed sonographic abnormalities are hydrocephalus, spina bifida (including meningocoele or meningomyelocoele), microcephaly and anencephaly.[17,27,28,58,59] Other diagnoses include macrocephaly, holoprosencephaly, Dandy–Walker malformation, porencephaly, iniencephaly, arachnoid cyst, agenesis of the corpus callosum and aneurysm of the vein of Galen.[17,18,20,27,28,58,59] The sensitivity of ultrasound in detection of abnormalities of the fetal central nervous system appears to vary widely between 50% and 96%.[18,27,28,59] In some studies abnormalities of the head and neck are grouped together making comparisons difficult.[26]

The highest detection rates are achieved for anencephaly and open neural tube defects (Table 3.1). Many studies report detection rates of 100% for anencephaly[17,18,20,27,59] with no false-negatives. This is not universally the case and the Italian study, referred to above, reported a detection rate of 66% with only 4 out of 37 lesions detected before 24 weeks' gestation.[28] However, while this should be taken as a note of caution, many cases are detected early in pregnancy by a combination of ultrasound and maternal serum alphafetoprotein screening[60,61] but this is not always the case for routine ultrasonography where all neural tube defects were detected in 18- to 20-week scans in the absence of maternal serum alphafetoprotein screening.[18–20] The effectiveness of ultrasound in diagnosing spina bifida has improved greatly in the last two decades. Series reported in the early 1980s show sensitivities ranging from 30% to 87% with specificities of 96% to 99%, positive predictive values of 80% to 92% and negative predictive values of 99%.[61,62] The overall detection rate from five studies of routine ultrasonography[18–20,24,59] in recent years was 80%.[63] In high-risk populations, recent studies have reported sensitivities of 90 to 100%.[64–66] This increased detection rate has been due to improved equipment and expertise and, most importantly, due to recognition of the intracranial findings associated with fetuses with spina bifida. In transverse section, the head is irregular with pointing of the frontal region owing to scalloping of the bones which is known as the 'lemon' sign.[67] The

Table 3.1
Detection of fetal abnormalities of the central nervous and cardiovascular systems

	Chitty et al 1991[18]	Shirley et al 1991[20]	Luck 1992[19]	Crane et al 1994[24]	Levi et al 1991[59]	Total % diagnosed
Central nervous system abnormalities						
Anencephaly	6/6	10/10	7/7	3/3	6/6	100
Spina bifida, meningocoele	5/5	3/3	2/2	4/5	4/7	56
Encephalocoele	2/2	1/1	1/1			100
Hydrocephaly	3/3	1/2			4/15	38
Porencephaly					0/1	40
Holoprosencephaly	2/3		1/1		0/1	75
Others	2/2			2/2	3/6	33
Total	20/21	15/16	11/11	9/10	17/36	76.6
Cardiovascular abnormalities						
Atrial and/or ventricular septal defects	1/2	1/1	2/3	0/21	0/27	7.4
Single atrium or ventricle	1/3		4/8		2/5	43.8
Transposition of the great arteries		0/1	0/3		0/5	0
Other complex heart	5/6	4/7	3/11	5/19	1/35	40.6
Total	7/11	5/9	9/25	5/40	3/72	18.5

Only studies which differentiate between women scanned and abnormalities detected before 24 weeks' gestation are included, i.e. routine anomaly scanning. This table lists selected abnormalities only and does not give all the abnormalities reported in the papers. The term 'other' may include some of the specific abnormalities listed in some of the papers.

cerebellum may be apparently absent sonographically (as a result of being very low or hypoplastic) or may be bowed in shape with an anterior concavity which is the 'banana' sign.[67] Using these signs in high-risk populations nearly all fetuses with open spina bifida can be identified before 20 weeks' gestation.[68,69] These signs are thought to be due to downward traction on the brain stem, and spina bifida occurring in their absence is generally associated with a simple meningocoele which carries a good prognosis. There are no reliable data available for the sensitivity of ultrasound for detection of spina bifida in a low-risk population using these signs only (i.e. detection rates prior to maternal serum alphafetoprotein being available) but good results should be possible.

Whilst the overall rates of detection of fetal hydrocephalus using ultrasound varied between 65% in the Italian study[28] and 97% in the Belgian Multicentric Study,[27] detection from its routine use (i.e. before 22 weeks) was remarkably different (6% and 35% respectively). This reflects the diverse aetiology of this condition and the fact that the sonographic features may not be apparent until the late second or early third trimester (or indeed postnatally in some cases). While significant dilatation of the lateral and third ventricles can easily be demonstrated, borderline ventriculomegaly in the second trimester can be more difficult to assess and interpret. Detection rates for other intracranial abnormalities, e.g. holoprosencephaly, hydranencephaly, Dandy–Walker malformation and porencephalic cysts have been reported but the numbers in general are small. Holoprosencephaly was detected in 6 out of 20 cases (30%) in the Italian study[28] and 2 out of 3 cases (66%) in the Luton study.[18] Porencephaly was detected in 2 out of 5 cases (40%) in the Belgian study.[27]

Microcephaly is similarly a heterogenous condition with many different causes. As with hydrocephalus it may not become apparent until the late second or early third trimester. The early Belgian study reported an overall detection rate of 66% (4 of 6)[59]

while the Italian study showed a rate of 31.4% (11 of 35) based on larger numbers[27] but fewer than half of the diagnoses made occurred before 24 weeks' gestation, demonstrating a very poor detection rate for microcephaly based on the routine fetal anomaly scan. Unless the head-to-abdomen circumference ratio is markedly reduced, serial scans are generally necessary to make the diagnosis with confidence.

Cardiovascular abnormalities

Congenital heart defects are the most common neonatal defects with a reported incidence of 8 per 1000.[70] Many of these defects (circa 50%) are critical and require intervention in the early neonatal period.[71] Routine prenatal detection of such defects, while preparing the parents for the prognosis, would also allow for antenatal transfer to a centre with paediatric cardiac facilities thereby ensuring optimum neonatal condition for surgery. It has been shown that the prognosis for an infant with congenital heart disease can improve if it is detected prenatally instead of after birth.[72]

Detection rates for cardiovascular abnormalities from five studies of routine ultrasound screening are shown in Table 3.1. There is great variation in the reported sensitivities of routine screening ultrasonography for fetal heart defects; 3.8% in the Italian study,[27] 28% in the Austrian study,[24] 43% in the RADIUS study,[20] 67% in the Spanish study[25] and 71% in the Belgian study.[58] As these studies were investigating the use of sonography for detection of all fetal abnormalities, and were mainly multicentre studies, the exact criteria used for diagnosis of congenital heart defects were not specified. However, several studies have evaluated inclusion of the 4-chamber view in routine screening for congenital heart defects. In a low-risk population of 5347 women Achiron et al[73] detected 48% of congenital heart lesions prenatally by obtaining the 4-chamber view between 18 and 24 weeks (mean 21 weeks). When they failed to obtain this view at the first scan, a repeat scan at 24 weeks was arranged. When the scan was extended to visualization of the great vessels, 78% of cardiac abnormalities were detected. Vergani et al[74] reported that inclusion of the 4-chamber view in the routine ultrasound examination increased the prenatal detection rate of congenital heart defects from 47% to an impressive 81%. Tegnander et al[71] compared detection rates for congenital heart defects in 4435 fetuses with no special attention to the heart and in 7459 fetuses after inclusion of the 4-chamber view. The detection rate improved from 18% in the former group to 26% in the latter for critical heart defects. These scans were performed at 18 weeks' gestation and the authors pointed out that some congenital heart defects (e.g. transposition of the great arteries, Fallot tetralogy, double outlet right ventricle, mild pulmonary stenosis, mild aortic stenosis and small ventricular septal defect) may have a normal 4-chamber view at that stage thereby partially explaining their relatively poor sensitivity. In addition, they were unable to obtain the 4-chamber view in 4% of fetuses at this gestation owing to poor image quality or difficult fetal position. The incidence of critical heart defects was much higher in this group than the overall study population. These results led the authors to conclude that good equipment, education, adequate time, the resources to arrange follow-up scans when the 4-chamber view has not been seen and inclusion of imaging the great vessels, are essential to a policy of routine screening based on the 4-chamber view at 18 weeks' gestation. This study carried out the best postnatal ascertainment and is probably most consistent with daily clinical practice in relation to screening ultrasonography and fetal cardiac abnormalities.

The alternative screening policy of indication-based ultrasonography has not yielded sensitivity results for congenital heart defects which are comparable with routine screening. In the RADIUS study,[21] 21% of complex cardiac lesions were detected in the control group for whom ultrasound was performed only if indicated in comparison to 43% in the routinely screened group as outlined above. Chambers et al[31]

reported that the greatest shortfall in diagnosis in their indication-based, fetal ultrasound policy in Edinburgh occurred among the cardiac defects. In that study, 31 of 38 isolated severe cardiac defects were not detected until after birth. Analysis of all cases of congenital heart disease detected at Guy's Hospital, London betwen 1980 and 1990 has shown that 80 to 85% of these were referred because of a suspected abnormality on routine screening.[75] During a 2.5-year period of assessment of routine screening in 10 district hospitals, Sharland & Allan demonstrated that 69% of cardiac abnormalities were detected as a result of routine screening (mainly using the 4-chamber view) while only 10% were identified as a result of referral for other high-risk factors (21% were overlooked).[75] The authors concluded that the incidence of congenital heart disease merited routine screening which could be performed safely, with good results and which led to diagnoses that were amenable to intervention or treatment. It was felt that if such screening was implemented effectively it would lead to significantly fewer newborn infants presenting to paediatric cardiology units and would allow planning for optimal postnatal care for sick infants. Further evidence to support this comes from the observation that in recent years there has been a significant fall in the number of neonatal cases of hypoplastic left heart syndrome seen at a specialized paediatric surgery referral centre.[76]

Urinary tract abnormalities

Congenital abnormalities of the urinary tract are common and the incidence, while difficult to determine exactly, appears to vary between 2 and 5 per thousand.[58,77] They are therefore less common than malformations of either the central nervous or cardiovascular systems. The majority of urinary tract congenital abnormalities are not lethal and many have an unknown natural history and may be clinically silent in early postnatal life.[78] The use of routine sonography in pregnancy has resulted in

Table 3.2
Detection of fetal abnormalities of the urinary tract and skeletal systems

	Chitty et al 1991[18]	Shirley et al 1991[20]	Luck 1992[19]	Crane et al 1994[24]	Levi et al 1991[59]	Total % diagnosed
Urinary tract abnormalities						
Obstructive uropathy	10/10	7/8	99/99	28/29	2/25	85.4
Renal agenesis	5/5		2/2		3/4	90.9
Unilateral	(1/1)					
Bilateral	(4/4)		(2/2)		(3/4)	
Renal dysplasia	5/8	0/1	4/4		4/11	54.2
Unilateral	(3/5)		(4/4)			
Bilateral	(2/3)	(0/1)				
Prune belly syndrome					3/3	100
Other	1/2			6/6	0/1	77.8
Total	21/25	7/9	105/105	34/35	12/44	82.5
Skeletal abnormalities						
Talipes	6/12	0/6	2/2*	2/24	3/14	22.4
Unilateral	(3/8)	(0/4)				
Bilateral	(3/4)	(0/2)				
Limb reduction defect	2/5	1/1	1/2	2/5	0/1	42.9
Skull anomaly	1/1				0/3	25
Spinal anomaly	3/3		1/1	0/1	0/2	57.1
Dwarfism	2/2	1/1	2/2		0/2	71.4
Other skeletal anomalies	3/4		0/1		1/1	66.6
Total	17/27	2/8	6/8	4/30	4/23	34.4

*Only severe cases reported.
Only studies which differentiate between women scanned and abnormalities detected before 24 weeks' gestation are included, i.e. routine anomaly scanning. This table lists selected abnormalities only and does not give all the abnormalities reported in the papers. The term 'other' may include some of the specific abnormalities listed in some of the papers.

early detection of many cases of urinary tract dilatation but there is often difficulty in predicting the clinical significance of the prenatal sonographic findings to the neonate. There is very little information regarding long-term follow-up in childhood to assess the significance in later life.

The sensitivity of ultrasound in detecting abnormalities of the urinary tract is reportedly good, 66% in the Belgian study,[59] 72% in the Austrian study,[25] 75% in the Italian study[28] and 91% in the Spanish study.[26] The diagnostic label of obstructive uropathy, hydronephrosis or upper urinary tract dilatation (not including mild pyelectasis) accounted for approximately 60% of all urinary tract abnormalities in the above series for which detection rates varied between 78% and 80% overall but fell sharply to between 14% and 58% for scans performed before 22 to 23 weeks' gestation (calculations based on 83 cases of obstructive uropathy in the Belgian 1984–1992 study[27] and 372 cases

of hydronephrosis in the Italian study[28]). There were 9 such cases in the Luton study with 100% detection,[18] 7 in the Ascot study with 100% detection but follow-up was suboptimal[19] and 7 in the Hillingdon study of which 6 (86%) were detected.[20] These results would all suggest that ultrasound is fairly sensitive for significant obstructive disease of the urinary tract but the full sonographic picture may not become obvious until the second half of pregnancy. However, the significance of the findings may not be clear until neonatal imaging is performed (on infants with and without antenatal sonographic findings) or until later into childhood or adult life and hence these figures are difficult to interpret meaningfully as there are no reliable, positive, predictive or specificity values.

While moderate-to-severe degrees of urinary tract dilatation are more readily detected leading to planned neonatal management, the interpretation of mild dilatation or pyelectasis has been much more difficult. Furthermore there is still considerable debate over the criteria used to diagnose dilatation of the renal pelvis at the time of the routine scan. It is established that fetal renal pelves measuring less than 5 mm in the anteroposterior diameter are normal while measurements greater than 10 mm may sometimes reflect pathology.[77,79] The significance of renal pelves measuring between 5 and 10 mm is far from clear and, while there are no gestational-age-based data, this finding is thought to be more serious the earlier in pregnancy it is detected from the beginning of the second trimester onwards. Langer et al[80] have reported prenatal and postnatal data from 2170 pregnant women in whom there were 95 fetuses (4.4%) with pyelectasis which was classified as mean renal pelvis dimension > 5 or 10 mm before or after 28 weeks' gestation. There was no urological abnormality in cases that had remained less than 10 mm throughout pregnancy. Chitty et al[81] have reviewed the outcome of over 400 fetuses found to have unilateral or bilateral dilatation of the renal pelvis between 5 and 10 mm in the second trimester. Over half the fetuses had some degree of dilatation detected on a postnatal, renal ultrasound scan, 12% had a pathological diagnosis (reflux, duplex system, pelvi-ureteric junction obstruction) and 4% required surgery in infancy.

Detection rates for unilateral and bilateral renal agenesis or dysplasia are of the order of 60 to 80%.[18,27,28] Podevin et al[82] in a recent French study reported a sensitivity value of 86% for dysplastic kidneys in their series of 142 urinary malformations which included 52 cases of suspected renal dysplasia (3 cases had renal agenesis on histological examination). Their detection rates for other malformations were similar to those cited above. This led the authors to conclude that there were clear benefits from routine screening for uropathies in terms of prenatal consultation between paediatric surgeon and parents, planning of postnatal care and selection of fetuses with potential renal failure and a high risk of pulmonary

hypoplasia to provide the option of termination of pregnancy.

Musculoskeletal abnormalities

This group of disorders includes skeletal dysplasias, arthrogryposis syndromes, talipes and club-hand, limb reduction defects, digit abnormalities and miscellaneous deformities of the spine, ribs, skull and long bones. Because they constitute a large heterogenous group of disorders, estimations of prevalence are difficult and have been reported to vary between 2.6 per 1000[60] to 14.3 per 1000.[59] Skeletal abnormalities can be the most difficult to detect and even when abnormal findings are observed their interpretation frequently does not lead to a definitive prenatal diagnosis. Sensitivity values can be readily assessed accurately as postnatal ascertainment is easier than with other disorders. Taken as a group, overall detection rates for musculoskeletal abnormalities have been reported as 23% in the Italian study,[28] 34% in the Belgian study[27] and 55% in the Luton study[18] (see Table 3.2 for further details).

Routine anomaly scanning includes assessment and measurement of the long bones, giving potential for the diagnosis of many serious skeletal dysplasias.[83,84] With routine ultrasound screening, skeletal dysplasias accounted for 42% (115 out of 271 cases) of all skeletal abnormalities in the Italian study[28] but only 19% in the Belgian study[27] which reported a far greater incidence of club-hand and -foot deformities. In these studies[27,28] detection rates varied from 37% for skeletal dysplasias overall to 100% for thanatophoric dwarfism but detection rates before 22 to 24 weeks were 4% for skeletal dysplasias as a group and 20% for thanatophoric dwarfism. Heterozygous achondroplasia is the most common, non-lethal, skeletal dysplasia with an estimated incidence of 1 per 25 000 of which 80 to 90% are sporadic.[85] The limb measurements may not deviate much from normal before 24 weeks' gestation[86,87] and hence the diagnosis cannot be definitively made before this time, resulting in the poor detection rates described above from routine screening. Modaff et al[88] have recently reported that of 28 infants referred with achondroplasia, who had prenatal ultrasound performed and had no family history to suspect the diagnosis, 12 (43%) were not recognized as having a fetal abnormality, confirming the view that achondroplasia is an acceptable false-negative diagnosis on routine scanning.

Finally, in the future, routine ultrasound may be used in conjunction with molecular screening for accurate determination of skeletal dysplasias. This is currently available for achondroplasia as the vast majority of subjects with this diagnosis have a single common mutation of the fibroblast growth factor receptor 3 (FGFR3).[89] Advances are currently being made in characterization of the molecular basis of other skeletal dysplasias[90,91] which may lead to improved diagnostic ability for these conditions in the future.

Facial abnormalities

Facial clefts occur in approximately 1 in 700 live births and account for 10% of all congenital anomalies.[92] Results for detection rates of facial abnormalities derived from routine screening from the Luton,[18] Ascot,[19] Hillingdon,[20] Belgian,[59] American[24] and Austrian[25] studies vary between 13 and 30% with an average rate of 20%. There are no reliable detection rates from routine screening of less common facial abnormalities such as hypo- and hypertelorism, microphthalmia and nasal abnormalities.

Respiratory tract abnormalities

The prevalence of malformations of the respiratory tract has been estimated at 4.3 per 1000.[59] The most common abnormality is congenital diaphragmatic hernia which occurs in about 1 in 2000 to 1 in 5000 births.[93] The differential diagnosis for congenital diaphragmatic hernia encompasses the various causes of cystic lung lesions which include congenital cystic adenomatoid malformation (CCAML), pulmonary

sequestration, bronchogenic cysts, bronchial atresia and teratomata.[94,95] Detection rates for some of these abnormalities are also shown in Table 3.3.

Published reports vary in their categorization of abnormalities (e.g. diaphragmatic hernia may be grouped alone or with gastrointestinal or respiratory abnormalities) making it difficult to compare detection rates for lung abnormalities. In the Spanish study, Carrera et al[26] reported a rate of 56% for lung abnormalities (excluding diaphragmatic hernia) from routine screening (i.e. before 22 weeks) which was increased to 85% (23 out of 27) when diagnosis at all gestation periods was considered. In the Luton study,[18] 7 out of 9 lung abnormalities were detected with 2 cases of pleural effusion missed (both of which were diagnosed in the third trimester). For diaphragmatic hernia, detection rates are between 70 and 80%[26,27] with good evidence to suggest that a worse prognosis is associated with lesions diagnosed antenatally in comparison to postnatally.[93] The diagnosis of congenital diaphragmatic hernia should lead to a thorough detailed scan of the fetus because of its association with other structural abnormalities and aneuploidy.

The majority of cystic lung lesions can be attributed to CCAML and are generally diagnosed at the time of routine scanning in the second trimester. Caution should be observed in predicting outcome for such lesions. In a series of 40 cases of cystic lesions of the fetal lung diagnosed in the second trimester, we have found that spontaneous improvement occurred in 21 cases (68%) with complete resolution in 5 cases (16%).[96] There was 1 perinatal death in this series and postnatal follow-up, at variable periods up to 3 years, suggests that outcome is much more favourable than previously reported.

Abdominal wall and gastrointestinal system abnormalities

Anterior abdominal wall defects are frequently detected by ultrasound after 12 weeks' gestation. While most studies report

Table 3.3
Detection of fetal abnormalities of the respiratory tract, abdominal wall and gastrointestinal systems

	Chitty et al 1991[18]	Shirley et al 1991[20]	Luck 1992[19]	Crane et al 1994[24]	Levi et al 1991[59]	Total % diagnosed
Respiratory tract abnormalities						
Cystic adenomatoid malformation	4/4	1/1	1/1			100
Diaphragmatic hernia	2/2	2/3	2/5	1/1	1/2	61.5
Pleural effusion	1/3					33.3
Others		1/1		1/4		40
Total	7/9	4/5	3/6	2/5	1/2	63
Abdominal wall and gastrointestinal abnormalities						
Omphalocoele	3/3	1/1	2/2	1/1	2/2	100
Gastroschisis	1/1	1/1	2/2		2/2	100
Small bowel obstruction/atresia	0/1	0/1	1/1	1/1	0/1	40
Anal atresia/imperforate anus					0/7	0
Oesophageal atresia/tracheo-oesophageal fistula	0/2		1/2	0/3	1/7	14.3
Others			1/1		1/14	13.3
Total	4/7	2/3	7/8	2/5	6/33	37.5

Only studies which differentiate between women scanned and abnormalities detected before 24 weeks' gestation are included, i.e. routine anomaly scanning. This table lists selected abnormalities only and does not give all the abnormalities reported in the papers. The term 'other' may include some of the specific abnormalities listed in some of the papers.

detection rates of 90% or greater[18,26,27] (see Table 3.3), this is not universally the case with detection rates of 50% reported in the Italian study.[28] Accurate prenatal diagnosis leading to tertiary referral for delivery and planned neonatal surgery is standard practice in the UK.

Detection rates for intestinal atresia vary between 40 and 50%[27,28] but the diagnosis is often not apparent until the third trimester. Detection rates before 22 weeks were as low as 6% in the Belgian study[28] presumably because the sonographic signs of dilated bowel loops and polyhydramnios are frequently not present until late in pregnancy. Prediction of postnatal outcome is difficult in these cases as the sonographic findings may be similar when there are very small or very extensive areas of atretic bowel. Anorectal atresia was presented separately in the Italian study.[27] There were 83 such cases of which none was detected sonographically.

Oesophageal atresia occurs in about 1 in 5000 live births.[97] It may be diagnosed if there is a persistent inability to visualize the fetal stomach on serial scans. However, there is an associated tracheo-oesophageal fistula in most cases which allows the stomach to fill via the trachea, and polyhydramnios which develops well after the time of the routine scan may occasionally be the only clue to the underlying pathology. In the Italian study, only 12 out of 98 cases (12%) of oesophageal atresia were detected.[28] In the Belgian study,[27] all gastrointestinal atresias were reported as one group. There were 2 cases of oesophageal atresia in the Luton study[18] and 1 case in the Ascot study,[18] none of which was diagnosed antenatally.

Financial implications of the routine fetal anomaly scan

Recent years have seen an expansion in the availability of routine, antenatal sonography for the detection of fetal anomalies. While the medical aspects of such routine sonography have been widely discussed, the financial implications have also stimulated much debate. This issue was highlighted in 1993 with publication of the findings from the RADIUS trial in the USA[21] which concluded that routine ultrasound screening would add considerably to the cost of health care without providing benefit in terms of perinatal outcome. As previously discussed, the RADIUS trial was the centre of much controversy at that time and was criticized for the limited sensitivity of ultrasound it reported. However, in an era in which clinical practice is increasingly exposed to financial accountability, the practice of routine antenatal sonography for diagnosis of fetal anomalies requires economic evaluation.

Routine, antenatal sonography can be described as efficient if the benefits it provides are deemed greater than its cost. The cost can be assessed in two ways; cost–benefit analysis and cost-effectiveness analysis.[98] The former assessment questions how much of society's resources should be directed, for example, at achieving a routine fetal anomaly scan for all. The answer to this question is complex and involves perinatal morbidity, perinatal mortality, costs averted such as long-term care for handicap, patients' wishes and the benefits of reassurance from a normal scan. These factors may be difficult to assess. Cost-effectiveness analysis is concerned with what is the best way of spending a particular budget to achieve a decided goal of, for example, providing a routine fetal anomaly scan for the population. This latter question is simpler as it does not require the financial evaluation of the benefits mentioned above. Neither analysis has been adequately performed although some of these issues have been addressed. DeVore[97] examined the cost effectiveness of ultrasound screening for fetal abnormalities in the tertiary and non-tertiary centres which participated in the RADIUS study. The diagnostic rate for the tertiary centres was 6.8 per 1000 which amounted to circa $30 000 per malformed fetus identified (based on $200 per scan). In the non-tertiary centres the diagnostic rate was 1.7 per 1000 resulting in a cost of circa $115 000 per malformed fetus identified. The author suggested that one way of reducing the overall cost would be to reimburse ultrasound providers with greater diagnostic skills.

There is no UK data concerning the financial implications of sonographic screening in pregnancy. The most reliable European data on this topic were reported from Finland by Leivo et al.[99] They evaluated the cost of a one-staged, ultrasound screening in pregnancy between 16 and 20 weeks' gestation in a study group of 4691 women with a randomly allocated control group of 4619 women from 1986–88. They calculated all costs to the hospital, the state, the woman, the woman's employer and overhead costs. Cost-effectiveness was estimated by dividing costs by the difference in perinatal deaths between the screened and control groups. In the screened group 12 fetuses with major malformation were found and 11 women elected to terminate the pregnancy. The gross cost of avoiding one perinatal death was $21 938 dollars which they felt was reasonable in both economic and human terms. They estimated that the cost of each ultrasound scan was $102 per patient but this resulted in savings of $182 per patient because of fewer inpatient and outpatient visits and fewer unnecessary, later ultrasound scans. If one applies this saving of $80 (without allowing for inflation) per patient to the UK for 700 000 deliveries per annum, it would represent a saving of $56 million annually. The authors concluded that second trimester ultrasound screening is cost effective and that longer, ultrasound examination time and more numerous, advanced examinations were rewarded by fewer perinatal deaths and a better cost-effectiveness ratio.

Conclusion

The use of routine ultrasound in pregnancy for detection of fetal anomalies requires further evaluation from both a clinical and economic viewpoint. While there is evidence that it can reduce perinatal mortality if congenital anomalies are appropriately identified, it is imperative that sonographers receive adequate training to achieve an accepted minimum standard of practice.

Because there are currently no such standards, centres should be obliged to audit their screening programme to allow for continuous evaluation of their detection rates. Congenital malformation registers, with data recording to at least 1 year of life, would provide for greater ascertainment of abnormalities postnatally. It is difficult, if not impossible, to estimate the value in financial terms of providing a routine, fetal anomaly service for the population but the data that are available suggest that its cost–benefit advantages and cost-effectiveness justify the practice. Research into the psychological consequences of prenatal diagnosis by ultrasound, and false-positive and false-negative diagnoses, is needed. Consideration should be given to alternative screening policies using first, second and third trimester scanning in combination with biochemical screening methods. Finally, although diagnostic ultrasound during pregnancy appears to be safe, we should remain vigilant about the possibility of subtle adverse effects.

References

1. Bakketeig LS, Jacobsen G, Brodtkorb CJ. Randomised controlled trial of ultrasonography screening in pregnancy. Lancet 1984; ii:207–211.
2. Eik-Nes SH, Okland O, Aure JC, Ullstein M. Ultrasound screening in pregnancy: a randomised controlled trial. Lancet 1984; i:1347.
3. Ewigman BG, LeFevre M, Hesser J. A randomized trial of routine prenatal ultrasound. Obstet Gynecol 1990; 76:189–194.
4. McClure N, Dorman JC. Early identification of placenta praevia. Br J Obstet Gynaecol 1990; 97:959–961.
5. Saari-Kemppainen A, Karjalainen O, Ylostalo P, Heinonen OP. Ultrasound screening and perinatal mortality: controlled trial of systematic one-stage screening in pregnancy. Lancet 1990; 336:387–391.
6. Larson T, Falck Larson J, Petersen S, Greisen G. Detection of small-for-gestational-age fetuses by ultrasound screening in a high risk population: a randomised controlled study. Br J Obstet Gynaecol 1992; 99:469–474.
7. Bucher HC, Schmidt JG. Does routine ultrasound scanning inprove outcome in pregnancy? Meta-analysis of various outcome measures. BMJ 1993; 307:13–17.
8. Alberman E. Perinatal mortality. In: Turnbull A, Chamberlain G, eds. Obstetrics. Edinburgh: Churchill Livingstone; 1989:1111–1119.
9. Kalter H, Warkany J. Congenital malformations (first of two parts). N Engl J Med 1983; 308:424–431.
10. Kalter H, Warkany J. Congenital malformations (second of two parts). N Engl J Med 1983; 308:491–497.
11. Kalter H. Five-decade international trends in the relation of perinatal mortality and congenital malformations: stillbirth and neonatal death compared. Int J Epidemiol 1991; 20:173–179.
12. DeCrespigny LC, Warren P, Buttery B. Should all pregnant women be offered an ultrasound examination? Med J Aust 1989; 151:613–615.
13. Members of the joint study group on fetal abnormalities. Recognition and management of fetal abnormalities. Arch Dis Child 1989; 64:971–976.
14. Thacker SB. Quality of controlled clinical trials. The case of imaging ultrasound in obstetrics: a review. Br J Obstet Gynaecol 1985; 92:437–444.
15. Lys F, DeWals P, Borlee-Grimes I, Billiet A, Vincotte-Mols M, Levi S. Evaluation of routine ultrasound examination for the prenatal diagnosis of malformation. Eur J Obstet Gynaecol Reprod Biol 1989; 30:101–109.
16. Levi S, Crouzet P, Schaaps JP et al. Ultrasound screening for fetal malformations. Lancet 1989; i:678.
17. Rosendahl H, Kivinen S. Antenatal detection of congenital malformations by routine ultrasonography. Obstet Gynecol 1989; 73:947–951.
18. Chitty LS, Hunt GH, Moore J, Lobb MO. Effectiveness of routine ultrasonography in detecting fetal abnormalities in a low risk population. BMJ 1991; 303:165–169.
19. Luck CL. Value of routine ultrasound scanning at 19 weeks: a four year study of 8849 deliveries. BMJ 1992; 304:1474–1478.
20. Shirley IM, Bottomley F, Robinson VP. Routine radiographer screening for fetal abnormalities in an unselected low risk population. Br J Radiol 1992; 65:564–569.
21. Ewigman BG, Crane JP, Frigoletto FD, LeFevre ML, Bain RP, McNellis D and the RADIUS Study Group. Effect of prenatal ultrasound screening on perinatal outcome. N Engl J Med 1993; 329:821–827.
22. Romero R. Routine obstetric ultrasound. Ultrasound Obstet Gynecol 1993; 3:303–307.
23. DeVore GR. The routine antenatal diagnostic imaging with ultrasound study: another perspective. Obstet Gynecol 1994; 84:622–626.
24. Crane JP, LeFevre ML, Winborn RC et al. A randomized trial of prenatal ultrasonographic screening: Impact on the detection, management and outcome of anomalous fetuses. Am J Obstet Gynecol 1994; 171:392–399.
25. Bernaschek G, Stuempflen I, Deutinger J. The value of sonographic diagnosis of fetal malformations: different results between indication-based and screening-based investigations. Prenatal Diagnosis 1994; 14:807–812.

26. Carrera JM, Torrents M, Mortera C, Cusi V, Munoz A. Routine prenatal ultrasound screening for fetal abnormalities: 22 years' experience. Ultrasound Obstet Gynecol 1995; 5:174–179.

27. Levi S, Schaaps JP, De Havay P, Coulon R, Defoort P. End-result of routine ultrasound screening for congenital anomalies: The Belgian Multicentric Study 1984–92. Ultrasound Obstet Gynecol 1995; 5:366–371.

28. Baronciani D, Scaglia C, Corchia C, Torcetta F, Mastroiacovos P. Ultrasonography in pregnancy and fetal abnormalities: screening or diagnostic test? IPIMC 1986–1990 Register Data. Prenat Diagn 1995; 15:1101–1108.

29. Sabbagha RF, Sheikh Z, Tamura RK et al. Predictive value, sensitivity, and specificity of ultrasonic targeted imaging for fetal anomalies in gravid women at high risk for birth defects. Am J Obstet Gynecol 1985; 152:822–827.

30. Manchester DK, Pretorius DH, Avery C et al. Accuracy of ultrasound diagnoses in pregnancies complicated by suspected fetal anomalies. Prenat Diagn 1988; 8:109–117.

31. Chambers SE, Geirsson RT, Stewart RJ, Wannapirak C, Muir BB. Audit of a screening service for fetal abnormalities using early ultrasound scanning and maternal serum α-fetoprotein estimation combined with selective detailed scanning. Ultrasound Obstet Gynecol 1995; 5:168–173.

32. Cullen MT, Green J, Whetham J, Salafia C, Gabrielli S, Hobins JC. Transvaginal ultrasonographic detection of congenital anomalies in the first trimester. Am J Obstet Gynecol 1990; 163:466–476.

33. Timor-Tritsch HE, Monteagudo A, Peisner DB. High frequency transvaginal sonographic examination for the potential malformation assessment of the 9-week to 14-week fetus. J Clin Ultrasound 1992; 20:231–238.

34. Bronshtein M, Yoffe N, Blumfield Z. Detection of fetal abnormalities by ultrasonography: Which sonogram, when, and by whom, to whom and how many? Ultrasound Obstet Gynecol 1991; 1(Suppl 1):125.

35. Economides DL, Braithwaite JM, Armstrong MA. First trimester fetal abnormality screening in a low risk population. Proc British Congress Obstet Gynecol 1995; Dublin abstract: 4-55.

36. Achiron R, Tadmor O. Screening for fetal abnormalities during the first trimester of pregnancy: transvaginal versus transabdominal sonography. Ultrasound Obstet Gynecol 1991; 1:186–191.

37. Waldenstrom U, Nilsson S, Fall O. Effects of routine one stage ultrasound screening in pregnancy: a randomised controlled trial. Lancet 1988; ii:585–588.

38. Morrison JJ, Rennie JM. Changing the definition of perinatal mortality. Lancet 1995; 346:1038.

39. Morrison JJ. Prediction and prevention of preterm labour. In: Studd J, ed. Progress in obstet gynecol, vol 12. Edinburgh: Churchill Livingstone; 1996:65–82.

40. Sandelowski M. Channel of desire: Fetal ultrasonography in two use-contexts. Qual Health Res 1994; 4:262–266.

41. Crang-Svalenius E, Dykes A-K, Joregensen C. Women's informed choice of prenatal diagnosis: Early ultrasound examination – routine ultrasound examination – age-independent amniocentesis. Fetal Diag Ther 1996; 11:20–25.

42. Marteau T, Slack J, Kidd J, Shaw R. Presenting a routine screening test in antenatal care: practice observed. Public Health 1992; 106:131–141.

43. Marteau T, Plenicar M, Kidd J. Obstetricians presenting amniocentesis to pregnant women: practice observed. J Reprod Inf Psychol 1993; 11:3–10.

44. Smith DK, Marteau TM. Detecting fetal abnormality: serum screening and fetal anomaly scans. Br J Midwifery 1995; 3:133–136.

45. Lele PP. Review: safety and potential hazards in the current applications of ultrasound in obstetrics and gynaecology. Ultrasound Med Biol 1979; 5:307–320.

46. Economides DL, Braithwaite JM. Safety of ultrasound in obstetrics. Contemp Rev Obstet Gynaecol 1996; 8:11–14.

47. Tarantal AF, Hendericks AG. Evaluation of the bioeffects of prenatal ultrasound exposure in the cynomolgus macaque. 2. Growth and behaviour during the first year. Teratology 1989; 39:149–162.

48. Salvesen KA, Vatten LJ, Jacobson G et al. Routine ultrasonography in utero and subsequent vision and hearing at primary school age. Ultrasound Obstet Gynecol 1992; 2:243–247.

49. Salvesen KA, Bakketeig LS, Eik-nes SH, Undeheim L, Okland O. Routine ultrasonography in utero and school performance at age 8–9 years. Lancet 1992; 339:85–91.

50. Salvesen KA, Vatten LJ, Eik-nes SH, Hugdahl K, Bakketeig LS. Routine ultrasonography in utero and subsequent handedness and neurological development. BMJ 1993; 307:159–162.

51. Newnham JP, Evans SF, Michael CA, Stanley FJ, Landau LI. Effects of frequent ultrasound during pregnancy: a randomised controlled trial. Lancet 1993; 342:887–891.

52. Newnham JP, Evans SF, Michael CA, Stanley FJ, Landau LI. Effects of frequent ultrasound during pregnancy. Lancet 1993; 342:1360–1361.

53. Visser GHA, de Vries JIP, Mulder EJH, Ververs IAP, van Geijn HP. Effects of frequent ultrasound during pregnancy. Lancet 1993; 342:1359–1360.

54. MacDonald W, Newnham J, Gurrin L, Evans S. Effect of frequent prenatal ultrasound on birthweight. follow up at 1 year of age. Lancet 1996; 348:482.

55. Bude RO, Rubin JM. Power Doppler sonography. Radiology 1996; 200:21–23.

56. Calman KC. Safe use of diagnostic ultrasound. A communication to all doctors from the Chief Medical Officer, Department of Health, November 1994.

57. Merritt CRB, Kremkau FW, Hobbins JC. Diagnostic ultrasound: bioeffects and safety. Ultrasound Obstet Gynecol 1992; 2:366–374.

58. Pitkin RM. Screening and detection of congenital malformation. Am J Obstet Gynecol 1991; 164:1045–1048.

59. Levi S, Hyjazi Y, Schaaps JP, Defoort P, Coulon R, Buekens P. Sensitivity and specificity of routine antenatal screening for congenital anomalies by

ultrasound: the Belgian multicentric study. Ultrasound Obstet Gynecol 1991; 5:366–371.

60. Roberts CJ, Hibbard BM, Roberts EE, Evans KT, Laurence KM, Robertson IB. Diagnostic effectiveness of ultrasound in detection of neural tube defect. The South Wales experience of 2509 scans (1977–1982) in high risk mothers. Lancet 1983; ii:1068–1069.

61. Hogge WA, Thiagarajah S, Ferguson JE, Schnatterly PT, Harbert GM. The role of ultrasonography and amniocentesis in the evaluation of pregnancies at risk for neural tube defects. Am J Obstet Gynecol 1989; 161:520–524.

62. Allen LC, Doran TA, Miskin M, Rudd NL, Benzie RJ, Sheffiels LJ. Ultrasound and amniotic fluid alpha-fetoprotein in the prenatal diagnosis of spina bifida. Obstet Gynecol 1982; 60:169–173.

63. Chitty LS. Ultrasound screening for fetal abnormalities. Prenat Diagn 1995; 15:1241–1257.

64. Richards DS, Seeds JW, Katz VL, Lingley LH, Albright SG, Cefalo RC. Elevated maternal serum alphafetoprotein with normal ultrasound: is amniocentesis always appropriate? A review of 26069 screened patients. Obstet Gynecol 1988; 71:203–207.

65. Gough JD. Ultrasound, antenatal and neonatal screening. In: Wald NJ, ed. Oxford: Oxford University Press; 1984:432–433.

66. Watson WJ, Chescheir NC, Katz VL, Seeds JW. The role of ultrasound in evaluation of patients with elevated maternal serum alpha-fetoprotein: a review. Obstet Gynecol 1991; 78:123–128.

67. Nicolaides KH, Gabbe SG, Campbell S, Guidetti R. Ultrasound screening for spina bifida: cranial and cerebellar signs. Lancet 1986; ii:72–74.

68. Thiagarayah S, Henke J, Hogge WA, Abbitt PL, Breeden N, Ferguson JE. Early diagnosis of spina bifida: the value of cranial ultrasound markers. Obstet Gynecol 1990; 76:54–57.

69. Van den Hof MC, Nicolaides KH, Campbell J, Campbell S. Evaluation of the lemon and banana signs in 130 fetuses with open spina bifida. Am J Obstet Gynecol 1990; 162:1000–1003.

70. Mitchell SC, Korones SB. Congenital heart disease in 56 109 births. Incidence and natural history. Circulation 1971; 43:323–332.

71. Tegnander E, Eik-Nes SH, Johansen OJ, Linker DT. Prenatal detection of heart defects at the routine fetal examination at 18 weeks in a non-selected population. Ultrasound Obstet Gynecol 1995; 5:372–380.

72. Davis GK, Farquhar CM, Allan LD, Crawford DC, Chapman MG. Structural cardiac abnormalities in the fetus: reliability of prenatal diagnosis and outcome. Br J Obstet Gynaecol 1990; 97:27–31.

73. Achiron R, Glaser J, Gelernter I, Hegesh J, Yagel S. Extended fetal echocardiographic examination for detecting cardiac malformations in low risk pregnancies. BMJ 1992; 304:671–674.

74. Vergani P, Mariani S, Ghidini A et al. Screening for congenital heart disease with the four-chamber view of the fetal heart. Am J Obstet Gynecol 1992; 167:1000–1003.

75. Sharland GK, Allan LD. Screening for congenital heart disease prenatally. Results of a 2.5 year study in the South East Thames region. Br J Obstet Gynaecol 1992; 99:220–225.

76. Allan LD, Cook A, Sullivan I, Sharland GK. Hypoplastic left heart syndrome: effects of fetal echocardiography on birth prevalence. Lancet 1991; 337:959–961.

77. Fowlie A, McHugo J. The urinary tract. In: Dewbury K, Meire H, Cosgrove D, eds. Ultrasound in obstetrics and gynaecology. Edinburgh: Churchill Livingstone; 1993:313–344.

78. Livera LN, Brookfields DSK, Egginton JA, Hawnaur JN. Antenatal ultrasonography to detect fetal renal abnormalities: a prospective screening programme. BMJ 1989; 198:1421–1423.

79. Arger PH, Coleman BG, Mintz MC et al. Routine fetal genitourinary tract screening. Radiology 1985; 156:485–489.

80. Langer B, Sineoni U, Montoya Y, Casanova R, Schlaeder G. Antenatal diagnosis of upper urinary tract dilation by ultrasonography. Fetal Diagnosis and Therapy 1996; 11:191–198.

81. Chitty LS, Chudleigh P, Campbell S, Pembrey M. The clinical significance of mild fetal pyelectasis. Ultrasound Obstet Gynaecol 1996; 8:157.

82. Podevin G, Mandelbrot L, Vuillard E, Oury JF, Aigrain Y. Outcome of urological abnormalities prenatally diagnosed by ultrasound. Fetal Diagnosis and Therapy 1996; 11:181–190.

83. Escobar LM, Bixler D, Weaver DD, Padilla LM, Golichowski A. Bone dysplasias: the prenatal diagnostic challenge. Am J Med Genet 1990; 36:488–494.

84. Kurtz AB, Needelman L, Wapner RJ et al. Usefulness of a short femur in the in utero detection of skeletal dysplasias. Radiology 1990; 177:197–200.

85. Oberlaid F, Danks DM, Jensen F, Stace L, Rosshandler S. Achondroplasia and hypochondroplasia. Comments on frequency, mutation rate, and radiologic features in skull and spine. J Med Genet 1979; 16:140–146.

86. Filly RA, Golbus MS, Cary JC, Hall JG. Short limbed dwarfism: ultrasonographic diagnosis by mensuration of fetal femoral length. Radiology 1981; 138:653–656.

87. Griffin DR, Chitty LS. The skeleton. In: Dewbury K, Meire H, Cosgrove D, eds. Ultrasound in obstetrics and gynaecology. Edinburgh: Churchill Livingstone; 1993:379–403.

88. Modaff P, Horton VK, Pauli RM. Errors in the prenatal diagnosis of children with achondroplasia. Prenat Diagn 1996; 16:525–530.

89. Bellus GA, Hefferon TW, Ortiz de Luna RI et al. Achondroplasia is defined by recurrent G380R mutations of FGFR3. Am J Hum Genet 1995; 56:368–373.

90. Hastabacka J, de la Chapelle A, Mahtani MM et al. The diastrophic dysplasia gene encodes a novel sulfate transporter: positional cloning by fine-structure linkage disequilibrium mapping. Cell 1994; 28:1073–1087.

91. Bellus GA, McIntosh I, Smith EA et al. A recurrent mutation in the tyrosin kinase domain of the fibroblast growth factor receptor 3 causes hypochondroplasia. Nature Genet 1995; 10:357–359.

92. Pearce JM. Miscellaneous abnormalities. In: Dewbury K, Meire H, Cosgrove D, eds. Ultrasound in obstetrics and gynaecology. Edinburgh: Churchill Livingstone; 1993:417–433.

93. Cannon C, Dildy GA, Ward R, Varner MW, Dudley DJ. A population-based study of congenital diaphtagmatic hernia in Utah: 1988–1994. Obstet Gynecol 1996; 87:959–963.

94. Griffin DR, Chitty LS. The thorax. In: Dewbury K, Meire H, Cosgrove D, eds. Ultrasound in obstetrics and gynaecology. Edinburgh: Churchill Livingstone; 1993:405–416.

95. King SJ, Pilling DW, Walkinshaw S. Fetal echogenic lung lesions: prenatal ultrasound diagnosis and outcome. Pediatr Radiol 1995; 25:208–210.

96. Morrison JJ, Chitty LS, Clark T, Sultan S, Maxwell D, Rodeck CH. Natural history cystic lung lesions in the fetus. Ultrasound Obstet Gynaecol 1996; 8:185.

97. David TJ, O'Callaghan SE. Oesophageal atresia in the south-west of England. J Med Genet 1975; 12:1–11.

98. Shackley P. Economic evaluation of prenatal diagnosis: a methodological review. Prenat Diagn 1996; 16:389–395.

99. Leivo T, Tuominen R, Saari-Kemppainen A, Ylostalo P, Karjalainen O, Heinonen OP. Cost-effectiveness of one-stage ultrasound screening in pregnancy: a report from the Helsinki ultrasound trial. Ultrasound Obstet Gynecol 7:309–314.

CHAPTER 4

First trimester detection of fetal anomalies

Peter Twining

Introduction

The improvement in ultrasound technology and the development of transvaginal scanning has revolutionized assessment of the first trimester fetus.[1-4] There are many advantages to first trimester scanning and these are outlined in Table 4.1.

It has been established that up to 2.8% of pregnancies will be non-viable between 10 and 13 weeks of gestation and that chromosomal abnormalities may be present in 45 to 70% of cases.[5] It is also likely that the early detection of a non-viable pregnancy and the elective evacuation of retained products of conception is more cost effective and potentially safer than emergency surgery in a patient presenting during miscarriage.[5]

Multiple pregnancy can be reliably diagnosed in the first trimester and using the 'lambda sign' chorionicity can also be assessed as it is well recognized that in monochorionic twin pregnancies the prevalence of antenatal and perinatal complications is much higher.[6]

Accurate dating of pregnancy is important as up to 30% of women attending an antenatal clinic have uncertain or unreliable menstrual dates.[5] Dating is valuable not only for estimating the date of delivery but also as a baseline for both first trimester and second trimester biochemical screening for Down's syndrome. Recent studies suggest a sensitivity of 62% (with a 5% false-positive rate) for the first trimester detection of Down's syndrome using free beta human chorionic gonadotrophin (HCG) and pregnancy associated plasma protein A (PAPP-A)[7] which is similar to the sensitivity of biochemical screening in the second trimester.

The early detection of fetal abnormalities has a number of advantages, not least of which is the fact that a suction termination of pregnancy can be carried out if the mother elects not to continue with the pregnancy.[3,4] In this way the physical and psychological morbidity associated with second trimester abortion may be reduced.[3] It is known that the level of psychological morbidity following a second trimester termination is similar to that following spontaneous perinatal loss and is of the order of 25%.[4]

It is now becoming increasingly clear that an increased nuchal translucency measurement is associated with a high risk of chromosomal disease, particularly trisomy 21[8,9] (see Chapter 14). A recent large multicentre study revealed a sensitivity of 84% for the first trimester detection of Down's syndrome using nuchal translucency scanning and maternal age.[10] In addition there is now increasing evidence that an increased nuchal translucency measurement is also associated with structural abnormalities, particularly cardiac anomalies,[11-13] and also rare genetic syndromes.[14,15] Fetuses with an increased nuchal translucency measurement and a normal karyotype should therefore have detailed transvaginal scanning in the first trimester and also detailed scanning at 20 weeks to look for structural abnormalities and also major cardiac defects. Further follow-up scans may also be indicated.

The first trimester diagnosis of fetal abnormalities is therefore important, although there are a number of disadvantages to this technique (Table 4.2).

It is clear that transvaginal scanning is far superior to transabdominal scanning in the first trimester diagnosis of fetal abnormalities.[16,17] Indeed, Achiron and Tadmor demonstrated an improved sensitivity for fetal anomaly detection from

---

Table 4.1
Advantages of first trimester scanning

1 Establishing fetal viability and excluding early pregnancy complications
2 Confirming multiple pregnancy and determining chorionicity
3 Accurate dating for estimated date of delivery and as a baseline for both first and second trimester biochemical screening
4 Early detection of fetal abnormalities
5 Termination of pregnancy may be carried out as a suction curettage
6 Nuchal translucency measurement for the detection of chromosomal disease, and as a marker for other syndromes and structural abnormalities, especially cardiac anomalies

---

Table 4.2
Disadvantages of first trimester diagnosis of fetal anomalies

1 Difficulties in technique of transvaginal fetal scanning
2 Inability to detect all abnormalities due to the natural history of some anomalies
3 Significance of minor anomalies unclear at present
4 Pitfalls in first trimester diagnosis of fetal anomalies
5 No pathological confirmation of diagnosis
6 High spontaneous loss rate in fetuses with major abnormalities

29 to 57% when comparing transabdominal and transvaginal scanning.[16]

Similarly, Economides and Braithwaite improved fetal anomaly detection from 35 to 65% using transabdominal and transvaginal scanning respectively.[17] There are, however, technical difficulties in using transvaginal scanning to demonstrate fetal anomalies. Scanning before 12 weeks' gestation is unsatisfactory as assessment of fetal anatomy is often incomplete.[18] Indeed Whitlow and Economides have proposed 13 weeks' gestation as the optimal gestational age to examine fetal anatomy and measure nuchal translucency.[19] Probe manoeuvrability is superior with transabdominal scanning and orientation and training are faster and easier.[4] There may also be problems with unfavourable fetal position, fibroids, contraction of the uterus and limited time caused by the patient's anxiety.[20] In addition, a chaperone is required for transvaginal scanning.

Although a large number of fetal anomalies can be detected in the first trimester[1-3] there are certain conditions which have variable onset or only present later in gestation and so will not be detectable on first trimester scanning. Rottem has proposed a classification of fetal anomalies based on their natural history[21] (Table 4.3). Class I are abnormalities in the primordium of an organ and occur very early in pregnancy. They can be detected at a constant gestational age during the first trimester. Class II are transient conditions and are usually the result of an abnormal accumulation or distribution of fluid in the fetal body involving the lymphatic, urinary or central nervous systems. Although these findings do not necessarily constitute a fetal abnormality per se, their presence may indicate an underlying chromosomal defect or they may constitute a prelude to an anomaly developing in another system. Class III anomalies have a variable onset or are potentially unstable anomalies. Conditions with a variable onset include diaphragmatic hernia and hydrocephalus. Potentially unstable anomalies are defects that may disappear after they are initially diagnosed only to reappear a few days later. Examples include exomphalos, megacystis, and encephalocoele. Finally, Class IV anomalies

Table 4.3
Classification of fetal anomalies

Class I	**Early onset at constant gestational age** Anencephaly, spina bifida, holoprosencephaly, conjoined twins, cyclops deformity, facial cleft, osteogenesis imperfecta Type II, dextrocardia
Class II	**Transient conditions** Increased nuchal translucency, nuchal or axillary cystic hygromas, pericardial and pleural effusions, choroid plexus cysts, hydronephrosis, mesenteric cyst echogenic bowel
Class III	**Anomalies with variable onset or potentially unstable* anomalies** Congenital diaphragmatic hernia, hydrocephalus, talipes, Dandy–Walker malformation, coarctation of the aorta, pulmonary stenosis, Fallot tetralogy, aortic stenosis, ovarian cyst and atrioventricular heart block, obstructive uropathy, exomphalos*, megacystis* and encephalocoele*
Class IV	**Late onset anomalies** Agenesis of the corpus callosum, lissencephaly, porencephaly, microcephaly, arachnoid cysts, duodenal atresia, jejunal atresia, anal atresia, fetal tumours, endocardial fibroelastosis, hypertrophic cardiomyopathy, ventricular aneurysm

Reproduced with permission from Rottem S. IRONFAN: New time-oriented malformation work up and classification of fetal anomalies. Ultrasound Obstet Gynecol 1997;10:373–374.[21]

present late and either affect those organs that develop late, or are the end point in the natural history of abnormalities affecting those organs that develop early in pregnancy (Table 4.3). First trimester scanning therefore will be of value in detecting abnormalities in Class I and II; however, there will be major limitations in detecting anomalies in Class III and Class IV.

Another problem area which also affects second trimester scanning is the detection of minor anomalies such as mild renal pelvic dilatation, choroid plexus cysts, echogenic foci in the fetal heart, intra-abdominal cysts and umbilical cord cysts.[22-24] It is seen that many of these anomalies resolve by the second trimester but their significance is unclear and care must be taken in the interpretation of such ultrasound findings. Larger studies are required in order to determine the importance of such minor ultrasound findings in the first trimester.

In order that first trimester scanning can be carried out accurately it is important that there is a full understanding of embryological development. In this way some of the common pitfalls in first trimester diagnosis may be avoided. The normal midgut herniation of the bowel which occurs between 8 and 12 weeks' gestation should not be confused with an anterior abdominal wall defect.[25] Similarly, in the brain the normal single ventricle appearance of the rhombencephalon seen between 7 and 9 weeks' gestation should not be confused with holopros-encephaly.[26] A full understanding of normal embryological development is therefore essential prior to the interpretation of the ultrasound appearances of the first trimester fetus. In addition to an understanding of the normal development of the fetus, it is also important to be aware that certain fetal abnormalities seen in the second trimester will present in a different manner in the first trimester. A typical example is renal agenesis, which will demonstrate severe oligo-hydramnios at 18 to 20 weeks but may have normal liquor volume in the first trimester. The presence of normal liquor volume at 12 to 14 weeks therefore does not exclude renal agenesis or other major renal abnormalities.[3]

A major disadvantage to first trimester diagnosis of fetal anomalies is that there is often no pathological confirmation of the diagnosis as a suction termination of pregnancy is usually carried out. This is of importance as it has been shown that an accurate post-mortem examination may alter the sonographic diagnosis.[27] This has significance for clinical genetic counselling in terms of future pregnancies, as in order to provide the best genetic counselling in terms of recurrence risks and the best method of subsequent prenatal diagnosis it is important to have an accurate initial diagnosis.[2]

One further important point is that many pregnancies complicated with a serious malformation will abort spontaneously in the first or early second trimester. Whilst it may be helpful for parents to understand the reason for the pregnancy loss, this benefit must be weighed against potential harm which may result from making parents choose to terminate a wanted pregnancy which might have been lost spontaneously.[2]

It is clear therefore that there are many advantages and disadvantages to the first trimester diagnosis of fetal abnormalities. What is also clear, however, is the need for good quality equipment with a high frequency transvaginal transducer, experience in the technique of transvaginal sonography and a thorough knowledge of the embryological development of the first trimester fetus.

First trimester screening for fetal abnormalities

Routine scanning at 18 to 20 weeks' gestation is now well established in Europe (see Ch. 3). However, routine first trimester scanning for fetal anomalies using the transvaginal approach has not gained widespread acceptance and there are only a few screening studies available in the literature. As an alternative to routine mid-trimester scanning some workers have evaluated the use of booking scans in the first trimester

Table 4.4
Detection rates for first trimester scanning followed by mid-trimester scanning

Author	Type of Population	Number in study	Detection Rates % First Trimester Trans-abdominal	First Trimester Trans-vaginal	Second trimester	Third trimester	Missed Anomalies %
Constantine and McCormack 1991*[28]	LR	3565	14	–	14	36	36
Chambers et al 1995*[29]	LR	19 497	13	–	52	20	15
Achiron and Tadmor 1991[16]	HR	800	29	57	36	–	7
Yagel et al 1995[32]	HR	536	–	74	16	–	10
Hernadi and Torocsik 1997[20]	LR	3991	–	41	19	20	20
D'Ottavio et al 1997[31]	LR	3490	–	32	48	5	15
Economides and Braithwaite 1998[17]	LR	1632	35	65	18	–	17

*Booking scans and clinically indicated scans only. LR – low risk populations; HR – high risk populations.

together with alphafetoprotein estimation at 16 weeks and then selective scanning based on clinical indication.[28–30] The results of such studies reveal an overall detection rate of 13 to 14% using transabdominal scanning in the first trimester (Table 4.4). Dedicated first trimester screening studies using transvaginal scanning show detection rates in the range of 32 to 65% in low-risk populations,[17,20,31] and 57 to 74% in high-risk pregnancies.[16,32] In addition, two studies compared the detection rates of transabdominal scanning to transvaginal scanning and documented improvements in the detection rates from 29 to 57% and 35 to 65%.[16,17] These studies also demonstrated that second trimester scanning picked up additional anomalies with detection rates in the range of 16 to 48%. There was also a significant percentage of anomalies not seen until the third trimester and the neonatal period (Table 4.4). These studies therefore suggest that first trimester scanning, even in expert hands, is unlikely to replace routine mid-trimester screening for fetal abnormalities.

The type and range of anomalies detected in the first trimester differs from those seen in the second trimester with high incidences of severe intracranial anomalies such as anencephaly and exencephaly. In addition, cystic hygromata and hydrops are common findings as is an increased nuchal translucency. Other common anomalies seen are anterior abdominal wall defects, renal anomalies and skeletal dysplasias,[16,17,20,31–33] (Table 4.5).

Nuchal translucency screening for fetal abnormalities

There is increasing evidence that as well as being associated with a high risk of chromosomal disease[8–10] (see Ch. 14) an increased nuchal translucency measurement is also associated with structural anomalies and rare syndromes[13–15] (Table 4.6). The observed prevalence for some of the abnormalities such as anencephaly, holoprosencephaly, microcephaly, facial cleft, gastroschisis, renal abnormalities, bowel obstruction and spina bifida may not be different from that in the general population. However, the prevalence of major cardiac defects, diaphragmatic hernia, exomphalos, body stalk anomaly and fetal akinesia deformation sequence appears to be substantially higher than in the general population, indicating an association between these abnormalities and increased nuchal translucency thickness. Similarly, there may be an association between increased nuchal translucency and a wide range of skeletal dysplasias and genetic syndromes that are usually found in less than 1 in 10 000 pregnancies[14,15,34–43] (Table 4.6).

Fetuses with an increased nuchal translucency thickness and a normal karyotype should therefore undergo transvaginal scanning in the first trimester, and also transabdominal scanning at 20 weeks in order to look for major fetal

Table 4.5
Type of abnormalities detected using transvaginal scanning in the first trimester

Organ system	Number	Percentage of total	Anomaly	Number
Central nervous system	30	25	Anencephaly/exencephaly	16
			Ventriculomegaly	7
			Dandy–Walker syndrome	3
			Holoprosencephaly	2
			Encephalocoele	2
Neck	22	18	Cystic hygroma	22
Cardiac*	14	11.5	Tetralogy of Fallot	3
			Hypoplastic left heart	3
			Hypoplastic right heart	1
			Truncus arteriosus	1
			Ebstein's anomaly	1
			Ventricular septal defect	2
			Aortic stenosis	1
			Complex cardiac anomaly	2
Renal	14	11.5	Hydronephrosis	5
			Bladder outlet	
			Obstruction/megacystis	4
			Cystic renal disease	4
			Renal agenesis	1
Abdomen	12	10	Anterior abdominal wall defects	12
Body	9	7.5	Oedema/hydrops	9
Musculoskeletal	5	4	Skeletal dysplasias	5
Spine	4	3.3	Spina bifida	4
Face	2	1.5	Facial clefting	2

Combined data from 121 anomalies detected in studies from references[16,17,20,31–33]. Increased nuchal translucency, choroid plexus cysts and mild renal pelvic dilatation excluded from the analysis.
*11 out of the 14 cardiac anomalies were detected in study reference[32].

Table 4.6
Fetal abnormalities associated with an increased nuchal translucency thickness

Common conditions
Cardiac abnormalities
Diaphragmatic hernia
Exomphalos
Body stalk anomaly

Rare conditions
Skeletal dysplasias
  Achondrogenesis
  Camptomelic dysplasia
  Achondroplasia
  Thanatophoric dysplasia
  Jarcho–Levin syndrome
  Short rib polydactyly syndrome
  Ectrodactyly-ectodermal dysplasia
  Asphyxiating thoracic dystrophy
Genetic syndromes
  Noonan syndrome
  Smith–Lemli–Opitz syndrome
  Joubert syndrome
  Zellweger syndrome
  Myotonic dystrophy
  Spinal muscular atrophy
  Fryns syndrome
  Hydrolethalus syndrome
  Meckel–Gruber syndrome
  Roberts syndrome

abnormalities. It would also seem prudent to follow-up these fetuses into the third trimester specifically looking for evidence of skeletal dysplasias such as achondroplasia, and other rare conditions which may only present later in gestation.

Normal appearances (sonoembryology)

Gestational sac, yolk sac and fetal pole

The gestational sac may be recognized as early as 4 weeks and 1 day from the last menstrual period and should always be seen after 4 weeks and 4 days. Its diameter is about 2 mm and increases in size to measure 5 to 6 mm at 5 weeks.[44] The mean gestational sac diameter then increases by approximately 1 mm per day throughout the first trimester.[45] The yolk sac should be

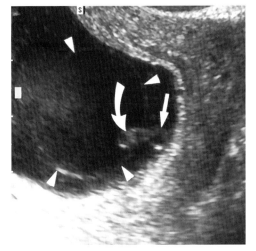

Fig. 4.1 Transvaginal scan of a 6-week pregnancy showing the embryo (curved arrow), yolk sac (straight arrow) and amniotic sac (arrowheads).

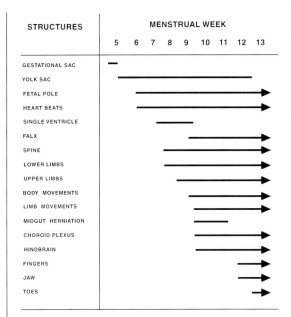

STRUCTURES	MENSTRUAL WEEK								
	5	6	7	8	9	10	11	12	13
GESTATIONAL SAC	▬								
YOLK SAC		▬▬▬▬▬▬▬▬▬▬							
FETAL POLE		▬▬▬▬▬▬▬▬▬▶							
HEART BEATS		▬▬▬▬▬▬▬▬▬▶							
SINGLE VENTRICLE		▬▬							
FALX			▬▬▬▬▬▬▶						
SPINE		▬▬▬▬▬▬▬▶							
LOWER LIMBS		▬▬▬▬▬▬▬▶							
UPPER LIMBS		▬▬▬▬▬▬▬▬▶							
BODY MOVEMENTS		▬▬▬▬▬▬▬▶							
LIMB MOVEMENTS			▬▬▬▬▬▶						
MIDGUT HERNIATION			▬▬						
CHOROID PLEXUS			▬▬▬▬▶						
HINDBRAIN			▬▬▬▶						
FINGERS			▬▶						
JAW			▬▶						
TOES			▬▶						

Fig. 4.2 Sequential appearance of embryonic structures and functions. (Reproduced with permission from Timor-Tritsch I, Farine D, Rosen M. A close look at early embryonic development with the high-frequency transvaginal transducer. Am J Obstet Gynecol 1988;159:676–681.)

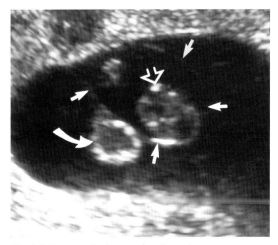

Fig. 4.3 Transvaginal scan of an 8-week pregnancy showing the embryo, amniotic sac and yolk sac lying outside the amniotic sac within the extraembryonic coelom (curved arrow – yolk sac, open arrow – embryo, small arrows – amniotic sac).

visible from 5 weeks' gestation and increases in size to a maximum mean diameter of 5 mm at 10 weeks' gestation. The majority of yolk sacs decrease in size before disappearing at around 12 weeks' gestation. Some yolk sacs, however, will increase in size before disappearing.[45] The fetal pole is usually visible towards the end of the 5th week and at 6 weeks the developing embryo appears as an echogenic line of about 5 mm tangentially touching and closely attached to the yolk sac[26] (Fig. 4.1). The fetal heartbeat should be demonstrated from 6 weeks' gestation (Fig. 4.2) and the heart rate is approximately 120 beats per minute. The amniotic sac is seen surrounding the developing fetus and the yolk sac lies outside the amniotic sac within the extra embryonic coelom (Fig. 4.3).

Central nervous system

The central nervous system develops from the neural tube and at 5 weeks' gestation the cephalic end separates into three primary brain vesicles: prosencephalon (forebrain), mesencephalon (midbrain) and rhombencephalon (hindbrain). At 6 weeks' gestation the secondary brain vesicles occur and the prosencephalon differentiates into the telencephalon and diencephalon, the mesencephalon remains unchanged and the rhombencephalon divides into the metencephalon and myeloencephalon.[46] Between 7 and 8 weeks the fetal cephalic pole is clearly distinguishable from the fetal torso.

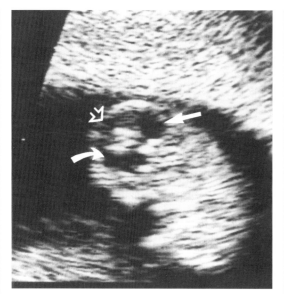

Fig. 4.4 Sagittal scan through the cephalic pole of an 8-week embryo showing the brain vesicles (curved arrow – prosencephalon, straight arrow – rhombencephalon. The mesencephalon – open arrow, lies between the prosencephalon and rhombencephalon).

On sagittal scanning the rudimentary brain vesicles can be demonstrated (Fig. 4.4) and on coronal scanning a single ventricle appearance can be seen representing the rhombencephalon[47] (Fig. 4.5). Towards the end of the 8th week the brain is divided by an echogenic line representing the falx cerebri and the biparietal diameter is approximately 8 mm.[46] The choroid plexuses appear soon after the falx as echogenic structures almost

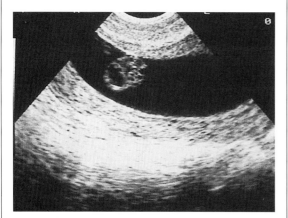

Fig. 4.5 Coronal scan through the cephalic pole of an 8-week embryo showing the single ventricle appearance of the rhombencephalon.

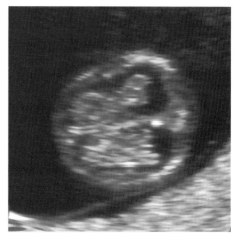

Fig. 4.6 Transverse scan through the head of a 10-week fetus showing choroid plexuses almost completely filling the fetal head.

completely filling the lateral ventricles[48] (Fig. 4.6). In the rhombencephalon the cerebellar hemispheres develop at the beginning of the 8th week as two laterally placed masses separated in the midline. During the 10th week the cerebellar hemispheres unite in the midline to form the definitive cerebellum[49] (Fig. 4.7). Ossification of the skull bones commences at 10 weeks and is complete at 11 to 12 weeks. The basic structure of the brain is therefore present at 11 to 12 weeks' gestation. The stages at which various intracranial structures can be demonstrated using transvaginal ultrasound are outlined in Figure 4.8.

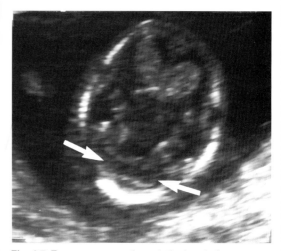

Fig. 4.7 Transverse scan through the head of an 11-week fetus showing the cerebellum (arrows).

Structure	*Menstrual age* (weeks)
	6 7 8 9 10 11 12 13
Cephalic pole	
Univentricular system	
Falx cerebri	
Biventricular system	
Choroid plexus	
Thalamus	
III ventricle	
Corpus callosum	
Cerebral peduncles	
Pons	
Cerebellum	
Cerebellar tentorium	
Hippocampus	
Posterior fossa (cisterna magna)	
IV ventricle	
Cerebral arteries	
Corpus striatum	
Calvarial skeleton	
Spinal skeleton	

Fig. 4.8 Sequential appearance of fetal neural structures during the first trimester. (Reproduced with permission from Achiron R, Achiron A. Transvaginal ultrasonic assessment of the early fetal brain. Ultrasound Obstet Gynecol 1991;1:336–344.)

The development of the spine is marked by the fact that at 5.5 weeks' gestation the neural folds are already fused, and the neural tube is already developed and covered by the neural crest and ectoderm.[44] Before 10 weeks the spine can be seen as hypoechogenic parallel lines (Fig. 4.9). After 10 weeks the spine starts to ossify (Fig. 4.10); however, ossification of the sacrum is not complete until 16 to 18 weeks' gestation.

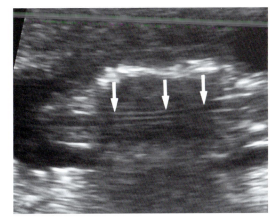

Fig. 4.9 Coronal scan through the spine of a 9-week fetus showing parallel hypoechogenic lines (arrows).

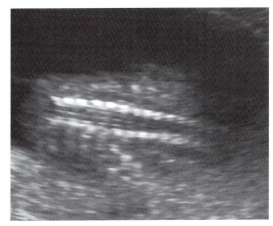

Fig. 4.10 Coronal scan through the spine of a 12-week fetus showing normal ossification.

The heart

The cardiovascular system begins to develop during the 3rd embryonic week and the fetal heartbeat can be discerned from the beginning of the 6th week. The heart gradually attains a tubular structure that resembles a trilocular cavity at the end of the 10th week. Formation of the septae, and arterial and venous connections are completed only after 8 weeks' gestation.[3] A 4-chamber view may be obtained at 10 weeks' gestation but it is seen in the majority of fetuses after 12 weeks' gestation and in all cases only after 13 weeks[19,50–54] (Fig. 4.11, Table 4.7). A full assessment of the fetal heart using transvaginal scanning in the first trimester is difficult due to the limitations of manoeuvreability of the transvaginal probe. Success rates vary between 43 and 95% at 13 weeks and 46 and 98% at 14 weeks.[52,54]

Table 4.7
Studies reporting the percentage of cases where the four chamber view of the heart was successfully visualized

Author	Gestational age (weeks)			
	10	11	12	13
Dolkart and Reimers[50]	–	30	90	100
Bronshtein et al[51]	–	16	36	90
Johnson et al[52]	27	58	71	73
Gembruch et al[53]	–	80	93	100
Whitlow and Economides[19]	9	83	96	98

Reproduced with permission from Souka A P, Nicolaides K H. Diagnosis of fetal abnormalities at the 10–14 week scan. Ultrasound Obstet Gynecol 1997;10:429–442.[1]

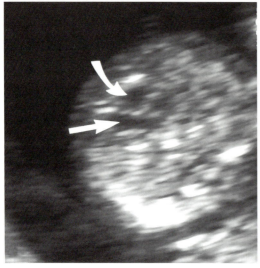

A

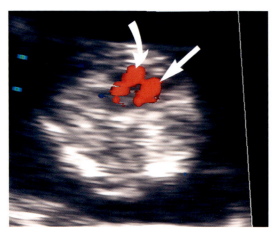

B

Fig. 4.11 (A) Transverse scan through the thorax of a 12-week fetus showing the 4-chamber view. Curved arrow – right ventricle, straight arrow – left ventricle. (B) Colour flow image showing filling of both ventricles (red jets). Curved arrow – right ventricle, straight arrow – left ventricle.

Urinary tract

The fetal kidneys can be identified as early as 9 weeks' gestation.[55] However, at 12 weeks' gestation the kidneys can be demonstrated in 86 to 99% of fetuses and at 13 weeks in 92 to 99%.[19,56] The upper limit of normal for the anteroposterior diameter of the renal pelvis is 3 mm[55] and normograms for renal size have also been reported for the first trimester.[56,57] In the first trimester the kidneys appear as oval echogenic structures on either

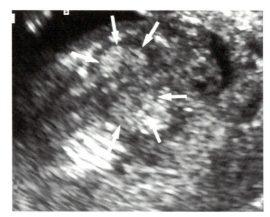

Fig. 4.12 Coronal scan of a 12-week fetus showing both kidneys – arrows.

side of the spine (Fig. 4.12) and the bladder is seen as a small echo free area within the pelvis. Colour flow Doppler is useful to confirm the location of the bladder (Fig. 4.13). Recent studies have shown that the bladder may be demonstrated in 88% of fetuses at 12 weeks' gestation and in 92 to 100% at 13 weeks' gestation.[56,57] The normal bladder diameter is approximately 5 to 6 mm in the first trimester.

Determination of the fetal gender is possible only after 12 weeks' gestation, as up to 6 weeks' gestation the external genitalia of the male and female are indifferent, and differentiation occurs between 8 and 11 weeks' gestation.[58] Female genitalia are visualized as two or four parallel lines that represent the labia major and minora. In addition, on sagittal scanning the clitoris is caudally directed. Male fetuses demonstrate a uniform, non-septated dome-shaped structure at the base of the fetal penis. The testes will not be demonstrated as they have not yet descended into the scrotum. Sagittal scanning will also reveal the cranially directed penis. Accuracy rates range from 87 to 90% for males and females respectively at 13 to 14 weeks' and 96 to 98% for males and females respectively at 15 to 16 weeks' gestation.[58]

The abdomen

During the 6th menstrual week, as the right and left lateral folds form, the dorsal part of

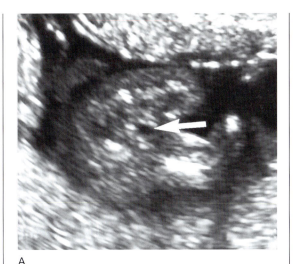

A

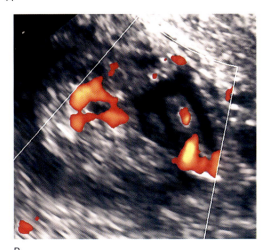

B

Fig. 4.13 (A) Transverse scan through the pelvis of a 12-week fetus showing bladder – straight arrow. (B) Power colour flow image of same fetus showing both umbilical arteries surrounding the bladder.

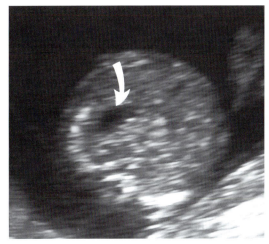

Fig. 4.14 Transverse scan through the abdomen of a 12-week fetus showing the stomach – curved arrow.

the yolk sac is incorporated into the embryo to form the primitive gut. The remaining yolk sac (secondary) pinches off the developing midgut loop, but remains connected to the gut by a stalk called the vitteline duct. Three distinct areas of primitive gut are identified – the foregut, the midgut and the hindgut.[3]

The foregut gives rise to the oesophagus, trachea, stomach, liver, gall bladder and biliary ducts. The stomach is identified as a sonolucent cystic structure in the left upper quadrant. It can be demonstrated as early as 8 weeks' gestation;[25] however, at 12 weeks it is seen in 97% of fetuses[19] (Fig. 4.14). It is thought that fetal swallowing does not begin until 12 to 13 weeks' gestation and so the fluid present in the fetal stomach before this time is likely to represent gastric secretions.[3]

The gall bladder emanates from the caudal part of the hepatic diverticulum at 7 weeks' gestation and bile starts to form at approximately 14 weeks.[3] The gall bladder is usually not detectable until 13 weeks' gestation when it is seen in 50% of fetuses. At 14 weeks it is normally seen in all cases.[59]

During the 7th week of gestation, due to extensive lengthening of the midgut and the enlargement of the liver, a portion of intestinal loop moves outside the abdomen and protrudes into the proximal umbilical cord (Fig. 4.15). Within the cord the midgut grows further and rotates clockwise through 90 degrees around the axis of the superior mesenteric artery.[3] This midgut herniation starts therefore from the 7th week and persists until the 11th week. It should spontaneously resolve by the 12th week.[25,60,61] Recent studies reveal that transverse measurements of the midgut herniation should not exceed 7 mm at any gestation and that no herniation should be present in a fetus with a crown rump length greater than 44 mm.[25,61]

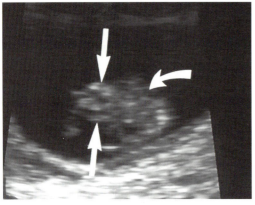

Fig. 4.15 Transverse scan through the abdomen of an 8-week fetus showing midgut herniation (straight arrows – midgut herniation, curved arrow – abdomen).

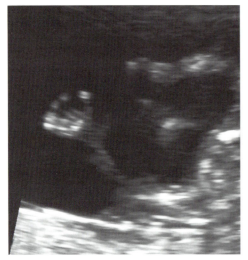

Fig. 4.16 Fetal fingers at 12 weeks' gestation.

Extremities

Limb buds are first seen by ultrasound at about the 8th week of gestation, the femur and humerus from 9 weeks' gestation, and tibia/fibula and radius/ulna from 10 weeks and digits of hands and feet from 11 weeks.[1,62] In early gestation the fetus tends to keep the hands open with fingers extended (Fig. 4.16) thus facilitating their visualization, unlike the second trimester when the hands are usually held in a flexed position. Similarly, the feet are held with heels almost touching and knees slightly flexed which also makes their visualization easier (Fig. 4.17).

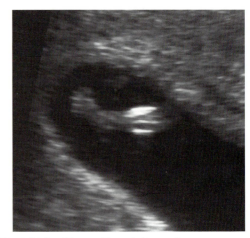

Fig. 4.17 Fetal foot at 12 weeks' gestation.

The face

The bones of the maxilla and mandible can be demonstrated as early as 9 to 10 weeks' and the orbits by 10 to 11 weeks' gestation. At 11 weeks the lenses of the eyes can be seen as tiny ring-like structures and may be demonstrated in all fetuses from the 14th week.[3] Between the 6th and 12th week the profile changes as at 7 weeks the forehead tends to dominate the face and the maxilla grows faster than the mandible. By 12 weeks the mandible catches up and reaches the size of the maxilla. The nose and lips finally form at 11 weeks and the palate at 12 weeks.[3] By 12 weeks the basic anatomy of the face is complete (Fig. 4.18).

Fetal abnormalities

CENTRAL NERVOUS SYSTEM ANOMALIES

Anencephaly/exencephaly

Anencephaly is the commonest anomaly to affect the central nervous system and results from failure of closure of the rostral portion of the neural tube which normally occurs during the 6th week of gestation.[63] The result is absence of the cranium (acrania) with complete but abnormal development of the brain. This condition is known as exencephaly and there is considerable

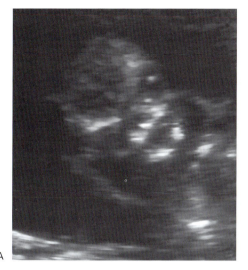

A

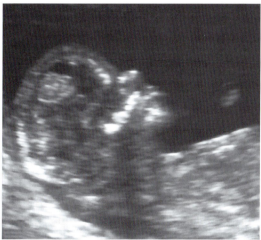

B

Fig. 4.18 (A) Coronal scan through 12-week fetus showing orbits, maxilla and mandible. (B) Sagittal scan showing fetal profile.

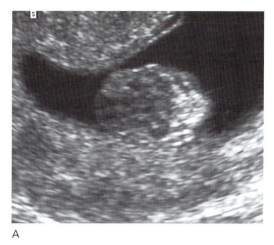

A

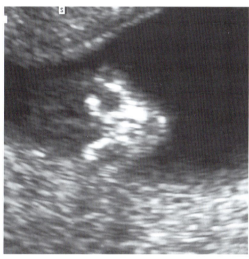

B

Fig. 4.19 Exencephaly. (A) Transverse scan through the head of a 12-week fetus showing abnormal brain and absence of the cranium (acrania). (B) Coronal scan showing normal orbits and absence of the skull.

evidence to show that prolonged exposure of the exencephalic brain to amniotic fluid and repeated mechanical trauma leads on to anencephaly.[64-66] Sonographically in exencephaly there is absence of the cranium but the brain may appear relatively normal (Fig. 4.19), or can appear as an abnormal mass of tissue floating above, or to either side of the head and this has been described as the 'Mickey Mouse' sign.[67,68] With progression to anencephaly one sees the characteristic 'frog's eyes' appearance with absence of the cranium and little brain tissue above the level of the orbits

(Fig. 4.20). The crown rump length is often reduced in cases of anencephaly due to the loss of brain tissue and a femur length measurement is a more accurate means of estimating gestational age. As skull ossification starts at 10 weeks' gestation the diagnosis of exencephaly or anencephaly cannot be made before this time and it would seem prudent to delay diagnosis until 12 weeks when skull ossification is likely to be complete in a normal fetus. In addition, transabdominal scanning may not have sufficient resolution to accurately diagnose anencephaly in the early first trimester.

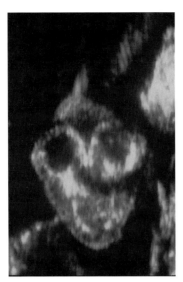

Fig. 4.20 Anencephaly. Typical frog's eyes appearance of anencephaly.

Achiron and Tadmor described three fetuses scanned transabdominally between 12 and 13 weeks which demonstrated a suspicious-looking cephalic pole. Transvaginal scanning revealed exencephaly in all three fetuses.[16] Goldstein et al also reported a fetus which appeared normal at 12 weeks but which was subsequently found to have anencephaly later in pregnancy.[64] In suspicious cases therefore it is recommended that standard transabdominal scanning be supplemented with transvaginal scanning to improve visualization of the fetus.

Recently a multicentre trial using transabdominal scanning only in the first trimester reported a detection rate of 74% for anencephaly; however, following an audit programme the detection rate increased to 100%.[69]

Encephalocoele

Encephalocoeles are herniations of the intracranial contents through a bony defect in the skull. If brain tissue is involved it is defined as an encephalocoele and if only meninges are involved it is called a cranial meningocoele.[70] In 75% of cases the encephalocoele is occipital. Lateral or parietal encephalocoeles should raise the possibility of amniotic band syndrome.

Sonographically the diagnosis is based on the demonstration of an occipital bony defect with varying degrees of brain herniation. As skull ossification starts at 10 weeks' gestation diagnosis is not possible before this time and the earliest reported diagnosis is at 13 weeks' gestation.[71] This case was followed-up however, and the encephalocoele disappeared at 15 weeks only to reappear again at 19 weeks, thus confirming that encephalocoele should be classified as an unstable abnormality (Table 4.3). van Zalen-Sprock also reported a case of encephalocoele at 13 weeks' gestation where earlier scanning at 11 weeks' gestation had shown two translucent areas in the occipital region suggestive of a septated cystic hygroma. Pathological examination at 13 weeks confirmed the diagnosis of encephalocoele.[72]

It is clear therefore that the sonographic appearances of encephalocoele are variable in the first trimester and can actually resolve to reappear at a later gestation. In addition, once an encephalocoele is diagnosed a search should be made for other anomalies, particularly enlarged cystic kidneys and polydactyly (Fig. 4.21), in order to confirm the diagnosis of Meckel–Gruber syndrome.[73] In theory at least it should be easier to visualize the large dense kidneys and polydactyly seen in Meckel–Gruber syndrome in the first trimester, due to the presence of normal liquor volume. In the second trimester there

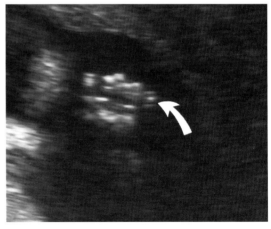

Fig. 4.21 Polydactyly. Coronal scan through the hand of a 14-week fetus showing polydactyly (curved arrow points to extra digit).

may be oligohydramnios which will hamper visualization of the encephalocoele and polydactyly. A number of prenatal diagnoses have been reported between 11 and 14 weeks' gestation.[74,75]

Hydrocephalus

Hydrocephalus is caused by an abnormal accumulation of cerebrospinal fluid within the ventricular system. It is usually caused by an obstruction of the ventricular system at the aqueduct (aqueduct stenosis) or posterior fossa (Dandy–Walker syndrome or Arnold–Chiari malformation secondary to spina bifida).

In the second trimester the diagnosis of ventriculomegaly is based on enlargement of the lateral ventricles with measurements greater than 10 mm indicative of ventriculomegaly. In the first trimester this sign is of little value as the ventricles almost completely fill the hemispheres (Fig. 4.6). What is more important is the morphology of the choroid plexus. Bronshtein and Ben-Shlomo reported thinning of the choroid plexus and the dangling choroid, as the earliest signs of fetal ventriculomegaly[76] (Fig. 4.22). However, these signs are present in a relatively small proportion of fetuses as prospective screening studies have shown. By pooling the data from three such studies it

is seen that ventriculomegaly was diagnosed in only 38% of fetuses in the first trimester, the remaining cases were detected at the mid-trimester scan.[16,20,32]

Dandy–Walker syndrome

The Dandy–Walker syndrome is characterized by absence of the cerebellar vermis and separation of the cerebellar hemispheres by a posterior fossa cyst which communicates with the fourth ventricle. It is thought the malformation originates before the 6th to 7th week of gestation.[3] Sonographically there is a large posterior fossa cyst separating the cerebellar hemispheres (Fig. 4.23).

A number of cases have been reported in the first trimester, one of which was associated with triploidy.[77–79]

Spina bifida

Spina bifida is caused by failure of closure of the neural tube and most commonly affects the lower lumbar and lumbo-sacral region. In the second trimester there are specific ultrasound signs within the fetal head which have a high specificity for the detection of spina bifida. These signs include the 'lemon'

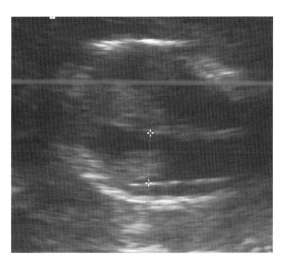

Fig. 4.22 Ventriculomegaly. Transverse scan through the head of a 13-week fetus showing moderate ventriculomegaly.

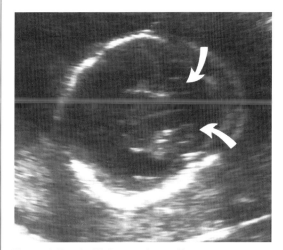

Fig. 4.23 Dandy–Walker syndrome. Transverse scan through the head of a 14-week fetus showing absence of the vermis and separation of the cerebellar hemispheres (curved arrows point to cerebellar hemispheres) (same fetus as in Fig. 4.24).

shaped head, 'banana' cerebellum and ventriculomegaly.[80]

The earliest reported diagnosis of spina bifida is at 10 weeks' gestation;[81] however, it is becoming clear that the intracranial signs seen in the second trimester may also be present in the first trimester and may precede the demonstration of the spinal defect by 1 to 2 weeks.[3,82,83]

In a large screening study using transvaginal scanning Blumenfeld et al detected all 10 cases of neural tube defect and in the 6 cases of lumbo-sacral spina bifida the 'banana' and 'lemon' signs were present. In one case scanned at 10 weeks there was a sacral irregularity but the cerebellum appeared normal, at 12 weeks there was a 'banana' sign and at 15 weeks a sacral meningocoele was detected and a 'lemon' sign was also seen in the head. These findings suggest that the signs within the head may evolve and precede the demonstration of a definite defect in the spine.[82] Sebire et al also reported the 'lemon' sign in three fetuses with spina bifida between 12 and 14 weeks.[83] The same group also reported the results of a multicentre screening study of transabdominal scanning at 10 to 14 weeks' gestation. None of the 29 cases of spina bifida were detected using transabdominal scanning in the first trimester, but 28 of the 29 were detected at mid-trimester scanning.[83]

In a further large screening study using transvaginal scanning, two out of five spina bifida cases were not detected during the first trimester scan.[20]

These results would indicate that transabdominal scanning may not have sufficient resolution to detect the subtle intracranial signs of spina bifida in the first trimester and that transvaginal scanning is required to diagnose this condition. However, even in expert hands some cases may be missed.

Holoprosencephaly

Holoprosencephaly is caused by failure of the forebrain to divide into the lateral ventricles. The result is a monoventricle and

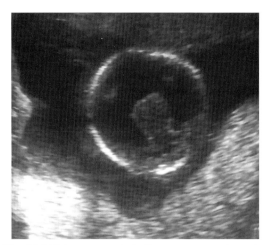

Fig. 4.24 Holoprosencephaly. Transverse scan through same fetus as in Figure 4.23 showing monoventricle with fused thalami.

in the most severe alobar form both thalami are fused and protrude into the single ventricular cavity. There is a high association with facial abnormalities, other major abnormalities and chromosomal disease, particularly trisomy 13. Sonographically the diagnosis is made by demonstrating a single ventricular cavity with fused thalami protruding into the monoventricle. There is a rim of cortex anteriorly but this may be difficult to demonstrate in the first trimester (Fig. 4.24).

A number of cases have been diagnosed in the first trimester usually with transvaginal scanning.[78,84-86]

Agenesis of the corpus callosum

The corpus callosum begins to develop at 11 to 12 weeks' gestation and its formation is complete by 18 weeks' gestation. In view of this fact prenatal diagnosis in the first trimester has not been reported.[3]

Cystic hygroma

Cystic hygroma is a congenital malformation of the lymphatic system producing large swellings that occur on the postero-lateral aspect of the fetal neck. They are usually multiseptate and the hallmark of a true cystic hygroma is the presence of the midline nuchal septum[87,88] (Fig. 4.25). There is a high

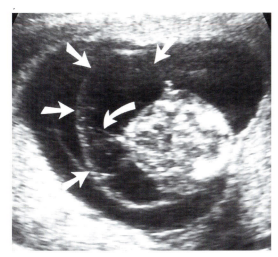

Fig. 4.25 Cystic hygroma. Transverse scan through fetal neck. Classic appearance of septated cystic hygroma (straight arrows outline cystic hygroma, curved arrow points to midline septum).

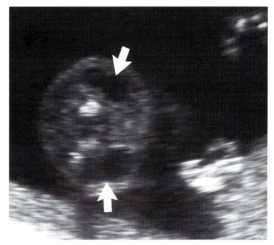

Fig. 4.26 Non-septated cystic hygroma. Transverse scan through fetal neck. The cystic spaces are seen on either side of the fetal neck (arrows).

incidence of chromosomal disease, predominantly Turner's syndrome but also trisomy 21 and trisomy 18. However, about 20% of fetuses with a cystic hygroma will have a normal karyotype.[89,90] There is also an association with generalized hydrops which carries a poor prognosis.[91]

Bronshtein et al have proposed classifying cystic hygromata into septated and non-septated types and state that the two different types have different outcomes and different rates of associated abnormalities[92,93] (Table 4.8). Septated hygromas have the

Table 4.8
Differences between septated and non-septated cystic hygromata

	Septated cystic hygroma	Non-septated cystic hygroma
Incidence	0.3%	1.1%
Earliest week of detection	9	13
Transient	41%	96%
Abnormal karyotype	80%	4%
Associated anomalies	40%	6%
Hydrops	40%	4%
Survival rate	6%	90%
Location	Posterior nuchal	Bilateral

Reproduced with permission from Bronshtein M, Blumenfeld Z. Transvaginal sonography – detection of findings suggestive of fetal chromosomal anomalies in the first and early second trimesters. Prenat Diagn 1992;12:587–593. Copyright John Wiley & Sons Limited.[93]

classical appearance (Fig. 4.25), however non-septated appear as cystic spaces on either side of the fetal neck (Fig. 4.26).

It is also known that cystic hygromata can completely resolve whether the karyotype is normal or abnormal.[90,94,95]

CARDIAC ABNORMALITIES

Congenital cardiac abnormalities are one of the commonest congenital malformations with an incidence of approximately 8 per 1000 live births.[52] Although fetal echocardiography in specialized centres can detect up to 85% of cardiac abnormalities[96,97] routine screening using the 4-chamber view at 18 to 20 weeks' gestation has a much lower detection rate in the range of 15 to 26%.[98–101]

Gembruch et al made the first diagnosis of a major cardiac defect in the first trimester using transvaginal scanning in 1990,[102] and since that time a number of studies have been reported using this technique[52–54,103–106] (Table 4.9). Most of the studies are from high-risk groups with associated anomalies present in 62 to 100% of cases. There are also high rates of chromosomal disease ranging from 36 to 54%. The commonest syndromes associated are trisomy 21, trisomy 18 and Turner's syndrome.[53,103,107] In these high-risk studies

Table 4.9
Data from studies using transvaginal sonography in the first trimester to detect cardiac abnormalities

Author	Number of patients in study	Type of population	Number of cardiac anomalies detected	Sensitivity %	False-positive rate %	Associated abnormalities %	Chromosomal disease %
Johnson et al 1992[52]	302	HR/LR	3	–	–	–	–
Bronshtein et al 1993[103]	12 793	HR/LR	47	76	5	62	36
Gembruch et al 1993[53]	114	HR	12	92	–	85	54
Achiron et al 1994[54]	1000	HR	8	–	–	100	12
Achiron et al 1994[105]	660	LR	3	50	0	0	–
Yagel et al 1997[106]	6294	HR/LR	66	64	4	6	10

HR – high risk; LR – low risk.

the sensitivity for detecting cardiac defects ranges from 64 to 92%.[53,103,106] The only low-risk study published to date reported a sensitivity of 50%.

In the study by Yagel et al, patients were assigned to two groups: one group had early transvaginal scanning looking for cardiac anomalies and then mid-trimester scanning, and the second group had mid-trimester scanning only.[106] Transvaginal scanning detected 64% of cardiac anomalies and mid-trimester scanning a further 17%; a total of 81%. Mid-trimester scanning alone detected 78% of cardiac defects. The authors concluded that transvaginal fetal echocardiography should always be followed by a mid-trimester scan in order to pick up the 17% of cardiac anomalies that would not have been evident in the first trimester.[106]

One of the reasons that cardiac defects are not seen in the first trimester is that some lesions tend to undergo progression in utero. It is well established that ventricular outflow tract obstruction such as aortic stenosis seen in the first half of pregnancy can progress in utero to produce the hypoplastic left heart syndrome later in gestation.[108–110] Thus, in some forms of the hypoplastic left heart syndrome, the left ventricle can be of normal size or even dilated in early pregnancy. Indeed a number of conditions such as myocardial hypertrophy, hypoplasia of one cardiac chamber and/or great artery in the presence of outflow tract obstructions (pulmonary stenosis/atresia, aortic stenosis/atresia, aortic coarctation and Fallot tetralogy) may be discernible only in the

second or third trimester.[3,106,111,112] Other conditions that may present in the second half of pregnancy include endocardial fibroelastosis, cardiac rhabdomyoma, hypertrophic cardiomyopathy and ventricular aneurysm[106] (Table 4.10). There are other defects which, because of their small size, are difficult to demonstrate during fetal endocardiography. A typical example is ventricular septal defect. In the study by Yagel et al only 10% of cases were detected using transvaginal scanning in the first trimester with an overall detection rate of 35%.[106]

In view of these difficulties Gembruch et al have proposed a sequential approach to fetal echocardiography in the first trimester supplemented with colour flow mapping.[111]

The position of the heart and its correlation to other intrathoracic and intra-abdominal organs must be documented first. A short transabdominal scan is often helpful in determining fetal orientation and the

Table 4.10
Cardiac anomalies that may present in the second or third trimester

Endocardial fibroelastosis
Cardiac rhabdomyoma
Hypertrophic cardiomyopathy
Ventricular aneurysm
Pulmonary stenosis
Aortic stenosis
Aortic coarctation
Fallot tetralogy
Hypoplasia of one cardiac ventricle secondary to outflow tract obstruction
Ventricular septal defect
Atrial septal defect

laterality of heart and stomach. Then the inflow of the pulmonary veins into the left atrium and venous inflow into the right atrium are demonstrated. Colour flow Doppler is useful for this part of the scan. The 4-chamber view is then assessed and finally the left and right outflow tracts and the origin and crossing of the great arteries. The aortic arch and ductus should also be visualized.[111] In this way a full assessment of cardiac anatomy is made. However, there are a number of technical difficulties in first trimester fetal echocardiography. First, the imaging planes are limited by a narrow focal range, unfavourable fetal position and lack of manoeuvreability of the transducer. Spatial orientation is more difficult and before 13 weeks' gestation the heart is very small, making subtle defects difficult to diagnose because of limited resolution. In addition, the low spatial resolution of colour flow Doppler in the presence of a high fetal heart rate make it difficult to obtain sharply divided blood flow patterns[111] (Figs 4.11, 4.27). Even though there are difficulties in the technique, in specialist centres a large number of cardiac anomalies can be diagnosed in the first trimester and these are outlined in Table 4.11.

Although the first trimester detection of cardiac abnormalities is an exciting area, most authors state that the technique should be limited to the high-risk group. Such cases

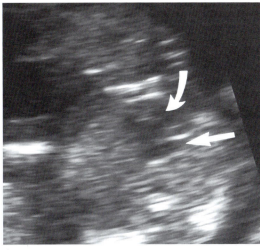

A

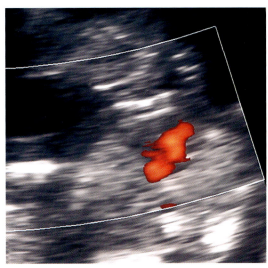

B

Fig. 4.27 Hypoplastic left heart. (A) Transverse scan through the heart of a 14-week fetus showing normal right ventricle (curved arrow) but small left ventricle (straight arrow). (B) Colour flow Doppler image showing flow into the right ventricle but absence of flow into the left side of the heart.

Table 4.11
Cardiac anomalies detected in the first and early second trimester using transvaginal scanning

Hypoplastic left ventricle
Hypoplastic right ventricle
Single ventricle
Single atrium
Ventricular septal defect
Atrioventricular septal defect
Tricuspid regurgitation
Fallot tetralogy
Double outlet right ventricle
Aortic coarctation
Truncus arteriosus
Transposition
Ectopia cordis
UHL disease
Pericardial effusion
Dextrocardia

*Data derived from First trimester cardiac studies:
References[53,103,104,105,106].*

---

include fetuses with other anomalies such as nuchal oedema, increased nuchal translucency, cystic hygroma, hydrops, omphalocoele, situs inversus or bradycardia, high-risk families with one or more first degree relatives with cardiac defects and diabetic mothers.[53,54,106,111]

It should also be noted that although high sensitivities for the detection of cardiac anomalies are reported in studies from specialist centres and from studies specifically looking for cardiac defects,[53,54,106,111] when studies from low risk populations and screening studies for fetal anomalies are analyzed the detection rates for cardiac anomalies are in the range of 0 to 18%.[16,17,31,33]

All authors also state that first trimester fetal echocardiography should always be followed by mid-trimester fetal scanning.[106,112]

URINARY TRACT ABNORMALITIES

Renal agenesis

Bilateral renal agenesis has an incidence of 1 in 4000 live births[3] and in the second trimester presents as severe oligohydramnios with absence of the kidneys and bladder. In the first trimester, however, liquor volume may be normal, potentially making the diagnosis of renal agenesis easier. Bronshtein et al reported eight cases of renal agenesis diagnosed in the first trimester.[113] In four cases liquor volume was normal prior to 17 weeks' gestation and in two cases a cystic structure compatible with the bladder was seen in the fetal pelvis. All eight fetuses demonstrated hypoechogenic masses in the flanks which were subsequently demonstrated to be the adrenal glands (normal kidneys in the first trimester are echogenic) (Fig. 4.12).[113] The demonstration of a bladder in fetuses with renal agenesis could be explained by retrograde filling or the presence of a small midline urachal diverticulum. Additional techniques that may be used to confirm renal agenesis include colour flow Doppler to demonstrate absence of the renal arteries.[33]

In summary therefore there are three possible ultrasound appearances in early pregnancy all of which are compatible with bilateral renal agenesis:

1. Absence of echogenic masses (kidneys) in the fetal flanks without sonographic signs of an ectopic kidney.
2. Hypoechogenic masses (adrenals) in the fetal flanks in association with absence of the bladder and oligohydramnios.

3. Hypoechogenic masses (adrenals) in the fetal flanks in association with a small urinary bladder and normal liquor prior to 17 weeks' gestation. Failure to visualize the bladder should also raise the possibility of bladder extrophy or bilateral multicystic dysplastic kidneys.[3]

Cystic renal disease

Multicystic dysplastic kidney

This abnormality usually results from obstruction to the developing kidney in the early first trimester.[3] The result is a kidney replaced by multiple cysts of varying sizes often associated with a dense central stroma. The condition is bilateral in 20% of cases.

Bronshtein et al detected two cases of multicystic dysplastic kidney in a screening programme for the detection of fetal malformations. One case was diagnosed at 12 weeks', the second at 15 weeks' gestation.[55] Yagel et al also detected both cases of multicystic dysplastic kidney in the first trimester in their screening study[132] and Economides and Braithwaite picked up one case in a screening study involving a low-risk population.[17] In a further screening study involving an unselected population Hernadi and Torocsik failed to detect all three cases of multicystic dysplastic kidneys in the first trimester. Two were detected at mid-trimester scanning and the third case in the third trimester.[20]

Infantile polycystic kidney disease

This autosomal recessive condition has an incidence of one in 50 000 live births.[1] This condition is usually diagnosed in the second or even third trimester and presents as bilaterally enlarged echogenic kidneys associated with oligohydramnios and an absent bladder.[3] It is well established that the kidneys may appear normal in the first and second trimester and so the condition cannot be excluded following a normal mid-trimester scan.[114]

Bronshtein et al reported a single case of infantile polycystic kidneys which demonstrated enlarged, hyperechogenic kidneys (too good looking kidneys) at 12

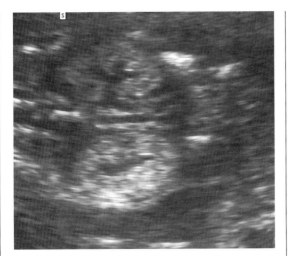

Fig. 4.28 Echogenic kidneys. Coronal scan through a 15-week fetus showing bilaterally enlarged echogenic kidneys. The fetus had polydactyly and an encephalolocoele and a diagnosis of Meckel–Gruber syndrome was made.

weeks' gestation.[114] The same authors reported two further cases of enlarged echogenic kidneys associated with other anomalies which were subsequently found to have the Meckel–Gruber syndrome[55] (Fig. 4.28).

Hydronephrosis

The renal pelvis can be demonstrated as early as 9 weeks' gestation as a central hypoechogenic dot within the normally echogenic kidney. The anteroposterior diameter of the renal pelvis has an upper limit of normal of 3 mm in the first trimester.[55]

Bronshtein et al reported 27 fetuses with hydronephrosis detected in the first trimester. Six cases progressed to a significant hydronephrosis and two of these cases required surgery due to compromised renal function of the affected kidney. Ten cases showed complete resolution in utero and the remaining eleven cases were lost to follow-up. Down's syndrome was diagnosed in one of the six babies with significant hydronephrosis in the neonatal period.[55]

In the screening study by Yagel et al, six cases of hydronephrosis were detected in the first trimester. One case progressed to a pelvi-ureteric junction obstruction and the other five cases resolved in utero.[32]

Low urinary tract obstruction

Bladder outlet obstruction can be diagnosed in the first trimester by demonstration of dilatation of the bladder (megacystis) which may be associated with oligohydramnios[115,116] or liquor volume may be normal.[117,118] The main causes are posterior urethral valves in the male and urethral atresia in females.[3] In the first trimester, bladder outlet obstruction produces hydronephrosis in only 40% of cases and this may be due to the relatively high compliance of the renal parenchyma at this stage of pregnancy.

Sebire et al reported 15 cases of megacystis in the first and early second trimester. Longitudinal bladder diameters were greater than 8 mm in all cases (upper limit of normal is 6 mm).[119] There were three cases of chromosomal anomalies, one trisomy 21, one trisomy 13 and an unbalanced translocation of chromosomes 14 and 20. In all cases when the bladder diameter exceeded 16 mm, there was progression to severe obstructive uropathy. In addition, there was resolution to normal in the majority of fetuses with bladder diameters in the range of 8 to 12 mm[119] (Fig. 4.29).

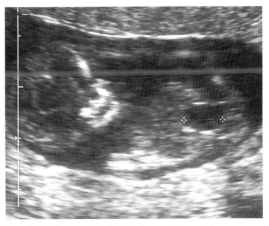

Fig. 4.29 Megacystis. Sagittal scan through the abdomen of a 12-week fetus showing dilatation of the bladder. Longitudinal diameter was 8 mm-calipers, follow-up scans showed resolution to a normal sized bladder in the second trimester.

Minor renal anomalies

A number of minor renal anomalies have been reported in the first trimester and these include mild renal pelvic dilatation,[120] unilateral renal agenesis, pelvic kidney and duplex kidney.[121] The outcome for these conditions is good.

ABNORMALITIES OF THE GASTROINTESTINAL TRACT

Duodenal atresia

There are a few case reports of early diagnosis of duodenal atresia. The diagnosis is based on the double bubble sign of fluid within the stomach and also the proximal duodenum.[3] Patrikovsky made the diagnosis at 14 weeks' gestation,[122] and Zimmer and Bronshtein diagnosed a case at 15 weeks' gestation. The latter authors also described three other cases of a double bubble sign visualized at 15 weeks which disappeared on repeated scans 10 to 15 min later. The authors concluded the appearances were due to normal intestinal peristalsis and suggested that repeat scan could differentiate the transitory nature of intestinal peristalsis from the constant dilated appearance of duodenal atresia.[123] Tsukerman et al reported a case of duodenal atresia at 12 weeks' gestation, however this was also associated with oesophageal atresia[124] (Fig. 4.30).

As in the second trimester, duodenal atresia has an important association with trisomy 21.[3]

Omphalocoele

Omphalocoele is the most common congenital midline defect in the anterior abdominal wall resulting from primary failed fusions of the lateral folds. The result is herniation of abdominal contents into a sac which is composed of the parietal peritoneum, the amniotic membrane and Wharton's jelly.[3] The umbilical cord is inserted into the upper region of the sac. The defect may contain bowel loops, and if large the liver, spleen or stomach (Fig. 4.31). There is a high association with chromosomal

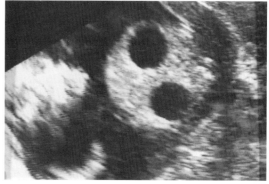

A

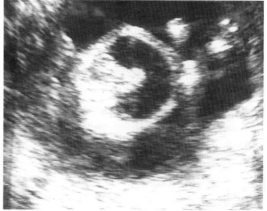

B

Fig. 4.30 Duodenal and oesophageal atresia. (A) Transverse scan through a 14-week fetus showing typical 'double bubble' appearance. (B) Coronal scan through the fetal abdomen showing the typical 'C' shaped appearance of duodenal and oesophageal atresia.

disease and also other major fetal abnormalities.[125] An increased nuchal translucency thickness is also associated with omphalocoele.[15]

Omphalocoele should always be differentiated from the normal midgut herniation which occurs between the 7th and 11th week of gestation and has usually resolved by the 12th week.[60,61] Recent reports suggest that the midgut herniation should not exceed 7 mm in diameter at any gestation and that no herniation should be present in a fetus with a crown rump length greater than 44 mm[61] (Fig. 4.15).

There are a number of features which may be helpful in differentiating omphalocoele from the midgut herniation.

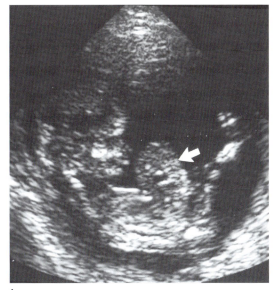

A

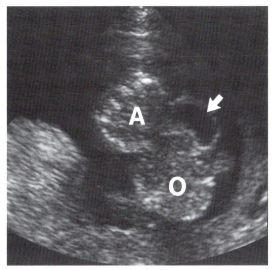

B

Fig. 4.31 Omphalocoele. (A) Sagittal scan through 14-week fetus showing large omphalocoele containing liver (arrow). (B) Transverse scan showing a large omphalocoele containing stomach (arrow) and liver. Note that the omphalocoele (O) is larger than the abdomen (A).

1. Echogenicity – physiological herniation contains only bowel loops which may be recognizable as a heterogeneous echogenic structure compared with the pathological herniations in which the eviscerated liver produces a characteristic uniform and homogeneous pattern (Fig. 4.31).

2. Size – the diameter of the physiological midgut herniation should not exceed 7 mm, whereas in omphalocoele the herniated mass is usually larger.

3. Abdominal diameter – in midgut herniation the herniated mass is usually smaller in diameter than the remainder of the abdomen (Fig. 4.15), whereas in omphalocoele the extra-abdominal mass is usually larger than the abdominal diameter (Fig. 4.31).

4. Time – persistent evisceration of abdominal contents after 12 weeks' gestation or a fetus with a crown rump length greater than 44 mm usually represents a true omphalocoele.[3]

Gastroschisis

Gastroschisis is a para-umbilical ventral defect usually located to the right of the midline. Gastroschisis results from early compromise of the right umbilical vein or the omphalomesenteric artery which causes mesodermal and endodermal ischaemic injury to the abdominal wall. At about 7 weeks' gestation the normal midgut herniation should occur; however, in gastroschisis there is rupture of the fetal abdomen on the right paramedian side instead, at the site of the previous ischaemic damage.[3] Gastroschisis is differentiated from omphalocoele by the lack of a sac so that the bowel loops float freely in the amniotic fluid and also the umbilical cord inserts normally.[3]

There are only a few first trimester diagnoses of gastroschisis. In the screening study of D'Ottavio et al one case was diagnosed[31] and Guzman, and Kushnic et al reported cases at 13 weeks and 12 weeks respectively.[126,127] In addition, Bonilla-Musoles et al reported two cases and using colour flow Doppler demonstrated the normal cord insertion in both.[33]

Body stalk anomaly

Although not strictly speaking a gastrointestinal anomaly, a major component of this condition is a large abdominal wall defect. Other features include severe kyposcoliosis, a short umbilical cord, amputation defects of the limbs, facial clefting and encephalocoele.[1] Recent reports demonstrate evidence of amnion rupture with the upper part of the fetal body being in the amniotic cavity and the lower half in the coelomic cavity.[128–130]

In a recent screening study Hernandi and Torocsik reported two cases of body stalk anomaly detected at 12 and 13 weeks' gestation respectively.[20]

Abdominal and umbilical cord cysts

Intra-abdominal cysts have been reported in the first trimester.[23,131] Zimmer and Bronshtein reported four cases between 11 and 15 weeks' gestation. Two cases were thought to represent a dilated fetal bladder and there was associated bilateral hydronephrosis. These patients opted for a termination of pregnancy. The other two cases resolved spontaneously by 20 weeks' gestation and the exact nature of the cysts was not established.[23] McMalla et al reported a fetus at 8 weeks' gestation with two large cysts almost completely filling the abdomen. Two weeks later repeat scanning showed absent fetal heart motion with total disappearance of the abdominal cysts and the presence of two cysts in the umbilical cord.[131] It was postulated that the abdominal cysts had migrated to the umbilical cord and represented omphalomesenteric cysts. The cysts may have been large enough to compromise blood flow to the developing fetus, leading to its death.[131]

It would appear therefore that abdominal cysts in the first trimester can have a variable outcome and careful follow-up is essential. Large cysts may have more significance whereas smaller cysts may resolve spontaneously.

Umbilical cord cysts appear to have a good prognosis without any major associations. The majority seen in the first trimester between 8 and 9 weeks' gestation resolve by 12 to 14 weeks and long term follow-up reveals a normal outcome.[24,132]

THORACIC ABNORMALITIES

Diaphragmatic hernia

The development of the diaphragm is usually complete by the 9th week of gestation and in the presence of a defective diaphragm herniation of abdominal viscera into the thoracic cavity is likely to occur at about 10 to 12 weeks, when the intestines return to the abdominal cavity from the umbilical cord.[1] However in some cases intra-thoracic herniation of viscera may be delayed until the second or even third trimester of pregnancy.[133]

The diagnosis of diaphragmatic hernia is usually made at 20 weeks' gestation; however, the diagnosis has been reported as early as 12 weeks.[134] The main sonographic signs are mediastinal shift of the heart associated with herniation of the stomach and/or other intra-abdominal organs into the thorax. There is associated chromosomal disease or other structural anomalies in up to 50% of cases and the survival rate following postnatal surgery is also approximately 50%.[1]

In a recent screening study Bronshtein et al documented the timing of visceral herniation in 15 cases of diaphragmatic hernia. In seven cases herniation was seen at 14 to 16 weeks' gestation. In a further two cases diaphragmatic hernia was diagnosed at 21 and 23 weeks, and herniation was delayed until 26 to 28 weeks in the remaining six fetuses.[133] The outcome for the six cases diagnosed after 26 weeks was good with all six surviving following neonatal surgery. The two fetuses diagnosed at 21 and 23 weeks both died following surgery from respiratory insufficiency. The seven fetuses diagnosed early underwent termination of pregnancy and four of the seven had either chromosomal disease or other abnormalities.[133] These findings indicate that late herniation carries a better prognosis than early diagnosis of diaphragmatic hernia and that diaphragmatic hernia may not be diagnosed in the first or even second trimester. It should be noted therefore that a normal first or mid-trimester fetal anomaly scan does not exclude diaphragmatic hernia.

A recent study has demonstrated an association with increased nuchal translucency and diaphragmatic hernia in the first trimester of pregnancy.[135] Sebire et al found that 37% of fetuses with a diaphragmatic hernia had had an increased nuchal translucency measurement earlier in pregnancy. This finding may also be an important prognostic sign as the fetuses with an increased nuchal translucency included 83% of babies that resulted in neonatal death but only 22% of survivors.[135]

SKELETAL ABNORMALITIES

Skeletal dysplasias

Skeletal dysplasias are a heterogeneous group of growth disorders of bone and cartilage which are characterized by deformation and reduction of various segments of the skeletal system. The prevalence of these anomalies varies from 2.3 to 7.6 per 10 000 births and 1.5 per 10 000 births for lethal skeletal dysplasias.[136]

There have been a number of case reports of individual skeletal dysplasias in the first trimester and these have included: achondrogenesis,[137,138] thanatophoric dysplasia,[139] osteogenesis imperfecta,[140] asphyxiating thoracic dystrophy,[39] Roberts syndrome,[38] and short-rib polydactyly syndrome.[141] In addition, first trimester screening studies have also reported skeletal dysplasias such as achondroplasia,[20] hypophosphatasia,[31] amelia,[32] osteogenesis imperfecta[31] and thanatophoric dysplasia.[32]

There have been very few screening studies attempting to detect skeletal dysplasias; however, in a recent report of high-risk cases Gabrelli et al were able to detect only two out of five cases in the first trimester (one case of recurrent osteogenesis imperfecta and one with recurrent achondrogenesis).[136] In the series of skeletal anomalies reported by Bronshtein et al only two skeletal dysplasias were reported, one case of osteogenesis imperfecta and one proximal femoral deficiency.[142]

It is of interest that many skeletal dysplasias reported are associated with an increased nuchal translucency measurement and this may be a useful clue to the diagnosis (Table 4.6). The main sonographic findings are shortened, bowed or fractured long bones.[1] It seems probable that first trimester scanning for skeletal dysplasias is unlikely to be as accurate as mid-trimester scanning; however, an increased nuchal translucency thickness may be a useful marker for these conditions.[15]

ABNORMALITIES OF THE HANDS AND FEET

Although the fetal finger buds can be imaged as early as 9 or 10 weeks of gestation, a thorough examination of all fingers is possible at 12 to 13 weeks. In the first trimester the fetus tends to keep the hands open with fingers extended (Fig. 4.16).[143] In a recent study Bronshtein et al reported 25 fetuses with abnormalities of the fingers. The conditions included polydactyly (Fig. 4.21), syndactyly, overlapping fingers, cleft hand, adactyly and adduction of the thumb.[143] The authors noted a family history in only 10% of cases and 60% of affected fetuses were found to have a malformations syndrome or chromosomal disease.

The fetal feet may be visualized from 12 weeks' gestation and both feet are held with the heels almost touching and knees slightly flexed. Talipes has been reported as early as 13 weeks' gestation (Fig. 4.32);[144,145] however, in the study by Bronshtein et al 13 cases of talipes were detected in the first trimester but a 3 further cases were thought to develop later in pregnancy. Two cases were diagnosed at 20 to 21 weeks' gestation and the third in the neonatal period. All three cases had had normal scans in the first trimester.[142] Once again these findings indicate that a normal first trimester scan does not exclude the possibility of an anomaly developing later in pregnancy.

ABNORMALITIES OF THE FACE

Facial clefting is the commonest facial abnormality with an incidence of approximately 1 per 1000 live births.

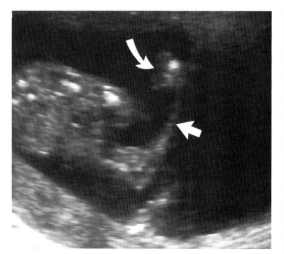

Fig. 4.32 Talipes. Coronal scan through lower limb of a 12-week fetus showing talipes (straight arrow – tibia/fibula, curved arrow – foot).

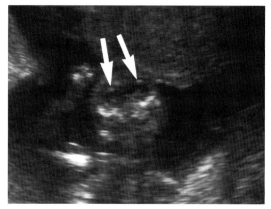

Fig. 4.33 Hypotelorism. Coronal scan through the orbits of a 13-week fetus showing marked hypotelorism associated with holoprosencephaly (arrows point to both orbits).

Bronshtein et al reported 11 cases of facial clefting detected using transvaginal scanning at 13 to 16 weeks' gestation.[146] Five cases were associated with other anomalies – two cases of ectrodactylyectodermal dysplasia syndrome, one holoprosencephaly, one Meckel–Gruber syndrome and one trisomy 18. Only one case of facial clefting was missed in the series, producing a sensitivity of 92%.[146]

Abnormalities of the orbits are difficult to demonstrate; however, severe anomalies associated with holoprosencephaly have been reported. Cullen et al reported a case of hypotelorism (Fig. 4.33) in his study of first trimester pregnancies[147] and van Zalen-Sprock detected cyclopia at 12 weeks' gestation in a fetus with holoprosencephaly.[84]

TWIN PREGNANCY

Twins are the most prevalent type of multiple pregnancy with a spontaneous incidence of 1 in 80 pregnancies. Nigeria has the highest rate of twins at 1 in 20 to 25 pregnancies and Japan the lowest rate at 1 in 150 pregnancies.[148] There are two types of twins: dizygotic, which result from multiple ovulation and monozygotic (identical) which are the result of cleavage of a single fertilized ovum. Thirty percent of all twin pregnancies are monozygotic and have a frequency of 4 per 1000 conceptions.[149] The incidence of multiple births has increased since the introduction of infertility treatment and in vitro fertilization techniques, and also as more women are delaying childbirth. There is a natural increase in twin pregnancy in older women.[148] The perinatal mortality of twin pregnancies is six times that of singleton pregnancies.[149] This accounts for 12.6% of the perinatal mortality, but twins account for only 2.5% of the population.[148]

Embryology

In dizygotic twins there is multiple ovulation and fertilization. Each zygote arrives at the uterus and implants at around 6 to 7 days post-conception and development then proceeds in a fashion similar to that of a singleton pregnancy.[148] Monozygotic twins, however, arise at different times post-conception, resulting in a variety of clinical presentations. The main difference between these two types of twins involves the placenta. Zygosity therefore refers to the type of conception and chorionicity denotes the type of placentation.

There are two types of placenta encountered in twin pregnancies: the dichorionic and the monochorionic. All dizygotic twins are dichorionic and

Table 4.12
Summary of embryology of monozygotic twinning

Timing of cleavage (days from ovulation)	Number of fetuses	Type of placenta	Number of amniotic sacs	Number of yolk sacs
1–3*	Two	Dichorionic	Two	Two
4–8*	Two	Monochorionic	Two	Two
8–10	Two	Monochorionic	One	Two
13–16	Conjoined	Monochorionic	One	One

*Implantation occurs 6–7 days.
Reproduced with permission from Monteagudo A, Haberman S, Timor-Tritsch. The diagnosis of multiple pregnancy. In: Ultrasound in early pregnancy. Edited by Jurkovic D, Jauniaux E. Published by Parthenon Publishing Group, London.[148]

diamniotic. Monozygotic twins on the other hand may be dichorionic or monochorionic, and the monochorionic placentas may be diamniotic or mono-amniotic depending on the time after fertilization that the zygote divides[148] (Table 4.12).

In 30% of monozygotic twins, division of the zygote occurs within the first 3 days after fertilization. This results in the formation of two blastocysts and a dichorionic-diamniotic placenta.

In 70% of monozygotic twins, the zygote divides between 4 and 8 days after fertilization, i.e. post-implantation but before the development of the amniotic cavity. The result is a monochorionic-diamniotic placenta.

When the zygote divides between 8 and 13 days after fertilization and the amniotic cavity has developed the result is a monochorionic-mono-amniotic placenta.

Finally, if the zygote divides between days 13 and 16, this late division will result in conjoined twins (Table 4.12).[148]

Sonographic appearances

The number of gestational sacs of a multiple pregnancy can be established by the 5th week of gestation using transvaginal scanning; however, the number of fetuses cannot be determined until the 6th week. By 5.5 weeks the yolk sacs can be counted; however, using the number of yolk sacs to determine the number of fetuses can be misleading due to the rare cases of conjoined twins (Table 4.12). If only one fetus is seen within each gestational sac the pregnancy is dichorionic-diamniotic. If two fetuses are seen within one chorionic sac the amnionicity

cannot be determined until the 8th week when the amniotic sacs should be clearly demonstrated. If two amniotic sacs are seen (one around each fetus) the pregnancy is monochorionic-diamniotic. If a single sac is seen around both fetuses the pregnancy is monochorionic-mono-amniotic[148] (Fig. 4.34).

Between 10 and 14 weeks the 'lambda' sign may be visible, i.e. a projection of placental tissue between the inter-twin membrane[150] (Fig. 4.35). This sign usually indicates a dichorionic pregnancy, but the absence of this sign does not exclude a dichorionic pregnancy.

After 14 weeks one can count the placentas – two placentas indicates a dichorionic pregnancy. However, dichorionic placentas can fuse to produce the appearance of a single placenta.

The sex of the fetuses is important as fetuses of different sex are always dizygous and so dichorionic and diamniotic. If the fetuses are the same sex they may still be dizygous or monozygous.

Measuring the thickness of the separating membrane is of value as a membrane measuring 2 mm or more is reported to be 95% predictive of dichorionic twins.[451–153] Determining the chorionicity of twin pregnancy is important due to the increased rate of pregnancy complications and increased perinatal mortality in monochorionic twins.[149]

Complications in twin pregnancies

Growth discordancy

Growth discordancy is normally detected in the late second or third trimester of

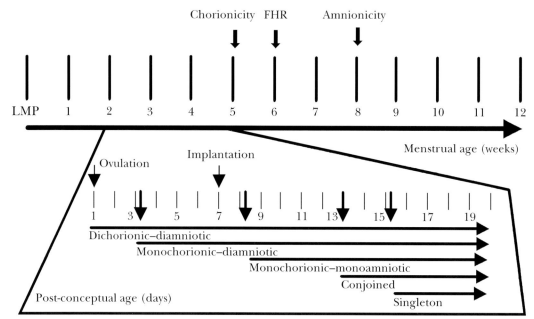

Fig. 4.34 Summary of the sonoembryology and embryology of twinning. The upper half of the drawing depicts the gestational age (menstrual weeks) at which, with transvaginal sonography, the chorionicity, fetal heart rate (FHR) and amnionicity can be established. The lower inset shows that if division of the zygote occurs during the first 3 days post-conception, a dichorionic-diamniotic twin pregnancy will result. If division occurs around the time of implantation, a monochorionic-diamniotic twin pregnancy will result. If division occurs around day 8 to 10 post-conception, a monochorionic-monoamniotic twin pregnancy will result. If separation occurs around day 13 to 16 post conception, conjoined twins will result. No separation can occur beyond 15 days post-conception (see Table 4.12). (Reproduced with permission from Monteagudo A, Haberman S, Timor-Tritsch I E. The diagnosis of multiple pregnancy in the first trimester. In: Jurkovic D, Jauniaux E, eds. Ultrasound in early pregnancy. London: Parthenon Publishing Group.)

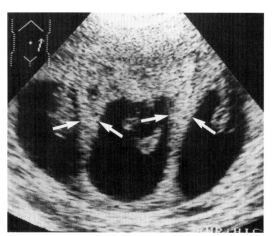

Fig. 4.35 Lambda sign. Triplet pregnancy with placental tissue protruding into the intertwin membranes (arrows). This sign normally indicates dichorionic placentation. In this case it is trichorionic placentation.

pregnancy; however, it can occur in the first trimester. Weissman et al reported five cases of growth discordancy at 6 to 11 weeks'

gestation. Growth discordancy was defined as a difference in crown rump length corresponding to 5 days or more. In all five smaller fetuses there were major abnormalities including diaphragmatic hernia, ventriculomegaly, schizencephaly, aortic stenosis and sacral agenesis. The authors concluded that the first trimester growth discordant twin is at increased risk of fetal anomalies.[154]

Twin-twin transfusion syndrome

Although this condition normally presents in the second and third trimester of pregnancy with the 'stuck twin' phenomenon, it has been reported in the first trimester. Sharma et al reported a subjective impression of reduced liquor around the smaller twin and increased liquor around the larger twin in a monochorionic-diamniotic twin pregnancy at 13 weeks' gestation. Follow-up scans confirmed the diagnosis.[155]

Acardiac twin

A case of acardiac twin pregnancy has been reported in the first trimester;[156] however, most cases are detected at mid-trimester scanning. This condition is only seen in monochorionic twins.

Conjoined twins

This rare complication of monochorionic twins has been reported in the first trimester on a number of occasions.[157–159] The earliest gestation at which the condition was suspected is 8 weeks' gestation.[159]

References

General

1. Souka A P, Nicolaides K H Diagnosis of fetal abnormalities at the 10–14 week scan. Ultrasound Obstet Gynecol 1997;10:429–442.
2. Chitty L S, Pandya P P Ultrasound screening for fetal abnormalities in the first trimester. Prenat Diagn 1997;17:1269–1281.
3. Weissman A, Achiron R Ultrasound diagnosis of congenital anomalies in early pregnancy. In: Ultrasound and Early Pregnancy. Jurkovic D, Jauniaux E, eds. London: Parthenon Publishing Group; 1996.
4. Economides D L Early pregnancy screening for fetal abnormalities. Ultrasound Obstet Gynecology 1999;13:81–83.
5. Pandya P P, Snijders R J M, Psara N, Hilbert L, Nicolaides K The prevalence of non-viable pregnancy at 10–13 weeks of gestation. Ultrasound Obstet Gynecol 1996;7:170–173.
6. Finberg H J The 'twin peak' sign: reliable evidence of dichorionic twinning. J Ultrasound Med 1992;11:571–577.
7. Wald N J, Hackshaw A K Combining ultrasound and biochemistry in first trimester screening for Down's Syndrome. Prenat Diagn 1997;17:821–829.
8. Nicolaides K H, Azar G, Byrne D, Mansur C, Marks K Fetal nuchal translucency: ultrasound screening for chromosomal defects in the first trimester of pregnancy. BMJ 1992;304:867–869.
9. Pandya P P, Snijders R J M, Johnson S P, Brizot M, Nicolaides K M Screening for fetal trisomies by maternal age and fetal nuchal translucency thickness at 10–14 weeks of gestation. Br J Obstet Gynaecol 1995;102:957–962.
10. Snijders R J M, Nobles P, Sebire N J, Souka A P, Nicolaides K H UK Multicentric project on the assessment of risk for trisomy 21 by maternal age and fetal nuchal translucency at 10–14 weeks of gestation. Lancet 1998;352:343–346.
11. Hyett J, Moscoso G, Papapanagiotou G, Perdu M, Nicolaides K H Abnormalities of the heart and great vessels in chromosomally normal fetuses with increased nuchal translucency thickness at 10–13 weeks of gestation. Ultrasound Obstet Gynecol 1996;7:245–250.
12. Hyett J, Perdu M, Sharland G K, Snijders R J M, Nicolaides K H Increased nuchal translucency at 10–14 weeks gestation as a marker for major cardiac defects. Ultrasound Obstet Gynecol 1997;10:242–246.
13. Hyett J, Perdu M, Sharland G K, Snijders R, Nicolaides K H Using fetal nuchal translucency to screen for major cardiac defects at 10–14 weeks gestation: population based cohort study. BMJ 1999;318:81–85.
14. Bilardo C M, Pajkrt E, deGraff I M, Mol B W J, Bleker O P Outcome of fetuses with enlarged nuchal translucency and normal karyotype. Ultrasound Obstet Gynecol 1998;11:401–406.
15. Souka A P, Snijders R J M, Novakov A, Soares W, Nicolaides K H Defects and syndromes in chromosomally normal fetuses with increased nuchal translucency thickness at 10–14 weeks of gestation. Ultrasound Obstet Gynecol 1998;11:391–400.
16. Achiron R, Tadmor O Screening for fetal anomalies during the first trimester of pregnancy: transvaginal versus transabdominal sonography. Ultrasound Obstet Gynecol 1991;1.
17. Economides D L, Braithwaite J M First trimester ultrasonographic diagnosis of fetal structural abnormalities in a low risk population. Br J Obstet Gynaecol 1998;105:53–57.
18. Braithwaite J M, Armstrong M A, Economides E L. Assessment of fetal anatomy at 12–13 weeks of gestation by transabdominal and transvaginal sonography. Br J Obstet Gynaecol 1996;103:82–85.
19. Whitlow B J, Economides D L The optimal gestational age to examine fetal anatomy and measure nuchal translucency in the first trimester. Ultrasound Obstet Gynecology 1998;11:258–261.
20. Hernadi L, Torocsik M Screening for fetal anomalies in the 12th week of pregnancy by transvaginal sonography in an unselected population. Prenat Diagn 1997;17:753–759.
21. Rottem S Ironfan: a new time-orientated malformation work-up and classification of fetal anomalies. Ultrasound Obstet Gynecol 1997;10:373–374.
22. Lazanakis M, Whitlow B J, Economides D L The significance of choroid plexus cysts, 'golf ball' sign and pyelectasis in the first trimester pregnancy. J Obstet Gynecol 1997;17:532.
23. Zimmer E Z, Bronshtein M Fetal intra-abdominal cysts detected in the first and early second trimester by transvaginal sonography. JCU 1991;19:564–567.
24. Sepulveda W, Leible S, Ulloa A, Ivankovic M, Schnapp C Clinical significance of first trimester umbilical cord cysts. J Ultrasound Med 1999;18:95–99.
25. Blaas H-G, Eik-Nes S, Keserud T, Hellevik L R Early development of the abdominal wall, stomach and heart from 7–12 weeks of gestation: a longitudinal

ultrasound study. Ultrasound Obstet Gynecol 1995;6:240–249.

26. Timor-Tritsch I E, Farine D, Rosen M C A close look at early embryonic development with the high-frequency transvaginal transducer. Am J Obstet Gynecol 1988;159:676–681.

27. Medeira A, Norman A, Haslam J Clayton-Smith J, Donnai D Examination of fetuses after induced abortion for fetal abnormality – a follow up study. Prenat Diagn 1994;14:381–385.

First trimester screening (See also references 16, 17, 20)

28. Constantine G, McCormack. Comparative audit of booking and mid trimester ultrasound scans in the prenatal diagnosis of congenital anomalies. Prenat Diagn 1991;11:905–914.

29. Chambers S E, Geirrson R T, Stewart R J, Wannapirak C, Muir B B Audit of a screening service for fetal abnormalities using early ultrasound scanning and maternal serum alpha feto protein estimation combined with selective detailed scanning. Ultrasound Obstet Gynecology 1995;5:168–173.

30. Long G, Sprigg A A comparative study of routine versus selective fetal anomaly ultrasound scanning. Journal of Medical Screening 1998;5:6–10.

31. D'Ottavio G D, Meir Y J, Rustico M A, et al. Screening for fetal anomalies by ultrasound at 14 and 21 weeks. Ultrasound Obstet Gynecol 1997;10:375–380.

32. Yagel S, Achison R, Ron M, Revel A, Anteby E Transvaginal ultrasonography at early pregnancy cannot be used alone for targeted organ ultrasonographic examination in a high risk population. Am J Obstet Gynecol 1995;172:971–975.

33. Bonilla-Musoles F M, Raga F, Ballester M J, Serra V Early detection of embryonic malformations by transvaginal and colour doppler sonography. Ultrasound Med 1994;13:347–355.

Nuchal translucency screening for fetal abnormalities (See also references 11–15)

34. Hewitt B Nuchal translucency in the first trimester. Aust N Z J Obstet Gynecol 1993;33:389–391.

35. Ammala P, Salonen R First Trimester diagnosis of hydrolethalus syndrome. Ultrasound Obstet Gynecol 1995;5:60–62.

36. Cha'ban F K, Splunder P V, Los F J, Wladimiroff J W Fetal outcome in nuchal translucency with emphasis on normal fetal karyotype. Prenat Diagn 1996;16:537–541.

37. Hosli I M, Tercanli S, Rehder H, Holzgreve W Cystic hygroma as an early first trimester marker for recurrent Fryns' Syndrome. Ultrasound Obstet Gynecol 1997;10:422–424.

38. Petrikovsky B M, Gross B, Bialer M, Solamanzadeh K, Simlau E Prenatal diagnosis of pseudothalidomide syndrome in consecutive pregnancies of a consanguinous couple. Ultrasound Obstet Gynecol 1997;10:425–428.

39. Ben Ami M, Perlitz Y, Haddard S, Matilsky M

Increased nuchal translucency associated with asphyxiating thoracic dysplasia. Ultrasound Obstet Gynecol 1997;10:297–298.

40. Reynders P S, Pauker S P, Benacerraf B R First trimester isolated fetal nuchal lucency: significance and outcome. J Ultrasound Med 1997;16:101–105.

41. Hafner E, Schuchter K, Liebhart E, Philipp K Results of routine fetal nuchal translucency measurement at weeks 10–13, in 4233 unselected pregnant women. Prenat Diagn 1998;18:29–34.

42. van Vugt J M G, Tinnemans BW S, van Zalen-Sprock R M Outcome and early childhood follow up of chromosomally normal fetuses with increased nuchal translucency at 10–14 weeks gestation. Ultrasound Obstet Gynecol 1998;11:407–409.

43. Fukada Y, Yasumizu T, Takizawa M, Amemiya A, Hoshi K The prognosis of fetuses with transient nuchal translucency in the first and early second trimester. Acta Obstet Gynecol Scand 1998;76:913–916.

Normal appearances (sonoembryology)

44. Timor-Tritsch I E, Peisner D, Raju S Sonoembryology: an organ-oriented approach using a high frequency vaginal probe. JCU 1990;18:286–298.

45. Blaas H G, Eik-Nes S H, Bremnes. The growth of the human embryo. A longitudinal biometric assessment from 7–12 weeks of gestation. Ultrasound Obstet Gynecol 1998;12:346 354.

46. Achiron R, Achiron A Transvaginal ultrasonic assessment of the early fetal brain. Ultrasound Obstet Gynecol 1991;1:336–344.

47. Timor-Tritsch I E, Monteagudo A, Warren W Transvaginal ultrasonographic definition of the central nervous system in the first and early second trimesters. Am J Obstet Gynecol 1991;164:497–503.

48. Blass H-G, Eik-Nes S, Kiserud T, Hellevik L R Early development of the forebrain and midbrain: a longitudinal ultrasound study from 7 to 12 weeks of gestation. Ultrasound Obstet Gynecol 1994;4:183–192.

49. Blass H-G, Eik-Nes S, Kiserud T, Hellevik L R Early development of the hindbrain: a longitudinal ultrasound study from 7–12 weeks of gestation. Ultrasound Obstet Gynecol 1995;5:151–160.

50. Dolkhart L A, Reimers F T Transvaginal fetal echocardiography in early pregnancy: normative data. Am J Obstet Gynecol 1991;165:688–691.

51. Bronshtein M, Sugler E, Eschcoli Z, Zimmer E Z Transvaginal ultrasound measurements of the fetal heart and 11 to 17 weeks of gestation. Am J Perinatol 1992;9:38–42.

52. Johnson P, Sharland G, Maxwell D, Allan L The role of transvaginal sonography in the early detection of congenital heart disease. Ultrasound Obstet Gynecol 1992;2:248–251.

53. Gembruch U, Knopfle G, Bald R, Hausmann M Early diagnosis of fetal congenital heart disease by transvaginal echocardiography. Ultrasound Obstet and Gynecology 1993;3:310–317.

54. Achiron R, Weissman A, Rotstein Z, Lipitz S, Mashiach S, Hegesh J Transvaginal echocardiagraphic examination of the fetal heart between 13 and 15 weeks gestation in a low-risk population. J Ultrasound Med 1994;13:783–789.

55. Bronshtein M, Yoffe N, Brandes J M, Blumenfeld Z First and early second-trimester diagnosis of fetal urinary tract anomalies using transvaginal sonography. Prenat Diagn 1990;10:653–666.

56. Rosati P, Guariglia L Transvaginal sonographic assessment of the fetal urinary tract in early pregnancy. Ultrasound Obstet Gynecol 1996;7:95–100.

57. Bronshtein M, Kushnir O, Ben-Rafael Z, et al. Transvaginal sonographic measurement of fetal kidneys in the first trimester of pregnancy. JCU 1990;18:299–301.

58. Bronshtein P M, Rottem S, Yoffe N, Blumenfeld Z, Brandes J M Early determination of fetal sex using transvaginal sonography: technique and pitfalls. JCU 1990;18:302–306.

59. Bronshtein M, Weiner Z, Abramovici H, Filmar S, Erlik Y, Blumenfeld Z Prenatal diagnosis of gall bladder anomalies: report of 17 cases. Prenat Diagn 1993;13:851–861.

60. Schmidt W, Yarkoni S, Crelin E S, Hobbins J C Sonographic visualisation of physiologic anterior abdominal wall hernia in the first trimester. Obstet Gynecol 1987;69:911–915.

61. Bowerman R A Sonography of fetal midgut herniation: normal size criteria and correlation with crown-rump length. J Ultrasound Med 1993;5:251–254.

62. van Zalen-Sprock R M, Brons J T J, van Hugt J M G, van der Harten M J, van Geijn H C Ultrasonographic and radiologic visualisation of the developing embryonic skeleton. Ultrasound Obstet Gynecol 1997;9:392–397.

Fetal abnormalities: Anencephaly/exencephaly

63. van Zalen-Sprock R M, van Vugt J M, van Geijn H P First and early second trimester diagnosis of anomalies of the central nervous system. J Ultrasound Med 1995;14:603–610.

64. Goldstein R B, Filly R A, Callen P W Sonography of anencephaly: pitfalls in early diagnosis. JCU 1989;17:397–402.

65. Wilkins-Haug L, Freedman W Progressions of exencephaly to anencephaly in the human fetus – an ultrasound perspective. Prenat Diagn 1991;11:227–233.

66. Timor-Tritsch I E, Greenbaum E, Monteagudo A, Baxi L Exencephaly-anencephaly sequence: proof by ultrasound imaging and amniotic fluid cytology. Journal of Maternal and Fetal Medicine 1996;5:182–185.

67. Nishi T, Nakano R First trimester diagnosis of exencephaly by transvaginal ultrasonography. J Ultrasound Med 1994;13:149–151.

68. Chatzipapas I K, Whitlow B J, Economides D L The 'Mickey Mouse' sign and the diagnosis of anencephaly in early pregnancy. Ultrasound Obstet Gynecol 1999;13:196–199.

69. Johnson S P, Sebire N J, Snijders R J M, Tunkel S, Nicolaides K H Ultrasound screening for anencephaly at 10–14 weeks of gestation. Ultrasound Obstet Gynecol 1997;9:14–16.

Encephalocoele

70. Cullen M T, Athanassiadis A P, Romero R Prenatal diagnosis of anterior parietal encephalocoele with transvaginal sonography. Obstet Gynecol 1990;75:489–491.

71. Bronshtein M, Zimmer E Z Transvaginal sonographic follow up on the formation of fetal cephalocoele at 13–19 weeks gestation. Obstet Gynecol 1991;78:528–530.

72. van Zalen-Sprock M M, van Hugt J M G, van der Harten H J, van Geijn H P Cephalocoele and cystic hygroma: diagnosis and differentiation in the first trimester of pregnancy with transvaginal sonography. Report of two cases. Ultrasound Obstet Gynecol 1992;2:289–292.

73. Salonen R, Paavola P Meckel Syndrome. J Med Genet 1998;35:497–501.

74. Sepulveda W, Sebire N J, Souka A, Snijders R J M, Nicolaides K H Diagnosis of the Meckel–Gruber Syndrome at eleven to fourteen weeks gestation. Am J Obstet Gynecol 1997;176:316–319.

75. Braithwaite J, Economides D L First trimester diagnosis of Meckel–Gruber syndrome by transabdominal scanning in a low risk case. Prenat Diagn 1995;15:1168–1170.

Hydrocephalus

76. Bronshtein M, Ben-Shlomo I Choroid plexus dysmorphism detected by transvaginal sonography: the earliest sign of fetal hydrocephaly. JCU 1991;19:547–553.

77. Achiron R, Achiron A, Yagel S First trimester transvaginal sonography diagnosis of Dandy–Walker malformation. JCU 1993;21:62–64.

78. Gembruch U, Baschat A A, Reusche E, Wallner S J, Greive M First trimester diagnosis of holoprosencephaly with a Dandy–Walker malformation by transvaginal ultrasonography. J Ultrasound Med 1995;14:619–622.

79. Ulm B, Ulm M R, Deutinger J, Bernaschek G Dandy–Walker malformation diagnosed before 21 weeks of gestation: associated malformations and chromosomal abnormalities. Ultrasound Obstet Gynecol 1997;10:167–170.

Spina bifida

80. Nicolaides K H, Campbell S, Gabee S G, Guiditi R Ultrasound screening for spina bifida: cranial and cerebellar signs. Lancet 1986;2:72–74.

81. Bernard J P, Suarez B, Rambaud C, Muller F, Ville Y Prenatal diagnosis of neural tube defect before 12 weeks' gestation: direct and indirect ultrasonographic semeiology. Ultrasound Obstet Gynecol 1997;10:406–409.

82. Blumenfeld Z, Siegler E, Bronshtein M The early diagnosis of neural tube defects. Prenat Diagn 1993;13:863–871.

83. Sebire N J, Noble P L, Thorpe-Beeston J G, Snijders R J M, Nicolaides K H Presence of the 'lemon' sign in fetuses with spina bifida at the 10–14 week scan. Ultrasound Obstet Gynecol 1997;10:403–405.

Holoprosencephaly

84. van Zalen-Sprock M M, van Vugt I M G, van der Harten H M, Nieuwint A W M, van Geijn H P First trimester diagnosis of cyclopia and holoprosencephaly. J Ultrasound Med 1995;14:631–633.

85. Bronshtein M, Weiner Z Early transvaginal sonographic diagnosis of alobar holoprosencephaly. Prenat Diagn 1991;11:459–462.

86. Gonzalez-Gomez F, Salamanca A, Padilla M C, Camara M, Sabatel R M Alobar holoprosencephalic embryo detected via transvaginal sonography. Eur J Obstet Gynecol Reprod Biol 1992;47:266–270.

Cystic hygroma

87. Chervenak F A, Isaacson G, Blakemore K J Fetal cystic hygroma: cause and natural history. N Engl J Med 1983;309:822–825.

88. Cullen M T, Gabrielli S, Green J J Diagnosis and significance of cystic hygroma in the first trimester. Prenat Diagn 1990;10:643–651.

89. Trauffer P M L, Anderson C, Johnson A, Helger S, Morgan P, Wapner R J The natural history of euploid pregnancies with first trimester cystic hygromas. Am J Obstet Gynecol 1994;170:1279–1284.

90. Abramowitcz J S, Warsof S L, Doyle D L, Smith D, Levy D L Congenital cystic hygroma of the neck diagnosed prenatally: outcome with normal and abnormal karyotype. Prenat Diagn 1989;9:321–327.

91. Johnson M P, Johnson A, Holygreve W First trimester simple hygroma, etiology and outcome. Am J Obstet Gynecol 1993;168:156–161.

92. Bronshtein M, Rottem S, Yoffe N, Blumenfeld Z. First trimester and early second-trimester diagnosis of nuchal cystic hygroma by transvaginal sonography: diverse prognosis of the septated from the non septated lesion. Am J Obstet Gynecol 1989;161:78–82.

93. Bronshtein M, Blumenfeld Z Transvaginal sonography – detection of findings suggestive of fetal chromosomal anomalies in the first and early second trimesters. Prenat Diagn 1992;12:587–593.

94. Chodirker B N, Harmon C R, Greenberg C R Spontaneous resolution of a cystic hygroma in a fetus with Turners Syndrome. Prenat Diagn 1988;8:291–296.

95. Rottem S, Bronshtein M, Thaler I, Brandes J M First trimester transvaginal sonographic diagnosis of fetal anomalies. Lancet 1989;1:444–445.

Cardiac abnormalities (See also references 52, 53, 54)

96. Vergani P, Mariani S, Ghidini A, et al. Screening for congenital heart disease with the four chamber view of fetal heart. Am J Obstet Gynecol 1992;167:1000–1005.

97. Stumpflen I, Stumpflen A, Wimmer M, Bernaschek. Effect of detailed fetal echocardiography as part of routine prenatal ultrasonographic screening on detection of congenital heart disease. Lancet 1996;348:854–857.

98. Todros T, Faggiano F, Chiappa E, Gagliotti P, Mitola B, Sciarrone A Accuracy of routine ultrasonography in screening heart disease prenatally. Prenat Diagn 1997;17:901–906.

99. Stoll C, Alembik Y, Dott B Evaluation of prenatal diagnosis of congenital heart disease. Prenat Diagn 1993;13:453–461.

100. Levi J S, Hyjazi Y, Schaaps J P, Defoort P, Coulon R, Buekens P Sensitivity and specificity of routine antenatal screening for congenital anomalies by ultrasound: the Belgian multicentre study. Ultrasound Obstet Gynecol 1991;1:102–110.

101. Tegnander E, Eik-Nes S, Johansen O J, Linker D T Prenatal detection of heart defects at the routine fetal examination at 18 weeks in a non-selected population. Ultrasound Obstet Gynecol 1995;5:372–380.

102. Gembruck U, Knopfle G, Chatterjee M, Bald R, Hausmann M First trimester diagnosis of fetal congenital heart disease by transvaginal two dimensional and doppler echocardiography. Obstet Gynecology 1990;75:496–498.

103. Bronshtein M, Zimmer E Z, Gerlis L M, Lorber A, Drugan A Early ultrasound diagnosis of fetal congenital heart defects in high risk and low risk pregnancies. Obstet Gynecol 1993;82:225–229.

104. Bronshtein M, Zimmer E Z, Milo S, Ho S Y, Lorber A, Gerlis L M Fetal cardiac abnormalities detected by transvaginal sonography at 12–16 weeks gestation. Obstet Gynecol 1991;78:374–378.

105. Achiron R, Rotstein Z, Lipitz S, Mashiach S, Hegesh J First trimester diagnosis of fetal congenital heart disease by transvaginal ultrasonography. Obstet Gynecol 1994;84:69–72.

106. Yagel S, Weissman A, Rotstein Z, et al. Congenital heart defects. Natural course and in utero development. Circulation 1997;96:550–555.

107. Gembruch U, Baschat A A, Knopfle G, Hausmann M Results of chromosomal analysis in fetuses with cardiac anomalies as diagnosed by first and early second-trimester echocardiography. Ultrasound Obstet Gynecol 1997;10:391–396.

108. Allan L D, Sharland G, Tynan M J The natural history of the hypoplastic heart syndrome. Int J Cardiol 1989;25:341–343.

109. Marasini M, De Caro E, Pongiglione G, Ribaldone D, Caponetto S Left heart obstructive disease: changes in the echocardiagraphic appearance during pregnancy. JCU 1993;21:65–68.

110. Achiron R, Weissman A, Matitiahu A, Lipitz S, Rotstein Z, Hegesh J Endocardial fibroelastosis secondary to critical aortic stenosis: natural course and evaluation in utero. Ultrasound Obstet Gynecol 1994;203 (Supplement 1):354, Abstract.

111. Gembruch U, Baschat A A, Knopfle G, Hausmann M First and early second trimester diagnosis of fetal cardiac anomalies. In: Wladimiroff J, Pilu G, eds. Ultrasound and the fetal heart. London: Parthenon Publishing Group.

112. Gembruch U Prenatal diagnosis of congenital heart disease. Prenat Diagn 1997;17:1283–1298.

Urinary tract abnormalities

113. Bronshtein M, Amit A, Achiron R, Noy I, Blumenfeld Z The early prenatal sonographic diagnosis of renal agenesis: techniques and possible pitfalls. Prenat Diag 1994;14:291–297.

114. Bronshtein M, Bar-Hana I, Blumenfeld Z Clues and pitfalls in the early prenatal diagnosis of late onset infantile polycystic kidney. Prenat Diagn 1992;12:293–298.

115. Bulic M, Podobnick M, Korenic B, Bistricki J First-trimester diagnosis of low obstructive uropathy: an indication of initial renal function in the fetus. JCU 1987;15:537–541.

116. Drugan A, Zador I, Bhatia R K, Sacks A J, Evans M First trimester diagnosis and early in utero treatment of obstructive uropathy. Acta Obstet Gynecol Scand 1989;68:645–649.

117. Stiller R J Early ultrasonic appearance of fetal bladder outlet obstruction. Am J Obstet Gynecol 1989;160:584–585.

118. Hoshino T, Ihara Y, Shirane H, Ota T Prenatal diagnosis of prune belly syndrome at 12 weeks of pregnancy: case report and review of the literature. Ultrasound Obstet Gynecol 1998;12:362–366.

119. Sebire N J, Von Kaisenberg C, Rubio C, Snijders R J M, Nicolaides K H Fetal megacystis at 10–14 weeks of gestation. Ultrasound Obstet Gynecol 1996;8:387–390.

120. Whitlow B J, Lazanakin M L, Kadir R A, Chatzipapas I, Economides D L The significance of choroid plexus cysts, echogenic foci in the heart and renal pyelectasis in the first trimester. Ultrasound Obstet Gynecol 1998;12:385–390.

121. Bronshtein M, Bar-Hava I, Lightman A The significance of early second trimester sonographic detection of minor fetal renal anomalies. Prenat Diagn 1995;15:627–632.

Abnormalities of the gastrointestinal tract

122. Petrikovsky B M First trimester diagnosis of duodenal atresia. Am J Obstet Gynecol 1994;171:569–570.

123. Zimmer E Z, Bronshtein M Early diagnosis of duodenal atresia and possible sonographic pitfalls. Prenat Diagn 1996;16:564–566.

124. Tsukerman G L, Krapiva G A, Kirillova I A First trimester diagnosis of duodenal stenosis associated with oesophageal atresia. Prenat Diagn 1993;13:371–376.

125. Snijders R J M, Brizot M L, Faria M, Nicolaides K H Fetal exomphalos at 10–14 weeks of gestation. J Ultrasound Med 1995;14:569–574.

126. Guzman E R Early prenatal diagnosis of gastroschisis with transvaginal ultrasound. Am J Obstet Gynecol 1990;162:1253–1254.

127. Kushnir O, Izquierdo L, Vigil D, Curet L B Early transvaginal diagnosis of gastroschisis. JCU 1990;18:194–197.

128. Daskalakis G, Sebire N J, Jurkovic D, Snijders R J M, Nicolaides K H Body stalk anomaly at 10–14 weeks of gestation. Ultrasound Obstet Gynecol 1997;10:416–418.

129. Ginsberg N E, Cadkin A, Strom C Prenatal diagnosis of body stalk anomaly in the first trimester of pregnancy. Ultrasound Obstet Gynecol 1997;10:419–421.

130. Shalev E, Eliyahu S, Battino S, Weiner E First trimester transvaginal sonographic diagnosis of body stalk anomaly. J Ultrasound Med 1995;14:641–642.

131. McMalla C, Lajinian S, DeSouza D, Rottem S Natural history of antenatal omphalomesenteric duct cyst. J Ultrasound Med 1995;14:639–640.

132. Skibo L K, Lyons E A, Levi C S First trimester umbilical cord cysts. Radiology 1992;182:719–722.

Diaphragmatic hernia

133. Bronshtein M, Lewit N, Sujov P O, Makhoul I R, Blazer S Prenatal diagnosis of congenital diaphragmatic hernia: timing of visceral herniation and outcome. Prenat Diagn 1995;14:695–698.

134. Lam Y H, Tang M H Y, Yuen S T Ultrasound diagnosis of fetal diaphragmatic hernia and complex congenital heart disease at 12 weeks gestation – a case report. Prenat Diagn 1998;18:1159–1162.

135. Sebire N J, Snijders R J M, Davenport M, Greenough A, Nicolaides K H Fetal nuchal translucency thickness at 10–14 weeks gestation and congenital diaphragmatic hernia. Obstet Gynecol 1997;90:943–946.

Skeletal abnormalities

136. Gabrielli S, Falco P, Pilu G, Perolo A, Milano V, Bovicelli L Can transvaginal fetal biometry be considered a useful tool for early detection of skeletal dysplasias in high-risk patients. Ultrasound Obstet Gynecol 1999;13:107–111.

137. Soothill P W, Vuthiwong C, Rees H Achondrogenesis Type II diagnosed by transvaginal ultrasound at 12 weeks gestation. Prenat Diagn 1993;13:523–528.

138. Fisk N, Vaughan J, Smidt M, Wigglesworth J Transvaginal ultrasound recognition of nuchal oedema in the first trimester diagnosis of achondrogenesis. JCU 1991;19:586–590.

139. Benaceraff B R, Lister J E, DuPonte B L First trimester diagnosis of fetal anomalies. A report of three cases. J Reprod Med 1988;33:777–780.

140. Dimaio M S, Barth R, Koprivnikar K E, et al. First trimester prenatal diagnosis of osteogenesis imperfecta Type II by DNA analysis and sonography. Prenat Diagn 1993;13:589–596.

141. Hill L M, Leary J Sonographic diagnosis of short rib polydactyly dysplasia at 13 weeks. Prenat Diagn 1998;18:1198–1201.

142. Bronshtein M, Keret D, Deutch M, Liberson A, Bar Chava I Transvaginal sonographic detection of skeletal anomalies in the first and early second trimesters. Prenat Diagn 1993;13:597–601.

143. Bronshtein M, Stahl S, Zimmer E Transvaginal sonographic diagnosis of fetal finger abnormalities in early gestation. J Ultrasound Med 1995;14:591–595.

144. Bronshtein M, Zimmer E Z Transvaginal ultrasound diagnosis of fetal club foot at 13 weeks, menstrual age. JCU 1989;17:518–520.

145. Rottem S, Bronshtein M Transvaginal sonographic diagnosis of congenital anomalies between 9 weeks and 16 weeks, menstrual age. JCU 1990; 18:307–314.

Abnormalities of the face

146. Bronshtein M, Blumenfeld I, Kohn J, Blumenfeld Z Detection of cleft lip by early second trimester transvaginal sonography. Obstet Gynecol 1994;84:73–76.

147. Cullen M T, Green J, Whetham J, Salafia C, Gabrielli S, Hobbins J Transvaginal ultrasonographic detection of congenital anomalies in the first trimester. Am J Obstet Gynecol 1990;163:466–476.

Twin pregnancy

148. Monteagudo A, Haberman S, Timor–Tritsch I E The diagnosis of multiple pregnancy in the first trimester. In: Jurkovic D, Jaunıaux E, eds. Ultrasound in Early Pregnancy. London: Parthenon Publishing Group 1996.

149. Bajoria R, Kingdom J The case for routine determination of chorionicity and zygosity in multiple pregnancy. Prenat Diagn 1997;17:1207–1225.

150. Sepulveda W, Sebire N J, Hughes A, Odibo A, Nicolaides K H The lambda sign at 10–14 weeks gestation as a predictor of chorionicity in twin pregnancies. Ultrasound Obstet Gynecol 1996;7:421–423.

151. Townsend R R, Simpson G F, Filly R A Membrane thickness in ultrasound prediction of chorionicity in twin gestations. J Ultrasound Med 1988;7:327–332.

152. Vayssiere C F, Nazbanon H, Camus E P, Hillion Y E, Nisand I F Determination of chorionicity in twin gestations by high frequency abdominal ultrasonography: counting the layers of the dividing membrane. Am J Obstet Gynecol 1996;175:1529–1533.

153. Winn N H, Gabrielli S, Reece S, Robert E A, Salafia J A, Hobbin J C Ultrasonographic criteria for the prenatal diagnosis of placental chorionicity in twin gestations. Am J Obstet Gynecol 1989;161:1540–1542.

154. Weissman A, Achiron R, Lipitz S, Blickstein I, Mashiach S The first trimester growth discordant twin: an ominous prenatal finding. Obstet Gynecol 1994;84:110–114.

155. Sharma S, Gray S, Guzman E R, Rosenberg J C, Shen-Schwartz S Detection of twin-twin transfusion syndrome by first trimester ultrasonography. J Ultrasound Med 1995;14:635–637.

156. Shaleu E, Zalel Y, Ben-Ami M, Weiner E First trimester ultrasonic diagnosis of twin reversed arterial perfusion sequence. Prenat Diagn 1992;12:219–222.

157. Meizner I, Levy A, Kaltz M, Glezerman M Early ultrasonic diagnosis of conjoined twins. Harefuah 1993;124:741–744.

158. Skupski D W, Streltzoff J, Hutson J M, Rosenwaks Z, Cohen J, Chervenak F Early diagnosis of conjoined twins in triplet pregnancy after in vitro fertilisation and assisted hatching. Ultrasound Med 1995;14:611–615.

159. Lam Y H, Sin S Y, Lam C, Lee C P, Tang M H Y, Tse H Y Prenatal sonographic diagnosis of conjoined twins in the first trimester: two case reports. Ultrasound Obstet Gynecol 1998;11:289–291.

CHAPTER 5

Disorders of amniotic fluid

R. Bryan Beattie

Background

In the distant past the amniotic fluid was thought to be a source of nourishment for the fetus[1] but its main functions seem to be the preservation of euthermia, to provide a protective environment for safe fetal movement and development and to play an important role in lung development. It also has anti-bacterial properties. More importantly disorders of amniotic fluid volume seem to reflect both fetal health and perinatal outcome and therefore they warrant a thorough understanding.

Normal pregnancy

The amniotic sac forms about 12 days after fertilization as a cleft near the embryonic plate which deepens and becomes enclosed by amnion as it fuses with the body stalk and then later the chorion. Amniotic fluid volume is dependent upon various mechanisms responsible for inflow to and outflow from the amniotic cavity. The latter is normally an enclosed space in normal pregnancy until spontaneous or artificial rupture near term. In early pregnancy significant amounts of amniotic fluid are present before substantial fetal urine production and fetal swallowing are present and it is speculated that active transport of solute by the amnion may result in passive movement of water across a chemical gradient into the amniotic cavity. Certainly before 20 weeks' gestation the fluid is isotonic and its composition approximates that of maternal plasma.[2,3] In late pregnancy fetal urine production and swallowing are the two major pathways for production and clearance of amniotic fluid (Fig. 5.1) and the net volume turnover is in excess of 95% of the total in late pregnancy with an approximate turnover time of one day. Certainly proteins injected into the amniotic cavity have a daily clearance rate of about 63%[4] and isotopically labelled water has a turnover volume in excess of one volume daily which probably represents diffusion exchange of water molecules rather than net volume movements.[5] After 24 weeks levels of urinary excretion products such as urea, creatinine and uric acid are 2 to 3 times higher than in fetal plasma. Electrolytes such as sodium, potassium and chloride are, however, about 70 to 80% of fetal plasma

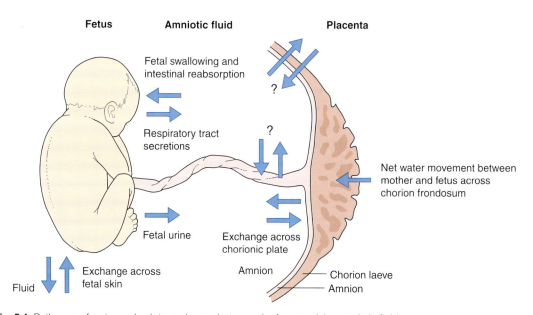

Fetus   Amniotic fluid   Placenta

Fetal swallowing and intestinal reabsorption

Respiratory tract secretions

Fetal urine

Exchange across chorionic plate

Exchange across fetal skin

Fluid

Amnion

Net water movement between mother and fetus across chorion frondosum

Chorion laeve

Amnion

Fig. 5.1 Pathways of water and solute exchange between the fetus and the amniotic fluid.

levels whereas protein levels peak at 32 weeks and then decline towards term.[6] There are also increasing amounts of solid materials such as vernix, fetal squames, lanugo and hair[7] and the osmolality becomes hypotonic[8] such that by term it is 92% of that of the maternal serum.

The gestational changes in pregnancy are exhibited in Figure 5.2 which shows a rising amniotic fluid volume in the first and second trimester (200 ml at 16 weeks) which peaks at 32 to 34 weeks (1000 ml) and then declines in late third trimester (150 ml/week 38 to 43 weeks). There is wide variation, however, in the volume of amniotic fluid, the accepted methods for measuring amniotic fluid volume and definitions of abnormal amniotic fluid volume. At 32 to 36 weeks volumes of more than 1500 to 2000 ml (polyhydramnios) or less than 500 ml (oligohydramnios) are associated with fetal abnormalities and adverse perinatal outcome.[9,10] Whilst polyhydramnios in the second trimester resolves spontaneously in up to 50% of cases with normal perinatal outcome,[11] oligohydramnios rarely resolves spontaneously and is invariably associated with poor perinatal outcome.[12]

Pressure measurements in normal singleton pregnancy have been used to produce a gestation specific nomogram which shows a sigmoid regression curve with advancing gestation which plateaus in the mid trimester. There is no relationship to multiple pregnancy, amniotic fluid index,

maternal age, parity, fetal sex or subsequent preterm delivery and the authors suggest that it may be useful in therapeutic amnioinfusion or amnioreduction.[13] In pregnancies complicated by polyhydramnios the pressure is elevated (exceeding the upper limit in 53% cases) and correlates positively with the depth of the deepest pool and negatively with fetal PO2 and pH. In those complicated by oligohydramnios the pressures were lower than the mean (below the lower limit in 33% cases).[13]

Fetal urine production

Fetal urine production has been recognized as the major source of amniotic fluid since the times of Hippocrates and micturition occurs as early as 8 to 11 weeks' gestation.[14] Ultrasound assessment of hourly fetal urine production shows a biphasic directly proportional linear relationship with advancing gestation with accelerated urine production after 30 to 32 weeks (Fig. 5.3). The urine production rate per kg body weight also increases from about 110 ml/kg/24 hr at 25 weeks to almost double this at 190 ml/kg/24 hr at 39 weeks.[15] At term the daily urine production rate is maximal at about 500 to 600 ml/day before falling with prolonged pregnancy with consequent reduction in liquor volume.[16]

It is therefore likely that any pathological process causing reduction in the renal production of urine or mechanical

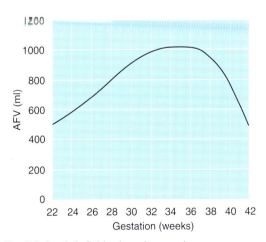

Fig. 5.2 Amniotic fluid volume in normal pregnancy.

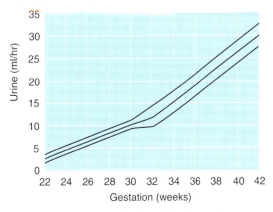

Fig. 5.3 Hourly urine production in the human fetus.

obstruction to renal outflow or micturition will lead to oligohydramnios. Low urinary flow rates and oligohydramnios are frequently observed in intrauterine growth retardation (IUGR)[9,17] and severe renal tract anomalies such as renal agenesis, cystic dysplasia and urinary tract obstruction are also invariably associated with anhydramnios or oligohydramnios.[18]

Polyhydramnios is rarely due to increased urinary flow rates and fetal urine production has been shown to be similar to normal pregnancy rates in such cases.[19] In diabetic pregnancies fetal hyperglycaemia might be expected to cause increased glucose excretion into the fetal urine with increased urinary production. Kurjak and colleagues found that only about 30% have urinary production rates more than 95th centile[20] and indeed others have found normal urinary production rates in diabetic pregnancies complicated by polyhydramnios.[17]

Fetal swallowing

Fetal swallowing begins almost simultaneously with fetal urine production at about 8 to 11 weeks, with reported late pregnancy volumes from 200 to 450 ml/day to 1500 ml/day.[14,21] Some tracheal fluid from the lungs will also be swallowed, however, such that the total volume of fluid swallowed may be considerably more.[22] Swallowing usually occurs during fetal breathing though fetal breathing is usually suppressed prior to the onset of labour.[22] Other factors such as alterations in fetal plasma osmolality also affect the periodicity and extent of fetal swallowing.[23] Pathological conditions affecting the neurological, muscular and mechanical components of fetal swallowing are responsible for about 30% of cases of polyhydramnios in late pregnancy.[24] A review of almost 2000 cases of polyhydramnios in human pregnancy identified oesophageal abnormalities in 27% cases and abnormal fetal swallowing mechanisms in a further 18%.[25] Animal studies in fetal monkeys with oesophageal

ligation have been shown to result in polyhydramnios.[26]

Fetal lung fluid production

Whilst accurate quantitation has not been possible there is substantial evidence that there is production of fetal lung fluid which is excreted into the amniotic cavity. Liley injected contrast media into the amniotic cavity and none was found in the fetal or neonatal lungs of almost all the 800 fetuses studied.[5] Other observations such as the infrequent observation of meconium aspiration despite meconium stained liquor, the presence of pulmonary phospholipids in amniotic fluid and ultrasound evidence of accumulation of fluid in the trachea and bronchial tree in cases of laryngeal atresia would also support this view. Whilst animal studies suggest that active transport of chloride ions across the epithelial lining of the fetal lungs from the lung capillaries to the alveolar lumen mediates excretion of lung fluid, the proportional contribution that this makes to amniotic fluid volume in normal pregnancy remains unquantified and although the osmolality is similar to fetal plasma the chloride concentration is higher.[27,28,29]

Fetal skin

In the first half of pregnancy the highly permeable fetal skin is thought to allow transport of water into the amniotic cavity prior to keratinization at about 24 weeks' gestation when significant transport of water and solutes ceases and there is a well recognised relationship between transepidermal water loss in very preterm and preterm neonates compared with those at full term.[30] Small lipid soluble molecules such as carbon dioxide may, however, continue to be transported throughout the whole of pregnancy and are not affected by keratinization to the same extent.

Fetal membranes and other sources

The amnion and chorion provide a large surface area for transport of water and solutes[31] and transfer of solute followed by inward passive diffusion of water is the most likely source of amniotic fluid in early pregnancy. In late pregnancy, however, there is a net outward transfer of water across the amnion (estimated at about 300 ml/day in late pregnancy) whilst net electrolyte transfer is thought to be inwards.[5] Changes within the structure and molecular biology of the membranes have been demonstrated in oligohydramnios and polyhydramnios where the thickness of the amniotic epithelial cell layer thickness is reduced or increased respectively.[32] Scanning electron microscopy has also shown a proportional decrease and increase in intracellular canals in the amnion. There is, however, dispute as to whether altered membrane transport is a primary cause or a secondary response to disordered amniotic fluid volume particularly in cases of polyhydramnios.[33]

The thick layer of Wharton's Gel and the relatively small surface area of the umbilical cord make it an unlikely source of amniotic fluid exchange though the large surface area of the fetal side of the chorionic plate and its rich underlying blood supply would facilitate such a role and certainly this has been suggested in the past.[34] Despite the fact that fetal sweat glands are present in larger numbers than later in life it is not known whether there is any *sweating* in utero[30,5] and other potential small sources of fetal fluid such as nasal and buccal secretions warrant consideration.

Regulation of amniotic fluid volume

The tight control of amniotic fluid within limits of 0.5 to 2.0 l in human pregnancy is supported though not proven by animal studies. The proposed mechanisms of regulation include alterations in chorioamnion membrane permeability,[35] alterations of fetal urine regulation via hormones such as arginine, vasopressin, adrenaline and cortisol[30,36] and alterations in fetal swallowing.[5] Maternal factors such as osmolality have been shown to affect fetal hydration which may in turn affect amniotic fluid volume but this remains entirely speculative. Certainly there is a close positive correlation between maternal plasma and amniotic fluid volume in normal pregnancy and that correction of subnormal maternal plasma volume in oligohydramnios restores the amniotic fluid volume.[37]

Ultrasound evaluation of amniotic fluid volume

Subjective and objective assessment of amniotic fluid volume remains an important part of antenatal fetal surveillance. Although both methods are useful when performed by an experienced observer, objective methods are important in providing useful comparative data in multicentred studies and when multiple observers are involved in the care of the same pregnancy.

Subjective assessment of oligohydramnios depends on the absence of cord free pockets of liquor and crowding of fetal small parts whereas in polyhydramnios there are multiple large pockets and a free floating fetus with free limb movements. The simplest objective method of assessment is the measurement of the vertical length of the largest cord free pool and although this is subject to variation by changes in fetal position it does provide a reasonable guide to liquor assessment. Perinatal mortality is increased at the extremes of liquor volume with a bimodal distribution which is maximal below 20 mm or above 80 mm. Intervention on the basis of oligohydramnios seems appropriate at values less than 20 mm.

The amniotic fluid index (AFI) which was first described in 1987[38] is the most robust method of assessing amniotic fluid volume and should be adopted as the standard technique in assessing liquor volume. It is more reliable than single pocket techniques[39] and is less prone to inter- and intra-observer error.[40] Furthermore it has been shown to be directly correlated with true amniotic fluid volume (approximately 1 cm for each 50 ml).[41] It has been found to be clinically valuable in estimating the amniotic fluid volume in patients with premature rupture of the membranes[42] and those on indomethacin therapy.[43]

The technique involves dividing the abdomen into four quadrants based on the umbilicus. The transducer is placed vertically in each quadrant in turn perpendicular to the floor and the largest vertical pool of liquor is measured. The sum of the four measurements (in centimetres) equates to the amniotic fluid index and gestational nomograms are available for normal pregnancy (Fig. 5.4). Abnormalities of liquor volume such as polyhydramnios and oligohydramnios can then be defined as an AFI > 90th centile or <10th centile respectively though Phelan and his colleagues used absolute gestation independent values of 25 cm and 5 cm respectively.[38,44]

The main causes of oligohydramnios are rupture of the membranes, renal agenesis or obstructive uropathy, and reduced renal

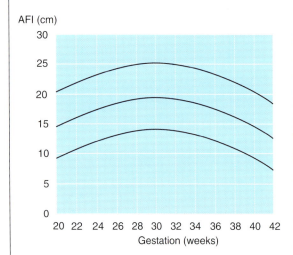

Fig. 5.4 Amniotic fluid index reference range. (Reproduced with permission from Ninosu.)

perfusion and chronic fetal urine under production as a consequence of hypoxic redistribution of fetal blood flow. In the mature fetus with a normal renal tract and no evidence of ruptured membranes, oligohydramnios usually implies fetal hypoxia and is often an indication for delivery. Certainly this has been recognised in scoring systems of fetal wellbeing such as the Biophysical Profile Score[45] with the liquor volume being the most predictive parameter for perinatal mortality.

Oligohydramnios

Oligohydramnios can be defined as an amniotic fluid volume of less than 400 ml[46] or an AFI < 5.0 cm.[38,40] It is associated with a high perinatal mortality and morbidity and in scoring systems of fetal wellbeing oligohydramnios has been shown to be the most important predictor of subsequent perinatal outcome.[39] It typically presents in the third trimester with renal impairment, such as renal agenesis, or diminished urinary output as the final common pathway for the development of oligohydramnios.[47] Intrapartum complications include cord compression, meconium stained liquor, variable decelerations and other CTG abnormalities with the pregnancy outcome inversely related to the amniotic fluid volume.[39] Similarly in prolonged pregnancy oligohydramnios represents an important marker for adverse outcome and delivery should be considered. As a labour ward admission test numerous investigators have shown that amniotic fluid assessment can identify the at-risk fetus[48,39] with a view to continuous fetal heart rate surveillance in labour and thus stratify the process of fetal monitoring in labour and also the distressed fetus requiring immediate delivery. Similarly assessment of amniotic fluid volume may identify a group of women who would benefit from amnioinfusion which has been shown to reduce the incidence of abnormal CTG patterns and intervention for fetal distress with better cord pH values at birth in cases of oligohydramnios.[49,50]

Second trimester oligohydramnios is generally associated with a poor perinatal outcome with a favourable outcome in 18% in the absence of premature rupture of the membranes[51] and only a moderate improvement to 25% when it was present.[52] Various mechanically induced fetal abnormalities have been reported in association with second trimester oligohydramnios and include a 10 to 15% risk of cranial, facial, and skeletal abnormalities[53,54] and a 17% risk of pulmonary hypoplasia.[55,56]

Patients referred to the ultrasound department with suspected oligohydramnios on clinical grounds (subjective impression of small uterus with easily palpable fetal parts or subnormal symphysis-fundal height) should have a careful review of their antenatal history with particular attention to the possibility of ruptured membranes and clinical and ultrasound evaluation of growth. The classical history of leaking clear fluid may well be absent and a speculum examination should be performed to look for liquor in the posterior fornix. The patient should be instructed to cough to visualize any liquor being expelled through the cervical os. Any fluid in the posterior fornix should be tested by nitrazine sticks (which detect the alkaline pH of liquor), a 'fern test' using microscopy to evaluate a dried slide sample of the aspirated liquor (which shows a ferning pattern due to sodium chloride crystals), and more recently products such as the Mast Amni-check which are highly accurate in identifying amniotic fluid.

The sonographer should then make a subjective and objective assessment of liquor volume, biometry and a detailed anomaly scan with particular attention being paid to the fetal renal tract. Imaging may need to be enhanced by amnioinfusion[2] or colour Doppler. Karyotyping is an important consideration based on amniocentesis (of infused fluid if necessary), CVS, fetal blood or even urine.[57] Even if the findings are entirely normal there is value in repeating the assessment 2 weeks later as a means of ensuring normal growth velocity and that there has been no deterioration in liquor volume. If oligohydramnios is confirmed in the absence of ruptured membranes or fetal abnormality, then weekly ultrasound scans are appropriate for fetal surveillance and should include serial growth assessment, liquor volume, umbilical artery Doppler studies and after 26 weeks biophysical profile scores. These are high-risk pregnancies and should be subsequently managed at consultant level preferably by a specialist with an interest in fetal medicine.

One of the main determinants of neonatal outcome regardless of the underlying aetiology is pulmonary hypoplasia since fetal breathing of quantities of amniotic fluid is necessary for normal lung development. Various antenatal attempts to predict pulmonary hypoplasia have been unsuccessful and include measurement of the fetal chest circumference and lung length on ultrasound; however, their predictive value is poor. Prophylactic treatment by serial amnioinfusion has, however, been advocated and evaluated in pregnancies complicated by oligohydramnios. There is merit in therapy not only in reducing pulmonary hypoplasia by serial infusions prior to delivery but also intrapartum therapy which reduces the incidence of variable decelerations, intervention for fetal distress, fetal acidosis at delivery and meconium aspiration and ventilation at birth.[41,50,58]

Preterm premature rupture of the membranes

Preterm premature rupture of the membranes accounts for about 30% of all preterm deliveries and complicates about 6% of all pregnancies. In the USA it is the commonest indication for NICU admission and a major cause of neonatal death.[59] The aetiology is largely unknown but it may be associated with cervical incompetence, unstable lie or polyhydramnios. Local infection may also be a significant factor along with placental abruption. Ultrasound prediction of amniotic fluid volume is an important predictor of the interval to delivery,[60,61] intra-uterine infection[60,62] and general fetal wellbeing.[63] In the presence of a normal liquor volume on admission following PPROM the patient is four times more likely to be undelivered within a week and there is a lower risk of subsequent caesarean section, low Apgar score and perinatal death.[61] Chorioamnionitis is also six to seven times more likely in the presence of oligohydramnios or an unreactive CTG[62,64] and one can argue that amniocentesis in such cases would be appropriate to confirm or exclude intra-uterine infection.[60]

Making the diagnosis can often be quite difficult with either an atypical history or little objective evidence on which to base it. Sterile speculum examination followed by the use of the 'fern test' based on salt crystal formation or nitrazine sticks which change to black in the presence of an alkali pH are recognized to have an unacceptable false-positive and false-negative rate. Recently the availability of a sensitive dipstick 'Mast Amni-Check'[65] has improved the reliability of diagnosis. It is based on the fact that insulin growth binding factor protein-1 is found in amniotic fluid at levels 100 to 1000 times the level in maternal serum and is not normally found in cervical or vaginal secretions with intact membranes. The test uses immunochromotography and can detect levels of down to 100 μg/l IGBFP-1. False-negative results may, however, occur if the membrane rupture has been over 12 hours previously due to proteases in vaginal secretions.

Once the diagnosis of PPROM has been made it is appropriate to assess the mother at the time of the initial speculum examination by looking for any vaginal discharge, taking a high vaginal (and possibly endocervical) swab, a white cell count and perhaps a C-reactive protein along with observations of maternal pulse and temperature, and an examination of the abdomen for uterine tenderness and contractions. In the absence of infection it is no longer necessary to keep the patient in hospital. Patients can be instructed on how to take their own pulse and temperature such that they can monitor themselves 2–4 times daily with 1–2 weekly visits to the hospital for white cell counts and ultrasound scans. This approach has been employed with some success in our own unit in women of varied educational and cultural backgrounds. Patients are given clear thresholds for presenting themselves to the hospital and are also advised on the significance of other symptoms such as abdominal pain, fever or purulent vaginal discharge. The role of steroids for prophylaxis against respiratory distress syndrome is, however, controversial since they may mask fetal infection and increase the risk of neonatal infection and the stress of PPROM alone may enhance surfactant production. Overall the benefits in significantly reducing the risk of respiratory distress syndrome would, however, seem to justify its use in PPROM.[66] The main obstetric risks of PPROM are intra-uterine infection, premature labour and pulmonary hypoplasia.

Polyhydramnios

Historical teaching suggests that a clinical diagnosis of polyhydramnios should be based on observations made by two independent observers on at least 2 occasions or the recovery of more than 1500 ml liquor at amniotomy. Polyhydramnios can, however, be more appropriately defined as an amniotic fluid volume of more than 2000 ml[46] or an AFI > 25 cm.[38,44] It is associated with a high perinatal mortality and morbidity[44,46,67] and is typically a disorder of late pregnancy. It occurs in about 1 in 250 singleton pregnancies and about 5 to 10% of multiple pregnancies. It is frequently associated with structural fetal abnormalities such as neural tube defects, anterior abdominal wall defects and upper GIT obstruction or atresias together with impaired swallowing in fetuses with chromosomal anomalies such as trisomy 13 and 18. The mechanism in diabetes is controversial with some investigators ascribing the polyhydramnios to increased production by the amnion or fetal polyuria whilst others dispute this.[68] Other possible aetiological considerations include fetal toxoplasmosis and cytomegalovirus infection, rhesus disease and hydrops fetalis from any cause.

Polyhydramnios usually presents in the second half of pregnancy with a history of being large for dates, abdominal discomfort or uterine contractions. In 90% cases it presents as a slowly developing chronic condition but in 10% cases severe acute polyhydramnios may develop. Acute polyhydramnios is usually found in early pregnancy and maternal symptoms may occur due to the mechanical effects of the rapidly enlarging uterus on the diaphragm (breathlessness), the pelvic veins (vulval and leg oedema) and rarely the ureters (oliguria). There is thus a substantial risk of premature delivery and considerable perinatal mortality and morbidity as a consequence. Acute polyhydramnios may be associated with monozygous twin pregnancies and large placental chorioangiomas.

The appropriate clinical examination includes measurement of symphysis fundal height and the abdominal palpation when the impression of the tenseness of the abdomen, difficulty in palpating fetal parts and fetal heart auscultation are suggestive of polyhydramnios. It is important to assess any uterine contractions and if present then a short 20-minute cardiotocograph will provide an objective assessment of their frequency. The antenatal notes should be reviewed to confirm whether it is a single or multiple pregnancy, whether there has been elevated maternal serum alphafetoprotein (MSAFP) and whether there are any risk factors for carbohydrate intolerance. The urine should be tested for glucose and a random blood glucose or glucose tolerance test should be considered. Ultrasound examination should include a subjective and an objective assessment of liquor volume, a detailed anomaly scan with reference to anomalies such as neural tube defects which

are recognised causes of polyhydramnios and assessment of fetal growth. This is often difficult in the third trimester when the head may be deeply engaged and evaluation of the intracerebral anatomy is thus limited; however, transvaginal sonography may be useful in this situation.

Other important medical causes such as toxoplasmosis and cytomegalovirus infection and rhesus disease should also be excluded by maternal blood sampling. The ability to determine the cause of the polyhydramnios is heavily dependent on its extent due to limitations in ultrasound imaging in extreme cases and failure to identify fetal abnormalities prior to delivery.[69] If however the polyhydramnios is an isolated finding then therapeutic use of indomethacin should be considered.[43]

The suspected mechanism in neural tube and anterior abdominal wall defects is the transudation of fluid across exposed membranes or low levels of fetal antidiuretic hormone leading to fetal polyuria.[70] Upper GIT obstruction prevents swallowing with the most severe forms of polyhydramnios occurring in those cases with the highest level of obstruction.

Since there is often a propensity to preterm labour and preterm premature rupture of the membranes (PPROM), there may be merit in treating the polyhydramnios in order to prolong the pregnancy. Indeed in acute decompression of the uterus following rupture of the membranes, placental abruption may occur. The intra-amniotic pressure and myometrial tension are elevated and the fetal PO2 is reduced.[13] This may be facilitated either by serial amnioreduction using a 20 gauge needle under ultrasound guidance though with an increased risk of premature rupture of the membranes, premature labour (50% cases), abruption, infection and rapid reaccumulation. Alternatively medical therapy with indomethacin as a 100 mg suppository PR followed by 25 mg tid given orally is effective. This not only acts on the fetal kidneys by reducing fetal urine production but also by reducing chorion-amnion production and its other beneficial effect as a tocolytic agent. The main side effects, however, include gastritis in the mother and premature closure of the fetal ductus when used for prolonged periods after 32 weeks' gestation. Some centres in the USA monitor ductal blood flows using pulsed Doppler but this is probably unnecessary. The amniotic fluid volume should be carefully monitored in order to prevent overtreatment. It would also seem prudent to administer prophylactic steroids (2 doses of dexamethasone 12 mg at an interval of 24 hours repeated at 10-day intervals from 26 to 34 weeks' gestation). Following delivery there remains a substantial risk to the mother of primary postpartum haemorrhage and prophylactic infusion of an oxytocic agent should be considered (20 IU Syntocinon in 1000 ml Hartmann's solution).

Twin-twin transfusion syndrome

This rare cause of acute polyhydramnios occurs in a minority of monochorionic twins with abnormal communicating intraplacental vascular vessels. The donor is small, hypoperfused, anaemic and has poor urinary output with oligohydramnios or anhydramnios and indeed the amniotic membrane may be totally invisible to ultrasound assessment and this finding be wrongfully ascribed to a monoamniotic pregnancy. The donor may therefore be plastered to the uterine wall by its membranes – a so-called 'stuck twin'. The recipient, however, is hyperperfused, plethoric, discrepitantly larger and found in a polyhydramniotic sac (presumably on the basis of increased renal blood flow and polyuria). Fetal survival without treatment is poor at under 20% but improves to up to 70% with serial amnioreduction.[71] It has been observed that the reduction in amniotic fluid pressure associated with therapeutic amnioreduction leads to a consistent degree of cerebral hyperperfusion in the larger recipient twin and in our own institution

absent umbilical artery end diastolic velocities often return in the recipient following the procedure. In one series of 19 twin pregnancies complicated by TTTS and treated before 28 weeks' gestation, only 37% babies survived the neonatal period with intertwin disparity in fetal size and mean volumes of fluid drained being major determinants of survival.

Alternative therapeutic options also include selective feticide of the donor, hysterotomy and removal of the donor twin, laser or ultrasound ablation of the communicating vessels within the placenta.[72]

Assessment of fetal renal function

The San Francisco Fetal Treatment Group have performed a retrospective study to assess fetal renal function based on biochemical analysis of fetal urine.[73] In general it is known that after about 13 weeks fetal urine is an ultrafiltrate of fetal serum made hypotonic by selective tubular absorption of sodium and chloride. The levels of fetal urinary sodium and chloride fall during pregnancy and the finding of hypotonic as opposed to isotonic fetal urine confers a good prognosis in fetal renal disease. Similarly urinary osmolality has shown to be prognostically useful. Certainly absolute values of urinary sodium levels greater than 100 mmol/l, chloride levels greater than 90 mmol/l[74] or osmolarity greater than 210 mOsm imply insufficient tubular reabsorption and irreversible renal damage at birth. Operating by a totally different mechanism fetal urinary neutral amino acids also predict irreversible renal damage reflecting poor tubular capacity.[75] Further refinements in fetal selection for vesico-amniotic shunting include the use of gestation specific nomograms[76] and sampling each individual kidney.[77] It is not always possible to perform correct antenatal fetal selection[78,79] and other parameters indicative of impaired renal tubular reabsorption such as elevated urinary micromolecular proteins (mol. wt. < 70,000) have been proposed since albumen is normally the only protein found in fetal urine in mid-pregnancy.[80] Certainly this technique was shown to be of value in predicting subsequent outcome in 21 cases of fetal urinary tract obstruction whereas four cases were incorrectly classified using urinary electrolytes and osmolarity.[81]

Vesico-amniotic shunting

In pregnancies complicated by obstructive uropathy such as posterior urethral valves strict selection criteria must be applied before selection for shunting. These include a normal karyotype, no associated fetal abnormalities, urethral obstruction due to posterior urethral valves, oligohydramnios and a gestation under 32 weeks. Following shunt placement ultrasound follow-up should reveal bladder decompression and improvement or maintenance of liquor volume.[74]

Amnioinfusion

Amnioinfusion, the intra-amniotic injection of fluid under ultrasound guidance, is of value as both a diagnostic technique to enhance ultrasound imaging and also as a therapeutic one. In cases of severe oligohydramnios or anhydramnios it may be impossible to assess the fetal renal tract adequately and since renal agenesis is uniformly lethal, reliable diagnosis is essential to allow elective termination of pregnancy or to prevent unnecessary intervention in late pregnancy for a non-viable fetus. Whilst failure to identify a fetal bladder is highly suggestive, failure to identify the kidneys may not be adequate to make the diagnosis, especially with the risk of enlarged fetal adrenal glands occupying the renal fossae and being wrongly interpreted as kidneys. Certainly the use of colour Doppler ultrasound may be of value in identifying the fetal renal arteries if present and indeed power Doppler based on

flow velocity amplitude rather than velocity may improve the sensitivity further. Other useful options include amnioinfusion and installation of warmed saline into the fetal peritoneal cavity.[82]

Amnioinfusion not only improves the quality of the ultrasound examination[83] but may also help make the diagnosis of ruptured membranes in the period immediately following the instillation of fluid. The procedure is often complicated by either the failure to identify a cord free pocket of liquor to insert the needle or the accidental cannulation of the umbilical cord or its vessels. Again colour Doppler ultrasound should simplify this problem by accurate identification of the cord vessels. The therapeutic benefits of amnioinfusion include not only a reduction in pulmonary hypoplasia but also a reduction in limb deformities and facial abnormalities due to mechanical compression in the absence of the protective effects of normal quantities of liquor. In a series of 61 pregnancies treated by amnioinfusion at a median of 22 weeks, the procedure was successful in 95% cases, previously unsuspected anomalies were identified in 5 cases and a change in underlying diagnosis was made in 13% cases. Of 40 serial amnioinfusions performed on 9 women there were no skeletal abnormalities, 3 neonates survived, 5 of the 6 perinatal deaths that did occur did not have pulmonary hypoplasia, and the incidence of clinical chorioamnionitis was 2.2%.[84]

In the absence of any renal function there is currently not an option for renal dialysis in the newborn or renal transplantation though anencephalics have been used as a source of donor kidneys[85] with at least 81 cases reported to date.[86] The other main concerns about the long term outcome in prenatally diagnosed renal abnormalities is the risk of recurrent vesicorenal reflux, recurrent urinary tract infection and the development of hypertension.

References

1. Denman T. An introduction to the practice of midwifery. 1815 In London: Bliss & White.

2. King J C. Oligohydramnios. In: Charles D, Glover D D, eds. Current therapy in obstetrics, 1988, p 46. Philadelphia: B C Decker.

3. Vosburgh G H, Flexner L B, Cowie D B. The rate of renewal in women of water and sodium of the amniotic fluid as determined by tracer techniques. American Journal of Obstetrics and Gynecology, 1948;56:1156.

4. Gitlin D, Dumate J, Morales C, Noriega L, Arevalo N. The turnover of amniotic fluid protein in the human conceptus. American Journal of Obstetrics and Gynecology, 1972;113:632.

5. Liley A W. Disorders of amniotic fluid. In: Assali N S, ed. Pathophysiology of gestation, 1972; New York: Academic Press.

6. Mandelbaum B, Evans T N. Life in the amniotic fluid. American Journal of Obstetrics and Gynecology, 1969;104:365.

7. Hellman L M, Pritchard J A (14 ed.). New York: Appleton-Century-Crofts 1971.

8. Gillibrand. Changes in amniotic fluid volume with advancing pregnancy. Journal of Obstetrics and Gynaecology of the British Commonwealth, 1969;76:527.

9. Chamberlain P F, Manning F A, Morrison I, Marman C R, Lange I R. Ultrasound evaluation of amniotic fluid, volume I. The relationship of marginal and decreased amniotic fluid volumes to perinatal outcome. American Journal of Obstetrics and Gynecology, 1984a;150:245–249.

10. Chamberlain P F, Manning F A, Morrison I, Marman C R, Lange I R. Ultrasound evaluation of amniotic fluid, volume I. The relationship of increased amniotic fluid volumes to perinatal outcome. American Journal of Obstetrics and Gynecology, 1984b;150:250.

11. Zamah N M, Gillieson M S, Walters J H, Hall P F. Sonographic detection of polyhydramnios: A five year experience. American Journal of Obstetrics and Gynecology, 1982;143:523.

12. Bastide A, Manning F A, Harmon C, Lange I, Morrison I. Ultrasound evaluation of amniotic fluid: Outcome of pregnancies with severe oligohydramnios. American Journal of Obstetrics and Gynecology, 1986;154:895.

13. Fisk N, Tannirandron Y, Nicolini U, Talbert D, Rodeck C H. Amniotic pressure in disorders of amniotic fluid volume. Obstetrics and Gynecology, 1990;76:210–214.

14. Abramovich D R, Gordon A, Jandial L, Page K R. Fetal swallowing and voiding in relation to hydramnios. Obstetrics and Gynecology, 1979;54:15.

15. Lotgering F K, Wallenburg H C S. Mechanisms of production and clearance of amniotic fluid. Seminars of Perinatology, 1986;10:94.

16. Vorherr H. Placental insufficiency in relation to postterm pregnancy and fetal postmaturity. Evaluation of placental function and the management of the postterm gravida. American Journal of Obstetrics and Gynecology, 1975;123:67.

17. VanOtterlo L C, Wladimiroff J W, Wallenburg H C S. Relationship between fetal urine production and amniotic fluid volume in normal pregnancy and pregnancy complicated by pregnancy. British Journal of Obstetrics and Gynaecology, 1977;84:205.

18. Bain A D, Scott J S. Renal agenesis and severe urinary tract dysplasia. A review of 50 cases with particular reference to the associated anomalies. British Medical Journal, 1960;841.

19. Abromovich D R, Page K P. Pathways of water transfer between liquor amnii and the feto-placental unit at term. European Journal of Obstetrics and Gynaecology, 1973;3:155.

20. Kurjak A, Kirkinen P, Latin V, Ivankovic D. Ultrasonic assessment of fetal kidney function in normal and complicated pregnancies. American Journal of Obstetrics and Gynecology, 1981;141:266.

21. Pritchard J A. Deglutition by normal and anencephalic fetuses. Obstetrics and Gynecology, 1965;25:289.

22. Harding R, Bocking A D, Sigger J N, Wickham P J D. Composition and volume of fluid swallowed by fetal sheep. Q J Exp Physiol, 1984;69:487.

23. Ross M G, Shermin D J, Ervin M G. Stimuli for fetal swallowing: systemic factors. American Journal of Obstetrics and Gynecology, 1984;161:1559.

24. Scott J S, Wilson L K. Hydramnios as an early sign of oesophageal atresia. Lancet, 1957;2:569.

25. Moya F, Apgar V, St. James L, Berrien C. Hydramnios and congenital abnormalities. JAMA, 1960;173:1552.

26. Minei L J, Suzuki K. Role of fetal deglutition and micturition in the production and turnover of amniotic fluid in the monkey. Obstetrics and Gynecology, 1976;48:177.

27. Adamson T M, Boyd R D H, Platt H S, Strang L B. Composition of alveolar liquid in the fetal lamb. Journal of Physiology (London), 1969;204:159.

28. Adamson T M, Brodecky V, Lambert T F. The production and composition of lung fluid in the in utero foetal lamb. 1973. Cambridge, England: Cambridge University Press.

29. Olver R E, Schneeberger E E, Walters D V. Epithelial solute permeability, ion transport and tight junction morphology in the developing lung of the fetal lamb. Journal of Physiology (London), 1981;315:395.

30. Brace R A. Amniotic fluid volume and its relationship to fetal fluid balance: Review of experimental data. Seminars in Perinatology, 1986;10:103.

31. Abromovich D R, Page K R, Jandial L. Bulk flows through human fetal membranes. Gynecology Investigations, 1976;7:157.

32. Herbertson R M, Hammond M E, Bryson M J. Amniotic epithelial ultrastructure in normal, polyhydramnic and oligohydramnic pregnancies. American Journal of Obstetrics and Gynecology, 1986;68:74.

33. Brace R A. Amniotic Fluid Dynamics. In: Creasy R K, Resnik R, eds. Maternal Fetal Medicine: Principles and practice, 1989; pp 128–135. Philadelphia: WB Saunders Company.

34. Plentl A. A transfer of water across perfused umbilical cord. Proceedings of the Society of Experimental Biology in Medicine, 1961;107:622.

35. Lingwood B E, Wintour E M. Amniotic fluid volume and in vivo permeability of ovine fetal membranes. Obstetrics and Gynecology, 1984;64:368.

36. Kitterman J A, Ballard P L, Clements J A. Tracheal fluid in fetal lambs: Spontaneous decrease prior to birth. Journal of Applied Fetal Physiology, 1979;47:985.

37. Goodlin R C, Anderson J C, Gallagher T F. Relationship between amniotic fluid volume and maternal plasma volume expansion. American Journal of Obstetrics and Gynecology, 1983;146:505.

38. Phelan J P, Ahn M O, Smith C V. Amniotic Fluid Index measurements during pregnancy. Journal of Reproductive Medicine, 1987;32:627.

39. Rutherford S E, Phelan J P, Smith C V. The four quadrant assessment of amniotic fluid volume: an adjunct to antepartum fetal heart rate testing. Obstetrics and Gynecology, 1987a;70:533.

40. Rutherford S E, Phelan J P, Smith C V. The four quadrant assessment of amniotic fluid volume: intraobserver and intraobserver variation. Journal of Reproductive Medicine, 1987b;32:597.

41. Strong T, Hetzler G, Paul R H. Amniotic fluid volume increase after amnioinfusion of a fixed volume. American Journal of Obstetrics and Gynecology, 1990a;162:746.

42. Smith C V, Greenspoon J, Phelan J P, Platt L D. The clinical utility of the nonstress test in the conservative management of patients with preterm spontaneous premature rupture of the membranes. Journal of Reproductive Medicine, 1987;32:1.

43. Cabrol D, Landesman R, Muller J. Treatment of polyhydramnios with prostaglandin synthetase inhibitors (indomethacin). American Journal of Obstetrics and Gynecology, 1987;157:422.

44. Phelan J P, Martin G I. Polyhydramnios: Fetal and neonatal implications. Clinics in Perinatology, 1989a;16:987.

45. Manning F A 1981.

46. Cunningham F G, McDonald P C, Gant N F. Disorders of the amnion and amniotic fluid volume. In: Williams Obstetrics, 1989; p 553. New York: Appleton and Lange.

47. Phelan J P. The postdate pregnancy: an overview. Clinics in Obstetrics and Gynaecology, 1989b; 32:221.

48. Phelan J P, Sarno A P, Ahn M O. The Fetal Admission Test. In 36th Annual Clinical Meeting of the American College of Obstetricians and Gynecologists, 1989c; Atlanta.

49. Nageotte M P, Freeman R K, Garite T J, Dorchester W. Prophylactic intrapartum amnioinfusion in patients with preterm premature rupture of the membranes. American Journal of Obstetrics and Gynecology, 1985;153:557.

50. Sadovsky Y, Amon E, Bade M E, Petrie R H. Prophylactic amnioinfusion during labour complicated by meconium: a preliminary report. American Journal of Obstetrics and Gynecology, 1989;161:613.

51. Garite T J. Premature rupture of the membranes: the enigma of the obstetrician. American Journal of Obstetrics and Gynecology, 1985;151:1001.

52. Landy J H, Isada N B, Larsen J W. Genetic implications of idiopathic hydramnios. American Journal of Obstetrics and Gynecology, 1987;157:114.

53. King J C, Mitzner W, Butterfield A B, Queenan J T. Effect of induced oligohydramnios on fetal lung development. American Journal of Obstetrics and Gynecology, 1986;154:823.

54. Nimrod C, Varela-Bittings F, Machin G. The effect of very prolonged membrane rupture on fetal development. American Journal of Obstetrics and Gynecology, 1984;148:540.

55. Nimrod C, Davies D, Iwanicki S. Ultrasound prediction of pulmonary hypoplasia. American Journal of Obstetrics and Gynecology, 1986;68:495.

56. Perlman M, Williams J, Hirsch M. Neonatal pulmonary hypoplasia after prolonged leakage of amniotic fluid. Archives of Disease in Childhood, 1976;51:349.

57. Platt A A, Devore G R, Lopez E. Role of amniocentesis in ultrasound detected fetal malformations. Obstetrics and Gynecology, 1986;68:153.

58. Miyasaki F, Navarez F. Saline amnioinfusion for relief of repetitive variable decelerations: a prospective randomised study. American Journal of Obstetrics and Gynecology, 1985;153:301–316.

59. ACOG Premature rupture of the membranes. In Technical Bulletin, 1988 115. Washington DC: American College of Obstetricians and Gynecologists.

60. Garite T J, Freeman R K, Linzey E M, Braly P. The use of amniocentesis in patients with premature rupture of the membranes. Obstetrics and Gynecology, 1979;54:226.

61. Vintzileos A M, Campbell W A, Nochimson D J, Weinbaum P J. Degree of oligohydramnios and pregnancy outcome in patients with premature rupture of the membranes. Obstetrics and Gynecology, 1985;67:579.

62. Vintzileos A M, Campbell W A, Nochimson D J, Weinbaum P J. The use of the nonstress test in patients with premature rupture of the membranes. American Journal of Obstetrics and Gynecology, 1986b;155:149.

63. Clark S L. Managing PPROM: a continuing controversy. Contemporary Obstetrics and Gynecology, 1989;33:49.

64. Vintzileos A M, Campbell W A, Nochimson D J, Weinbaum P J. Qualitative amniotic fluid volume verus amniocentesis in predicting infection in preterm premature rupture of the membranes. Obstetrics and Gynecology, 1986a;67:579.

65. Mast. Mast Amni-Check. Mast Group Limited, Mast House, Derby Road, Bootle, Merseyside L20 1EA, UK. 1995.

66. Crowley P, ed. Corticosteroids after preterm prelabour rupture of membranes, 1995; London: BMJ Publishing Group.

67. Phelan J P, Park Y W, Ahn M O, Rutherford S E. Polyhydramnios and perinatal outcome. Journal of Perinatology, 1990;4:347.

68. Wladimiroff J W, Barentsen R, Wallenburg H C S, Drogendijk A C. Fetal urine production in a case of diabetes associated with polyhydramnios. Obstetrics and Gynecology, 1975;45:100.

69. Hill L, Breckle R, Thomas M L, Fries J K. Polyhydramnios: ultrasonically detected prevalence and neonatal outcome. Obstetrics and Gynecology, 1987;69:21.

70. Wallenburg H C, Wladimiroff J W. The amniotic fluid: polyhydramnios and oligohydramnios. Journal of Perinatal Medicine, 1977;5:233.

71. Mahoney B, Petty C, Nyberg D, Luthy D, Hictok D, Hirsch J. The 'stuck twin' phenomenon: ultrasonographic findings, pregnancy outcome and management with serial amniocentesis. Obstetrics and Gynecology, 1990;77:537–540.

72. Delia J, Cruikshank D, Keye W. Fetoscopic neodymium: YAG laser occlusion of placental vessels in severe twin-twin transfusion syndrome. Obstetrics and Gynecology, 1990;75:1046–1053.

73. Appelman Z, Golbus M S. The management of fetal urinary tract obstruction. Clinics in Obstetrics and Gynaecology, 1990;29:483–489.

74. Cromblehome T, Harrison M, Golbus M. Fetal intervention in obstructive uropathy: prognostic indicators and efficacy of intervention. American Journal of Obstetrics and Gynecology, 1990;162:1239–1244.

75. Lenz S, Lund-Hansen T, Bang J. A possible prenatal evaluation of fetal renal function by amino acid analysis on fetal urine. Prenatal Diagnosis, 1985;5:259–267.

76. Nicolini U, Fisk N, Rodeck C H, Beacham J. Fetal urine biochemistry: an index of renal maturation and renal dysfunction. British Journal of Obstetrics and Gynaecology, 1992;99:46–50.

77. Nicolini U, Rodeck C H, Fisk N M. Shunt treatment for fetal obstructive uropathy. Lancet, 1987;2:1338–1339.

78. Reuss A, Wladimiroff J W, Pijpers L. Fetal urinary electrolytes in bladder outlet obstruction. Fetal Therapy, 1987;2:148–153.

79. Wilkins I A, Chitkara U, Lynch L. The nonpredictive value of fetal urinary electrolytes: preliminary report of outcomes and correlations with pathologic diagnosis. American Journal of Obstetrics and Gynecology, 1987;157:694–698.

80. Holzgreve W, Aydinli K, Evans M, Miny P, eds. Fetal Genitourinary Tract Abnormalities, 1992. Carnforth, Lancashire: Parthenon Publishing Group.

81. Holzgreve W, Lison A, Bulla M. Protein analysis to determine fetal kidney function (Abst). American Journal of Obstetrics and Gynecology, 1991;164 (suppl): 336.

82. Haeusler M, Ryan G, Robson S, Lipitz S, Rodeck C H. The use of saline solution as a contrast medium in suspected diaphragmatic hernia and renal agenesis. American Journal of Obstetrics and Gynecology, 1993;168:1486–1492.

83. Quetel T A, Meijdes A A, Salman F A, Rodriguez M M T. Amnioinfusion: an aid in the ultrasonographic evaluation of severe oligohydramnios in pregnancy. American Journal of Obstetrics and Gynecology, 1992;167(2):333–336.

84. Strong T, Hetzler G, Sarno A, Paul R. Prophylactic intrapartum amnioinfusion: a randomised clinical trial. American Journal of Obstetrics and Gynecology, 1990;162:1370–1374.

85. Holzgreve W, Beller F K, Buchholz B. Kidney transplantation from anencephalic donors. New England Journal of Medicine, 1989;316:1069–1070.

86. Anencephaly. New England Journal of Medicine, 1990;322:669–674.

CHAPTER 6

Cranial abnormalities

Sarah A. Russell

Embryology

Introduction

It is helpful for the sonographer to have a basic understanding of the development of the brain. Knowledge of the timescale of central nervous system development helps the sonographer to answer queries regarding any potential harmful effects from medication (teratogens), the likelihood of adverse impact being maximal during the period of organogenesis prior to 12 weeks' gestation. Armed with this knowledge, it becomes easier to understand why various abnormalities often occur together and to recognize these patterns. Gestational age will influence which abnormalities may be diagnosed – unless a part of the brain has developed fully, it is not possible for us to recognize and diagnose an abnormality of that region.

Furthermore, studies comparing ultrasound with other imaging modalities, in particular computed tomography and magnetic resonance imaging (MRI), suggest that there is not a direct temporal relationship between the embryologic development of the brain and our ability to image that development contemporaneously.[1] For example, comparative studies between MRI and neuroanatomy between 9 and 24 weeks' gestation show that there is up to a 5-week lag in the ability of MRI to demonstrate the development seen in neuroanatomy.[2]

Therefore, when attempting firm diagnosis with ultrasound it is important to know when a particular anatomical structure should always be recognizable on scan rather than the earliest documented sighting. Reliance on the latter will lead to false-positive diagnoses. For example, the cerebellar vermis does not fully form until 19 weeks' gestation and therefore inferior vermian agenesis, an important diagnosis prognostically, may not be made with confidence until this time. Complete vermian agenesis, however, is recognizable earlier. It is through understanding human embryology that the anatomy we observe on ultrasound becomes vital.

The sequence of development[2,3] will be described in weeks related to last menstrual period, i.e. menstrual dates, and not from time of conception.

Week 5

This is the week following the first missed period. During this week, the primitive streak forms within the trilaminar embryo progressing to form the neural plate which then curves in to form the neural groove.

Week 6

The neural groove folds in and starts to fuse to form the neural tube starting in the region that becomes the cervical cord with the top two-thirds of the tube forming the brain and the bottom third forming the cord. The top end of this tube (rostral or anterior neuropore) closes first, followed by the bottom end (caudal or posterior neuropore) 2 to 3 days later (Fig. 6.1). The lumen of the tube forms the ventricular system and the central canal, with the substance of the tube thickening and folding to become the brain and cord. Three primary brain vesicles differentiate, namely the forebrain (prosencephalon), the midbrain (mesencephalon) and the hindbrain (rhombencephalon). This differentiation into the three vesicles will not occur if the rostral neuropore fails to close. The optic vesicles (which later form the retina and optic nerves) develop prior to closure of the neuropore.

Insults occurring before the end of the 6th week result in anencephaly (failure of closure of the rostral neuropore) or neural tube defect (failure of closure of the caudal neuropore).

Week 7

Each of the three primary vesicles of the brain subdivide and each has its own portion of the ventricular system (Fig. 6.2). The forebrain (prosencephalon) divides into two parts. The telencephalon forms the cerebral

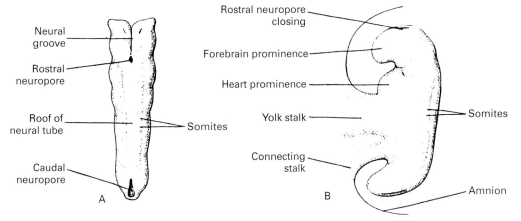

Fig. 6.1 23-day-old embryo (6^{+2} gestational age). (Reproduced from Moore KL, Persaud TVN. The developing human – clinically oriented embryology. 6th ed. Philadelphia: WB Saunders; 1998.)

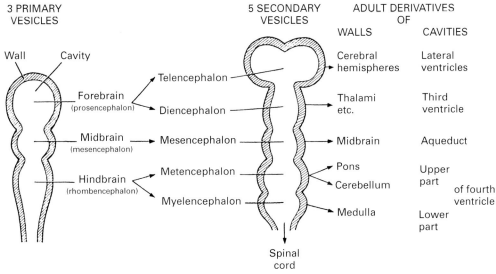

Fig. 6.2 Brain vesicles and derivatives. (Reproduced from Moore KL, Persaud TVN. The developing human – clinically oriented embryology. 6th ed. Philadelphia: WB Saunders; 1998.)

hemispheres, the caudate and the putamen and the accompanying lateral ventricles. The diencephalon forms the thalami, hypothalamus and the globus pallidus and the accompanying third ventricle.

The midbrain (mesencephalon) forms the midbrain and the accompanying aqueduct of Sylvius.

The hindbrain (rhombencephalon) divides into two parts. The metencephalon forms the pons and cerebellar hemispheres and vermis and the myelencephalon forms the medulla. Both contribute to the fourth ventricle.

During this week the eyes, nasal pits and mouth begin to develop. Insults occurring before the end of the 7th week result in abnormalities of midline development, principally holoprosencephaly and agenesis of the corpus callosum.

Week 8 to term

By this stage, differentiation has occurred to form the basic template of the structure of the brain; subsequently during pregnancy there is further growth and development.

Sulcation

The mature brain is characterized by multiple gyri (ridges) and sulci (grooves). The surface of the fetal brain is featureless until the development of the Sylvian or lateral sulcus during the 5th month. From 23 to 25 weeks, the brain becomes increasingly folded, with the appearance from 27 weeks of the central (rolandic), interparietal and superior temporal fissures. Secondary and tertiary sulci develop from 32 to 33 weeks' gestation. Insults during this process will result in abnormalities of sulcation, e.g. lissencephaly and schizencephaly.

Neuronal migration

Between 9 and 10 weeks' menstrual age, radial glial fibres develop, extending from the germinal matrix lining the ventricles to the brain surface. Neurones migrate along these fibres to form the cerebral cortex in an orderly fashion in layers. Insults occurring during this process will result in neuronal migration disorders and heterotopias. These are very difficult disorders to recognize and diagnose in utero; frequently they are only diagnosed in families with an a priori risk.

Teratogens

Teratogens may be chemical, as in ingested drugs, or environmental, as in infection or irradiation.[4] The impact of the insult will depend on gestational age of the pregnancy at the time of the insult and on the mechanism of action of the drug. In general terms, any organ is most vulnerable at the time of highest cell division. For the human fetus, the most vulnerable period is between 5 to 11 weeks' menstrual age but different organ systems have their own critical period. For the human brain, this is between 5 and 18 weeks although it remains sensitive to insult throughout pregnancy. Major structural abnormality is likely to result from an insult prior to 10 weeks and a functional or minor structural abnormality from later insults.

Environmental teratogens are infection and irradiation. For an infectious agent to cause problems the mother has to be infected and the fetus affected via the transplacental route. Infection, most commonly viral, can cause microcephaly, eye abnormality (microphthalmia, retinal dysplasia, glaucoma, cataracts), calcification and mental retardation. High-level irradiation causes microcephaly and mental retardation.

Ingested drugs that cause developmental and structural abnormalities of the brain may be prescribed or connected with drug abuse and misuse. The most common drugs with known teratogenetic properties are listed in Table 6.1. These agents can cause multisystem abnormality but only those relating to the central nervous system are listed. The reader is directed to other more comprehensive texts for more detailed information.

Conclusion

There are a number of agents that can affect development and growth of the neural axis. The most vulnerable period for the brain is from 5 to 18 weeks but it remains sensitive to insult throughout fetal life. Advice given is to avoid unnecessary medication during the whole of pregnancy and for women, particularly those on anticonvulsants, to be referred to a specialist prior to conception for advice on treatment regimens.

Table 6.1
Teratogens and the brain

Phenytoin	Craniofacial abnormalities, microcephaly, mental retardation
Sodium valproate	Ten-fold increase of neural tube defect, facial clefting
Methotrexate	Folate antagonist, used in rheumatoid arthritis, neural tube defect
Antimalarials	Mefloquine (Lariam), no definite pattern as yet, potential central nervous system anomalies
Warfarin	Microcephaly, mental retardation
Retinoic acid	Used in acne, toxic at low doses, neural tube defect, facial clefting
Alcohol	Microcephaly, mental retardation, ocular abnormalities
Vasoactive drugs, e.g. heroin, cocaine	Agenesis of the corpus callosum, septo-optic dysplasia, schizencephaly, hydranencephaly, ventriculomegaly, porencephaly, infarction

Normal variants, pitfalls and artefacts

Introduction

A serious risk in prenatal diagnosis is that of the false-positive diagnosis, the consequences of which are unnecessary parental anxiety at best and, at worst, management decisions reached on the basis of the erroneous sonographic findings leading to the termination of a normal pregnancy. Risk management mandates that we do everything in our power to minimize the occurrence of a false-positive diagnosis whilst recognizing that no screening technique enjoys 100% accuracy. Factors to bear in mind when aiming to reduce risk in this context are listed in Table 6.2.

Errors in interpretation of fetal brain images may be categorized into three areas: firstly, those caused by the equipment; secondly, those caused by patient characteristics; thirdly, those caused by the operator. Diagnostic errors are of two main types: the first is to fail to make an observation (an error of omission); the second (an error of interpretation) is to misinterpret a scan finding. Interpretation and diagnostic errors are equally serious from the patient's perspective.

The equipment

Pitfalls and errors originate if the operator uses suboptimal or incorrect machine settings, most commonly gain, or selects an inappropriate probe for the area or feature to be examined.

If the overall gain is set too low, then it is possible to incorrectly assign the ventricular

Table 6.2
Ultrasound risk management

A reproducible and structured examination
Objective, critical observation and evaluation
Knowledge of normal through embryology and practical experience
Self-knowledge – knowing individual limitations
Continued professional development and education

wall margin when taking the atrial measurement.[5] The cerebral hemispheres are hypoechoic which compounds the problem. It is the medial wall of the lateral ventricle which is most difficult to assign; the lateral one is usually clearly indicated as the choroid plexus abuts it owing to the effect of gravity. The consequence of this error is to incorrectly diagnose ventriculomegaly, a false-positive diagnosis. To avoid this, ensure that the midline of the brain lies as parallel as possible to the maternal skin, and hence the probe surface, as possible. This will help you to identify the ventricular wall by utilizing the specular reflection from the ventricular wall which renders it more visible.[6]

Probe selection is important, especially when assessing the near-field. If you have chosen a probe with a small footprint (e.g. a sector or vector format), then examination of the near-field is compromised and this problem should be overcome by selecting a curved array or linear format. Combine a small footprint with too high gain settings or maternal obesity (resulting in near-field reverberation artefact) and you will be unable to adequately assess structures close to the maternal skin surface. With fetal cranial assessment, the undesirable consequence would be to miss pathology in the near-field hemisphere, giving the opportunity for a false-negative diagnosis. Utilization of multiple focal zones improves resolution at the expense of decreased frame rate. Many machines have the facility to magnify or zoom the image which can also improve resolution and image clarity.

The patient

Patient obesity which leads to reverberation artefact may seriously compromise the diagnostic ability of the ultrasound scan.[7] It is possible, however, to influence the image quality and it is therefore important to endeavour to optimize the image. The machine characteristics which have most impact on image quality in this situation are operating frequency and log compression. Switch to a lower frequency to increase the depth of beam penetration, being aware that the trade-off is one of reduced resolution. Reduce the log compression by 5 to 10 dB which will further enhance visualization. The other technique to employ is to roll patients onto their side which can have a dramatic impact on image quality by reducing the depth of maternal soft tissues traversed by the ultrasound beam. Finally, when discussing scan abnormality, it is reasonable to indicate to obese patients that their body habitus does have an adverse impact on the sensitivity and diagnostic power of ultrasound.

The operator

Sonographers have the most significant impact on image quality and interpretation through their knowledge and examination technique. The unskilled operator is potentially the single most dangerous component of any ultrasound examination. It is essential in fetal diagnosis that the sonographer is fully conversant with normal brain anatomy and with its embryological development.

In the assessment of the fetal brain this means knowing that it is normal for the brain to be monoventricular until 10 weeks and that the skull vault does not fully ossify until 12 to 13 weeks (Fig. 6.3). This will prevent the sonographer from making the false-positive diagnoses of holoprosencephaly and acrania or anencephaly respectively. The cerebellum changes its appearance with time; as the vermis does not complete development until 19 weeks partial vermian agenesis should not be diagnosed before this gestation.[8] Complete agenesis, in contrast, may be evident earlier.

There are several linear structures that traverse the cisterna magna in the normal fetus (Fig. 6.4) – these are normal and not pathological.[9] Knowledge of anatomy will also prevent the sonographer from misassigning the deep perforating veins in the frontal white matter as the ventricular wall. When measuring head size, it is preferable to use head circumference to biparietal diameter as the former takes account of head shape. This will prevent the misdiagnosis of microcephaly in cases with dolicocephaly, and macrocephaly in those

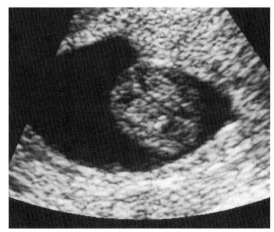

A

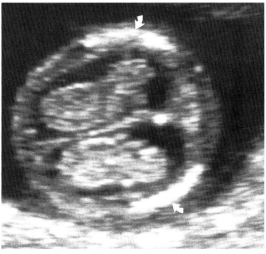

B

Fig. 6.3 (A) Vaginal scan of fetus at 11 weeks, showing no ossification of the skull vault. (B) Vaginal scan at 13 weeks showing ossification of the vault (arrows).

with brachycephaly. Technique is also important, for example in assessment of the posterior fossa using the transcerebellar view, a false-positive diagnosis of mega cisterna magna or Dandy–Walker variant may be made if the image plane is too steeply inclined. An oblique axial section through the skull base may give the impression of an echogenic mass in the middle cranial fossa. This is, in fact, the petrous ridge and is not abnormal but the result of an inclined section obtained by the sonographer.

If the presenting part is deep in the maternal pelvis and the usual techniques of

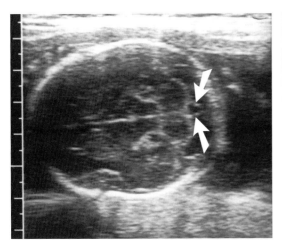

Fig. 6.4 Arachnoid septae (arrows) traversing the cisterna magna in a 19-week fetus.

bladder filling and the Trendelenburg manoeuvre have failed, do not hesitate to proceed to vaginal scanning (Fig. 6.5).[10]

Pitfalls and artefacts exist in ultrasound of the fetus. It is important that both the sonographer and the patient are aware of the limitations they impose on the accuracy and sensitivity of the technique.

Normal anatomy

Head shape and size

The fetal head is egg-shaped, being broader posteriorly and symmetric without irregularity of contour. Ossification of the skull vault is complete by 12 weeks' gestation with the sutures remaining visible throughout pregnancy. The skin overlying the vault is thin, measuring 1 to 2 mm thickness increasing slightly posteriorly (nuchal thickness) to a maximum which varies with gestational age. At 12 weeks, the maximum is 3 mm[11] and at 19 weeks, 5 to 6 mm.[12] The soft tissues are of uniform echotexture with no discrete cystic spaces. The recognition of an intact skull vault after 12 weeks' gestation excludes anencephaly.

Head size is assessed by the biometric measurements of biparietal diameter and head circumference. Gestational age may be confirmed using these measurements until

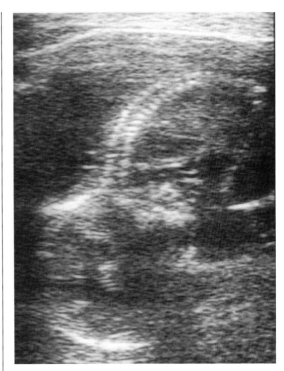

A

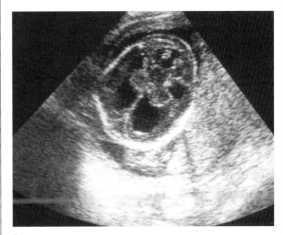

B

Fig. 6.5 Deep cephalic presentation at 17 weeks' gestation. (A) Transabdominal image, poor image quality and definition. (B) Endovaginal image showing ventriculomegaly and Dandy–Walker complex.

the mid-second trimester after which femur length is the more reliable measure. For assessment of head growth the head circumference is preferred to the biparietal diameter as the former takes account of the head shape and is therefore more reliable. With all biometric measurements it is good practice to refer to established nomograms whose origin is known and whose study population is similar to your own.

Brain structure

There are two components to the assessment of the brain by ultrasound. The first is to confirm, by critical observation of the image, that early embryological development has proceeded normally with the assumption that normal brain shape indicates normal brain structure and development. The second is to be familiar with the changes in the brain that occur with advancing gestational age and how these impact upon the ultrasound image. The brain may be divided into supratentorial structures (cerebral hemispheres, ventricular system and midline structures) and infratentorial structures (cerebellar hemispheres, vermis and fourth ventricle) and achieving a diagnosis of abnormality requires the sonographer not only to detect that there is an abnormality present but to also define which parts of the brain are involved.

To maximize the sonographer's ability to make such a diagnosis, a systematic approach to evaluation of brain structure is essential.[5,13,14] There are three axial image planes through the fetal brain which allow for an effective screen for normality. Studies show that 95% of all central nervous system abnormalities may be detected using this approach.[13] The planes are illustrated in Figure 6.6. The first transthalamic view (A) is that used for measuring biparietal diameter; the second transventricular view (B) is obtained superior and parallel to plane (A) at the level of the ventricular atrium; the third transcerebellar view (C) is inclined inferiorly through the posterior fossa. Table 6.3 lists which of the three planes best demonstrates each area of the brain.

The following text describes the landmarks which define each image plane and the parts of the brain best demonstrated, and provides a list of the types of abnormality which can be recognized, or conversely excluded, by careful scrutiny of each image plane.

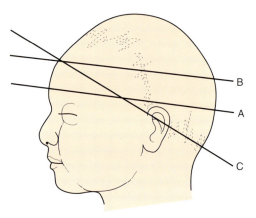

Fig. 6.6 Diagram of the sagittal view of the fetal head showing the three image planes used in the assessment of fetal cranial anatomy: A, transthalamic; B, transventricular; C, transcerebellar.

Table 6.3
Landmarks of the brain and associated image plane

Brain area	Image plane
Midline structures	Transthalamic (A), transcerebellar (C)
Supratentorial ventricular system	Transthalamic (A), transventricular (B)
Cerebral hemispheres	Transthalamic (A), transventricular (B)
Posterior fossa	Transcerebellar (C)
Head size and shape	Transthalamic (A)

Transthalamic image plane (A)

This is the image section obtained for measurement of the biparietal diameter (Fig. 6.7). The cavum septum pellucidum is sited anteriorly in the midline and is recognized as a small 'box' bordered laterally

Table 6.4
Transthalamic image plane (A)

Landmarks to check for normality
Cavum septum pellucidum
Third ventricle
Paired thalami
Sylvian fissure

Anomalies to detect, or exclude, on this view are
Midline developmental abnormalities
Agenesis of the corpus callosum
Holoprosencephaly
Midline cystic abnormalities (e.g. arachnoid cysts, vein of Galen aneurysm)
Ventricular enlargement involving the third ventricle
Gross abnormality of the cerebral hemispheres
Focal abnormality of the cerebral hemispheres

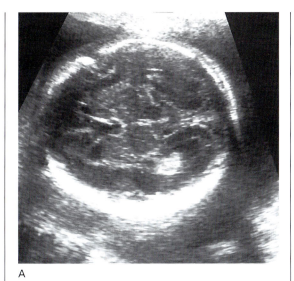

A

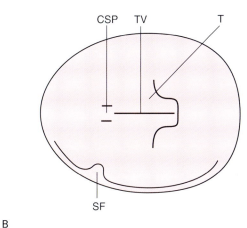

B

Fig. 6.7 Transthalamic image plane (A). (A) The ultrasound image. (B) Diagram illustrating the landmarks: CSP, cavum septum pellucidum; T, thalami; TV, third ventricle; SF, Sylvian fissure.

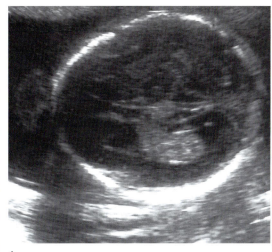

A

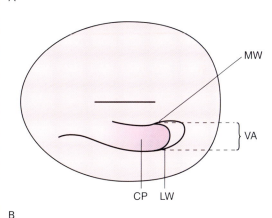

B

Fig. 6.8 Transventricular image plane (B). (A) The ultrasound image. (B) Diagram illustrating the landmarks: CP, choroid plexus; VA, ventricular atrium; MW & LW, medial and lateral walls of the lateral ventricle.

by two fine parallel linear echoes; the posterior and anterior borders are not defined. It is demonstrable in 95% of fetuses.[13] Posterior to the cavum septum pellucidum lie the paired hypoechoic thalami separated in the midline by the potential space of the third ventricle. The third ventricle is separate to, and distinguishable from, the cavum septum pellucidum. The cerebral hemispheres are hypoechoic and featureless; the Sylvian fissure is recognizable as an indentation of the cerebral mantle on its outer surface mid-way anteroposteriorly.

Transventricular image plane (B)

The plane for this image lies superior and parallel to the transthalamic biparietal diameter image (Fig. 6.8). The technique for measurement is well described and is obtainable in 99% of sonographic studies, thereby providing a reliable and reproducible landmark structure.[13,15] The ventricular atrium is stable in size throughout gestation from 15 weeks to term, with a mean measurement first reported as 7.6 mm ± 0.6 mm standard deviation, giving a measurement of 10 mm as +4 SD above the mean.[16] Ventriculomegaly is diagnosed when the atrium measures 11 mm and above.

Ventricular symmetry is assumed in the routine assessment of the atria using the ventricular atrial measurement.[14] Asymmetry has been recognized and reported as occurring in one large study in only 21 cases (0.3%) out of 7200 patients.[17] The majority of cases (71%) had enlargement of the left lateral ventricle and persistence of the discrepancy was observed in 75%. The outcome was good with 85% normal outcome. The cerebral hemispheres should be symmetric in thickness and shape.

In the late first, early second trimester (before 16 weeks), the dominant features on images of the cerebral hemispheres are the highly echogenic choroid plexi (Fig. 6.3) which fill each of the lateral ventricles. The cerebral hemispheres are themselves featureless and hypoechoic with both ventricular and arachnoid surfaces being indistinct unless perpendicular to the ultrasound beam when they produce a strong, specular echo. The cerebral hemispheres themselves have a very smooth, featureless surface contour.

By mid-second trimester (18–20 weeks), folding (sulcation) of the cerebral hemispheres begins with the definition of the lateral sulcus or Sylvian fissure (Fig. 6.7). The cerebral tissue becomes less hypoechoic and there is greater clarity of the cerebral borders with the ventricular walls becoming more clearly defined and the arachnoid surface distinct (Fig. 6.9). The lateral ventricles remain static in size (mean 6.5 mm, +3 SD = 10 mm) with the brain developing around them, as with a template. Towards term,

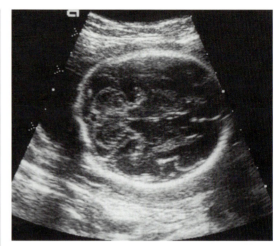

Fig. 6.9 25-week fetus showing high reflectivity of the arachnoid surface.

there is progressive sulcation of the brain, particularly from 28 weeks' gestation, and this development is recognized as increased folding of the cerebral mantle. The third ventricle becomes more readily visible, defined laterally by its walls which are echogenic, linear and separated by 1 to 2 mm.

Transcerebellar image plane (C)

This view is obtained starting from image plane (A) by fixing anteriorly on the cavum septum pellucidum and angling inferiorly posteriorly through the posterior fossa (Fig. 6.10A). The cerebellum consists of paired, round hemispheres connected by an echogenic midline bridge, the vermis. The cisterna magna lies posterior to the vermis and is crescentic in shape, necessarily for it follows the posterior contour of the cerebellum. The cisterna magna is measured in the midline from the posterior aspect of the vermis to the internal surface of the occipital bone and should measure between 4 and 10 mm. The posterior fossa structures can be reliably imaged in 90% of fetuses between 15 and 25 weeks' gestation.[13] In, or near to, the midline within the cisterna magna several fine echogenic lines may be observed (Fig. 6.4C); these are seen in 92%

Table 6.5
Transventricular image plane (B)

Landmarks to check for normality
Ventricular atrium
Symmetry of the cerebral hemispheres

Anomalies to detect, or exclude, on this view are
All those associated with ventriculomegaly
Neural tube defects
Holoprosencephaly
Agenesis of the corpus callosum
Hydrocephalus of all aetiologies
Porencephaly
Tumours

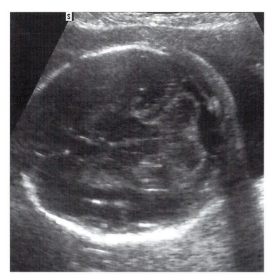

A

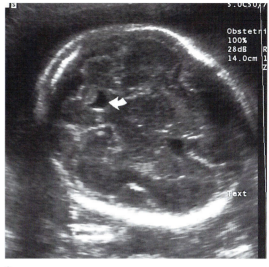

C

Fig. 6.10 Transcerebellar image plane (C). (A) The ultrasound image. (B) Diagram illustrating the landmarks: CH, cerebellar hemispheres; CV, cerebellar vermis; CM, cisterna magna; CSP, cavum septum pellucidum. (C) The fourth ventricle in a 26-week fetus (arrow).

CSP   CH

CV

CM

B

| Table 6.6 |
| Transcerebellar image plane (C) |

Landmarks to check for normality
Cisterna magna
Cerebellar vermis
Cerebellar hemispheres
Fourth ventricle

Anomalies to detect, or exclude, on this view are:
Arnold–Chiari type 2 malformation
Cerebellar vermian dysgenesis
Dandy–Walker complex
Mega cisterna magna
Aneurysm of the vein of Galen
Midline arachnoid cysts

scans between 15 and 38 weeks' gestation. These are thought to represent arachnoid septae and are not of pathological significance.[9]

The cerebellar hemispheres are recognized on ultrasound as discrete structures from 12 to 13 weeks' gestation with the vermis recognizable approximately 1 week later. Initially the hemispheres are hypoechoic with echogenic margins but, with increasing development of the folds of the surface (known as folia), they become increasingly echogenic with a characteristic stripey appearance (Fig. 6.11) by the late second trimester. Formation of the vermis itself is not complete until 19 weeks and it is consistently echogenic on ultrasound.[8] The fourth ventricle is a fluid-filled, triangular structure, sited anterior to the vermis in the midline (Fig. 6.10C). The vermis always interposes between it and the cisterna magna from 19 weeks when vermian development is complete.

Additional views

With practice and skill, the fetal brain may be imaged in a variety of planes in addition to those described above by imaginative use of the ultrasound probes and by altering maternal position from supine to decubitus. Parasagittal and midline sagittal views are

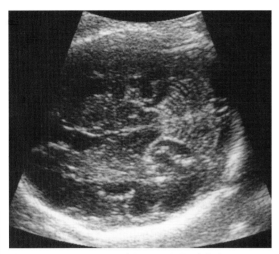

Fig. 6.11 Development of the cerebellar folia in a 29-week fetus showing as echogenic stripes on the surface of the cerebellum.

helpful for evaluation of the nearside lateral ventricle (Fig. 6.12) and for demonstration of the corpus callosum (Fig. 6.12). Studies have shown that the near-field ventricle can be readily demonstrated, and the ventricular size can be measured in 77% of fetuses with a further 19% seen with some difficulty. Coronal views are most readily obtained through the anterior fontanelle and elegantly demonstrate the anatomy (in the same way as the neonatal brain is assessed), particularly the ventricles confirming symmetry (Fig. 6.12) and, again, the presence of the corpus callosum (Fig. 6.12). Endovaginal scanning can be contributory in cases with a deep cephalic presentation (Fig. 6.5), affording greater visualization in all three trimesters.[10] These additional views provide further information and reassurance about both normality and abnormality.

The sonographic approach to central nervous system abnormalities

General principles

In the assessment of any central nervous system abnormality there are a few general principles that are important in helping to establish the prognosis and hence help the parents to reach a decision regarding management.

Firstly, look closely at the whole of the brain structure to establish how many abnormalities are present; remember that midline abnormalities such as Dandy–Walker malformation and agenesis of the corpus callosum often go together. Secondly, look at the rest of the fetus to search for any associated abnormalities in other body systems. Thirdly, consider offering a karyotype procedure to determine the fetal chromosomes; the risk of aneuploidy is increased if there are multiple systems involved or if certain central nervous system abnormalities, including Dandy–Walker malformation, holoprosencephaly and encephalocoele, are diagnosed.

Finally, it is important to establish the exact diagnosis either following delivery or termination. In the latter circumstance, external assessment of the abortus by clinical geneticists will help to detect soft markers of genetic and syndromal disorders. Radiographs (supine and lateral of whole body, separate anteroposterior views of both hands and feet) and a thorough post-mortem study by a perinatal pathologist should be offered to the parents. These three components will maximize the opportunity to reach a sound diagnosis and will greatly assist in counselling of the parents regarding recurrence risk and enable recommendations to be made for screening in any subsequent pregnancy. It is important to raise these issues sensitively with the parents, and ideally, this is done at the time of initial decision-making rather than at the time of admission for termination or following the termination itself.

Introduction

When an abnormality is found during the scan, define which anatomical regions of the brain have been affected using the three image planes described in the section on normal anatomy. Once the anatomical region(s) is(are) defined, read the

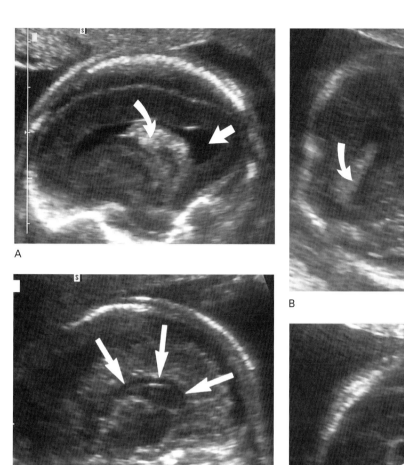

A

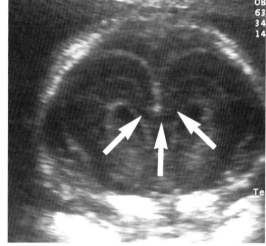

B

C

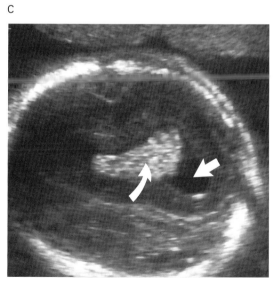

D

E

Fig. 0.12 Normal appearances. (A) Parasagittal view through the lateral ventricle in a 19-week fetus. Choroid plexus – curved arrow, occipital horn – straight arrow. (B) Coronal view of a 19-week fetus demonstrating ventricular symmetry – curved arrows point to choroid plexuses. (C) Midline sagittal view of a 19-week fetus showing the corpus callosum – arrows. (D) Coronal view of a 19-week fetus demonstrating the corpus callosum – arrows. (E) Oblique scan demonstrating contralateral choroid plexus and ventricle. choroid plexus – curved arrow, occipital horn – straight arrow.

corresponding section(s) below to find the possible structural anomalies described and illustrated. Frequently, more than a single anatomical site is involved in the abnormality which will therefore be referred to in each corresponding anatomical section. It should be possible to make a provisional diagnosis at this point. Then refer to the detailed information in the following section for each abnormality listed in alphabetical order. This last pathological section describes each condition in detail, together with any associated abnormalities that should be sought on scan. Further diagnostic tests are given followed by the prognosis.

Abnormalities of the midline structures – image planes A, C

The abnormalities recognizable and covered in this section are:

Agenesis of the corpus callosum
Holoprosencephaly   } supratentorial
Arachnoid cyst
Aneurysm of the vein
of Galen
Dandy–Walker   } infra-
malformation   tentorial
Inferior vermian dysgenesis

The cavum septum pellucidum, third and fourth ventricles, the corpus callosum and the cerebellar vermis all lie in the midline and are recognized on planes A and C. Developmental abnormalities of the midline structures are symmetric. If the cavum septum pellucidum, third and fourth ventricles, paired thalami and the cerebellar vermis can all be demonstrated using image planes A and C, then the operator may exclude a midline developmental abnormality.

Midline developmental abnormalities may first be suspected when measuring the biparietal diameter and there is failure to demonstrate the cavum septum pellucidum. When the cavum septum pellucidum cannot be identified, next measure the ventricular atrium and examine the cerebral hemispheres. The ventricular atrium should

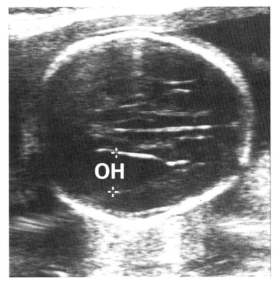

Fig. 6.13 Axial view of fetus with agenesis of the corpus callosum showing colpocephaly with focal dilatation of the occipital horns and pointed frontal horns at 20 weeks. OH, occipital horns.

measure ≤ 10 mm and is mildly increased in **agenesis of the corpus callosum** (Figs 6.13, 6.14) and usually very large in holoprosencephaly. Try to obtain views through the anterior fontanelle in coronal and midline sagittal planes (like a neonatal headscan) to look for the corpus callosum (Fig. 6.12) which is a hypoechoic linear structure with fine echogenic borders. The cerebral mantle itself is complete in agenesis of the corpus callosum with no focal defects; this is helpful in the differentiation from the more severe midline abnormality of holoprosencephaly. Next, follow the lateral ventricles anteriorly; in agenesis of the corpus callosum they remain clearly separate but in **holoprosencephaly** (Fig. 6.15), there is a monoventricle with free communication between the frontal horns across the midline. All forms of holoprosencephaly have symmetric focal defects of the cerebral mantle so if holoprosencephaly is now suspected, look at the cerebral hemispheres to search for focal defects to allow categorization into the three subgroups of holoprosencephaly. This is important to establish for prognosis. The head circumference in fetuses with holoprosencephaly is often small

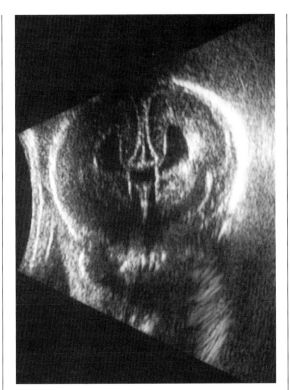

Fig. 6.14 Coronal views in a fetus with agenesis of corpus callosum showing wide separation of the frontal horns ('steerhorn') and a high rising third ventricle at 20 weeks.

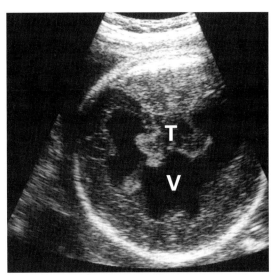

Fig. 6.15 32-week fetus with semi-lobar holoprosencephaly. Coronal view of the fetal brain showing a monoventricle (V) and fused thalami (T). This fetus had a bilateral facial cleft.

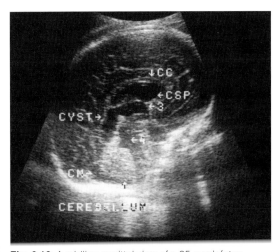

Fig. 6.16 A midline sagittal view of a 35-week fetus demonstrating an arachnoid cyst at the posterior end of the third ventricle.

(microcephaly) and accompanying abnormalities, particularly of the face, are frequent.

If there is a large, fluid-filled structure (a **cyst**) in the midline, related to the third ventricle and the cerebral structures (including the cavum septum pellucidum), which looks essentially normal, check for blood flow in the cyst, using Doppler to look for venous signals. This is facilitated by colour flow but duplex Doppler will suffice. If there is no demonstrable blood flow, then this is likely to be an **arachnoid cyst** (Fig. 6.16). Should Doppler reveal blood flow within the cyst, this will be an **aneurysm of the vein of Galen**. The third and lateral ventricles may increase in size because of obstruction from either an arachnoid cyst or from an aneurysm of the vein of Galen.

The midline structural abnormalities of **Dandy–Walker malformation** and **inferior vermian dysgenesis** are discussed in the section on the posterior fossa.

Supratentorial ventricular system – image planes A, B

The abnormalities recognizable and covered in this section are:

Isolated ventriculomegaly – symmetric and asymmetric
Holoprosencephaly and agenesis of the corpus callosum
Neural tube defects including anencephaly

Infection
Porencephaly
Choroid plexus cysts.

The lateral and third ventricles are supratentorial structures. The atrium of the lateral ventricle should measure less than 10 mm and the third ventricle is maximally 1 to 2 mm in the coronal plane.

Ventriculomegaly is simply diagnosed by measuring the ventricular atrium, 11 mm and above is abnormal at any gestation (Fig. 6.17). The challenge in the assessment of these cases is to determine the underlying aetiology as it is this which primarily determines the prognosis.

There are several observations to make when evaluating these cases:

The measurement of the atrium in mm.
How many ventricles are affected?
Is the enlargement symmetric?
Is the brain structure normal, in particular the midline and posterior fossa?

Ventriculomegaly is readily diagnosed but try to scan both hemispheres by using coronal and parasagittal views. Look for associated structural abnormality; this most commonly affects the midline structures (e.g. agenesis of the corpus callosum and holoprosencephaly), not forgetting that abnormality in the posterior fossa (e.g.

Arnold–Chiari 2 and neural tube defects and Dandy–Walker complex) can be associated with supratentorial ventriculomegaly. Ventriculomegaly may only be defined as isolated when other central nervous system or extra-central nervous system abnormalities have been confidently excluded by scan.

Large ventricles, symmetrically dilated, with echogenic walls can be an indication of **infection** or an **intraventricular bleed** secondary to a blood clotting disorder. Blood clotting disorders in the fetus are usually a secondary event; the underlying insult may be infection (e.g. parvovirus, cytomegalovirus) or maternal antibodies that cross the placenta (e.g. platelet antibodies in auto-immune thrombocytopaenia). If there has been an associated, intracerebral bleed (often unilateral or asymmetric), this can result in **porencephaly** of the lateral ventricles. This is characterized by asymmetric ventricles with a 'punched-out' focal loss of brain tissue at the site of a previous intracerebral bleed. The area of tissue loss is filled with cerebrospinal fluid extending into the defect from the lateral ventricle with a resulting irregular contour to that ventricle.

Cerebral mantle – image planes A, B

The abnormalities recognizable and covered in this section are:

Anencephaly and acrania
Holoprosencephaly
Infection
Bleed and porencephaly
Lissencephaly and schizencephaly
Tumour.

The normal appearance of the cerebral mantle is described in the relevant sections on image planes A and B. If the brain tissue or cerebral mantle looks abnormal, decide whether it is symmetric or asymmetric, focal or generalized.

Cerebral abnormalities may be congenital or acquired. Congenital abnormalities are **anencephaly**, **holoprosencephaly** and **schizencephaly/lissencephaly**, and these

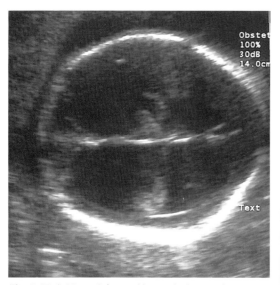

Fig. 6.17 A 20-week fetus with ventriculomegaly.

abnormalities will have been determined from conception and established by 12 weeks' gestation. The acquired abnormalities are **tumour**, **infection** and **porencephaly** and are the result of an insult or pathological process damaging what was previously a normal brain.

Symmetric abnormalities

If the skull vault is absent after 12 weeks' gestation and the cerebral mantle asymmetric and/or disorganized, the most likely diagnosis is **anencephaly** (Fig. 6.18). This condition has a varied appearance and is considered, in appearance and prognosis, to be the same as **acrania**.

If the cerebral mantle is symmetric but incomplete, consider **holoprosencephaly**. This will be confirmed by the presence of a monoventricle and abnormalities of the midline structures (see above).

If the cerebral mantle is symmetric but complete with very echogenic ventricular walls (normal or large atrial measurement), consider **infection**. Infection may cause low platelets in the fetus and cause intracerebral or intraventricular haemorrhage. Recent haemorrhage is echogenic and becomes increasingly hypoechoic with time and occupies space. This can cause displacement of the midline structures. Bleeds into the cerebral mantle eventually break down and cause destruction of brain tissue. The space is then filled by cerebrospinal fluid and forms a **porencephalic cyst** which, by definition, communicates with the lateral ventricle. Bleeds into the ventricles cause a chemical ventriculitis which manifests on scan as increased echogenicity of the ependymal lining of the ventricles. This ventriculitis, together with blood degradation products within the ventricle itself, can cause an obstructive hydrocephalus, which is recognized as ventriculomegaly on scan.

Asymmetric abnormalities

Brain **tumours** may look very similar to a recent or evolving **bleed** and should be included in the differential diagnosis. Features more in favour of the lesion being a tumour are a progressive increase in size, vascularity and poorly defined borders.

Schizencephaly and lissencephaly are disorders of sulcation and neuronal migration. **Schizencephaly** is recognized by the presence of clefts in the cerebral mantle which extend through from the ventricle to the arachnoid surface. They are frequently bilateral but asymmetric. **Lissencephaly** is the failure of normal sulcation and is frequently associated with heterotopias of the neurones. The neurones normally migrate into seven layers during development in an ordered configuration; if this process is interrupted or prevented (as may occur in schizencephaly and lissencephaly), the function of the brain is severely affected. Heterotopia is not a condition readily diagnosed on ultrasound but should be suspected in the presence of disorders of sulcation. The only ultrasound feature that may be observed is of an irregular contour to the ventricular wall. As the fetal brain has a smooth contour until 26 weeks' gestation, lissencephaly is a very difficult diagnosis to make prenatally. Both these conditions are often seen in association with midline structural abnormality, in particular agenesis of the corpus callosum, and all are easier to define on MRI performed postnatally.

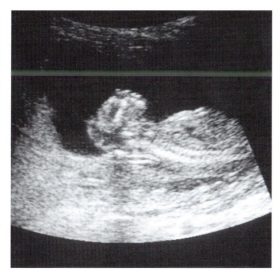

Fig. 6.18 Anencephaly, sagittal profile view, showing absence of the vault and of normal cerebral development at 14 weeks' gestation.

Posterior fossa – image plane C

The abnormalities recognizable and covered in this section are:

Arnold–Chiari 2 and neural tube defects
Mega cisterna magna
Dandy–Walker malformation
Inferior vermian dysgenesis
Cerebellar hypoplasia.

When examining the posterior fossa on view B, it is important to look critically at the size of the cisterna magna as this is frequently the best pointer to abnormality. Should the cisterna magna be effaced, then Arnold–Chiari 2 is the likely diagnosis. If the cisterna magna is large, examine the vermis as it is likely that this is abnormally developed and Dandy–Walker malformation or variant may be present. Mega cisterna magna is essentially a diagnosis of exclusion once the observer is satisfied that there is no underlying cerebellar abnormality or posterior fossa arachnoid cyst to account for its dominant appearance. Charts exist to allow assessment of cerebellar hemisphere size.

Effacement of the cisterna magna

In the **Arnold–Chiari 2** malformation there is hypoplasia of the bony posterior fossa of the skull combined with descent of the brain stem and cerebellar structures into the widened foramen magnum and upper cervical spine. This is recognized on ultrasound as effacement of the cisterna magna with accompanying distortion (the so-called 'banana' sign) of the cerebellum. It is best not to rely on recognizing a 'banana' configuration as the cerebellum may adopt a number of differing shapes in this condition and has been observed to be most prominent before 24 weeks' gestation. The Arnold–Chiari 2 malformation is pathognomonic of a neural tube defect and it is therefore mandatory to examine the spine in detail to locate the associated **neural tube defect**, its precise level, the number of segments affected, the contents of any sac and the location of the cord end. Arnold–Chiari 2 is seen in more than 95% of open neural tube defects.

Enlargement of the cisterna magna

A **mega cisterna magna** is defined as one which measures more than 10 mm from the posterior aspect of the cerebellar vermis to the inside of the occipital bone. Mega cisterna magna may only be diagnosed when the sonographer is satisfied that there is no underlying abnormality of the vermis and fourth ventricle. In normal fetuses there should be an echogenic vermis in the midline which clearly separates the fourth ventricle from the cisterna magna. In **Dandy–Walker malformation** there is complete vermian agenesis with clear communication in the midline between the ventricle and cisterna magna; there is always associated cerebellar hypoplasia.

During development, the superior portion of the cerebellar vermis is seen first with complete development of the inferior portion not being complete until 19 weeks' gestation. **Inferior vermian dysgenesis** is recognized after this gestation as a prominent 'key-hole' notch in the inferior portion of the vermis. This is a subtle observation with serious prognosis and, if suspected, should be confirmed by a specialist centre.

Cerebellar hypoplasia

When assessing size, it is important to be sure of the length of gestation either from certain menstrual dates or from first trimester biometry. This should minimize the opportunity for false-positive diagnosis. Small cerebellar hemispheres are seen in association with a number of central nervous system abnormalities, including Dandy–Walker malformation and microcephaly, or can be observed as an isolated phenomenon.

Head size and shape – image planes A, B, C

The abnormalities recognizable and covered in this section are:

Micro- and macrocephaly
Brachycephaly
Dolicocephaly
Clover-leaf and strawberry-shaped skull

Lemon-shaped skull
Encephalocoele.

The diagnosis of a small or large head circumference is made when the plotted measurement lies below the 3rd or above the 97th centile for gestational age, as established by last menstrual period or early scan biometry. **Microcephaly** is found in any condition which retards normal growth of the underlying brain and is therefore a hallmark of infection, chromosomal abnormality and of underlying structural brain abnormality (e.g. holoprosencephaly, some neural tube defects), conditions which should be sought by further targeted scanning and from the patient's history. Search also for complete integrity of the skull vault as microcephaly is found in cases of **encephalocoele**, a condition where there is a defect in the skull vault with herniation of brain and/or meninges through the vault defect (see below).

Macrocephaly is the term given to fetuses found to have a disproportionately large head measuring above the 97th centile. This disproportion may arise from a fundamental abnormality with the fetus such as triploidy or some cases of dwarfism (e.g. heterozygous achondroplasia). In other cases, there is an underlying abnormality of the brain which causes the disproportionately large head circumference. Examples of this would be obstructive ventriculomegaly (hydrocephalus) of whatever cause or a brain tumour. Clearly, resolution of the finding of macrocephaly requires a thorough examination both of the brain and the remainder of the fetus.

Dolicocephaly and brachycephaly are abnormalities of skull shape which are not always associated with abnormal outcome. **Dolicocephaly**, when the skull is elongated in axial section, is most commonly seen in cases with oligohydramnios. The important role for the sonographer in this circumstance is to look for any underlying fetal cause for the oligohydramnios. **Brachycephaly** occurs when the biparietal diameter is large in comparison to the head circumference. Brachycephaly may be observed in normal fetuses but a search should be made for underlying structural abnormality. Brachycephaly has been described as a feature of chromosomal abnormality and its detection should prompt a search for both structural and soft markers elsewhere in the fetus.

Other head shapes described in chromosomal abnormality are the **clover-leaf and strawberry-shaped head**. Although seen in trisomy 18, this shape may also indicate an abnormality in sutural development as occurs in conditions such as the craniosynostoses (e.g. Apert syndrome) or short-limbed dwarfs (e.g. thanatophoric).

The **lemon-shaped skull** is seen in association with neural tube defects and can be a useful indicator to the sonographer to diligently search the posterior fossa for an Arnold–Chiari 2 malformation and the spine for a neural tube defect. The underlying mechanism for the lemon shape in this context is not clearly understood. The chances are, however, that the fetus is normal (it is in 9 out of 10 cases) and no cause found for the lemon shape. The positive predictive value of the 'lemon' sign for neural tube defect in a low-risk population (prevalence 1 in 1000) is approximately 6%.

All the head shape anomalies described above have an intact skull vault. There are two abnormalities which are associated with a skull vault defect, an **encephalocoele** and **iniencephaly**. The vault defect in an **encephalocoele** is most commonly midline in the occipital region and is associated with herniation, through the defect, of brain and/or meninges. More difficult encephalocoeles to detect are those that are small and occur in the frontal region or are not in the midline. Recognition of an encephalocoele should prompt a thorough examination of the remainder of the fetus as this is an abnormality that is linked to both chromosomal and syndromal abnormality.

The extremely rare condition of **iniencephaly** affects the junction between the skull base and the cervical spine. There is hyperextension of the neck such that the occiput touches the upper thoracic or lower cervical region of the spine. This is a fixed deformity and is invariably associated with intracranial structural abnormality such as occipital encephalocoele or Dandy–Walker malformation. It is crucial to differentiate iniencephaly from the **star-gazing breech**. In this latter condition the fetus assumes a breech position with hyperextension of the neck but without any associated intracranial abnormality such as is seen in iniencephaly. The importance in differentiation lies in the different prognosis and in determining management.

Abnormal appearances

Agenesis of the corpus callosum

The corpus callosum is a bundle of fibres which connects the two cerebral hemispheres across the midline. It comprises four sections which develop from 7 weeks' gestation beginning with the most anterior portion called the genu. Subsequently, and sequentially, the body and splenium develop with the rostrum (continuous with the genu extending inferiorly and then posteriorly) being the last section to develop. The corpus callosum has formed in its entirety by 20 weeks (Fig. 6.12) after which gestation, diagnosis can be achieved with accuracy. Insults during development that occur prior to 12 weeks result in complete agenesis with partial agenesis (dysgenesis) after this gestation.

The hallmarks of complete agenesis of the corpus callosum in ultrasound diagnosis are colpocephaly, i.e. focal dilatation of the posterior horns of the lateral ventricles (Figs 6.13, 6.19), absent cavum septum pellucidum – seen to be absent on BPD image plane (A), and a high-riding third ventricle – filling the void left by the absent cavum septum pellucidum and corpus callosum (Figs 6.14, 6.20).

The features which alert the sonographer to this condition are mild ventriculomegaly and absence of the cavum septum pellucidum observed during the second trimester, screening sonogram using the standard, three axial image assessment.[18]

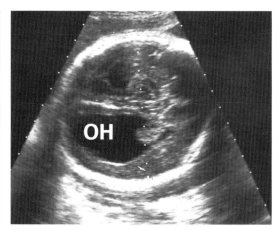

Fig. 6.19 Agenesis of the corpus callosum – note marked colpocephaly. OH, dilated occipital horns.

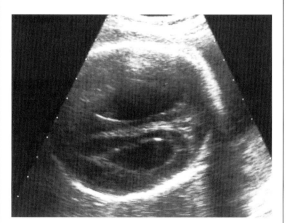

Fig. 6.20 Agenesis of the corpus callosum – note wide separation of lateral ventricles.

When abnormality of the corpus callosum is suspected, midline sagittal and coronal views of the corpus callosum through the fetal anterior fontanelle should be obtained to confirm the abnormality. On the coronal views, the frontal horns assume an abnormal position being more laterally placed with a 'steerhorn' configuration[18] (Figs 6.12D, 6.14). This occurs owing to the commisural fibres, normally contained within the corpus callosum and crossing the midline, turning posteriorly and parallel to the midline as the bundles of Probst along the superomedial border of the lateral ventricles. Partial agenesis of the corpus callosum, in which the splenium is absent, is more difficult to diagnose as the cavum septum pellucidum is present in the milder forms, leaving ventriculomegaly alone as the sonographic feature.[18,19] In our experience, it is usually a diagnosis that relies on postnatal confirmation with ultrasound.

Post-mortem studies in fetuses and postnatal follow-up of survivors with agenesis of the corpus callosum have shown association with other structural abnormalities (central nervous system 85% and non-central nervous system 62%[20]), genetic syndromes, inborn errors of metabolism and with aneuploidy (7–17%,[18,19,21] particularly trisomy 8 and 18). As these factors generally adversely influence prognosis, it is mandatory to perform a full structural survey and to offer a karyotype procedure before full counselling. Agenesis of the corpus callosum is reported to be present in as many as 10% of cases presenting with isolated, mild ventriculomegaly. The most common associated anomalies are of the central nervous system (see Table 6.7). There is a recognized association with midline lipomata; fetal series suggest that this is not readily diagnosed prior to the third trimester with the earliest recorded documentation at 26 weeks' gestation.[18,22]

Prognosis depends on the sonographic findings and on the results of chromosomal analysis. Chromosomal abnormality, when present, overrides all other findings and alone determines the prognosis. The most common chromosomal abnormalities seen in cases with agenesis of the corpus callosum are trisomies 8, 13 and 18. Whilst the majority of cases with trisomies 13 and 18 will have additional structural abnormalities on scan, those with trisomy 8 are isolated.[18,21] In the presence of normal chromosomes, those cases with the best prognosis have no other abnormalities found on scan. In this isolated group, the likelihood of a normal outcome is reported as approximately 85%.[21] In contrast, in the presence of additional abnormality on scan only 13% had a developmentally normal outcome.[21] Poor prognostic indicators suggested from analysis of prenatal scans are a high-riding third ventricle and a wide inter-hemispheric fissure.[18] Morbidity is highest in the presence of associated structural abnormality, heterotopias or a genetic syndrome (see Table 6.7); the last two are not reliably discernible on prenatal ultrasound. Those cases with the worst prognosis are those with other anomalies presenting in early childhood with mental retardation and seizures. Some series have suggested[19] that sonographically isolated agenesis of the corpus callosum carries a better prognosis in males than females; this reflects the fact that some of the genetic syndromes are found only in females, the male form being lethal.

In summary, when agenesis of the corpus callosum is found on scan, the sonographer must diligently search for other abnormalities and offer chromosome analysis. In the presence of additional structural or chromosomal abnormality, the outlook is poor with serious morbidity to be expected. Under these circumstances, termination of pregnancy is an option. In isolated agenesis of the corpus callosum, the prognosis is better with an 85% chance of normality. Parents in this group must, however, be warned of the possibility of neuronal migration disorders and of syndromal abnormality which are not

---

Table 6.7
Structural brain anomalies associated with agenesis of the corpus callosum

Integral feature of holoprosencephaly
Midline arachnoid cysts and lipomata
Neuronal migration disorders – lissencephaly, heterotopias
Dandy–Walker complex
Arnold–Chiari 2 malformation
Encephalocoele

Syndromes associated with agenesis of the corpus callosum
*Acrocallosal syndrome
Aicardi syndrome
*Andermann syndrome
Apert syndrome
Dandy–Walker complex
Fetal alcohol syndrome
Frontonasal dysplasia
Joubert's syndrome
*Lissencephaly
Neu–Laxova syndrome
Oro–facial–digital 1 syndrome
Rubenstein–Taybi syndrome
Shapiro syndrome

*Autosomal recessive.

reliably identified on scan but both of which carry serious prognostic impact.

Anencephaly and exencephaly sequence

Anencephaly is the most severe form of neural tube defect and is lethal. It results from failure of closure of the rostral neuropore and is recognized by failure of development of the skull vault (Fig. 6.18). The underlying brain tissue is disorganized, often asymmetric and incompletely formed. Ossification of the skull vault is normally present after 12 weeks' gestation and anencephaly should not be diagnosed before this time (Fig. 6.3). Exencephaly,[2,3] the absence of the skull vault with cerebral tissue present and also called acrania, is generally accepted as the precursor of anencephaly. Studies of the human fetus, now more clearly visualized with vaginal scanning in the first trimester, have shown pictorially this sequence in vivo.[24]

Other fetal anomalies that affect development of the fetal head, and are considered in the differential diagnosis of anencephaly, are the amniotic band syndrome and, one of the complications of monozygotic twinning, the acardiac, acephalic pump twin. In the amniotic band syndrome, there may be disruption of the formation of the face and skull vault. This is usually asymmetric and a search of the rest of the fetus will usually demonstrate multiple other abnormalities such as 90° scoliosis, abdominal wall defect and amputation abnormalities of the limbs. In the acardiac, acephalic twin, the fetus has a single umbilical artery with flow of the blood into the fetus through the artery. The fetal heart is rudimentary (frequently one or two chambers) with normal formation of the lower fetal trunk and limbs. The upper limbs are frequently rudimentary and the head and neck absent (Fig. 6.21). Both these differential diagnoses carry a lethal prognosis. The importance of recognizing either as the diagnosis, rather than anencephaly, is in counselling regarding recurrence risk. Anencephaly carries the same risk of recurrence in subsequent pregnancies as the other neural tube defects, namely 2 to 3% after one and 6% after two affected pregnancies. The amniotic band syndrome is a random occurrence and the acardiac, acephalic twin is an abnormality unique to monozygotic twinning and both therefore have no increased risk of recurrence.

If the parents decide to continue with an anencephalic pregnancy, for example in the presence of a normal co-twin, there is a risk of development of polyhydramnios and therefore of preterm labour. In our experience, parents have asked whether it is possible for the anencephalic fetus' organs to

---

Table 6.8
Characteristic findings in anencephaly

Absence of the skull vault and skin covering
'Frog's eye' appearance of fetal face owing to the absent skull vault
Failure of normal development of the cerebral hemispheres
Disorganization of brain tissue that is present
Widening (dysraphism) of the upper cervical spine
4:1 female to male predominance
Raised maternal serum alphafetoprotein.

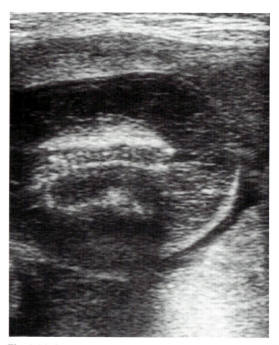

Fig. 6.21 A monochorionic twin pregnancy with a hydropic, acardiac, acephalic twin. Coronal view of the trunk; no normal limbs were demonstrated.

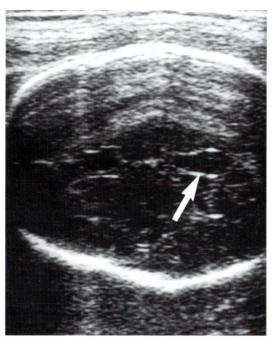
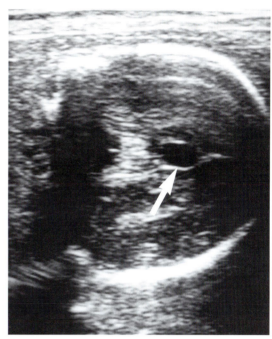

A

B

Fig. 6.22 Aneurysm of the vein of Galen. (A) Axial image showing a fluid-filled midline structure posteriorly. (B) Coronal image of same fetus showing the midline aneurysm (Arrows point to aneurysm).

be used for transplantation following delivery. Advice taken from our paediatric and transplant surgeon colleagues indicates that the organs are not considered suitable for transplantation and we no longer raise this issue in counselling.

Aneurysm of the vein of Galen

The primary defect in this abnormality is an arteriovenous malformation at the posterior end of the third ventricle. It is located supratentorially in the midline (Fig. 6.22) and is readily differentiated from an arachnoid cyst (also occurring at this site) by duplex or colour flow Doppler (Fig. 6.23).[25] A low flow signal is obtained from the turbulent blood flow within the enlarged (aneurysmal) venous side of the vascular malformation. This diagnosis is rarely made before the third trimester, presumably reflecting the fact that this is a dynamic abnormality whose appearance will alter with increasing flow and shunting as gestation advances. As the lesion increases in size and the vascular shunt becomes significant

haemodynamically, the fetus can develop high output cardiac failure (94% of newborns[26]). This is manifest by cardiomegaly, right heart failure with hepatic venous congestion and, latterly, hydrops. A fetus presenting in the third trimester with hydrops should have a critical evaluation of the intracranial contents to exclude aneurysm of the vein of Galen as the underlying cause.

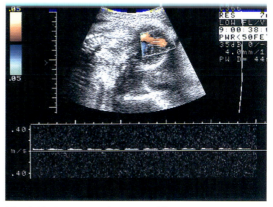

Fig. 6.23 Aneurysm of the vein of Galen; colour flow Doppler study.

In the past, the prognosis, even with prenatal diagnosis, has been dismal with very few survivors.[27] The reason for the high mortality rate is rapidly developing hydrops and uncontrollable heart failure. Cases may spontaneously thrombose the arteriovenous malformation and develop a secondary consumptive coagulopathy with death resulting from a disseminated intravascular coagulopathy. Other causes of morbidity are cerebral ischaemia and leukomalacia secondary to the huge vascular shunt.

Reliable prenatal diagnosis and interventional neuroradiology with intravascular embolization techniques have the potential to alter the prognosis of this condition.[26] Centres report successful embolization and good neurologic outcome in two-thirds of cases.[26] To achieve good outcome the prenatal assessment must be thorough and include mapping of the intracranial vessels feeding and draining the malformation, and a full fetal echocardiogram.[26,28] Features on prenatal scan which are associated with poor prognosis are hydrops, abnormal texture of the brain (hyperechoic owing to oedema[28]) and retrograde flow in the descending aorta during diastole. Those fetuses likely to do well are those in whom there is no evidence of a high output state.[28] Delivery, location, mode and timing must be co-ordinated between the obstetric and neurosurgical team to permit early neonatal stabilization and to avoid early surgical intervention.

Arachnoid cyst

Arachnoid cysts are avascular and usually lie in the midline. Most commonly they are related to the posterior end of the third ventricle (Fig. 6.16) and therefore are supratentorial within the interhemispheric fissure[27] or lie posterior to the cerebellar vermis (Fig. 6.24) in the posterior fossa.[29] Rarely, they are eccentric and can lie in the subarachnoid space overlying the cerebral hemispheres. This distribution is in contrast to paediatric series when the eccentric location, particularly related to the Sylvian fissure, is more common.[30] The differential

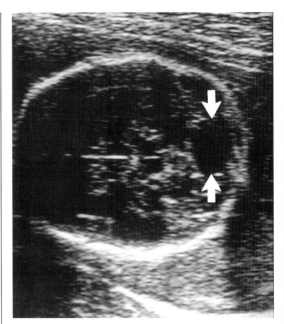

Fig. 6.24 A 24-week fetus with an arachnoid cyst in the posterior fossa (arrow).

diagnosis of an arachnoid cyst will depend on its location. Those related to the third ventricle may be differentiated from an aneurysm of the vein of Galen by interrogation with colour flow Doppler; the former will show no flow. In the posterior fossa, the differential diagnosis is from a variant of the Dandy–Walker malformation[29] and correctly diagnosing the presence of an arachnoid cyst in this location relies on establishing the integrity of the cerebellar vermis.

In the evaluation of an arachnoid cyst, and establishing prognosis, there are three main objectives. The first is to examine closely for the presence of other anomalies, particularly of midline brain development (e.g. agenesis of the corpus callosum), as the addition of any single other structural problem will adversely influence the prognosis. Second, assessment of the size of the ventricular system, by measuring the atrium, is necessary to look for associated obstructive hydrocephalus, as this is a further adverse prognostic sign. Finally, look for variation in size of the cyst with advancing gestation; if this increases, then obstructive hydrocephalus is more likely to develop and will have both prognostic and perinatal management implications. Obstructive hydrocephalus is most likely to occur with posterior fossa cysts.

There are case reports of chromosomal abnormality (trisomy 18[27]) therefore amniocentesis may be indicated should there be other abnormalities on scan. Ultrasound forms the pivot of the assessment, primarily in establishing the diagnosis from the differential, and sequentially in gauging the change with time to identify the onset of obstructive hydrocephalus. Indications for an early delivery would be rapidly increasing ventriculomegaly or head circumference. Both timing and mode of delivery should be discussed with the local neurosurgeons and neonatal team. Delivery should occur where there is the opportunity to perform postnatal evaluation with ultrasound and other cross-sectional imaging (computed tomography or MRI) as indicated clinically. Access to a neurosurgical unit is advisable to arrange follow-up and intervention (cyst-peritoneal shunting or fenestration of hydrocephalus) as indicated clinically. Morbidity is dependent on size, rate of growth and location. The benefit of prenatal diagnosis is of early postnatal evaluation and the opportunity for surveillance with early intervention if necessary aiming to minimize neurological damage.

Cerebellar hypoplasia

The cerebellum controls reflex and voluntary motor function including posture, gait, ocular movement, memory, motivational behaviour and learning. The most common abnormalities affecting the cerebellum are the Dandy–Walker malformation and inferior vermian agenesis, which are discussed separately below. Cerebellar hypoplasia may, however, be observed on scan with no accompanying vermian abnormality (Fig. 6.25). Causes of hypoplasia are listed in Table 6.9.

In summary, when cerebellar hypoplasia is observed, it is important to examine closely the vermis for dysgenesis. If the vermis is judged to be normal, then the list

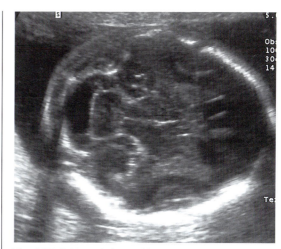

Fig. 6.25 A 20-week fetus with cerebellar hypoplasia.

Table 6.9
Causes of cerebellar hypoplasia
Viral infection
Teratogens
Multiple genetic syndromes – Joubert's syndrome
In utero ischaemic event
Arnold–Chiari 2 in neural tube defects
Chromosomal abnormality – trisomy 18

given in Table 6.9 should be investigated. A full history should establish both the drug history and family history to look for features suggesting an inherited disorder. Maternal blood should be tested for viral antibody levels to reveal evidence of a recent infection. The prognosis will necessarily be determined by the underlying aetiology and can vary from asymptomatic to severe developmental delay and early death (see Table 6.10).

Choroid plexus cysts

Choroid plexus cysts are frequently found during a second trimester screening examination. They are hypoechoic cystic

Table 6.10
Clinical symptoms in cerebellar hypoplasia
Moderate-to-severe developmental delay
Ataxia, broad-based gait
Hypotonia
Nystagmus, intention tremor, titubation
Seizures
Microcephaly

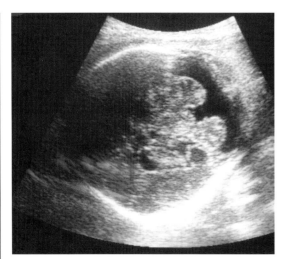

Fig. 6.26 Dandy–Walker malformation – complete vermian agenesis in a 32-week fetus with a large cisterna magna. This fetus also had trisomy 21.

structures contained within the body of the choroid plexus, are of variable diameter and may be unilateral, bilateral, simple or septated (Fig. 6.27). They were first documented in 1984[31] and were linked with chromosomal disorders in 1986.[32] Studies of low-risk populations give a prevalence of 0.5 to 1% and an overall risk of aneuploidy of approximately 1%.[33,34] The chromosomal abnormality most strongly associated with choroid plexus cysts is the lethal trisomy 18 with sporadic cases of trisomy 21, triploidy and Klinefelter's reported.[35–40] There are no reports linking choroid plexus cysts with any

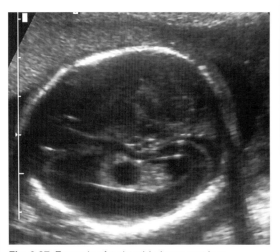

Fig. 6.27 Example of a choroid plexus cyst in a 20-week fetus.

other fetal abnormality. The majority (95%[41]) are isolated. The cysts do not cause any local damage or effect and the majority (96%) will resolve on scan by 26 weeks' gestation. The size, laterality, time taken to resolve, persistence or complexity have not been shown to be independently predictive of trisomy. Factors that do increase the probability of aneuploidy are structural abnormality and increased maternal age.

The presence of isolated choroid plexus cysts in a low-risk population increases the likelihood of trisomy 18 nine-fold and, if in association with a structural abnormality, increases the base-line risk almost 1800-fold.[41] A recent review of the literature[41] recommends the use of maternal age with calculated risks tabulated for choroid plexus cysts that are isolated or in association with additional sonographic abnormality (see Ch. 14).

Dandy–Walker complex

Dandy–Walker malformation was first described in 1914.[42] Dandy–Walker malformation is characterized by failure of development of the cerebellar vermis with resulting communication between the fourth ventricle and the cisterna magna with an associated midline cyst and cerebellar hypoplasia (Fig. 6.26). It is recognized on views of the posterior fossa (image plane C) with small cerebellar hemispheres that are displaced laterally together with absence of the echogenic vermis in the midline. Barkovich has proposed that Dandy–Walker malformation, Dandy–Walker variant (inferior vermian agenesis) (Figs 6.28A & B) and mega cisterna magna (Fig. 6.29) are all steps along a continuum of abnormality of the posterior fossa and that these conditions should be grouped under the umbrella term, Dandy–Walker complex.[43] In this section Dandy–Walker malformation and inferior vermian agenesis, both characterized by vermian abnormality, will be discussed. Mega cisterna magna is discussed on page 125.

Dandy–Walker complex is associated with chromosomal abnormality in 15 to 45% of cases,[44–46] in particular the trisomies 13, 18 and 21, therefore karyotype should be

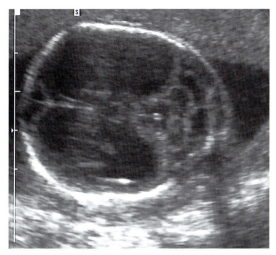

A

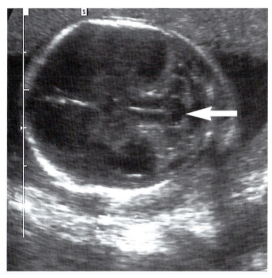

B

Fig. 6.28 Inferior vermian agenesis in a 20-week fetus. (A) The superior portion of the vermis is present. (B) The inferior defect (arrow).

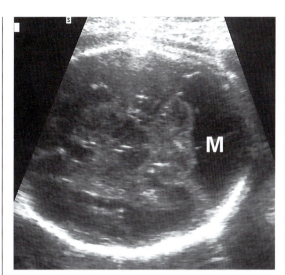

Fig. 6.29 Mega cisterna magna (M) in a 22-week fetus, normal at postnatal assessment.

age postnatally. This is important to consider in parent counselling.

The most common central nervous system abnormalities documented in the literature are listed in Table 6.11 and are found in approximately 45% of cases prenatally. These commonly occur in the midline and are more frequent in cases with complete vermian agenesis (57 vs 35%). Non-central nervous system anomalies are seen in 66% of cases overall but are, in contrast, more common in inferior vermian agenesis (81% vs 46%).[46]

There may be maldevelopment of other midline brain structures (see Table 6.11) and it is important to specifically exclude these by a thorough scan of the brain and vault. Dysgenesis of the corpus callosum (Fig. 6.30) is reported in up to 25% postnatally. Abnormalities of neuronal migration or sulcation (heterotopias, lissencephaly, seen in 5 to 10% postnatally) cannot be reliably excluded by ultrasound in the second trimester.

discussed and offered. The presence of additional central nervous system or other system abnormality increases this risk. Ventriculomegaly is found in approximately one-third of cases,[45,46] is less frequently seen in cases with complete vermian agenesis and is inversely related to risk of chromosomal abnormality (21% in cases with ventriculomegaly vs 54% without).[45,46,47] In our experience, ventricular enlargement does not always develop in utero with its appearance being delayed until 6 months of

Table 6.11

Other central nervous system abnormalities associated with Dandy–Walker malformation

Holoprosencephaly
Agenesis of the corpus callosum
Occipital encephalocoele
Neuronal migration disorders
Ventriculomegaly

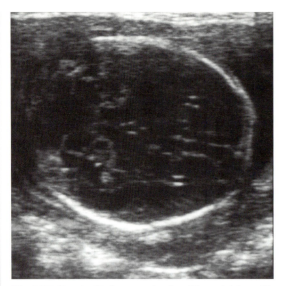

Fig. 6.30 Dandy–Walker complex in a 20-week fetus with agenesis of the corpus callosum.

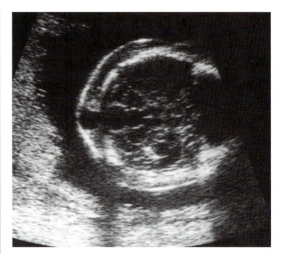

Fig. 6.31 Dandy–Walker complex in a 20-week fetus with a midline occipital defect and encephalocoele.

The two main features which impact on prognosis are karyotype and the presence of additional abnormalities on scan. Should a chromosomal abnormality be found, the prognosis for this will override that for the Dandy–Walker malformation alone. Series report a termination rate 57 to 68% and a 40% risk of fetal or neonatal death in the non-terminated cohort.[45,46] Of the liveborn survivors, there is a high risk of abnormality and significant morbidity with only 1 of 9[46] and none of 6[45] with follow-up being developmentally normal.

Dandy–Walker malformation may be a feature of a genetic syndrome or disorder such as Meckel–Gruber[48] (Fig. 6.31), Aicardi, Walker–Warburg, or Joubert's syndrome. It is important to identify a specific syndrome as this can influence both prognosis and recurrence risk. Involvement of clinical geneticists in establishing the differential diagnosis and in counselling can be very helpful.

Estimation of recurrence risk depends on establishing the exact diagnosis either following termination or delivery. Should there be death during the fetal or neonatal period, post-mortem studies are recommended. External examination of the fetus or neonate by a clinical geneticist is helpful to look for subtle morphological markers of genetic disease. Finally, imaging of the brain postnatally, by ultrasound initially, is advised to confirm the antenatal findings. Good views of the posterior fossa may be obtained by scanning in the axial plane through the squamous temporal bone just posterior to the neonate's ear. MRI is necessary to look for any associated neuronal migration disorders as these cannot be reliably identified or demonstrated by ultrasound. Their presence should be suspected if ultrasound shows abnormality of the sulcation pattern on postnatal ultrasound scan or if there is an irregular border to the ventricular wall.

In summary, when Dandy–Walker complex is diagnosed, the prognosis depends on the presence of other abnormalities and on the karyotype. Referral for detailed ultrasound is advised together with chromosome analysis.

Encephalocoele

An encephalocoele is characterized by a defect in the skull and dura through which

Table 6.12
Symptoms found in survivors
Developmental delay
Motor delay
Seizures
Spasticity
Porencephaly
Hydrocephalus

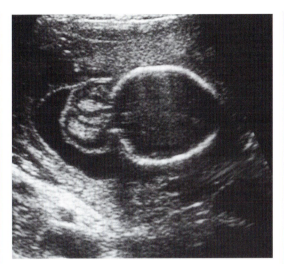

Fig. 6.32 Example of a 16-week fetus with an occipital encephalocoele containing herniated brain and echogenic choroid.

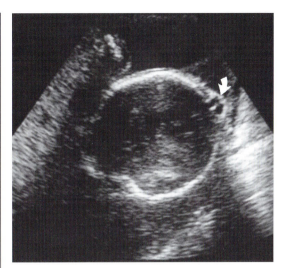

Fig. 6.33 Example of a 19-week fetus with an encephalocoele containing meninges only (meningocoele) (arrow points to meningocoele).

the meninges herniate with or without skin covering (Fig. 6.32). The meningeal sac can contain brain tissue and in 85% of cases occurs in the midline, particularly the occiput; it may be eccentric in the parietal region in approximately 12%.[49–51] A sac containing brain tissue is classically an encephalocoele, one containing cerebrospinal fluid only is more correctly a meningocoele (Fig. 6.33). A bone defect will be recognized on scan in 80% of cases. The majority of encephalocoeles are skin covered and will therefore be detected more commonly on a screening ultrasound than on maternal serum alphafetoprotein screening. Detection of an encephalocoele has been documented on vaginal scanning from as early as 13 weeks' gestation.[57] The differential diagnosis for an occipital encephalocoele includes cystic hygroma (this has no vault defect and contains no brain tissue) or a high cervical meningocoele.

A frontal encephalocoele may be mistaken for a nasal teratoma but both conditions are exceedingly rare and both carry a poor prognosis. True frontal encephalocoeles are associated with hypertelorism, facial abnormalities, heterotopias and agenesis of the corpus callosum.

In the presence of an encephalocoele there is a risk of associated structural abnormality

Table 6.13
Cranial abnormalities associated with encephalocoeles
Microcephaly
Ventriculomegaly
Agenesis of the corpus callosum
Dandy–Walker malformation
Arnold–Chiari 2 malformation
Lemon-shaped skull

both intra- and extracranially of 60 to 80% in prenatal series[49,50] and 50% in postnatal studies.[51] The literature suggests a 13 to 44% risk of chromosomal abnormality[49,50] and therefore karyotype should be discussed and offered. Encephalocoeles may be one component of a genetic syndrome or condition of which the most common are Meckel–Gruber syndrome and Walker–Warburg syndrome (Fig. 6.34). It is important to recognize these syndromes as many are autosomal recessive conditions with a risk of recurrence of 1 in 4. As they can be recognized on ultrasound, there is the opportunity to offer targeted screening in subsequent pregnancies.

Prognosis, and hence management, will depend on the site, size and content of the encephalocoele, karyotype, associated abnormalities and ease of surgical reduction and repair. Should the chromosomes be abnormal, this will be the determining

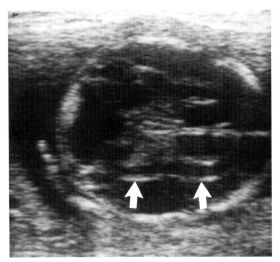

Fig. 6.34 Axial view of a 26-week fetus with Walker–Warburg syndrome showing lissencephaly and a huge subarachnoid space (arrows).

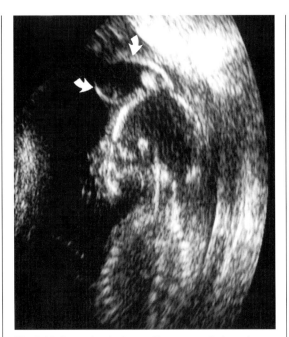

Fig. 6.35 Example of a fetus with an encephalocoele involving the vertex of the skull (arrows).

prognostic factor. If there are associated abnormalities, clinical geneticists should be consulted for their advice as to the likelihood of a syndrome unifying the scan features that will allow them to give a prognosis and risk of recurrence. Good prognostic indicators are defects that are anterior (Fig. 6.35), contain no brain and have no other anomalies identified. Poor prognostic features on scan are encephalocoeles that are posterior and large or those that contain brain and are associated with other system anomalies (Fig. 6.32). Prenatal series report low survival rates of 21%,[49,50] with significant developmental delay in the survivors compared with an overall survival rate in a postnatal series of 71%.[51] In the postnatal series, the survival rates and morbidity in survivors varied most strongly with anatomical site. Anterior defects had 100% survival and 50% morbidity compared with 55% and 83% respectively for posterior defects.[51]

In summary, following the identification of an encephalocoele, it is important to accurately define site, content and the presence of other abnormalities. The increased risk of aneuploidy warrants the offer of amniocentesis. Those cases with the best prognosis are encephalocoeles that are small and contain no brain and there are no

features to suggest microcephaly. Poor prognostic features are a large size, significant brain herniation, abnormality of the underlying brain, microcephaly and ventriculomegaly. These features will increase the likelihood of mental handicap and poorer result following surgical repair postnatally.

Holoprosencephaly and septo-optic dysplasia

Holoprosencephaly is a failure of development of both midline structures and of the cerebral mantle that arises from the embryologic forebrain. Cleavage of the prosencephalon occurs in the 7th week of gestation and insults to the brain at this time will result in midline defects such as holoprosencephaly and septo-optic dysplasia. The hallmarks of holoprosencephaly on ultrasound are listed in Table 6.14.

The cerebral hemispheres are abnormal with defects in the mantle such that the ventricular system is not wholly enclosed by brain tissue (Fig. 6.36). As a result of abnormal development of the structures in

Table 6.14
Sonographic features of holoprosencephaly

Microcephaly and brachycephaly
Absent cavum septum pellucidum
Fused thalami
Ventriculomegaly
Monoventricle
Incomplete cerebral mantle
Facial abnormalities

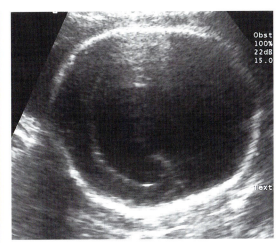

Fig. 6.37 Holoprosencephaly with a monoventricle.

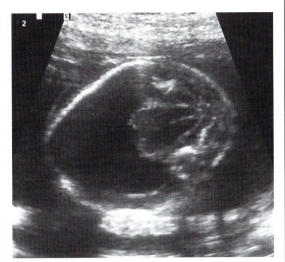

Fig. 6.36 Holoprosencephaly with fusion of the thalami; also note banana cerebellum indicating an associated neural tube defect.

the midline, the thalami and the third ventricle are also abnormal. There is often associated brachycephaly and microcephaly and abnormal facial development.[53,54] There is a high risk of aneuploidy in cases of holoprosencephaly, in particular trisomy 13. The diagnosis is usually made in the mid-second trimester but cases have been recognized on vaginal scanning as early as 15 weeks.[55]

Magnetic resonance studies in fetal or early neonatal life may aid in the recognition and diagnosis of holoprosencephaly but the technique is compromised by fetal movement and, despite multiplanar reconstruction, inflexibility.[56] In comparison with high resolution ultrasound in experienced hands, MRI has a limited application in the fetus.

Complete agenesis of the corpus callosum is classically described in holoprosencephaly. Cases have been reported[57,58] where the posterior portion of the corpus callosum (body and splenium) has developed and been demonstrated on magnetic resonance studies. Therefore the presence of the posterior corpus callosum does not appear to preclude the diagnosis of holoprosencephaly. Holoprosencephaly is classified into three groups depending on the severity of the intracranial findings. The most severe form is alobar holoprosencephaly (Fig. 6.37), in which there is fusion of the thalami, absent third ventricle, absent falx cerebri with the cerebral mantle covering only the most rostral (anterior) portion of the large monoventricle. The alobar form has the most severe of the mid-facial developmental anomalies, most commonly cyclops, ethmocephaly (proboscis) through to cebocephaly (single nostril) with hypotelorism (see Ch. 15). This form is lethal.[59]

The lobar form is the least severe type with partial development of the falx and interhemispheric fissure (Fig. 6.38), absent cavum septum pellucidum and corpus callosum and communication between the frontal horns across the midline but the third ventricle and thalami are often nearly normal. This lobar form will often have a normal face; hypotelorism will only be identified by referencing interorbital distances to gestational age-related charts.

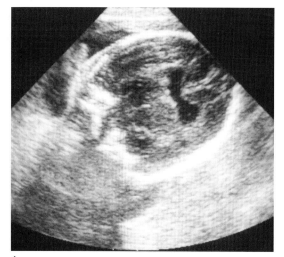

A

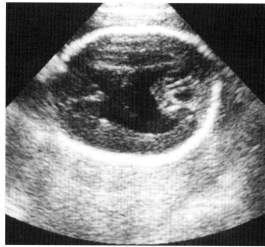

B

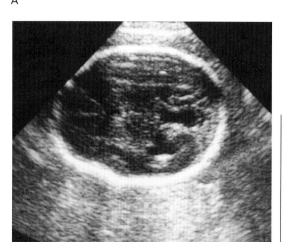

C

Fig. 6.38 20-week fetus with lobar holoprosencephaly. (A) Partial development of the falx, coronal view. (B) Free communication across the midline, axial view. (C) Normal thalami and third ventricle.

The intermediate form is the semi-lobar type with partial development of the inter-hemispheric fissure and posterior portion of the falx, partial separation of the thalami and a small third ventricle (Fig. 6.15). Facial abnormality (cebocephaly, median cleft lip) is common in this group. Lobar and semi-lobar forms of holoprosencephaly are compatible with survival.

Septo-optic dysplasia is a condition very similar to lobar holoprosencephaly. There is hypotelorism, septo-optic nerve hypoplasia and an absent cavum septum pellucidum. Additional abnormalities are pituitary malfunction in two-thirds and schizencephaly in approximately 50%.

Fetuses with the most severe forms of holoprosencephaly and associated facial defects (cyclopia, ethmocephaly, cebocephaly) will not survive. The lobar and semi-lobar types are frequently associated with developmental delay and with significant mortality in the semi-lobar group. The prognosis is poor for those who elect to continue with the pregnancy with 80% perinatal mortality rates in non-terminated cases. There are no reported normal survivors from prenatal series.[53,54]

In summary, holoprosencephaly is a severe developmental abnormality of the fetal brain, frequently associated with facial, systemic and chromosomal abnormality. Overall, the prognosis is poor with death or severe developmental delay probable. Parents should be offered chromosomal analysis and, should they elect termination of the pregnancy, post-mortem and genetic evaluation. Holoprosencephaly is linked with chromosomal abnormality, genetic syndromes and familial dominant forms although the majority of cases are sporadic.[60] Correct identification of the underlying aetiology is important in individual cases in order to accurately counsel regarding recurrence risk.

Infection

Intra-uterine infection is usually viral with cytomegalovirus, parvovirus and toxoplasmosis (a non-viral agent) being the most common agents. Maternal infection, often asymptomatic and therefore silent, occurs with variable transmission across the placenta. The fetus may be infected (have an antibody response) but is not always affected (symptomatic) by the agent or virus. Following maternal infection transmission rate to the fetus is approximately 40%.[61,62] Diagnosis may occur as a result of maternal symptomatology or following positive ultrasound findings which are suspicious for in utero infection (Table 6.15). Diagnosis is achieved by maternal serology, amniocentesis culture and polymerase chain reaction or by fetal blood sampling (lgM and culture). Studies of 16 pregnancies infected with cytomegalovirus showed that amniocentesis alone achieved a diagnosis in 75% while fetal blood sampling (lgM) picked up only 69%.[61]

In utero infection may manifest in a number of ways on ultrasound; series report positive findings in a variable proportion of affected fetuses ranging from 31 to 95% with multisystem abnormalities seen in nearly 50%.[61,63] Infection affecting the brain (42%) may manifest as haemorrhage, cerebral necrosis from ischaemia, calcification, or ventriculomegaly.[64] The most common presentation is haemorrhage, the mechanism being anaemia and thrombocytopaenia induced by the infectious agent resulting in an intracranial bleed. Haemorrhage may occur into the ventricles to cause a chemical

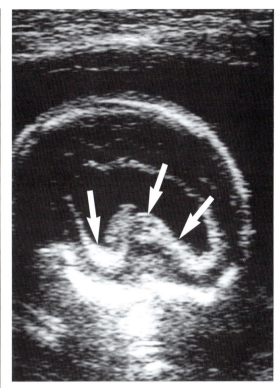

Fig. 6.39 Example of a 27-week fetus with proven cytomegalovirus infection. Parasagittal view of the lateral ventricle showing the increased echogenicity of the ependymal lining secondary to ventriculitis (arrows on the thickened ependyma).

ventriculitis (Fig. 6.39) and resulting obstructive hydrocephalus or may occur into the brain substance and ultimately break down to form a porencephalic cyst (Fig. 6.40). A bleed into the brain substance may mimic a tumour and it is the change in appearance with time of the haemorrhage that allows the distinction to be made. Infection occurring early may affect the process of neuronal migration and result in lissencephaly.[65] When any of the brain abnormalities described above are observed, the presence of cardiac abnormality (cardiomegaly, hydrops) and calcification elsewhere in the fetus, particularly the abdomen, should alert the sonographer to the possibility of infection.

The prognosis for fetuses with in utero infection is variable. If the infection is diagnosed as a result of abnormal ultrasound findings, this appears to pre-select those with the most severe manifestations. Outcome in

Table 6.15
Ultrasound findings in infection
Microcephaly
Ventriculomegaly
Intracerebral bleed
Porencephaly
Periventricular calcification
Intrahepatic calcification
Echogenic bowel
Cardiomegaly
Hydrops
In utero growth retardation

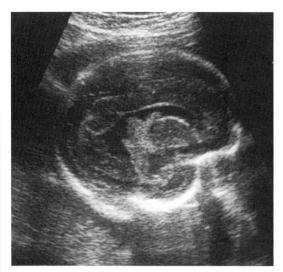

Fig. 6.40 A fetus with proven cytomegalovirus infection. Right parasagittal view at 29 weeks with development of a post-haemorrhagic porencephalic cyst and ventriculomegaly.

this group is poor with mortality rates of 63 to 100% and developmental impairment in any survivors.[65,66] Similarly, symptomatic newborns have a 30% mortality rate but those who are asymptomatic have a better prognosis with only 5 to 15% having developmental impairment.[61,66]

Treatment of in utero infection is controversial with little clear evidence of improvement in prognosis. The prognosis will depend on the gestational age at the time of the insult and the size and extent of the bleed. In general, the neurodevelopmental outcome for those cases with central nervous system abnormality diagnosed in utero is poor with in utero or neonatal death occurring in the majority and developmental impairment in the survivors.

In summary, there are features on ultrasound of the fetus which may suggest in utero infection. These are listed in Table 6.15 and may involve not only the brain but other systems, most notably the heart and abdomen. Diagnosis may be achieved by maternal and fetal serology or by amniocentesis. The prognosis for those diagnosed as a result of an abnormal scan is very poor with neonatal death or survival with developmental impairment the most common outcome.

Iniencephaly

This is an abnormality at the craniocervical junction which is recognized on scan as extreme retroflexion of the fetal head such that the occiput abuts the upper thorax or cervical spine (Fig. 6.41). This is a fixed deformity. Frequently the thorax and cranium may be imaged on the same plane owing to the extreme retroflexion. Associated, and intrinsically linked, with iniencephaly are abnormality of the posterior fossa (encephalocoele, Dandy–Walker complex) and the upper cervical spine (rachischisis) and spinal segmentation abnormality with resultant shortening. Abnormalities elsewhere in the fetus are found in the majority of cases (84%).[67] This condition is lethal in the vast majority of cases although survival in those with no associated brain abnormality and with skin covering has been reported.[68]

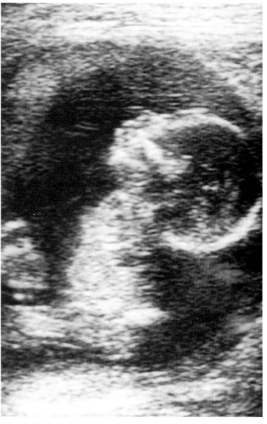

Fig. 6.41 Iniencephaly in a 17-week fetus. Sagittal view showing extreme retroflexion of the cervical spine.

Iniencephaly should be distinguished from hyperextension of the fetal head in the third trimester[69,70] in which the fetus has adopted a persistent breech presentation, spine posterior, cervical retroflexion and abnormal limb attitude (Fig. 6.42). This abnormal posture is reported as being present on radiographs in 12 to 15% of breech pregnancies.[70] This so-called 'star-gazing breech', in contrast to the fetus with iniencephaly, has a normal structure to the posterior fossa and cervical spine. If unrecognized and delivered vaginally, it is associated with a high risk of transection of the cervical cord and, when recognized prior to delivery, caesarean section is recommended.

In summary, iniencephaly is a lethal condition caused by the severe structural neurological abnormalities that are associated with it. It is important for the sonographer to be aware of the differential diagnosis of the star-gazing breech because of the serious implications for management and prognosis.

Lissencephaly and schizencephaly

These two disorders are grouped together as they are both abnormalities of sulcation. **Lissencephaly** (smooth brain) is a condition in which the brain fails to develop the normal gyri (ridges) and sulci (grooves) characteristic of the mature brain; the brain surface in lissencephaly is therefore smooth and featureless (Fig. 6.34). This is thought to be due to a disorder in the normal radial neuronal migration described in the section in normal anatomy. During fetal life, the lateral sulcus (Sylvian fissure) develops between the parietal and temporal lobes of the brain from 16 weeks but the cerebral hemispheres otherwise remain essentially featureless until 28 weeks, after which the folding process results in the characteristic pattern of the brain surface. There is progressive thickening of the cerebral cortex and the development of more sulci and accompanying gyri such that the brain surface looks more akin to the adult pattern by 36 weeks. Given this late development of the sulci and gyri in the normally developing brain, lissencephaly is a difficult and rare diagnosis to achieve prenatally but has been reported.[71,72] Prenatal use of MRI has been reported as contributing significantly to the recognition of neuronal migration disorders given the poor sensitivity of even high resolution ultrasound.[73]

Postnatally, ultrasound scans will demonstrate the abnormality but MRI is ultimately required to confirm the diagnosis and to fully evaluate the extent of the associated abnormalities.[2] Lissencephaly is associated with disorders of neuronal migration (heterotopias) and midline development and these pathologies together result in a poor prognosis with severe learning deficit and global developmental delay. The majority of syndromes (see Table 6.16) associated with lissencephaly have associated agenesis of the corpus callosum. There is an association between Miller–Dieker lissencephaly and abnormality

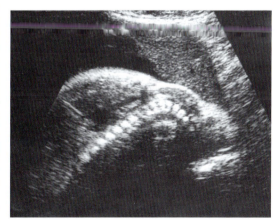

Fig. 6.42 Star-gazing breech in a 34-week fetus, sagittal view.

Table 6.16
Syndromes associated with lissencephaly
Type 1 Miller–Dieker Norman–Roberts Isolated
Type 2 Walker–Warburg Cerebro-oculomuscular
Unclassified Neu–Laxova

of chromosome 17 (monosomy 17p13) and therefore targeted chromosomal analysis is recommended.[72]

Schizencephaly (split brain) is a condition in which there is a complete cleft through the cerebral hemisphere, resulting in a free communication between the ventricular system and the subarachnoid space (Fig. 6.43). These clefts are lined by grey

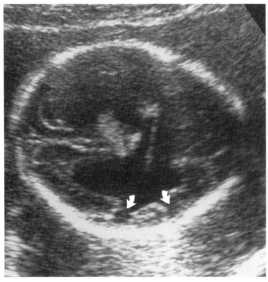

A

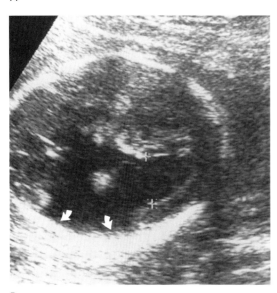

B

Fig. 6.43 Schizencephaly. 22-week fetus with asymmetric ventriculomegaly and cortical clefts. (A) Arrows point to two small cortical clefts. (B) Same fetus with a large cortical cleft in opposite hemisphere (arrows).

matter and therefore have an echogenic surface similar in appearance to the normal brain surface. The clefts are frequently asymmetric, may be unilateral and are most commonly located in the parietal lobe.[2] The cavum septum pellucidum is absent in 80 to 90% of cases. The underlying aetiology is thought to be vaso-occlusion and cocaine has been implicated in some cases. The prognosis ranges from a seizure disorder or hemiparesis (depending on the site of brain involved) with a unilateral, isolated cleft through to global developmental delay, seizures and motor abnormality in those with bilateral clefts. This condition is also associated with heterotopias.

MRI may be helpful in diagnosing and defining cases of lissencephaly and schizencephaly, which is difficult to recognize on ultrasound, especially prior to the third trimester. It also has the advantage of delineating additional structural abnormalities (e.g. midline defects) and neuronal migration disorders, both of which adversely influence prognosis.

Heterotopias are disorders of neuronal migration of the grey matter and are not recognizable on ultrasound scan but are known to be associated with a number of structural abnormalities that can be recognized. They are collections of grey matter in abnormal location as a result of failure of normal radial migration and are most commonly found in the sub-ependymal or periventricular region. Their importance lies in the adverse impact their presence has on prognosis and patients with heterotopias nearly always develop seizures.[2] Lissencephaly, schizencephaly, agenesis of the corpus callosum and holoprosencephaly are known to be associated with heterotopias.

In summary, these abnormalities of sulcation and neuronal migration are difficult, but not impossible, to detect prenatally. MRI of the fetus has a potential role in this group of fetuses, particularly in the context of known genetic risk. Identification of the abnormalities during fetal life is desirable given the poor prognosis and will maximize parental choice.

Mega cisterna magna

This is a diagnosis of exclusion. Mega cisterna magna is characterized by an enlarged cisterna magna which measures more than 10 mm from the posterior aspect of the vermis to the internal aspect of the skull vault[47] with no identifiable structural abnormality either supra- or infratentorially (Fig. 6.29).[74] The cisterna magna is readily demonstrated on the transcerebellar axial plane which can be achieved in the majority of cases between 15 and 28 weeks' gestation. This diagnosis may be falsely made if the plane used for the transcerebellar view is over-tilted and too near the coronal plane.

Before assigning a diagnosis of mega cisterna magna it is important to exclude inferior vermian agenesis (Fig. 6.28), Dandy–Walker complex (Fig. 6.27), or a posterior fossa cyst (Fig. 6.24) to be certain that the cerebellar hemispheres are of normal size and that the supratentorial brain structures are normal. The presence af any of these abnormal findings will adversely affect prognosis and require chromosomal and thorough ultrasound analysis. If in doubt, tertiary referral for assessment is recommended.

Should these criteria be satisfied, the prognosis for isolated mega cisterna magna is difficult to determine given the paucity of information in the literature. These scan appearances may be a variant of normal but it is prudent to exclude chromosomal and other structural abnormality.

Neural tube defects

Epidemiology

A neural tube defect is the most common form of central nervous system abnormality likely to be diagnosed by a sonographer. The incidence of neural tube defects is 1 to 2/1000 births and has shown a progressive decrease over the past 15 years. Approximately one-third of this reduction is attributable to antenatal screening and termination of affected fetuses; the remainder is due to an unexplained natural reduction. Figures from the Oxford study show a true reduction in prevalence in England and Wales from 3.4/1000 live and stillbirths in 1974 to just under 0.8/1000 in the 1990s.[75,76]

Neural tube defects have a multifactorial risk profile. The risk of a neural tube defect is increased or influenced by multiple factors, some of which are listed in Table 6.17.

Trials of folate supplementation have shown a 75% reduction in prevalence in women at high risk and is now recommended for a period of 6 months commencing 3 months pre-conception.[75,76]

There are several drugs which are **teratogens** that are known to increase the risk of neural tube defect. These are frequently folate antagonists.[4] The embryologic period of pregnancy, between 5 and 10 menstrual weeks, is the period of organogenesis and the vulnerable period for exposure.

Screening strategies for neural tube defects

Ninety percent of all neural tube defects are conceived in families with no prior history or recognizable risk factors, hence they arise de novo. This is an important factor when considering any screening strategy as one which only targets those perceived to be at risk will miss the majority of cases.

To date, there are two main approaches to

Table 6.17
Factors influencing likelihood of neural tube defect

Geography	Highest risk in the North-West and Ireland, reducing in the South-East
Family history	One affected child risk 2–3%, two affected children risk 6%, maternal neural tube defect 1.1%, maternal insulin-dependent diabetes mellitus 2%
Diet	Folate supplements (5 mg/day) from 3 months preconception for 6 months
Teratogens	Drugs taken in embryological period (see Table 6.18)

Table 6.18
Drugs which are teratogenic for neural tube defects

Anti-epileptics	Carbamazepine, sodium valproate (both anti-folates)
Anti-coagulants	Warfarin
Anti-psychotics	Lithium
Retinoic acid	
Etritinate	

neural tube defect screening polarized by the position held in England and Wales in comparison to that held in the USA. In England and Wales, the thrust in prenatal screening for all fetal abnormality is a thorough, second trimester, ultrasound scan and this scan is accepted by 95 to 96% of all pregnant women.[77,78] Studies have shown that ultrasound has the potential to detect about 98% of all central nervous system anomalies and 75% of all major structural anomalies.[77] As a result, the dependence on maternal serum alphafetoprotein as a tool for the detection of neural tube defects has significantly diminished in England and Wales. Maternal serum screening in the first trimester is being increasingly offered to optimize the detection of chromosomal abnormality, in particular trisomy 21. As alphafetoprotein is an integral part of all types of maternal serum screening, the potential remains for identifying mothers with elevated alphafetoprotein who are therefore at increased risk of fetal structural abnormality, including neural tube defects, abdominal wall defects, placental and cord anomalies. Maternal serum alphafetoprotein is normal in approximately 20% of cases of open neural tube defect.[79] Using a cut-off of 2.5 multiples of the median for maternal serum alphafetoprotein, this screening blood test will detect 80% of all open neural tube defects. Amniotic fluid acetylcholinesterase is elevated in 95.5% of neural tube defects and if both it and the alphafetoprotein are elevated in the amniotic fluid, the chances of the fetus having neural tube defects are 99.5%.[80] Given the accuracy and good negative predictive value of second trimester screening ultrasound in England and Wales, there is now no significant role for amniocentesis to quantify amniotic fluid levels of alphafetoprotein and acetylcholinesterase as a confirmatory test. Conversely, in the USA, where routine, second trimester scanning is not the norm, maternal serum alphafetoprotein does play a pivotal role in the selection of a high-risk group then referred for targeted ultrasound scan to specifically search for any underlying causative anomaly.

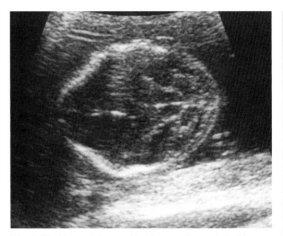

Fig. 6.44 18-week fetus with a lemon-shaped skull in association with a neural tube defect. There is also effacement of the cisterna magna owing to an Arnold–Chiari 2 malformation.

Diagnosis

The majority of spinal neural tube defects can be detected by careful evaluation of the fetal brain. First, the shape of the skull vault changes from being egg-shaped to lemon-shaped (Fig. 6.44) with indentation of the frontal bones bilaterally. This is seen in 98% of fetuses ≤ 24 weeks with open spina bifida giving a 82.2% positive and 99.5% negative predictive value.[81] Other workers have reported lower incidences of this sign ranging from 64 to 70% of cases with spina bifida.[82,83]

Second, there are pathognomonic changes seen in the posterior fossa (the Arnold–Chiari 2 malformation) owing to hypoplasia of the skull in this region, descent of the cerebellar hemispheres and effacement of the cisterna magna.[79] These changes result in deformity of the posterior fossa structures so that the cerebellum alters from its characteristic dumb-bell shape to a 'banana' shape (Fig. 6.45). It is, however, the observation of effacement of the cisterna magna that is the more reliable observation to make as the cerebellum may be distorted beyond the shape of a 'banana'. These cerebellar abnormalities are seen in 95% of cases with open spina bifida diagnosed ≤ 24 weeks.[81] No false-positive diagnoses have been reported with this sign, giving it a 100% positive and 99.7% negative predictive value ≤ 24 weeks.[82]

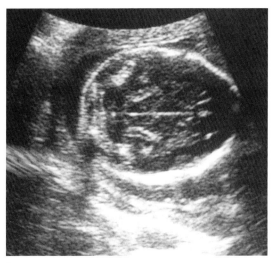

A

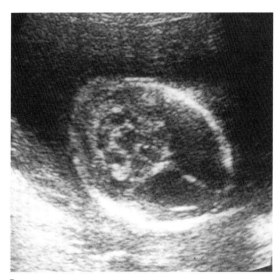

B

Fig. 6.45 Variable appearance of an Arnold–Chiari 2 malformation secondary to neural tube defects. (A) Effacement of the cisterna magna with little cerebellar distortion. (B) The 'banana' cerebellum. (C) More severe distortion of the cerebellum to a 'boomerang' shape.

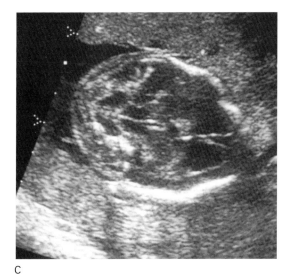

C

Third, there may be associated enlargement of the lateral ventricles (Fig. 6.46) identifiable by measurement of the ventricular atrium. This is seen in 61% of cases overall. There is, however, a variation in prevalence depending on gestational age at the time of ultrasound assessment. For fetuses scanned under 24 weeks, the prevalence is 44% rising to 94% after 24 weeks.[84] Finally, with progression through the pregnancy, microcephaly and/or enlarging ventricles may be observed. Whilst the main thrust of prenatal diagnosis with ultrasound remains directed at the 18- to

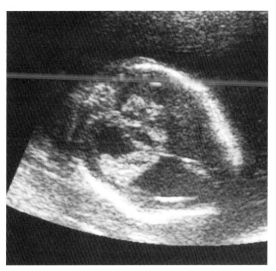

Fig. 6.46 Ventriculomegaly in association with neural tube defect and dangling choroid.

20-week scan, it has been demonstrated that a combination of abdominal and vaginal scanning can be effective in the detection of a neural tube defect before 17 weeks' gestation.[85] Blumenfeld at al stressed the reliance at this earlier gestation on the intracranial abnormalities which were identified in advance of the spinal lesion. It should also be noted, however, that the brain may be normal in the presence of a neural tube defect.

On the identification of the intracranial changes described above, it is mandatory to perform a thorough scan of the spine to identify the level and extent of the spina bifida and to search for any extra-central nervous system anomalies, including talipes. It is possible to accurately identify the number and level of the spinal segments involved and to identify the level at which the spinal cord ends.[86] The contents of the sac, and the presence or absence of skin covering, should also be sought as all these features assist in assessing the prognosis.

There is a risk of aneuploidy in cases with a neural tube defect, and identification of these cases is important for counselling regarding recurrence risk. In an isolated neural tube defect, the risk is reported as being 2%.[87] This increases to 24% in the presence of multiple structural anomalies found on ultrasound scan. The most common chromosomal abnormality found is trisomy 18.

Management

When a neural tube defect is diagnosed, it is essential to make observations and establish various facts to enable accurate counselling. This allows parents to make an informed choice and to decide whether to continue with the pregnancy or to opt for termination.

Prognosis is determined by a number of factors but grouping by the level of the lesion appears most predictive.[86] Cochrane et al suggest three broad groups – thoracolumbar, lumbar and sacral – taking the last, intact, spinal level as the classifier. The last, intact level in the spine predicts the level of ambulation achieved and the likelihood of bladder and bowel continence and of developing a kyphoscoliosis but does not predict the need for postnatal shunting nor the number of surgical interventions (Table 6.20).

Poor prognostic indicators are high lesions, especially those affecting multiple segments, microcephaly, enlarging ventricles and those with associated scolioses or gibbus and the presence of any other system abnormality.[88] The superior level of the defect will determine the level at which neurological deficit will occur. Finally, there remains dispute regarding which is the preferred mode of delivery for fetuses with a neural tube defect with proponents for both vaginal delivery and for pre-labour caesarean section.[89,90]

In summary, neural tube defects are successfully recognized in the second trimester in the majority of cases with the

---

Table 6.19
Ultrasound predictors

Level and number of segments
Skin covering
Head circumference and centile
Ventricular atrial size and variation with time
Talipes
Other system anomalies

Table 6.20
Prognosis in fetuses with neural tube defects (expressed as a percentage, *n* = 85)

Performance indicator	Thoracolumbar	Lumbar	Sacral
In normal school	36	40	46
Bladder control normal	0	0	17
Bladder social continence	70	–	83
Bowel continence	83	83	83
Number in wheelchair	90	45	17
Independent ambulation	0	7	57

emphasis on the intracranial abnormalities on recognition of the defect. Once a neural tube defect has been found, the sonographer must strive to define the extent of the lesion, its skin covering and the last intact segment of the spine. After these features have been defined, it becomes possible to give a broad prognosis regarding mental and physical handicap.

Porencephaly and haemorrhage

Porencephaly is a smooth-walled cavity within the cerebral cortex which communicates directly with the ipsilateral lateral ventricle. A porencephalic cyst is lined with white matter, is filled with cerebrospinal fluid and exerts no mass effect. It occurs following necrosis of the cerebral white matter. Porencephaly most commonly occurs secondary to an intra-uterine insult to the brain before the late third trimester (Figs 6.40, 6.47A) but cases of familial porencephaly have been recorded in the literature. The aetiology is variable with the most common causes listed in Table 6.21.

The prognosis is dependent on a number of factors. The size, extent and anatomical distribution of the porencephaly are the most important predictive features. Ten reported cases in a single series give an appalling prognosis with two terminations, three fetal or neonatal deaths and serious neurological damage in the five survivors.[27] The underlying aetiology and associated abnormalities are also determinants of morbidity. The clinical findings in survivors with porencephaly include seizures, hemiplegia, quadriplegia, blindness and mental retardation.

Porencephaly is frequently the sequel to intracerebral haemorrhage, but this is not the only underlying cause (see Table 6.21). Fresh haemorrhage is recognized on ultrasound as increased echogenicity. This changes with time and degradation of blood products to become hypoechoic (Fig. 6.47b). Haemorrhage may occur not only into the brain substance (giving rise to porencephaly) but also into the ventricular system or posterior fossa. Prognosis is determined by

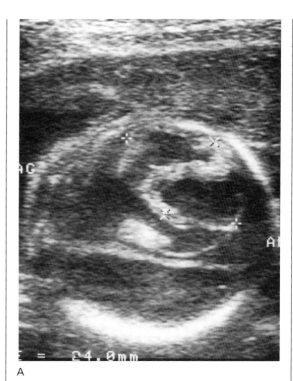

Fig. 6.47 (A) 25-week fetus with an intracerebral haemorrhage in the right parietal region with evolution of the haematoma which is of varied echogenicity. (B) 28-week fetus showing hypoechoic porencephaly (C, cystic areas).

site and extent of the bleed. It is therefore important to determine and document these factors during ultrasound assessment. Pooled data from several series show a poor outcome in 68% of all cases with bleeds in cerebral, ventricular and extra-axial sites.[93] Further subdivision of these cases shows the poor outcome for intraventricular bleeds

Table 6.21
Causes of porencephaly

Haemorrhage secondary to infection, thrombocytopaenia, maternal antibodies
Monochorionic twinning – twin-to-twin transfusion, death of co-twin
Vasoactive drugs, e.g. cocaine, heroin
Traumatic amniocentesis with penetration of the skull vault[91]
Fetal intravascular transfusion (embolic or hyperviscosity)[92]

Table 6.22
Genetic conditions with brain abnormality as a feature

Acrocephalosyndactyly, e.g. Apert syndrome
Aicardi syndrome
*Hydrolethalus syndrome
*Joubert's syndrome
*Meckel–Gruber syndrome
Miller–Dieker syndrome
Oro–facial–digital syndrome
Proteus syndrome
*Smith–Lemli–Opitz syndrome
Walker–Warburg syndrome
X-linked hydrocephalus
*Zellweger syndrome

Autosomal recessive.

(45%), parenchymal haemorrhage (92%), and extra-axial bleeds (88%). If intraventricular haemorrhage is subdivided further, those with the most favourable outcome (100% normal or mild sequelae) are in those with Grade 1 haemorrhage confined to the germinal matrix.[93]

The recognition of porencephaly or haemorrhage in utero should prompt a search for the underlying aetiology. Clearly, if related to interventional procedures, this will be evident from the history and serves to reinforce the need for direct and continuous ultrasound surveillance during all needling procedures during the pregnancy. In the absence of an iatrogenic cause, haematological, infectious and traumatic causes should be sought. However, whatever the underlying insult and aetiology, the prognosis for antenatally detected intracranial haemorrhage is poor for all groups other than Grade 1 ventricular bleeds.

Syndromes and genetic disorders

There are a number of genetic conditions and syndromes in which the first or dominant feature identified prenatally on ultrasound may be abnormality of the brain. The importance of recognizing these genetic conditions lies in the implications for counselling as many are autosomal recessive with a 1 in 4 risk of recurrence or autosomal dominant with variable expression or penetrance (Table 6.22).

Tumours

Primary brain tumours are exceedingly rare, are rapidly progressive and have an appalling prognosis. They are rarely diagnosed until the late second or third trimesters. Teratomas are the most common histologic type[94,95] with primitive neuroectodermal tumours and astrocytomas the next largest groups.[95,96] These tumours are usually supratentorial (67%) in location, have a varied sonographic appearance ranging from cystic through to solid and may change in appearance during the pregnancy (Fig. 6.48). They are eccentric in location, cause local mass effect and result in distortion of normal anatomy with obstructive hydrocephalus. The main differential diagnosis is from an intracerebral haemorrhage, a bleed characterized by change with time. In cases of intracranial haemorrhage, the blood is initially echogenic,

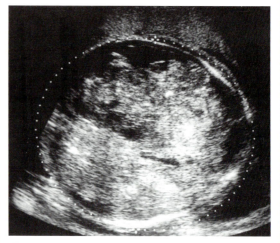

Fig. 6.48 29-week fetus with an intracerebral teratoma and gross macrocephaly. (Courtesy of Dr S. Rimmer.)

becoming less so with time until it appears purely cystic. A bleed becomes well marginated and can break down to communicate with the lateral ventricle to form a porencephalic cyst. Tumours, in contrast, are rapidly growing with poorly defined margins; haemorrhage may occur into the tumour which makes it more difficult to distinguish the two pathologies. Differentiation from vascular malformation is readily achieved by the use of colour Doppler. There is a slight male predilection (58%).[95]

Presentation of congenital brain tumours in the fetus is of a large, heterogenous mass and obstructive ventriculomegaly. In the newborn, the presenting features are of a large head, vomiting, seizures, hemiparesis and visual changes. Brain tumours carry a uniformly bad prognosis with neonatal death the likely outcome.[94–99] Median survival figures in the paediatric literature for congenital brain tumours are 3 weeks for teratomata, 5 months for primitive neuroectodermal tumours and 26 months for astrocytomata.[95]

Tumours of the choroid plexus may be benign (papilloma) or malignant (carcinoma). The prognosis for these tumours is poor as complete excision is rarely achieved, and local recurrence is common. They may occur in the lateral or third ventricle and may be recognized as a bulky choroid of heterogeneous echotexture or by identification of accompanying obstructive hydrocephalus. Both are more common in males.

Ventriculomegaly

Ventriculomegaly is a descriptive term for enlargement of the intracranial ventricular system. This is distinct from hydrocephalus which implies not only enlargement but also raised pressure within the system. Three standard deviations above the mean for normal atrial size is 10 mm and is taken as the upper limit of normal.[16] Ventriculo-megaly is defined as a ventricular atrium, at any gestation, which measures 11 mm or greater although in many series examining the outcome of ventriculomegaly 10 mm atria are included. The value of the 'dangling choroid' as a sign of ventriculomegaly is also favoured by some authors (Fig. 6.49). Ventriculomegaly is reported in 0.05 to 0.3% of all pregnancies[100] and is associated with central nervous system and non-central nervous system structural abnormality.[101–107] Associated central nervous system structural anomalies are seen in 14 to 67% of cases of ventriculomegaly[103–106] of which neural tube defects are the most common underlying pathology, accounting for 32 to 50% of the central nervous system anomalies.

Ventriculomegaly is associated with structural abnormality outside the central nervous system, chromosomal abnormality (3 to 12% including triploidy, trisomies 13, 18 and 21, translocations 7p and 9p[101,102,104,106]) and with fetal infection. Many of these can be identified on ultrasound, by chromosomal analysis and by serum screening for maternal and fetal infection. The diagnostic features of

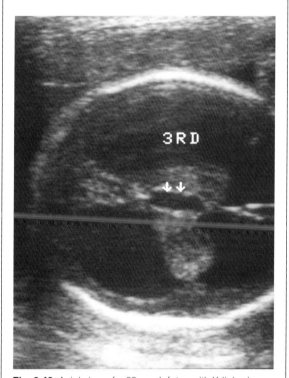

Fig. 6.49 Axial view of a 28-week fetus with X-linked ventriculomegaly showing enlargement of both lateral and third ventricles. There is a drooping choroid plexus in the dependent lateral ventricle (arrows point to dilated third ventricle).

Table 6.23
Congenital brain abnormality linked with ventriculomegaly

Holoprosencephaly
Agenesis of the corpus callosum
Dandy–Walker complex
Aneurysm of the vein of Galen
Arachnoid cyst
Arnold–Chiari 2 malformation in neural tube defects
Schizencephaly
Genetic syndromes and disorders

these abnormalities on ultrasound are described under the individual sections above.

Ventriculomegaly is also found in fetuses that have acquired an infection in utero, most commonly toxoplasmosis or cytomegalovirus (Fig. 6.39). Features of ventriculomegaly in association with infection that may suggest the underlying aetiology to the sonographer are asymmetry of ventricular size, blood in the ventricles or cerebral hemispheres (haemorrhage occurs as a result of secondary anaemia and thrombocytopaenia), a ventriculitis (increases echogenicity of the ependymal lining), and porencephaly (Fig. 6.40). Extracranial abnormality may also be found with calcification of the liver and with hydrops. The prognosis in these cases is poor and is discussed in more detail in the section on infection.

When ventriculomegaly is found on ultrasound scan of the fetus, it is important to exclude all the causes in Table 6.24 as they, if present, will determine the outcome. Once these causes have been excluded, the ventriculomegaly may then be divided into two broad groups. The first group is truly isolated ventriculomegaly. The second is ventriculomegaly that has no associated structural brain abnormality but may have other system abnormality. The management

Table 6.24
Features suggestive of infection in presence of ventriculomegaly

Ventricular asymmetry
Echogenic lining of the ventricles – ventriculitis
Blood in the ventricles
Porencephaly
Intracerebral bleed

of these two groups and how to attempt a prognosis are discussed below.

Comparison of outcome data from published series is confounded by variation in inclusion criteria. Earlier studies have included cases of ventriculomegaly that are secondary to evident major brain structural abnormality. Examples of this are given in Table 6.23. The presence of ventriculomegaly in the context of such abnormality is a secondary feature and it is the underlying structural abnormality which determines outcome. Inclusion of these cases in outcome series biases towards a less favourable outcome. With improvements in the sensitivity of ultrasound diagnosis, reflecting advances in technology and sonographers' skills and comprehension, the majority of these cases will be accurately identified and accurate prognosis given.

The managerial and prognostic dilemma predominates in cases identified with isolated ventriculomegaly or ventriculomegaly in association with anomalies in other body systems.[108,109,110] This section aims to aid the reader with the management of these two groups. When a fetus is identified as having ventriculomegaly, it is important to determine, by targeted ultrasound, the extent of the abnormalities. A careful search for central nervous system and other system anomalies is mandatory and chromosomal abnormality should be discussed and invasive testing offered given the increased risk of aneuploidy. The risk of aneuploidy in fetuses with ventriculomegaly is variable. Single series report incidences range from 3 to 27%[103,104] and literature review of pooled data indicates an incidence of 3 to 10%.[110] Risk may be further stratified to isolated ventriculomegaly with a risk of 3% rising to 36% in the presence of other anomalies. Information available to diagnosticians about the fetus after scan are gestational age at diagnosis, the size of the atrium, whether there are additional anomalies, fetal gender and, if amniocentesis has been performed, karyotype. In addition, if paired scans have been performed, change in size of the atrium with time will be known. Outcome is influenced by all of these factors.

Table 6.25

Guides to prognosis
Atrial size
Change with time
Other structural abnormality
Gender
Gestation at diagnosis
Chromosomes
Family history

Poor prognostic indicators
Large atria at diagnosis > 13 mm
Increase in size during the pregnancy
Diagnosis after 24 weeks
Male fetus
Positive family history

Good prognostic indicators
Atrial size stable and <13 mm
Decrease in size to normal
No other structural abnormality

The fetus identified on scan as having ventriculomegaly can be categorized further for the purposes of indicating prognosis. Having excluded chromosomal abnormality, fetuses with sonographically isolated ventriculomegaly have a good chance of survival (80%,[104] 70%[110]) but not of normal outcome (50%,[104] 41%[110]). These figures, however, take no account of change in ventricular atrium size with time nor of the severity of the ventriculomegaly at diagnosis.

Work in progress from our own unit[111] has analyzed the outcome for 104 fetal cases with ventriculomegaly after exclusion of cases of ventriculomegaly with sonographically identified, associated central nervous system anomalies. 31% opted for termination of the pregnancy and there were both fetal and postnatal deaths (7%). Of the remaining 65 cases, 40 (62%) were seen for detailed clinical and neurological assessment, and duration of follow-up was 6 weeks to 6 years (mean 31 months). Those fetuses whose ventriculomegaly resolved to normal values during pregnancy had a survival rate of 90% with normal development in 78%. Fetuses whose ventriculomegaly was stable during pregnancy also had 90% survival but fewer with normal development (56%). Finally, fetuses with progressive ventriculomegaly had a reduced survival rate of 77% and only 24% chance of normal development.

Furthermore, our data indicate that the length of postnatal follow-up is very important as we are now finding that some previously normal children are manifesting speech and learning difficulties after 3 years of age. Our analysis has shown that information available during the pregnancy from serial ultrasound scans, chromosomal analysis and family history can greatly assist in predicting prognosis to allow informed parental decisions regarding management.

In summary, following the identification of ventriculomegaly in utero, it is important to scrutinize the brain for underlying structural abnormality as this commonly occurs and it is the dominant prognostic indicator when present. It is also important to perform a full systemic review to look for other system anomalies, to exclude infection and to offer karyotype. Armed with these separate strands of information, it becomes possible to categorize the fetus into a good or bad prognostic group on the basis of ventricular size, change of ventricular atrium with time and associated other scan features, and counsel accordingly.

Magnetic resonance imaging

The advantages of MRI of the fetus are that it, in common with ultrasound, is non-invasive and does not involve the use of ionizing radiation. It affords the opportunity to visualize the anatomy and structure of the brain in detail. Its use was first described in pregnancy in 1983 but, since the earliest reports, there has not been wide application of the technique in fetal diagnosis. High-resolution ultrasound in skilled and experienced hands remains the gold standard. The early studies reported acquisition times of up to 60 minutes with intramuscular or intravenous fetal sedation proving necessary to reduce movement artefact. With advances in technology, new programmes and surface coils, fetuses can be imaged in 20 minutes without the use of sedation. This makes the examination comparable, in terms of time, with a level three sonogram although the cost, in general, remains higher.

Reported results of the power of MRI in fetal diagnosis reveal that it does have a contribution to make in some cases of fetal abnormality, particularly of the brain. It has been shown to add additional information in a significant number of cases (27%,[112] 55%[113]) and to change the counselling and management in a significant proportion (50%,[112] 39%[113]). The diagnosis made by ultrasound of the fetal abnormality was changed by the MRI examination in several cases. Many of these cases presented in the late third trimester, which is a time of gestation difficult to image and assess satisfactorily with ultrasound because of vault ossification and often deep cephalic presentation. Neither of these two factors poses a problem for MRI and may account for the apparent incorrect ultrasound diagnoses.

A further application of MRI in fetal diagnosis is as an alternative to post-mortem following termination or fetal or neonatal death.[114,115] Audit of uptake of post-mortem by bereaved parents following a perinatal death show acceptance figures of 53 to 58%.[116,117] Preliminary studies suggest that MRI, in common with ultrasound and radiographs, does provide a real, non-invasive alternative and may offer a diagnostic avenue for parents who decline post-mortem on their baby.

In summary, MRI does provide a viable adjunct to ultrasound in the diagnosis of fetal abnormality and is perhaps most powerful in imaging of the brain in fetal abnormality in terms of diagnostic yield. Authors of the larger series[118,119] do emphasize the complementary nature of this technique and that it does not offer a realistic alternative to ultrasound lacking, as it does, the ability to direct, target and focus the examination.

References

Embryology

1. Timor-Tritsch IE, Monteagudo A, Warren WB. Transvaginal ultrasonographic detection of the central nervous system in the first and early second trimesters. Am J Obstet Gynecol 1991; 164:497–503.

2. Barkovich AJ. Paediatric neuroimaging. New York: Raven Press; 1990.

3. Moore KL, Persaud TVN. The developing human – clinically oriented embryology. 6th ed. Philadelphia: WB Saunders; 1998.

4. Briggs GG, Freeman RK, Yaffe SJ. Drugs in pregnancy and lactation. Baltimore: Williams and Wilkins; 1990.

Normal variants and pitfalls

5. Nyberg DA. Recommendations for obstetric sonography in the evaluation of the fetal cranium. Radiology 1989; 172:309–311.

6. Heiserman J, Filly RA, Goldstein RB. The effect of measurement errors on the sonographic evaluation of ventriculomegaly. J Ultrasound Med 1991; 10:121–124.

7. Wolfe HM, Sokol RJ, Martier SM, Zador IE. Maternal obesity: a potential source of error in sonographic prenatal diagnosis. Obstet Gynecol 1990; 76:339–342.

8. Babcook CJ, Chong BW, Salamat MS, Ellis WG, Goldstein RB. Sonographic anatomy of the developing cerebellum: normal embryology can resemble pathology. AJR 1996; 166:427–433.

9. Knutzon RK, McGahan JP, Salamat MS, Brant WB. Fetal cisterna magna septa: a normal anatomic finding. Radiology 1991; 180:799–801.

10. Monteagudo A, Reuss ML, Timor-Tritsch IE. Imaging the fetal brain in the second and third trimesters using transvaginal sonography. Obstet Gynecol 1991; 77:27–32.

Normal anatomy

11. Nicolaides KH, Azar G, Byrne D, Mansur C, Marks K. Fetal nuchal translucency: ultrasound screening for chromosomal defects in the first trimester of pregnancy. BMJ 1992; 304:867–869.

12. Benacerraf BR, Frigoletto FD. Soft tissue nuchal fold in the second trimester fetus: standards for normal measurements compared with those in Down syndrome. Am J Obstet Gynecol 1987; 157:1146–1149.

13. Filly RA, Cardoza JD, Goldstein RB, Barkovich AJ. Detection of fetal central nervous system anomalies: a practical level of effort for a routine sonogram. Radiology 1989; 172:403–408.

14. Filly RA, Goldstein RB, Callen PW. Fetal ventricle: importance in routine obstetric sonography. Radiology 1991; 181:1–7.

15. Pilu G, Reece EA, Goldstein I, Hobbins JC, Bovicelli L. Sonographic evaluation of the normal developmental anatomy of the fetal cerebral ventricles: II. The atria. Obstet Gynecol 1989; 73:250–255.

16. Cardoza JD, Goldstein RB, Filly RA. Exclusion of fetal ventriculomegaly with a single measurement: the width of the lateral ventricular atrium. Radiology 1988; 169:711–714.

17. Achiron R, Yagel S, Rotstein Z, Inbar O, Mashiach S, Lipitz S. Cerebral lateral ventricular asymmetry: is this a normal ultrasonographic finding in the fetal brain? Obstet Gynecol 1997; 89:233–237.

Agenesis of the corpus callosum

18. Pilu G, Sandri F, Perolo A, et al. Sonography of fetal agenesis of the corpus callosum: a survey of 35 cases. Ultrasound Obstet Gynecol 1993; 3:318–319.

19. Vergani P, Ghidini A, Strobelt N, et al. Prognostic indicators in the prenatal diagnosis of agenesis of the corpus callosum. Am J Obstet Gynecol 1994; 170(3):753–758.

20. Parrish M, Roessmen U, Levinsohn M. Agenesis of the corpus callosum: a study of the frequency of associated malformations. Ann Neurol 1979; 6:349–352.

21. Gupta JK, Lilford RJ. Assessment and management of fetal agenesis of the corpus callosum. Prenat Diagn 1995; 15:301–312.

22. Bork MD, Smeltzer JS, Egan JFX, Rodis JF, DiMario Jr FJ, Campbell WA. Prenatal diagnosis of intracranial lipoma associated with agenesis of the corpus callosum. Obstet Gynecol 1996; 87(5) II Suppl:845–848.

Anencephaly and exencephaly

23. Casellas M, Ferrer M, Rovira M, et al. Prenatal diagnosis of exencephaly. Prenat Diagn 1993; 13:417–422.

24. Wilkins-Haug L, Freedman W. Progression of exencephaly to anencephaly in the human fetus – an ultrasound perspective. Prenat Diagn 1991; 11(1):227–233.

Aneurysm of the vein of Galen

25. Evans AJ, Twining P. Case report: in utero diagnosis of a vein of Galen aneurysm using colour flow Doppler. Clin Rad 1991; 44:281–282.

26. Rodesch G, Hui F, Alvarez H, Tanaka A, Las jaunias P. Prognosis of antenatally diagnosed vein of Galen aneurysmal malformation. Child's Nerv Syst 1994; 10:79–83.

27. Pilu G, Falco P, Perolo A, et al. Differential diagnosis and outcome of fetal intracranial hypoechoic lesions: report of 21 cases. Ultrasound Obstet Gynecol 1997; 9(4):229–236.

28. Yuval Y, Lerner A, Lipitz S, Rotstein Z, Hegesh J, Achiron R. Prenatal diagnosis of vein of Galen aneurysmal malformations: report of two cases with proposal for prognostic indices. Prenat Diagn 1997; 17(10):972–977.

Arachnoid cyst

29. Estroff JA, Parad RB, Barnes PD, Madsen JP, Benacerraf BR. Posterior fossa arachnoid cyst: an in utero mimicker of Dandy–Walker malformation. J Ultrasound Med 1995; 14(10):787–790.

30. Pelkey TJ, Ferguson II JE, Veille JC, Alston SR. Giant glioependymal cyst resembling holoprosencephaly on prenatal ultrasound: case report and review of the literature. Ultrasound Obstet Gynecol 1997; 9(3):200–203.

Choroid plexus cysts

31. Chudleigh P, Pearce JM, Campbell S. The prenatal diagnosis of transient cysts of the fetal choroid plexus. Prenat Diagn 1984; 4:135–137.

32. Bundy AL, Saltzman DH, Prober B, Fine C, Emerson D, Doubilet PM. Antenatal sonographic findings in trisomy 18. J Ultrasound Med 1986; 5:361–364.

33. Twining P, Zuccollo J, Clewes J, Swallow J. Fetal choroid plexus cysts: a prospective study and review of the literature. Br J Radiol 1991; 64:98–102.

34. Ostlere SJ, Irving HC, Lilford RJ. Fetal choroid plexus cysts: a report of 100 cases. Radiology 1990; 175:753–755.

35. Chinn DH, Miller EI, Worthy LM, Towers CV. Sonographically detected fetal choroid plexus cysts: frequency and association with aneuploidy. J Ultrasound Med 1991; 10:255–258.

36. Thorpe-Beeston JG, Gosden CM, Nicolaides KH. Choroid plexus cysts and chromosomal defects. Br J Radiol 1990; 63:783–786.

37. Nyberg DA, Kramer D, Resta RG, Kapur R, Mahony BS, Luthy DA. Prenatal sonographic findings of trisomy 18: review of 47 cases. J Ultrasound Med 1993; 12:103–113.

38. Nyberg DA, Resta RG, Luthy DA, Hickok DE, Mahony BS, Hirsch JH. Prenatal sonographic findings of Down's syndrome: review of 94 cases. Obstet Gynecol 1990; 76:370–377.

39. Snijders RJM, Shawa L, Nicolaides KH. Fetal choroid plexus cysts and trisomy 18: assessment of risk based on ultrasound findings and maternal age. Prenat Diagn 1994; 14:1119–1127.

40. Snijders RJM, Holzgreve W, Cuckle H, Nicolaides KH. Maternal age-specific risks for trisomies at 9–14 weeks' gestation. Prenat Diagn 1994; 14:543–552.

41. Gupta KS, Thornton JG, Lilford RJ. Management of fetal choroid plexus cysts. BJOG 1997; 104:881–886.

Dandy Walker complex

42. Dandy WE, Blackfan KD. Internal hydrocephalus: an experimental, clinical and pathological study. Am J Dis Child 1914; 8:406–482.

43. Barkovich AJ, Kjos BO, Norman D, Edwards MS. Revised classification of posterior fossa cysts and cystlike malformations based on the results of multiplanar MR imaging. Am J Roentgenol 1989; 153(6):1289–1300.

44. Cornford E, Twining P. The Dandy–Walker syndrome: the value of antenatal diagnosis. Clin Rad 1992; 45:172–174.

45. Ulm B, Ulm MR, Deutinger J, Bernaschek G. Dandy–Walker malformation diagnosed before 21 weeks of gestation: associated malformations and chromosomal abnormalities. Ultrasound Obstet Gynecol 1997; 10(3):167–170.

46. Chang MC, Russell SA, Callen PW, Filly RA, Goldstein RB. Sonographic detection of inferior vermian agenesis in Dandy–Walker malformations: prognostic implications. Radiology 1994; 193:765–770.

47. Nyberg DA, Mahony BS, Hegge FN, Hickok D, Luthy DA, Kapur R. Enlarged cisterna magna and the Dandy–Walker malformation: factors associated

with chromosome abnormalities. Obstet Gynecol 1991; 77:436–442.

48. Nyberg DA, Hallesy D, Mahony BS, Hirsch JH, Luthy DA, Hickok D. Meckel–Gruber syndrome. Importance of prenatal diagnosis. J Ultrasound Med 1990; 9(12):691–696.

Encephaloceles

49. Wininger SJ, Donnenfeld AE. Syndromes identified in fetuses with prenatally diagnosed cephaloceles. Prenat Diagn 1994; 14(9):839–843.

50. Goldstein RB, LaPidus AS, Filly RA. Fetal cephaloceles: diagnosis with US. Radiology 1991; 180(3):803–808.

51. Brown MS, Sheridan-Pereira M. Outlook for the child with a cephalocele. Pediatrics 1992; 90(6):914–919.

52. Bronshtein M, Zimmer EZ. Transvaginal sonographic follow-up on the formation of fetal cephalocele at 13–19 weeks' gestation. Obstet Gynecol 1991; 78(3) II:528–530.

Holoprosencephaly

53. Berry SM, Gosden C, Snijders RJM, Nicolaides KH. Fetal holoprosencephaly: associated malformations and chromosomal defects. Fetal Diagn Ther 1990; 5:92–99.

54. McGahan JP, Nyberg DA, Mack LA. Sonography of facial features of alobar and semilobar holoprosencephaly. Am J Roentgenol 1990; 154(1):143–148.

55. Stagiannis KD, Sepulveda W, Bower S. Early prenatal diagnosis of holoprosencephaly: the value of transvaginal ultrasound. Eur J Obstet Gynecol Reprod Biol 1995; 61:175–176.

56. Toma P, Costa A, Magnano GM, Cariati M, Lituania M. Holoprosencephaly: prenatal diagnosis by sonography and magnetic resonance imaging. Prenat Diagn 1990; 10(7):429–436.

57. Rubinstein D, Cajade-Law AG, Youngman V, Hise JM, Baganz M. The development of the corpus callosum in semilobar and lobar holoprosencephaly. Pediatr Radiol 1996; 26(12):839–844.

58. Sener RN. Anterior callosal agenesis in mild, lobar holoprosencephaly. Pediatr Radiol 1995; 25(5):385–386.

59. Fitz CR. Holoprosencephaly and septo-optic dysplasia. Neuroimaging Clin N Am 1994; 4(2):263–281.

60. Filly RA, Chinn DH, Callen PW. Alobar holoprosencephaly: ultrasonographic prenatal diagnosis. Radiology 1984; 151:455–459.

Infection

61. Donner C, Liesnard C, Content J, Busine A, Aderca J, Rodesch F. Prenatal diagnosis of 52 pregnancies at risk for congenital cytomegalovirus infection. Obstet Gynecol 1993; 82:481–486.

62. Tassin GB, Maklad NF, Stewart RR, Bell ME. Cytomegalic inclusion disease: intrauterine sonographic diagnosis using findings involving the brain. Am J Neuroradiol 1991; 12(1):117–122.

63. Drose JA, Dennis MA, Thickman D. Infection in utero: US findings in 19 cases. Radiology 1991; 178(2):369–374.

64. Twickler DM, Perlman J, Maberry MC. Congenital cytomegalovirus infection presenting as cerebral ventriculomegaly on antenatal sonography. Am J Perinatol 1993; 10(5):404–406.

65. Hewicker-Trautwein M, Trautwein G. Porencephaly, hydranencephaly and leukoencephalopathy in ovine fetuses following transplacental infection with bovine virus diarrhoea virus: distribution of viral antigen and characterization of cellular response. Acta Neuropathol 1994; 87(4):385–397.

66. Achiron R, Pinhas-Hamiel O, Lipitz S, Heiman Z, Reichman B, Mashiach S. Prenatal ultrasonographic diagnosis of fetal cerebral ventriculitis associated with asymptomatic maternal cytomegalovirus infection. Prenat Diagn 1994; 14:523–526.

Iniencephaly

67. Meizner I, Levi A, Katz M, Maor E. Iniencephaly: a case report. J Reprod Med 1992; 37(10):885–888.

68. Katz VL, Aylsworth AS, Albright SG. Iniencephaly is not uniformly fatal. Prenat Diagn 1989; 9(8):595–599.

69. Maekawa K, Masaki T, Kokubun Y. Fetal spinal-cord injury secondary to hyperextension of the neck: no effect of caesarean section. Develop Med Child Neurol 1976; 18:229–238.

70. Ballas S, Toaff R. Hyperextension of the fetal head in breech presentation: radiological evaluation and significance. Br J Obstet Gynecol 1976; 83:201–204.

Lissencephaly, Schizencephaly and Heterotopias

71. Holzgreve W, Feil R, Louwen F, Miny P. Prenatal diagnosis and management of fetal hydrocephaly and lissencephaly. Child's Nerv Syst 1993; 9(7):408–412.

72. Saltzman DH, Krauss CM, Goldman JM, Benacerraf BR. Prenatal diagnosis of lissencephaly. Prenat Diagn 1991; 11(3):139–143.

73. Okamura K, Murotsuki J, Sakai T, Matsumoto K, Shirane R, Yajima A. Prenatal diagnosis of lissencephaly by magnetic resonance imaging. Fetal Diagn Ther 1993; 8(1):56–59.

Mega cisterna magna

74. Mahony BS, Callen PW, Filly RA, Hoddick WK. The fetal cisterna magna. Radiology 1984; 153:773–776.

Neural tube defects

75. Murphy M, Seagroatt V, Hey K et al. Neural tube defects 1974–94 – down but not out. Arch Dis Child 1996; 75: F133–F134.

76. Department of Health. Folic acid and neural tube defects: guidelines on prevention. London: HMSO; 1992.

77. Chitty LS, Hunt GH, Moore J, Lobb MO. Effectiveness of routine ultrasonography in detecting fetal structural abnormalities in low risk population. BMJ 1991; 303:1165–1169.

78. Luck CA. Value of routine ultrasound scanning at 19 weeks: a four year study of 8849 deliveries. BMJ 1992; 304:1474–1478.

79. Nicolaides KH, Campbell S, Gabbe S, Guidetti R. Ultrasound screening for spina bifida: cranial and cerebellar signs. Lancet 1986; i:72–74.

80. Report of the UK collaborative study of alpha-fetoprotein in relation to neural tube defects. Lancet 1977; i:1323–1332.

81. Van den Hof MC, Nicolaides KH, Campbell J, Campbell S. Evaluation of the lemon and banana signs in one hundred and thirty fetuses with open spina bifida. Am J Obstet Gynecol 1990; 162:322–327.

82. Goldstein RB, Podrasky AE, Filly RA, Callan PW. Effacement of the fetal cisterna magna in association with myelomeningocele. Radiology 1989; 172:409–413.

83. Nyberg DA, Mack LA, Hirsch J et al. Abnormalities of fetal cranial contour in sonographic detection of spina bifida: evaluation of the 'lemon' sign. Radiology 1988; 167:387–392.

84. Babcook CJ, Goldstein RB, Barth RA, Damato NM, Callen PW, Filly RA. Prevalence of ventriculomegaly in association with myelomeningocele: correlation with gestational age and severity of posterior fossa deformity. Radiology 1994; 190(3):703–707.

85. Blumenfeld Z, Siegler E, Bronshtein M. The early diagnosis of neural tube defects. Prenat Diagn 1993; 13(9):863–871.

86. Cochrane DD, Wilson RD, Steinbok P, et al. Prenatal spinal evaluation and functional outcome of patients born with myelomeningocele: information for improved prenatal counselling and outcome prediction. Fetal Diagn Ther 1996; 11(3):159–168.

87. Hume Jr RF, Drugan A, Reichler A, et al. Aneuploidy among prenatally detected neural tube defects. Am J Med Genet 1996; 61(2):171–173.

88. Shurtleff DB, Luthy DA, Nyberg DA, Mack LA. The outcome of fetal myelomeningocele brought to term. Eur J Pediatr Surg Suppl 1994; 4(1):25–28.

89. Hogge WA, Dungan JS, Brooks MP, et al. Diagnosis and management of prenatally detected myelomeningocele; a preliminary report. Am J Obstet Gynecol 1990; 163(3):1061–1065.

90. Hill AE, Beattie F. Does Caesarean section delivery improve neurological outcome in open spina bifida? Eur J Pediatr Surg Suppl 1994; 4(1):32–34.

Porencephaly and intra-cranial bleeds

91. Eller KM, Kuller JA. Porencephaly secondary to fetal trauma during amniocentesis. Obstet Gynecol 1995; 85:865–867.

92. Dildy GA, Smith LG, Moise RJ, Cano LE, Hesketh DE. Porencephalic cyst: a complication of fetal intravascular transfusion. Am J Obstet Gynecol 1991; 165:76–78.

93. Vergani P, Strobelt N, Locatelli A, et al. Clinical significance of fetal intracranial hemorrhage. Am J Obstet Gynecol 1996; 175:536–543.

Tumours

94. Heckel S, Favre R, Gasser B, Christmann D. Prenatal diagnosis of a congenital astrocytoma: a case report and literature review. Ultrasound Obstet Gynecol 1995; 5(1):63–66.

95. Buetow PC, Smirniotopoulos JG, Done S. Congenital brain tumours: a review of 45 cases. AJNR 1990; 11:793–799.

96. Wienk MA, van Geijn HP, Copray FJA, Brons JTY. Prenatal diagnosis of fetal tumours by ultrasonography. Obstet Gynecol Survey 1990; 45(10):639–653.

97. Doren M, Tercanli S, Gullotta F, Holzgreve W. Prenatal diagnosis of a highly undifferentiated brain tumour – a case report and review of the literature. Prenat Diagn 1997; 17(10):967–971.

98. Pelkey TJ, Ferguson II JE, Veille JC, Alston SR. Giant glioependymal cyst resembling holoprosencephaly on prenatal ultrasound: case report and review of the literature. Ultrasound Obstet Gynecol 1997; 9(3):200–203.

99. McConachie NS, Twining P, Lamb MP. Case report: antenatal diagnosis of congenital glioblastoma. Clin Rad 1991; 44:121–122.

Ventriculomegaly

100. Serlo W, Kirkinen P, Jouppila P, Herva R. Prognostic signs in fetal hydrocephalus. Child's Nerv Syst 1986; 2:93–97.

101. Bromley B, Frigoletto FD Jr, Benacerraf BR. Mild fetal lateral cerebral ventriculomegaly: clinical course and outcome. Am J Obstet Gynecol 1991; 164:863–867.

102. Brown IM, Bannister CM, Rimmer S, Russell SA. The outcome of infants diagnosed prenatally as having cerebral ventriculomegaly. J Maternal Fetal Invest 1995; 5:13–19.

103. Goldstein RB, LaPidus AS, Filly RA, Cardoza J. Mild lateral cerebral ventricular dilation in utero: clinical significance and prognosis. Radiology 1990; 176(1):237–242.

104. Twining P, Jaspan T, Zuccollo J. The outcome of fetal ventriculomegaly. Br J Radiol 1994; 67(793):26–31.

105. Rosseau GL, McCullough DC, Joseph AL. Current prognosis in fetal ventriculomegaly. J Neurosurg 1992; 77(4):551–555.

106. Anhoury P, Andre M, Droulle P, et al. Dilatation of the cerebral ventricles diagnosed in utero. 85 case histories. J Gynecol Obstet Biol Reprod 1991; 20(2):191–197.

107. Kirkinen P, Serlo W, Jouppila P, Ryynanen M, Martikainen A. Long-term outcome of fetal hydrocephaly. J Child Neurol 1996; 11(3):189–192.

108. Patel MD, Filly AL, Hersh DR, Goldstein RB. Isolated mild fetal cerebral ventriculomegaly: clinical course and outcome. Radiology 1994; 192:759–764.

109. Bloom SL, Bloom DD, Dellanebbia C, Martin L, Lucas MJ, Twickler DM. The developmental outcome of children with antenatal mild isolated ventriculomegaly. Obstet Gynecol 1997; 90:93–97.

110. Gupta JK, Bryce FC, Lilford RJ. Management of

apparently isolated fetal ventriculomegaly. Obstet Gynecol Survey 1994; 49(10):716–721.

111. Arora A. Personal communication: work in progress. Outcome of fetal ventriculomegaly.

MRI

112. Yuh WT, Nguyen HD, Fisher DJ, et al. MR of fetal nervous system abnormalities. AJNR 1994; 15(3):459–464.

113. Levine D, Barnes PD, Madsen JR, Li W, Edelman RR. Fetal central nervous system anomalies: MR imaging augments sonographic diagnosis. Radiology 1997; 204(3):635–642.

114. Brookes JAS, Hall-Craggs MA, Sams VR, Lees WR. Non-invasive perinatal necropsy by magnetic resonance imaging. Lancet 1996; 348:1139–1141.

115. Editorial. Postmortem perinatal examination: the role of magnetic resonance imaging. Ultrasound Obstet Gynecol 1997; 9:145–147.

116. Editorial. Perinatal and infant postmortem examination – difficult to ask for but potentially valuable. BMJ 1995; 310:141–142.

117. Cartlidge PHT, Dawson AT, Stewart JH, Vujanic GM. Value and quality of perinatal and infant postmortem examinations: cohort analysis of 400 consecutive deaths. BMJ 1995; 310:155–158.

118. Resta M, Spagnolo P, Di-Cuonzo F et al. Magnetic resonance of the fetus. Part II: pathological features. Riv Neuroradiol 1994; 7(4):557–571.

119. Revel MP, Morel MP, Bessis R et al. In utero MRI of the fetus: a series of 40 cases. Rev Imag Med 1994; 6(2):91–100.

CHAPTER 7

Spinal abnormalities

Michael J. Weston

Introduction

Anomalies of the fetal spine, particularly spina bifida, are amongst the commonest fetal malformations detectable. All those who use ultrasound to look at the fetus should be aware of the signs of spina bifida that can be found in both the spine and the head. The UK and Ireland have the highest prevalences of neural tube defects in Europe. A prevalence of nearly 40 cases per 10 000 births was seen from the years 1980 to 1983,[1] though this has fallen to nearer 25 cases per 10 000 births in the years up to 1986.[2] In comparison the prevalence in continental Europe remained stable over the same time period at 11.5 cases per 10 000 births. There may be longer term fluctuations in the prevalence rates as data from the Eastern USA showed a peak of neural tube defects in the 1930s compared to both 1910 and 1970.[3] There has also been a seasonal variation in the incidence of neural tube defects reported with the highest peak said to occur in late summer.[4]

Anencephaly and spina bifida are the commonest neural tube defects and occur with a nearly equal frequency of 1 in 1000 births though there is some variation depending on geographic location and sex of the fetus.[5] Prevalence rates are becoming harder to compare because of the increasing impact of antenatal diagnosis and termination of pregnancy. However, a study in Atlanta showed that prenatal diagnosis and termination alone, whilst having a substantial impact on live births, could not account for the fall in their overall rate of neural tube defects from 1970 to 1991.[6]

The diagnosis of spinal abnormalities is closely linked with observation of anomalies in the head so that there is overlap between this chapter and Chapter 6 on cranial anomalies. However, there are a number of more subtle malformations such as occult spinal dysraphisms, diastematomyelia, lipomeningocoeles and scolioses that require detailed observation of the spinal anatomy itself if the diagnosis is to be made prenatally. These anomalies have a potentially huge impact on neurological and orthopaedic services as well as family life. It is to this end that considerable resources have been devoted to their prenatal detection, both through biochemical and ultrasound means. However, it is apparent that there have been quite marked regional variations in the effectiveness of prenatal diagnosis linked to different policies of prenatal screening.[2]

Embryology

The nervous system first appears as a rounded thickening of the ectoderm towards the cephalic end of the fetus. This elongates to form the neural plate and expands caudally in the direction of the primitive streak. Approximately 18 days after fertilization the neural plate furrows to form two lateral neural folds with a central neural groove. These neural folds continue to elevate and then approach each other in the midline to form an enclosed neural tube. This fusion commences in the region of the future neck and then extends in both cephalic and caudal directions, extending the length of the enclosed neural tube. As a result, the neural tube has two open ends communicating with the amniotic cavity, named the anterior and posterior neuropores. The anterior neuropore closes first at day 24 following fertilization and then the posterior neuropore closes at day 26 (approximately 5.5 weeks from the last menstrual period). This neural tube forms the brain and spinal cord, the lumen of the tube becoming the ventricular system of the brain and the central canal of the spinal cord. Failure of closure of the caudal neural tube (posterior neuropore) produces an exposed neural plate which leads to spina bifida. The earlier the failure of caudal fusion of the neural tube occurs, the higher the spina bifida and the worse the prognosis.[7–9]

There are alternative theories of how the neural tube closes. The sex bias of more males than females with lumbar neural tube defects and frontal encephalocoeles, and that of more females than males in cervical and thoracic neural tube defects suggests that there may be multiple closure sites rather than a steady zipping up outwards from a central point.[10] Each closure site would have its own sex bias. Rodents have an intermittent pattern of anterior neuropore closure. A similar pattern has been reported in a case report of a human fetus in which there were two distinct closure defects.[11] Neural tube defects are also thought to be concordant for type and level within sibship pairs and to have a higher recurrence rate in upper defects. This suggests the pathogenesis may be the same but the fetus may be more susceptible to neural tube defect during early rather than late tube closure.[12]

The vertebral column forms around the cord with chondrification of the vertebral bodies beginning in the 6th week and ossification 2 weeks later. There are three primary ossification centres in each vertebra: one in the vertebral body (the centrum) and two in the neural arch (one each at the base of each transverse process).[13] The ossification of the centra begins at the thoracolumbar junction and progresses in cephalic and caudad directions. The ossification of the neural arch proceeds independently to the centra. Neural arch ossification may have two or more patterns of ossification. One pattern suggests a craniocaudal spread of ossification from a mid-thoracic site with no systematic order of ossification above it. Another proposes three origins of ossification with there being spread of ossification cranially and caudally from each. In either case ossification of the lower lumbar spine and sacrum proceeds in a caudal direction. The rate of ossification in the female may be slightly more rapid than in the male.

Normal appearances and variants

Ultrasound assessment depends on the visualization of the ossification centres in the fetal spine. Each vertebra has three, one in the body (the centrum) and one at each lamina–pedicle junction (or base of the transverse process).[14] These can be rapidly and systematically examined at a routine 18- to 20-week anatomy scan. Three planes of imaging are commonly used: axial, coronal and parasagittal.[15] The axial plane shows all three ossification centres of a vertebra on the one image. If the fetus is lying prone with its back towards the transducer, the posterior centres appear to converge towards the midline; however, if the fetus is lying in a decubitus position with respect to the transducer, the posterior centres appear parallel to one another (Fig. 7.1).[14] In the coronal plane, the posterior centres give a characteristic railtrack appearance with the centres gradually widening apart towards the head, together with a slight expansion in the lumbar region before the centres converge in the sacrum (Fig. 7.2). The coronal image also allows determination of the level, as the twelfth rib can be seen adjacent to the twelfth thoracic vertebra (Fig. 7.3) and the S1 vertebra is level with the top of the iliac wing.[13] The parasagittal view demonstrates the ossification centre of the centrum and one of the posterior centres together. These show the normal steady curvature of the spine as well as a gradual tapering towards the sacrum. A true sagittal scan often shows only the ossification centre of the centrum as the overlying neural arch is insufficiently ossified. This plane can, with high quality equipment, allow visualization of the spinal cord and the more echogenic cauda equina (Fig. 7.4). At 18 weeks' gestational age the tip of the cord (conus medullaris) extends to the upper sacrum. With growth of the spine the conus medullaris will ascend gradually throughout pregnancy and infancy until it reaches its adult position at the L1–2 level.[16] The axial and sagittal planes also allow assessment of the integrity of the overlying skin. Assessment of the spine can be impossible if the fetus is consistently lying supine with its back away from the transducer. Likewise the integrity of the skin may be impossible to assess if the fetus has its back abutting the uterine wall or the

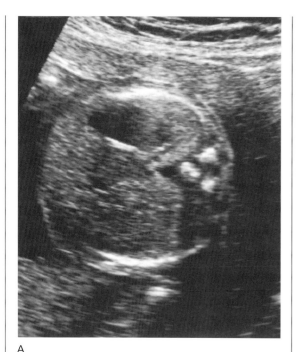

A

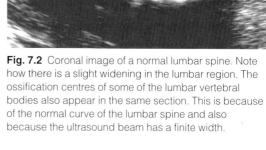

Fig. 7.2 Coronal image of a normal lumbar spine. Note how there is a slight widening in the lumbar region. The ossification centres of some of the lumbar vertebral bodies also appear in the same section. This is because of the normal curve of the lumbar spine and also because the ultrasound beam has a finite width.

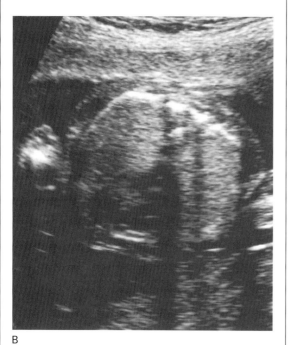

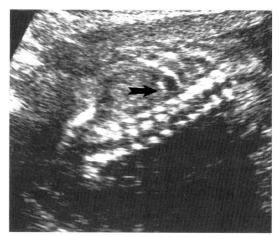

Fig. 7.3 Coronal image demonstrating the twelfth rib (arrow) which marks the level of the twelfth thoracic vertebra. In this instance the fifth lumbar vertebra is level with the top of the iliac wing.

B

Fig. 7.1 Axial views of the normal fetal spine demonstrating how the posterior ossification centres have a different appearance depending on their orientation relative to the transducer. (A) Fetus is lying decubitus. The posterior ossification centres appear parallel to each other. (B) Same fetus now with its back toward the transducer. The posterior ossification centres appear to converge.

placenta. If attempts to persuade the fetus to change position by agitation sound stimulus, altering the mother's position or bladder filling all fail, then it is best on a routine screen to rescan the fetus on another day. If the fetus is lying with the region of obscured interest near the cervix, then a transvaginal or transperineal scan may give the required information.[17]

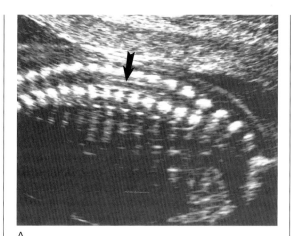

A

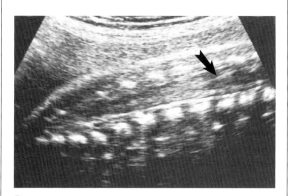

B

Fig. 7.4 (A) Parasagittal view of the spine at 18 weeks shows a short section of the spinal cord (arrow), where the cord is perpendicular to the beam. (B) Sagittal view of the spine at 32 weeks showing the hypoechoic conus medullaris (arrow), together with the more echogenic cauda equina extending below it.

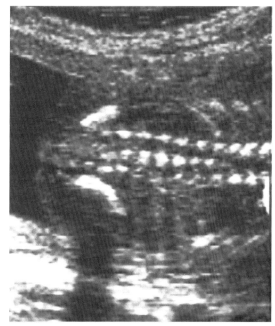

Fig. 7.5 Coronal image of normal spine at 18 weeks showing the sacral posterior ossification centres to be poorly ossified.

The ability to mentally build a picture of a three-dimensional structure from various two-dimensional images is a skill that all sonographers need to acquire. However, the technology exists to allow three-dimensional acquisition of ultrasound data. Early work suggests that such imaging improves the diagnostic accuracy in subtle malformations.[18] Three-dimensional images can be manipulated to give a surface appearance or a form of maximum intensity projection to show the bones. Clinicians and parents may benefit from these images as they allow a more recognizable structure to be observed. There are factors that reduce the quality of a three-dimensional image, it still being dependent on the quality of the original data acquisition, the lie of the fetus and whether or not the region of interest is abutting the placenta or other surface.

Normal variants

The sacrum may show incomplete ossification prior to 25 weeks' gestational age (Fig. 7.5).[19] The study by Budorick et al[13] showed that the gestational ages by which the neural arches had ossification as dense as the iliac wings in 100% of fetuses were as follows: L5, 16 weeks; S1, 19 weeks; S2, 22 weeks; S3, 24 weeks; S4, 25 weeks; and S5, 27 weeks. In other words, ossification progresses caudally at a rate of one level every 2 to 3 weeks after 16 weeks. This is of significance as imaging may need to be repeated at a later date in those fetuses at high risk for neural tube defect or sacral agenesis. In low-risk pregnancies, the finding of normal cranial anatomy is sufficient to avoid re-examination even if the distal sacrum is not yet ossified.

Potential pitfalls and artefacts

The unwary can misinterpret a normal fetal spine as having splaying in the thoracic region. This arises from inadvertently imaging through part of the fetal ribs in the parasagittal plane (Fig. 7.6). This trap can be avoided by examining the fetal spine in more than one plane to confirm the true position of the spinal ossification centres. The curvature of the fetal spine may also cause there to be too much craniocaudal tilt when trying to image axially. This can produce the appearance of splaying of the posterior elements, particularly in the lumbosacral region, and has been named 'pseudodysraphism'.[20] The beam spread or

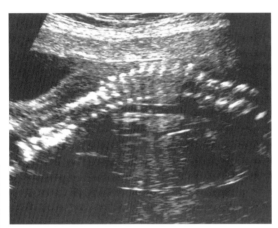

A

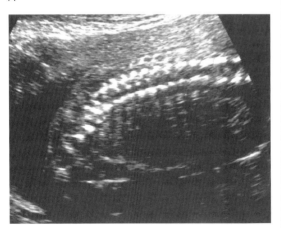

B

Fig. 7.6 (A) An artefactual appearance of splaying can be produced by the scan plane intersecting through part of the ribs. (B) Aligning the scan plane correctly shows the spine to be normal.

side lobe artefact can cause the appearance of false echoes extending out from bright reflectors such as the spinal ossification centres (Fig. 7.7). These may mimic the walls of a meningocoele but will prove to be artefacts when examined from a different angle.

These potential pitfalls are best avoided by careful attention to detail and by imaging in more than one plane from more than one direction. There is no substitute for examining the patient oneself rather than relying on someone else's images, particularly in cases of doubt.

Spina bifida

Aetiology and prevention

The great majority of spina bifida cases occur as isolated malformations and are believed to be multifactorial in origin.[21] They may involve a genetic predisposition together with other environmental agents. There are geographic and racial variations in prevalence as well as seasonal and yearly variations. Low parity, low socioeconomic class and relative infertility all have associations with an increased incidence of spina bifida.

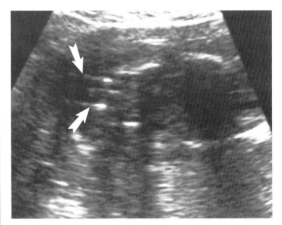

Fig. 7.7 Beam spread artefact. The posterior ossification centres are abnormally widened in this fetus with spina bifida. There appears to be the walls of a sac extending out from them (arrows). This is an artefact and can be revealed as such by scanning from a different perspective.

A few cases of spina bifida, particularly those with other anomalies also, are associated with specific causes. Abortuses with neural tube defects have a high rate of triploidy. Trisomies 13 and 18 may have spina bifida as part of their manifestations and there are also cases with partial duplications or deletions of chromosomal segments.[21]

Women with diabetes have a higher rate of malformations[22] than the general population and are said to have a risk of neural tube defect of 2%, although anencephaly is commoner than spina bifida. They have a particular risk for caudal regression syndrome.[23]

Obesity is now recognized as a separate risk for neural tube defects with the risk increasing with increasing maternal fatness. This is independent of potential confounding covariables such as maternal age, class, education, smoking and diet. There is also the suggestion that folic acid loses its protective benefit in overweight mothers.[24] A French study[25] has also shown that mothers who lose more than 2 kg in weight in the first month after conception have an increased rate of neural tube defect. They have postulated that it is the ketoacidosis associated with weight loss that is the risk factor.

The anti-epileptic drug sodium valproate in the first trimester of pregnancy causes an excess of spina bifida. American women taking the drug have a 1 to 2% chance of having an affected child.[26] There are also increased risks with carbamazepine and phenytoin and the British National Formulary[27] recommends doses of folic acid of the order of 5 mg daily to counteract this risk.

It has been shown that maternal overheating, either from exposure to hot baths or saunas[28] or from fevers,[29] in the first trimester is associated with an increased incidence of neural tube defects. However, because of the complexity of interaction of infection, fever and medication it is not possible to say which is responsible for the observed increased incidence.[30]

Other postulated risk factors have included parental occupation and recent miscarriage. A review of the published data on parental occupation[31] and a case control study on those with recent spontaneous abortion[32] failed to show any consistent relationship.

The main advance recently has been the discovery that multivitamin supplementation, and particularly folate in the periconceptual period, decrease the rate of neural tube defects, particularly in high-risk areas.[33,34] There is still argument over whether or not fortification of food with folate is required. Mothers who have had a baby with a neural tube defect are much more likely to be of lower socioeconomic status and consume less fruit, vegetables and cereals than controls.[35] Although this would appear to suggest the need for fortification of food there are other factors that are against it. Namely that neural tube defects have multifactorial causes and folate would not prevent all or even most neural tube defects, the dose of folate required in food is not known, folate might adversely affect those not at risk for neural tube defects and finally the rate of neural tube defects is declining anyway.[36] Consequently, best advice continues to be for expectant mothers to supplement their diet for 4 weeks prior to and during the early part of pregnancy.

Other trace elements are implicated in the aetiology of neural tube defects. Those living in houses with a high lead concentration in their drinking water have a greater chance of neural tube defects.[37] Lead either acts as a direct neurotoxin or by reducing the bioavailability of zinc from food. Zinc deficiency in turn impairs folate uptake. Others argue for[38] and against[39] zinc & folic whilst yet others believe it is homocysteine[40] that enables folate supplementation to work.

There is an information leaflet for prospective mothers on the use of folic acid supplementation produced by the Health Education Authority in the UK entitled 'Folic acid – what all women should know' (1996, ISBN 0 7521 0578 7).

Ultrasound features

Spina bifida can occur anywhere along the length of the spine but in the great majority of cases involves the lumbosacral region. A cohort of liveborn children between 1963 and 1968 showed 4% had sacral lesions, 59% had lumbar and lumbosacral lesions and the remaining 37% had thoracolumbar lesions.[41] A similar distribution comes from a series of 130 antenatally detected spina bifida with 23% being sacral, 64% lumbosacral, 12% thoracolumbar and 1% cervical.[42] Spina bifida cystica (Fig. 7.8) defines a sacular protrusion through a spinal defect and may be a meningocoele containing just cerebrospinal fluid (CSF) with a good prognosis (5% of total) or a myelomeningocoele containing neural elements as well as CSF (90–95% of total[43]) with a worse prognosis. Spina bifida can also be termed open (80%) or closed (20%). This

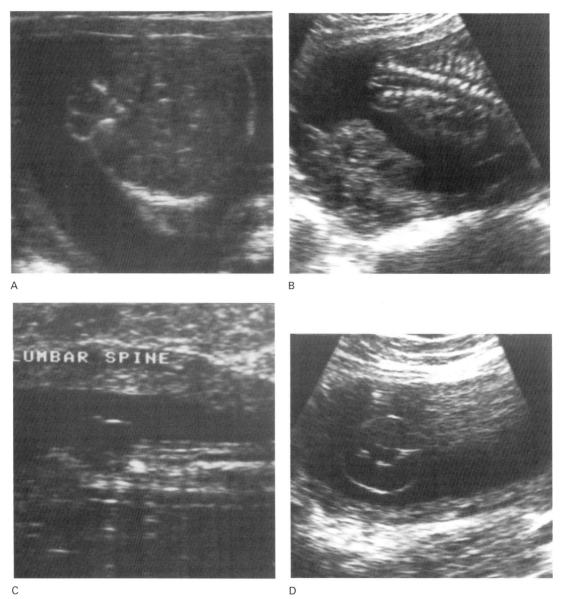

A

B

C

D

Fig. 7.8 Spina bifida cystica. (A) Axial view showing a cystic structure extending posteriorly from the spine. (B) Coronal view showing the pronounced splaying of the posterior ossification centres. (C) Sagittal view of the fetus also demonstrates the cyst. (D) Imaging plane cutting through the meningomyelocoele in isolation shows its structure.

has overlap with spina bifida cystica and can cause some confusion. An open defect is defined as either uncovered or covered with a fine translucent membrane (Fig. 7.9). A closed defect is covered either by skin or a thick, opaque membrane.[44] All spinal dysraphisms share the two features of a bony defect and caudal tethering of the spinal cord. They may be variably associated with other anomalies such as spinal cord lipoma, neurenteric cyst, intraspinal dermoid and kyphoscoliosis.

Even though the whole spine should be examined by ultrasound, it is reasonable to concentrate most effort on the lower spine where most defects are likely to occur. The axial plane will show abnormal widening of the posterior ossification centres to form an

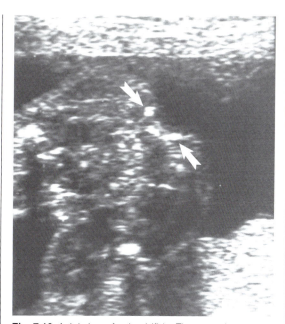

Fig. 7.10 Axial view of spina bifida. The posterior ossification centres (arrows) point outward from each other and are no longer parallel.

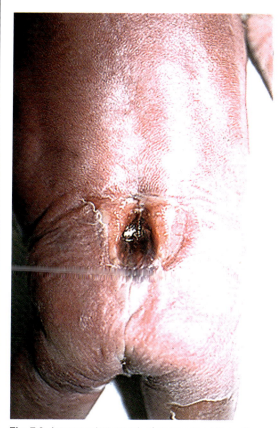

Fig. 7.9 Autopsy photograph of open spina bifida. The fine membrane that is often seen on antenatal ultrasound may collapse during delivery and not be readily appreciable at autopsy. (Courtesy of Dr Catherine Cullinane, Consultant Pathologist, St James's University Hospital, Leeds.)

open U or V shape (Fig. 7.10). The edges of these ossification centres can appear to have a sharper or more pointed edge than usual. This feature is lost if the defect is open and there has been secondary overgrowth of neural tissue consequent on its exposure to amniotic fluid (Fig. 7.11). The coronal plane will also show the abnormal splaying of the posterior ossification centres (Fig. 7.12) though care should be taken not to over-interpret the normal lumbar expansion. The loss of integrity of the overlying skin (Fig. 7.13) or the presence of a sacular protrusion can be seen in axial or sagittal planes. Modern machines can show a soft tissue defect and in some cases this is more readily demonstrable than any bony abnormality. A cystic meningeal sac often has a shimmering effect with movement of the fetus. Any loss of normal spinal curvature can be seen in the sagittal and coronal planes. The spinal defect can be readily found in cases where three or more vertebrae are involved but is more difficult for shorter lesions. In fact the features in the spine can be very subtle and it is not surprising that detection rates reported on older equipment and not using head signs

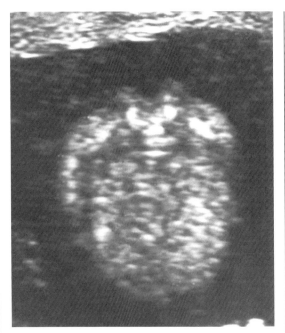

Fig. 7.11 Axial view of open spina bifida. The edges of the defect are raised owing to overgrowth of local tissue.

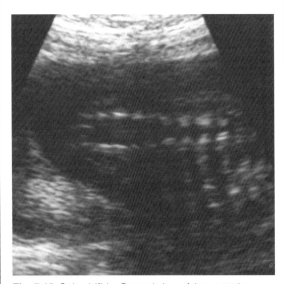

Fig. 7.12 Spina bifida. Coronal view of the posterior ossification centres showing splaying in the lumbar region over several levels. Note that these centres appear sharper than the normal ones in the thoracic region.

have been poor. Initial studies had detection rates of less than 40% with one study showing relatively inexperienced sonographers in the period 1977 to 1980 only achieving 33% sensitivity.[45]

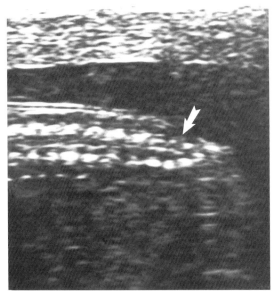

Fig. 7.13 Spina bifida. Sagittal view demonstrating a localized defect in the skin line (arrow).

All the spinal signs are most easily seen if the fetus is lying prone and does not have the placenta or uterine wall pressing against it. Normal fetal bladder filling and emptying as well as normal leg movements are to be expected and provide no help in excluding the diagnosis of spina bifida. Likewise, not all lesions found overlying the fetal spine will be due to spina bifida (Fig. 7.14).

Cranial signs

Fortunately for ultrasound users, spina bifida is associated with a number of signs that can be readily appreciated in the fetal head:

- small biparietal diameter for gestational age
- cerebral ventriculomegaly
- biconcavity of the frontal bones – the lemon-shaped head
- obliteration of the cisterna magna
- absent or abnormally shaped cerebellum – the 'banana' sign.

An early observation made in fetuses with spina bifida was the presence of a small biparietal diameter. Wald et al found the biparietal diameter to be smaller than normal in the second trimester in 20 fetuses with spina bifida,[46] and Roberts & Campbell

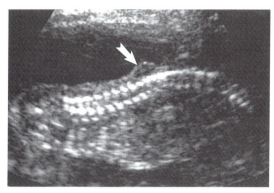

A

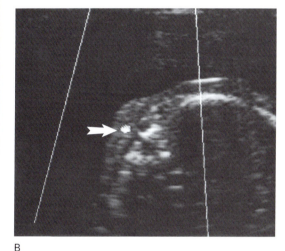

B

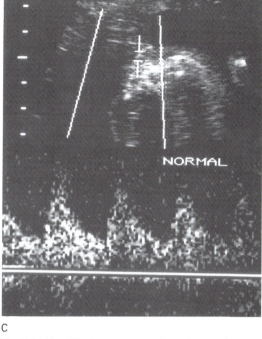

C

Fig. 7.14 Not all lesions seen over the spine are due to spina bifida. This small haemangioma was found on a routine 18-week anatomy scan. (A) Sagittal view showing a low echo lesion (arrow) protruding from the back. The adjacent spine is normal. (B) Axial view of the same region showing a small region of flow on colour Doppler (arrow). Note that the posterior ossification centres are normal. (C) Spectral Doppler trace showing low impedance flow as expected with a haemangioma.

showed this was not attributable to growth retardation.[47] Another series has shown that the biparietal diameter is reduced below the 5th centile in 43 out of 70 fetuses with spina bifida (61%), and head circumference in 26%.[48]

The finding of ventricular dilatation is another indicator of spina bifida: one-third of hydrocephalic fetuses will have spina bifida and around three-quarters of fetuses with spina bifida will have hydrocephalus by 24 weeks. The proportion of spina bifida with hydrocephalus has been reported as high as 100% in later cohorts.[49] The published data mostly refer to posterior and anterior ventricular hemisphere ratios though many extrapolate these results to the use of the ventricular atrial diameter as the determinant of hydrocephalus.

The 'lemon' sign was observed incidentally by Nicolaides and his co-workers as part of an investigation into why the fetal biparietal diameter was small in fetuses with spina bifida (Fig. 7.15).[48] It appears as a scalloping or biconcavity of the frontal bones seen on an axial view of the fetal cranium in the plane required for biparietal diameter measurement. It can be artefactually produced in normal fetuses by angling down anteriorly onto the fetal orbits but this should be readily recognized as such. A lemon-shaped cranium can be seen in 98% of fetuses with spina bifida before 24 weeks' gestational age, but only in 13% of those after 24 weeks.[24] Around 1% of normal fetuses thought at high risk for neural tube defect will show this as a false-positive sign; however, none of these normal fetuses show

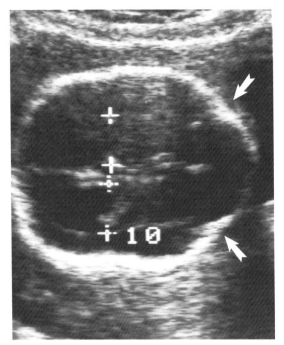

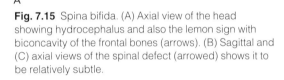

A

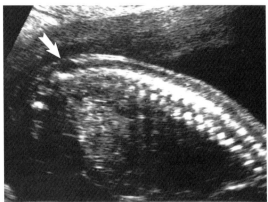

B

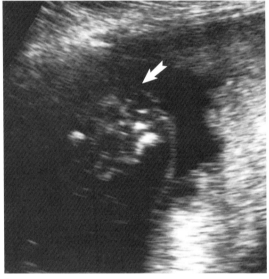

C

Fig. 7.15 Spina bifida. (A) Axial view of the head showing hydrocephalus and also the lemon sign with biconcavity of the frontal bones (arrows). (B) Sagittal and (C) axial views of the spinal defect (arrowed) shows it to be relatively subtle.

any other abnormal cranial feature.[42,50] The 'lemon' sign reliably differentiates which fetuses with hydrocephalus will have spina bifida.[51] Some reservations have been expressed regarding its use in a low-risk, general population rather than the high-risk series quoted above, as a lower positive predictive value will be present.[52] A proposed pathogenesis is that reduced intraspinal pressure or tethering of the cord at the site of the spina bifida causes downward displacement of the brain. The 'lemon' sign would arise as a result of decreased intracranial pressure and collapse of the soft frontal bones. Subsequently, the 'lemon' sign disappears in later pregnancy

either as a result of decreased deformability of the skull or from the developing hydrocephalus. This mechanism is challenged by the finding of the 'lemon' sign in fetuses with anomalies other than a neural tube defect, though an alternate hypothesis has not been put forward.[53]

The posterior fossa is abnormal in most fetuses with spina bifida. The signs are a consequence of an Arnold–Chiari malformation as part of the downward displacement of the brain described above. The cerebellum as it is displaced downward may become hypoplastic or it may disappear from the cranium. The cisterna magna becomes obliterated. The cerebellum

normally has a dumb-bell appearance
(Fig. 7.16), but in spina bifida its compression
in the posterior fossa as it is pulled down
gives rise to moulding of the cerebellar
hemispheres around the midbrain and a
curved appearance akin to a banana
(Fig. 7.17). The initial observation in a series
of 21 patients found the cerebellum to be
absent in 8 and banana-shaped in 12.[48]
Benacerraf et al in their survey of 23 fetuses
with spina bifida found 22 of them to exhibit
the 'banana' sign.[54] The one fetus with a
normal posterior fossa had a completely
skin-covered defect. Normal posterior fossas
have also been recorded in the presence of

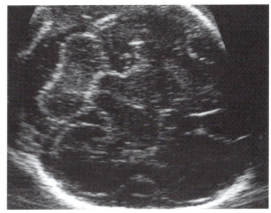

Fig. 7.16 Normal cerebellum. Axial view of the head with the plane of imaging tipped into the posterior fossa.

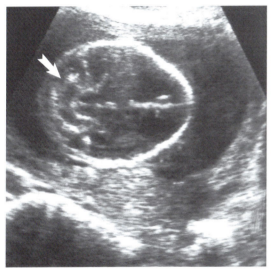

A

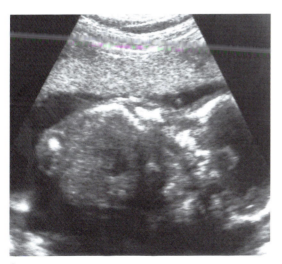

C

B

Fig. 7.17 Spina bifida. (A) Axial view of cerebellum (arrow) showing it has lost the normal dumb-bell shape and is now bowed like a banana. (B) Axial and (C) sagittal views of the high thoracic spina bifida. This fetus proved to have an abnormality of chromosome 9.

lipomeningocoeles and are to be expected with spina bifida occulta. The 130 fetuses with spina bifida evaluated by Van den Hof et al showed that cerebellar abnormalities were present in 95% of fetuses irrespective of gestation, but that before 24 weeks it was primarily the 'banana' sign (72%) and after 24 weeks it was absence of the cerebellum (81%).[42] A small, transcerebellar diameter indicates the presence of hypoplasia which is also associated with spina bifida (Fig. 7.18).

The presence of one of these abnormal cranial signs indicates the presence of a spinal defect; it does not have any correlation with the size of the defect. These cranial signs were initially reported in fetuses over 16 weeks' gestational age but it has been shown that the same signs can be seen using transvaginal ultrasound in fetuses of gestational age 12 to 17 weeks.[55] 8011 low-risk patients were assessed and 10 cases of neural tube defect found. Cerebellar dysmorphism (absent, small or banana shape) was found in all the 7 thoracic and lumbosacral lesions.

Abnormalities of the head are found in the majority of cases of spina bifida and in many cases are the important diagnostic clue to the presence of a subtle defect.[56] It is their recognition that has greatly improved the performance of ultrasound in detecting spina bifida and has enabled relatively rapid assessment of the neural axis in the routine, low-risk patient.

Associated anomalies

Chromosomal

Fetuses with spina bifida as their only structural anomaly have a significant rate of chromosomal anomaly. Data pulled from the records of 55 620 obstetric ultrasound examinations in Indianapolis showed 43 fetuses with isolated spina bifida in whom the karyotype was known. Seven of these 43 were abnormal, giving a rate of 16.3% compared to the expected rate of 0.3% based on maternal age alone.[57] Another series of 106 fetuses with neural tube defects (of which 62

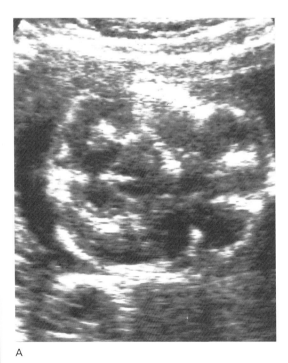

A

Fig. 7.18 Spina bifida. Two more examples (A and B) of abnormal posterior fossas with small, abnormally shaped cerebellums. Both were associated with spina bifida.

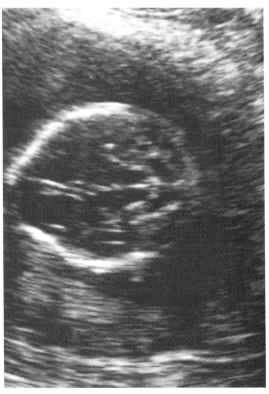

B

were spina bifida) found an overall aneuploidy detection rate of 5 to 6%, with a 2% risk in fetuses with isolated neural tube defects.[58] The majority of these were trisomy 18. Earlier reports suggesting even higher rates of chromosomal anomaly were probably biased by the small selected sample size.[59] Fetuses with other anomalies as well as spina bifida have a greater rate of karyotypic anomaly.

Neuromuscular

The commonest in utero finding in association with spina bifida is club-foot. There is also an incidence of congenital hip dislocation. Sonographic detection of absent leg movements or a fixed deformity may indicate a worse prognosis, although this is controversial. At least one study has shown that leg movement in utero cannot be used to predict how much motor function will be present after birth.[60]

Other systems

Associated anomalies have been reported in most other body systems. The commonest is the genitourinary tract. Hunt & Whitaker reported a series of 190 liveborns with neural tube defects in whom there were 17 renal anomalies. There were three renal ageneses, five horseshoe kidneys, eight ureteral duplications and one simple ureterocoele. The kidney anomalies were associated with a higher level of sensation loss, and the ureteral anomalies with a level in the sacral dermatomes.[61] Fetal mortality in fetuses with hydrocephalus is directly related to the presence of malformations outside the central nervous system.[49]

Prenatal screening

There has been a long-running debate on the most effective method of antenatal screening for neural tube defects. The options involve maternal serum alphafetoprotein (MSAFP), ultrasound, amniocentesis and various combinations of these three.

Alphafetoprotein (AFP) is a glycoprotein that is fetus specific as it is made first in the yolk sac and then in the fetal liver. Fetal serum levels peak at 12 to 13 weeks'

gestation. Normally amniotic fluid levels of AFP are low, although if there is an anomaly that causes a defect in normal fetal skin, there is passage of AFP into the amniotic fluid. MSAFP levels are also usually low, but rise gradually and peak at the 32nd week. Screening using MSAFP was pioneered in the UK.[62] Screening programmes optimally measure MSAFP between 15 and 20 weeks' gestational age and use a cut-off value of around 2.5 multiples of the median. Unfortunately, this cut-off level also includes a relatively large number of normal pregnancies giving it a low, positive, predictive value. There are other causes of elevated MSAFP other than neural tube defect, not the least of which is incorrect assignment of gestational age. Multiple pregnancy, fetal death, placental anomalies and fetal anterior abdominal wall defects also cause a raised MSAFP.[15,21] Consequently, a screening programme using MSAFP requires a second line test, either ultrasound or amniocentesis, to establish a diagnosis.

Amniocentesis is used to karyotype the fetus and to measure both amniotic fluid AFP and acetylcholinesterase. The latter is raised in open neural tube defects and almost specific. Amniocentesis carries a 0.5 to 1% risk of miscarriage so it cannot be used as a first-line screening tool.

American experience of MSAFP screening reported in the early 1980s showed that, using a cut-off of 2.5 multiples of the median, 80% of open neural tube defects could be diagnosed. Elevated values were found in up to 3.7% of pregnancies at least half of which had an obvious cause such as incorrect dates. Amniocentesis was required in 1% of all women screened and of those up to 13% had a neural tube defect.[21] This is an unacceptably high rate of amniocentesis.

Ultrasound has been shown to reliably diagnose neural tube defects in the high-risk cohort identified by MSAFP screening. Nadel et al found that ultrasound had 100% sensitivity for 51 consecutive fetuses with spina bifida, encephalocoele, gastroschisis and omphalocoele.[63] Using their lower limit of a calculated 95% confidence level for detection and applying it to those with an

MSAFP of 2 to 3.5 times the median would result in a woman having a risk of an undetected affected fetus of 0.01 to 0.15%. This is far lower than the risk of miscarriage from amniocentesis. Another study involved 20 211 patients, who had MSAFP measured, and resulted in 451 ultrasound examinations, but only 54 amniocenteses, with no loss of sensitivity.[64] A study from Glasgow showed that in 905 pregnancies with raised MSAFP, ultrasound alone detected 49 neural tube defects but missed one (98% sensitivity).[65] However, a more recent study conducted over a 6-year period showed that ultrasound detected all the cases of neural tube defect in those with raised MSAFP.[66] The same study also showed that MSAFP screening missed 10 neural tube defects in the same period. It can be concluded that ultrasound done by experienced operators is adequate to identify all neural tube defects in the high-risk population defined by MSAFP screening.

Routine sonography of all fetuses is offered in most centres in the UK, but this is not the case in the USA where argument on routine ultrasound screening still continues.[67] Proponents of ultrasound point to its better sensitivity than MSAFP screening, while opponents argue that ultrasound's sensitivity has only been shown to be good in high-risk cohorts preselected by MSAFP and that ultrasound screening would cost very much more than MSAFP screening. There are countries in which the necessary ultrasound expertise is not available and in these MSAFP performs much better than ultrasound.[68] A report from France in a region that does not have MSAFP screening but relies on ultrasound alone found that although all cases of anencephaly were detected, only 60% of spina bifida were.[69] The report concluded that their region needs an MSAFP programme as well as ultrasound. Finally, the experience reported from South Australia where both ultrasound and MSAFP are readily available showed that detection rates for spina bifida are best when results from both are pooled rather than just relying on one or the other.[70] This is in accord with experience in the Northern Region in the UK.[71]

In conclusion, prenatal screening for spina bifida is best when both routine ultrasound and MSAFP screening are available.[72] Different practices are constrained by the availability of the relevant expertise and adequate funds. Fortunately MSAFP screening has been given a lease of life by the advent of the 'triple test' for chromosomal anomalies of which it forms a part.

Prognosis and recurrence risk

Data on prognosis are nowadays skewed by the effectiveness of prenatal detection and because most parents opt for termination of pregnancy. Series from before prenatal screening was available show that the best prognosis occurs with the lowest level of lesion, closed lesions and lesions containing CSF only rather than neural elements.[41] Approximately 25% of fetuses with spina bifida will be stillborn. Early, aggressive, surgical treatment with closure of the defect results in more survivors in the neonatal period but these survivors will be more handicapped.[43] Only 17 out of 100 liveborns can expect to survive into their teens without operation. Intelligence depends on the presence or absence of hydrocephalus. Infants who do not require CSF shunting have a mean IQ of 104. If they require shunting and have no complications, mean IQ is 91, but if complications of shunting occur, the IQ mean is only 70.[73] Continence of urine and faeces is a problem. Lower urinary tract dysfunction is said to occur in 95%. An aggressive investigation plan with urodynamics, ultrasound and urinalysis followed by the use of intermittent, clean catheterization is advocated to preserve renal function.[74] The ability to walk may be achieved in many children in the first decade of life with the help of braces and calipers. However, as they grow older and heavier, they are more likely to become wheelchair bound. Divorce rates are twice as high among parents of children with spina bifida[21] (see also Ch. 6).

Recurrence rates are generally quoted as 5% after one affected pregnancy, 12% after two and 20% after three. The rates quoted in the USA are lower because of their lower overall prevalence of spina bifida.[21] Recurrence of a neural tube defect may not result in the same level and type of lesion as in the index case.

Management

If prenatal diagnosis of spina bifida is made before viability, it is appropriate to consider termination of the pregnancy. The likelihood of the parents opting for termination of pregnancy is in part related to the severity of the spina bifida, with one study showing that all fetuses with the lesion above the T9 level were terminated.[75] Adequate counselling must be available, not only before termination but also afterwards.[76] All fetuses with spina bifida require karyotyping. If a decision is made to continue the pregnancy, the fetus should be kept under regular ultrasound review to assess fetal growth and to monitor the development of any hydrocephalus. The presence of any other anomalies needs to be checked for thoroughly. The parents should be given the opportunity to visit the neonatal intensive care department and to meet the neonatologists and neurosurgeons before delivery so that an appropriate care and treatment plan can be made.

Obstetric management centres around the debate of whether elective caesarean section is required or not. Proponents of caesarean section claim it minimizes trauma to and infection of the lesion.[77] Proponents of vaginal delivery point to studies that find no difference between vaginal and caesarean delivery in neonatal morbidity and mortality, nor in developmental status at 1 year.[78]

Parents of spina bifida children in the UK may benefit from contacting The Association for Spina Bifida and Hydrocephalus (ASBAH) at ASBAH House, 42 Park Road, Peterborough PE1 2UQ (Tel. 01733 555988).

Variants

- *Rachischisis*. Complete cleft of the vertebral bodies and spinal cord.

- *Anterior sacral meningocoele*. Anterior herniation of spinal elements into the pelvis. This is usually occult and presents in the adult, predominantly in women.[79] It has been reported as a cause of obstructed labour. In the fetus, if a cyst is found in the pelvis, then commoner differential diagnoses would include ovarian cyst, enteric duplication cyst and meconium pseudocyst. A careful examination of the sacrum is required.

- *Lipomyelomeningocoele*. This usually presents as a fatty lump over the lumbosacral spine in association with spina bifida occulta. Open spina bifida may have fat within the sac as well as CSF and neural elements. It has been diagnosed prenatally by the finding of an echogenic mass within the spinal canal.[80] Splaying of the posterior elements of the spine may not necessarily be present. Surgery to the fatty lump is required as there is an incidence of tethering of the spinal cord at the lesion.

Diastematomyelia

Diastematomyelia is a mild form of spinal dysraphism in which there is a sagittal cleft in the spinal cord over a variable length with the cord reuniting below the cleft. It has been thought to be an occult lesion which presents in the infant or later. There has been an increasing number of prenatally diagnosed cases reported since the first description by Williams & Barth.[81-86]

Embryology

The occurrence of diastematomyelia is thought to relate to a persistence of the neuroenteric canal passing from Hensen's node, running in the midline of the embryonic plate and connecting the yolk sac with the amniotic cavity. Persistence would split the cord. The neuroenteric canal is also the precursor of the notochord which helps to explain the high incidence of associated vertebral anomalies.[82]

Ultrasound appearances

The ultrasound findings can be subtle. There should be localized widening of the posterior ossification centres when viewed coronally. A central, posterior, echogenic focus is found at this point of widening between the posterior ossification centres. This focus represents the bony spur or cartilaginous bar found dividing the cord, although in some cases the exact source of the echogenic focus is unclear. In these it is postulated that there may be fat between the two hemicords. In general, the echogenic focus is as bright as the adjacent ossification centres, in contradistinction to a lipomeningocoele where the echogenicity is a little less and the focus more diffuse.

Associations

Autopsy studies of myelomeningocoeles have shown diastematomyelia to coexist in 36%. Living children with surgically treated myelomeningocoele have a 5% incidence of diastematomyelia.[86] Kyphoscoliosis is also often present usually owing to associated hemivertebrae or block vertebrae (85% in one postnatal series). Skin manifestations are sometimes present above the affected area, such as excessive hair, naevus or lipoma.[83,87] There is an associated orthopaedic syndrome seen in 20% of affected children of a unilaterally weak, deformed, hypoplastic lower leg and foot,[82] of which club-foot is the likeliest manifestation to be seen in utero. It has been reported in association with maternal diabetes.[84]

Management and prognosis

Initial management requires the exclusion of any associated spina bifida. The integrity of the overlying skin and cranial signs of spina bifida should be checked. Amniocentesis to measure AFP is advocated to ensure that an open spina bifida is not inadvertently missed.[82] If there is no spina bifida, then it is not appropriate to advise termination. Babies with isolated diastematomyelia at birth may have entirely normal physical findings or may manifest cutaneous signs or the

orthopaedic syndrome. The degree of neurological deficit cannot be predicted in utero. Prenatal diagnosis allows early surgery to remove the dividing septum to prevent any neurological deterioration from tethering of the cord. Others advocate a watching policy for the first sign of neurological or musculoskeletal derangement and then to operate promptly to avoid further deterioration.[83]

Scoliosis – hemivertebrae

Longitudinal scanning of the fetal spine can demonstrate abnormal curvature. This is often caused by structural anomalies of the vertebrae which can result from failure of formation or failure of segmentation. Segmentation failures produce blocked vertebrae which in turn give rise to kyphosis or scoliosis and a shortening of the spine. Failure of formation of a part of the vertebra can produce hemivertebrae or butterfly vertebrae. A hemivertebra acts as a wedge in the spinal column and appears at the apex of the scoliosis.

Ultrasound appearances

Scoliosis is best recognized on longitudinal views. The angulation should be persistent despite fetal movement and changes in position (Fig. 7.19A). A coronal image through the anterior ossification centres may show displacement of one from the normal line of the others. This occurs at the apex of a curve (Fig. 7.19B). The axial view may demonstrate absence of part of the normal bony ring around the cord (Fig. 7.19C). The commonest site of vertebral anomalies is the lower thoracic region.[88] More than one vertebra or level may be affected. Anomalies of thoracic vertebrae have associated rib defects which can be seen if the plane of imaging is tangentially along the ribs.

Associations

Neural tube defects are the commonest defects associated with scoliosis (Fig. 7.20).

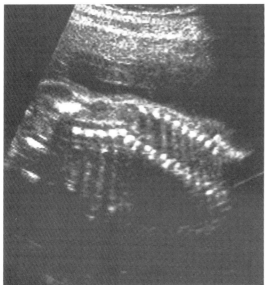

A

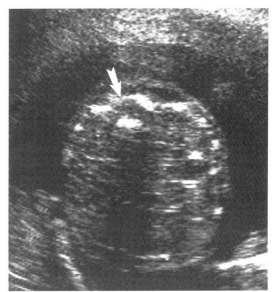

C

Fig. 7.19 Hemivertebra. (A) Coronal view showing angulation at the thoracolumbar junction. (B) Coronal view of the vertebral body ossification centres. The anomalous vertebra is displaced from the line of the others. (C) Axial view showing absence of part of the bony ring in this hemivertebra (arrow).

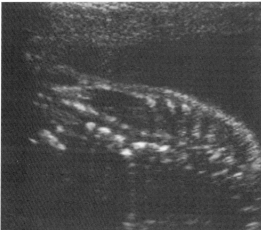

B

A series of 20 fetuses with scoliosis revealed 12 with a neural tube defect.[88] This high prevalence may have been an ascertainment bias as the cohort was collected retrospectively by examining the scans of fetuses with conditions known to be associated with scoliosis. In another study from the same group of authors, a related cohort of fetuses, in whom those with neural tube defects had been excluded, showed associated anomalies in 60%.[89] The commonest of these were renal. If the scoliosis is severe, then lethal associations such as anencephaly, limb–body wall

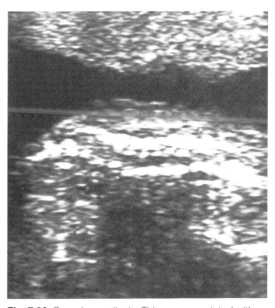

Fig. 7.20 Complex scoliosis. This was associated with a sacral spina bifida.

complex and amniotic band syndrome are more likely. If a vertebral anomaly is found, a systematic search should be made for the components of the VATER or VACTERL complex (Fig. 7.21). This consists of **V**ertebral defects, **A**nal atresia, **C**ardiovascular anomalies, **T**racheo-oesophageal fistula, o**E**sophageal atresia, **R**enal anomalies and radial ray **L**imb abnormalities. The Klippel–Feil deformity consists of a short neck and fusion of cervical vertebrae and in the antenatal group may be associated with a cervical myelomeningocoele.

Isolated vertebral anomalies are not associated with an abnormal karyotype.[89]

Management and prognosis

When a vertebral anomaly is mild and isolated, the prognosis is good.[15] Progression

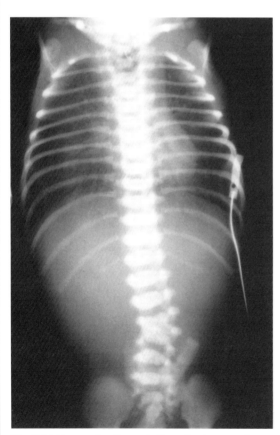

Fig. 7.21 Neonatal radiograph. There is absence of air in the abdomen because of oesophageal atresia and there are fused vertebrae in the lower lumbar spine. Both are part of the VATER association.

of the scoliosis may occur in childhood with advancing age and evaluation of the spine by an orthopaedic surgeon is required.[90] Approximately one-quarter will progress rapidly, another quarter does not progress and the remaining half progresses slowly.

The presence of associated anomalies reduces the survival to below 50%. If there is severe oligohydramnios, it is usually due to associated lethal renal disease, either agenesis or dysplasia, and mortality is 100%.[89]

There is a reported causal link between neural tube defects and scoliosis such that there is a 4% risk of neural tube defect in siblings of a child with congenital scoliosis.[91]

Sacral agenesis and caudal regression syndrome

Sacral agenesis and caudal regression syndrome are related in that the latter syndrome has variable spinal anomalies varying from partial sacral agenesis to complete absence of the lumbosacral spine. Ultrasound is the only reliable way of diagnosing these conditions antenatally as there is no open defect to raise the AFP and the chromosomes are usually normal. Caudal regression syndrome also has anomalies characteristically involving hypoplasia of the lower limbs. There may be genitourinary, gastrointestinal, cardiovascular and central nervous system abnormalities also, and in this aspect there is some overlap with the VATER constellation of anomalies.

Aetiology

Both sacral agenesis and caudal regression are strongly associated with maternal diabetes. The spectrum of anomalies is probably due to a generalized alteration in mesodermal cell migration in the primitive streak period.[92] Maternal metabolic derangement in diabetes may act through a diminished turnover of phosphoinositide or arachidonic acid.[93] These seem to have their effect in the first few weeks of pregnancy so diabetic control should be strict in this period, starting before conception. It has been estimated that caudal regression syndrome occurs 250 times more commonly in diabetic mothers. Up to 22% of fetuses with sacral agenesis will have diabetic mothers,[94] and 1% of fetuses born to diabetic mothers will have sacral agenesis.

Ultrasound appearances

The diagnosis of sacral agenesis should be made with knowledge of the normal rate of ossification of the sacral spine as discussed earlier in the chapter (Fig. 7.22). Notwithstanding this, the diagnosis has been correctly suspected at 9 weeks using transvaginal ultrasound by finding a shortened crown rump length in a diabetic mother.[95] Even so the diagnosis was not confirmed until 17 weeks' gestation.

In sagittal section the normal curve of the sacrum is lost and the spine appears shortened with an abrupt termination. If there is caudal regression, the lower limbs may be hypoplastic and the bladder may be large. In more severe cases the bones of the pelvis may be absent. A systematic search to look for associated abnormalities of club-foot, hip dislocation and scoliosis should be made. Also there may be anorectal atresia, tracheo-oesophageal fistula and genitourinary anomalies. Liquor volume should be preserved.

Differential diagnosis – sirenomelia

The condition of sirenomelia used to be thought to be part of the caudal regression sequence. The characteristic feature of this is the presence of single or fused lower limbs. Twickler et al[94] have provided evidence that caudal regression and sirenomelia are two different entities. In their series of seven patients, all those with caudal regression had two umbilical arteries, two hypoplastic lower limbs, non-lethal renal anomalies and imperforate or normal anus. Those with sirenomelia had renal agenesis, a single umbilical artery, a single or fused lower limb

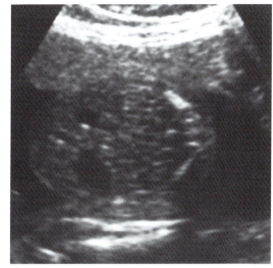

A

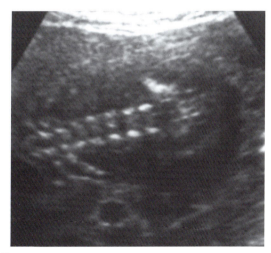

B

Fig. 7.22 Sacral agenesis. (A) axial and (B) coronal images of the sacrum in the fetus of a diabetic mother at 20 weeks' gestational age. There is poor ossification of the sacral vertebrae. There were no other anomalies and later scans showed normal ossification. This demonstrates the difficulty in differentiating delayed sacral ossification from agenesis.

and absence of the anus. The only common feature was the absence of varying amounts of the lower spine. Furthermore sirenomelia is not associated with maternal diabetes. The pathogenesis of sirenomelia has been proposed to be a vascular steal phenomenon with the single, aberrant, umbilical artery stealing blood supply from the lower torso and limbs. If there is oligohydramnios, it is more likely that the diagnosis will be sirenomelia than caudal regression. Amnioinfusion helps to better define the anatomy in this instance.[96]

Prognosis and management

The earlier in pregnancy that caudal regression is detected, the more likely it is that there will be major associated defects. The prognosis is ultimately governed by these associated defects and offering termination of pregnancy may be appropriate. Sacral agenesis has fewer associated anomalies than caudal regression and carries a greater chance of survival. Sirenomelia is uniformly fatal.

If the pregnancy is continued, then serial ultrasound scans to check growth and liquor volume are required. Surviving infants usually have normal intelligence but will require extensive urological and orthopaedic surgery. The long-term morbidity is of neurogenic bladder dysfunction leading to renal damage and disabling deficits of the lower limbs.[96] These children may have occult, correctable, intraspinal abnormalities such as a tethered cord. These should be actively sought as correction can improve bladder function.[97]

Iniencephaly

This is a rare, axial, dysraphic malformation diagnosed on the basis of three features: deficiency of the occipital bone, severe fixed retroflexion of the head and cervical rachischisis.[98] Some suggest that iniencephaly is a very severe form of the Klippel–Feil anomaly.

Ultrasound appearances

There are still a steady trickle of case reports of the antenatal diagnosis of iniencephaly.[99–102] Ultrasound will show the fetal occiput to be adjacent to the thoracic spine because of the profound fixed hyperextension. The spine will appear shortened with a kyphoscoliosis such that the head appears relatively large compared to the body. There may be associated anencephaly or myelomeningocoele. The earliest reported diagnosis was made at 13 weeks' menstrual age using transvaginal ultrasound.[103]

Associated anomalies

84% of cases of iniencephaly will have associated defects. There are many which can be listed: anencephaly, encephalocoele, hydrocephalus, microcephaly, holoprosencephaly, posterior fossa cysts, spina bifida, cyclopia, mandibular atresia, facial clefts, cardiac anomalies, genitourinary anomalies, diaphragmatic hernia, anterior abdominal wall defects, arthrogryposis, club-foot and single umbilical artery.[104,105]

Management and prognosis

Iniencephaly is almost invariably fatal. There have been a few reports of survivors in those who do not have severe associated defects.[100,101] Consequently management is dictated by the presence of associated anomalies and the severity of hyperextension. It is appropriate to offer termination of pregnancy when diagnosed before viability. If the pregnancy progresses to labour, then obstruction may result from an abnormal presentation caused by the hyperextension.

Sacrococcygeal teratoma

Sacrococcygeal teratoma is the most common congenital tumour and has an incidence of 1 in 40 000 live births.[106] The tumour has a predilection for females with 75% occurring in girls and 25% in boys.[107]

Embryology

Sacrococcygeal teratomas originate from an area of the primitive streak called the primitive knot or Hensen's node. As the mesoderm rapidly proliferates, the primitive streak comes to lie more and more caudally where the remnant of Hensen's node descends to the tip of the coccyx on its anterior surface.[108] Normally it undergoes degenerative changes and disappears but occasionally it persists and may give rise to a sacrococcygeal teratoma. The node contains pluripotential stem cells and so the tumour can contain tissues from the ectoderm, mesoderm and endoderm.[108]

Classification

Sacrococcygeal teratoma is classified into four types depending on the location and the amount of tumour that is intra-abdominal.

Type I describes tumours that are predominantly external with only a minimal presacral component. Type II tumours are predominantly external but have a significant intrapelvic extension. Type III tumours are also external but the major component is pelvic and intra-abdominal and Type IV tumours are totally intra-abdominal (Fig. 7.23).[107] The majority of sacrococcygeal teratomas (82%) are benign; however, malignancy rates are higher in the totally abdominal tumours (Type IV) at 38% compared to 8% for the totally external (Type I) tumours.[107]

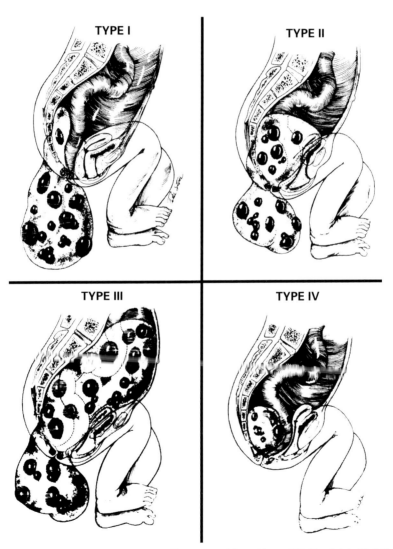

Fig. 7.23 Classification of sacrococcygeal teratomas. (Reproduced from Altman RP, Randolph JG, Lilly JR. Sacrococcygeal teratoma. American Academy of Paediatrics surgical section survey – 1973. Journal of Pediatric Surgery 1974; 9:389–398.)

Ultrasound appearances

Sonographically, a sacrococcygeal teratoma can be solid (Fig. 7.24), mixed cystic and solid or predominantly cystic (Fig. 7.25).[109,110–112] The cystic components are usually CSF spaces arising from choroid plexus elements within the tumour mass.[113] Demonstration of the intra-abdominal extension can be difficult but may be suggested if the bladder is displaced anteriorly or superiorly. Recent studies have shown that magnetic resonance imaging may be superior to ultrasound in assessing the intra-abdominal extension in Type II and Type III tumours.[114] Type IV tumours have been reported but the two cases described were predominantly cystic in nature.[108,115]

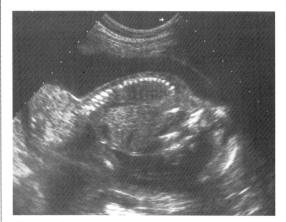

Fig. 7.24 Sacrococcygeal teratoma. A predominantly solid sacrococcygeal tumour.

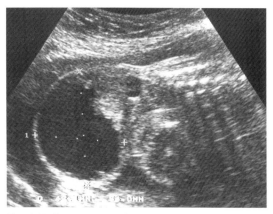

Fig. 7.25 Sacrococcygeal teratoma. A predominantly cystic tumour.

Associated abnormalities

Associated abnormalities are seen in up to 18% of cases[107] but no specific pattern has been reported. Anomalies described include anencephaly, spina bifida, cleft palate, and oesophageal and duodenal atresia.[116] Direct compression of the bladder may produce bladder outlet obstruction and bilateral hydronephrosis.[117] In addition, rapidly growing tumours can lead on to polyhydramnios, placentomegaly and hydrops. These findings may be caused by mechanical obstruction of the umbilical vessels by the tumour, chronic haemorrhage into the tumour causing fetal anaemia or from high output cardiac failure secondary to the high vascularity of certain tumours.[118]

Differential diagnosis

The differential diagnosis of a cystic, predominantly external, tumour (Type I) should include a meningomyelocoele; however, the absence of intracranial abnormalities should exclude the diagnosis. In the case of cystic intra-abdominal tumours there is a wide differential including ovarian cysts, haematometra, duplication cysts (see Ch. 11) and an anterior meningocoele. A recent report has documented a neuroectodermal cyst mimicking an intra-abdominal sacrococcygeal teratoma.[119]

Prognosis and management

When the initial diagnosis of sacrococcygeal teratoma is made, a careful ultrasound examination should be carried out to exclude associated anomalies.

Following this, the fetus should be monitored regularly during pregnancy to assess tumour growth and to detect the development of polyhydramnios or fetal hydrops.

The majority of fetuses with sacrococcygeal teratoma have a good outcome following surgery in the neonatal period. Most authors advise elective caesarean section if the tumour is large to avoid the complications of distocia and possible damage to the tumour which can lead to haemorrhage and neonatal complications.[106]

A small proportion of tumours are rapidly growing and progress to hydrops, polyhydramnios and fetal demise.[102,121] In addition, the fetal hydrops may also precipitate a pre-eclampsia-type condition in the mother with symptoms of vomiting, hypertension, peripheral oedema, proteinuria and pulmonary oedema. This condition is similar to the 'mirror syndrome' previously described in Rhesus disease in which the status of the mother begins to 'mirror' the condition of the fetus.[121] In this condition, premature delivery of the fetus may be necessary for maternal indications.[121]

As the outcome for this group of fetuses is so poor, certain groups have advocated either open fetal surgery[120–122] to remove the tumour or laser therapy to obliterate the feeding vessels to the tumour and to improve the fetal circulation.[123] In the absence of fetal intervention, the outcome for this group of fetuses is poor with a high, associated, maternal morbidity.

Surgery for sacrococcygeal teratoma is usually carried out early in the neonatal period as there is a risk of malignant transformation if surgery is delayed.

Acknowledgement

Figures 7.1A,B, 7.2, 7.3, 7.4A,B, 7.5, 7.6A,B, 7.7, 7.8A–D, 7.10, 7.11, 7.12, 7.13, 7.14A–C, 7.15A–C, 7.16, 7.17A–C, 7.18A,B, 7.19A–C, 7.20, 7.21 and 7.22A,B are © Medical Illustration, St James's University Hospital, Leeds.

References

Introduction

1. EUROCAT Working Group. Prevalence of neural tube defects in 16 regions of Europe, 1980–1983. Int J Epidemiol 1987; 16:246–251.
2. EUROCAT Working Group. Prevalence of neural tube defects in 20 regions of Europe and the impact of prenatal diagnosis, 1980–1986. J Epidemiol Community Health 1991; 45:52–58.
3. MacMahon B, Yen S. Unrecognised epidemic of anencephaly and spina bifida. Lancet 1971; i:31–33.
4. Fowlie A, Constantine G. The central nervous system. In: Dewbury K, Meire H, Cosgrove D, eds. Ultrasound in obstetrics and gynaecology. Edinburgh: Churchill Livingstone; 1993: 274.
5. Dolk H, De Wals P, Gillerot Y, et al. Heterogeneity of neural tube defects in Europe: The significance of site of defect and presence of other major anomalies in relation to geographic differences in prevalence. Teratology 1991; 44:547–559.
6. Roberts HE, Moore CA, Cragan JD, Fernhoff PM, Khoury MJ. Impact of prenatal diagnosis on the birth prevalence of neural tube defects, Atlanta, 1990–1991. Pediatrics 1995; 96:880–883.

Embryology

7. Langman J. Medical embryology. 3rd ed. Baltimore: Williams and Wilkins; 1975; 61–63.
8. Main DM, Mennuti MT. Neural tube defects: Issues in prenatal diagnosis and counselling. Obstet Gynecol 1986; 67:1–16.
9. Filly RA. Embryologic development of the brain. In: Callen PW, ed. Ultrasonography in obstetrics and gynecology. 3rd ed. Philadelphia: WB Saunders; 1994; 189–192.
10. Seller MJ. Sex, neural tube defects, and multisite closure of the human neural tube. Am J Med Genet 1995; 58:332–336.
11. Busam KJ, Roberts DJ, Golden JA. Clinical teratology counseling and consultation case report: Two distinct anterior neural tube defects in a human fetus: Evidence for an intermittent pattern of neural tube closure. Teratology 1993; 48:399–403.
12. Garabedian BH, Fraser FC. Upper and lower neural tube defects: An alternate hypothesis. J Med Genet 1993; 58:849–851.
13. Budorick NE, Pretorius DH, Grafe MR, Lou KV. Ossification of the fetal spine. Radiology 1991; 181:561–565.

Normal appearances

14. Gray DL, Crane JP, Rudloff MA. Prenatal diagnosis of neural tube defects: origin of midtrimester vertebral ossification centers as determined by sonographic waterbath studies. J Ultrasound Med 1988; 7:421–427.
15. Budorick NE, Pretorius DH, Nelson TR. Sonography of the fetal spine: Technique, imaging findings, and clinical implications. AJR 1995; 164:421–428.
16. Hawass ND, El-Badawi MG, Fatani JA, et al. Myelographic study of the spinal cord ascent during fetal development. AJNR 1987; 8:691–695.
17. Weber TM, Hertzberg BS, Bowie JD. Transperineal US: Alternative technique to improve visualization of the presenting fetal part. Radiology 1991; 179:747–750.
18. Mueller GM, Weiner CP, Yankowitz J. Three-dimensional ultrasound in the evaluation of fetal head and spine anomalies. Obstet Gynecol 1996; 88:372–378.
19. Filly RA, Simpson GF, Linkowski G. Fetal spine morphology and maturation during the second trimester. Sonographic evaluation. J Ultrasound Med 1987; 6:631–637.
20. Dennis MA, Drose JA, Pretorius DH, Manco-Johnson ML. Normal fetal sacrum simulating spina bifida: 'pseudodysraphism'. Radiology 1985; 155:751–754.

Spinal bifida: aetiology

21. Main DM, Mennuti MT. Neural tube defects: Issues in prenatal diagnosis and counselling. Obstet Gynecol 1986; 67:1–16.
22. Kalter H. Case reports of malformations associated with maternal diabetes: History and critique. Clin Genet 1993; 43:174–179.
23. Twickler D, Budorick N, Pretorius D, Grafe M, Currarino G. Caudal regression versus sirenomelia: Sonographic clues. J Ultrasound Med 1993; 12:323–330.
24. Prentice A, Goldberg G. Maternal obesity increases congenital malformations. Nutr Rev 1996; 54:146–150.
25. Robert E, Francannet C, Shaw G. Neural tube defects and maternal weight reduction in early pregnancy. Reprod Toxicol 1995; 9:57–59.
26. US Department of Health and Human Sciences, Public Health Service/Centers for Disease Control. Valproate: A new cause of birth defects – Report from Italy and follow up from France. MMWR 1983; 32:438.
27. British National Formulary 1996; 32:204. London: British Medical Association.
28. Milunsky A, Ulcickas M, Rothman KJ, Willett W, Jick SS, Jick H. Maternal heat exposure and neural tube defects. JAMA 1992; 268:882–885.
29. Sharma JB, Gulati N. Potential relationship between Dengue fever and neural tube defects in a northern district of India. Int J Gynaecol Obstet 1992; 39:291–295.
30. Lynberg MC, Khoury MJ, Lu X, Cocian T. Maternal flu, fever, and the risk of neural tube defects: A population-based case-control study. Am J Epidemiol 1994; 140:244–255.
31. Blatter BM, van der Star M, Roeleveld N. Review of neural tube defects: Risk factors in parental occupation and the environment. Environ Health Perspect 1994; 102:140–145.
32. Kurinczuk JJ, Clarke M. A case-control study to investigate the role of recent spontaneous abortion in the aetiology of neural tube defects. Paediatr Perinat Epidemiol 1993; 7:167–176.
33. Laurence KM, James N, Miller M, Tennant GB, Campbell H. Double blind randomised controlled trial of folate treatment before conception to prevent neural tube defects. BMJ 1981; 282:1509–1511.
34. Mulinare J, Cordero JF, Erickson JD, Berry RJ. Periconceptual use of multivitamins and the occurrence of neural tube defects. JAMA 1988; 260:3141–3145.
35. Friel JK, Frecker M, Fraser FC. Nutritional patterns of mothers of children with neural tube defects in Newfoundland. Am J Med Genet 1995; 55:195–199.
36. Gaull GE, Testa CA, Thomas PR, Weinreich DA. Fortification of the food supply with folic acid to prevent neural tube defects is not yet warranted. J Nutr 1996; 126:773S–780S.
37. Bound JP, Harvey PW, Francis BJ, Awwad F, Gatrell AC. Involvement of deprivation and environmental lead in neural tube defects: a matched case-control study. Arch Dis Child 1997; 76:107–112.
38. McMichael AJ, Dreosti IE, Ryan P, Robertson EF. Neural tube defects and maternal serum zinc and copper concentrations in mid-pregnancy: A case control study. Med J Australia 1994; 161:478–482.
39. Hambidge M, Hackshaw A, Wald N. Neural tube defects and serum zinc. Br J Obstet Gynaecol 1993; 100:746–749.
40. Mills JL, Scott JM, Kirke PN, et al. Homocysteine and neural tube defects. J Nutr 1996; 126:756S–760S.

Spina bifida: ultrasound features

41. Ames MD, Schut L. Results of treatment of 171 consecutive myelomeningoceles – 1963 to 1968. Pediatrics 1972; 50:466–470.
42. Van den Hof MC, Nicolaides KH, Campbell J, Campbell S. Evaluation of the lemon and banana signs in one hundred thirty fetuses with open spina bifida. Am J Obstet Gynecol 1990; 162:322–327.
43. Laurence KM. Effect of early surgery for spina bifida cystica on survival and quality of life. Lancet 1974; i:301–304.
44. Nyberg DA, Mack LA. The spine and neural tube defects. In: ultrasound of fetal anomalies. Chicago: Year Book Medical Publishers; 1990: 164.
45. Roberts CJ, Hibbard BM, Roberts EE, et al. Diagnostic effectiveness of ultrasound in detection of neural tube defect. Lancet 1983; ii:1068–1069.
46. Wald N, Cuckle H, Boreham J, Stirrat G. Small biparietal diameter of fetuses with spina bifida: implications for antenatal screening. Br J Obstet Gynaecol 1980; 87:219–221.
47. Roberts AB, Campbell S. Small biparietal diameter of fetuses with spina bifida: implications for antenatal screening. Br J Obstet Gynaecol 1980; 87:927–928.
48. Nicolaides KH, Campbell S, Gabbe SG, Guidetti R. Ultrasound screening for spina bifida: cranial and cerebellar signs. Lancet 1986; ii:72–74.
49. Nyberg DA, Mack LA, Hirsh J, Pagon RO, Shepard TH. Fetal hydrocephalus: sonographic detection and clinical significance of associated anomalies. Radiology 1987; 163:187–191.
50. Campbell J, Gilbert WM, Nicolaides KH, Campbell S. Ultrasound screening for spina bifida: Cranial and cerebellar signs in a high risk population. Obstet Gynecol 1986; 70:247–250.
51. Penso C, Redline RW, Benacerraf BR. A sonographic sign which predicts which fetuses with hydrocephalus have an associated neural tube defect. J Ultrasound Med 1987; 6:307–311.
52. Filly RA. The 'lemon' sign: a clinical perspective. Radiology 1988; 167:573–575.
53. Ball RH, Filly RA, Goldstein RB, Callen PW. The lemon sign: Not a specific indicator of myelomeningocele. J Ultrasound Med 1993; 12:131–134.
54. Benacerraf BR, Stryker J, Frigoletto Jr FD. Abnormal US appearance of the cerebellum (banana sign): indirect sign of spina bifida. Radiology 1989; 171:151–153.
55. Blumenfeld Z, Siegler E, Bronshtein M. The early diagnosis of neural tube defects. Prenat Diagn 1993; 13:863–871.
56. Thiagarajah S, Henke J, Hogge WA, Abbitt PL,

Breeden N, Ferguson JE. Early diagnosis of spina bifida: The value of cranial ultrasound markers. Obstet Gynecol 1990; 76:54–57.

57. Harmon JP, Hiett AK, Palmer CG, Golichowski AM. Prenatal ultrasound detection of isolated neural tube defects: Is cytogenetic evaluation warranted? Obstet Gynecol 1995; 86:595–599.

58. Hume Jr RF, Drugan A, Reichler A, et al. Aneuploidy among prenatally detected neural tube defects. Am J Med Genet 1996; 61:171–173.

59. Nyberg DA, Shepard T, Mack LA, et al. Significance of a single umbilical artery in fetuses with central nervous system malformations. J Ultrasound Med 1988; 7:265–273.

60. Warsof SL, Abramowicz JS, Sayegh SK, Levy DL. Lower limb movements and urologic function in fetuses with neural tube and other central nervous system defects. Fetal Ther 1988; 3:129–134.

61. Hunt GM, Whitaker RH. The pattern of congenital renal anomalies associated with neural tube defects. Dev Med Child Neurol 1987; 29:91–95.

Spina bifida: prenatal screening

62. UK collaborative study. Maternal serum alpha-fetoprotein measurement in antenatal screening for anencephaly and spina bifida in early pregnancy. Lancet 1977; i:1323–1332.

63. Nadel AS, Green JK, Holmes LB, Frigoletto Jr FD, Benacerraf BR. Absence of need for amniocentesis in patients with elevated levels of maternal serum alpha-fetoprotein and normal ultrasonographic examinations. N Engl J Med 1990; 323:557–561.

64. Katz VL, Seeds JW, Albright SG, Lingley LH, Lincoln-Boyea B. Role of ultrasound and informed consent in the evaluation of elevated maternal serum alpha-fetoprotein. Am J Perinatol 1991; 8:73–76.

65. Morrow RJ, McNay MB, Whittle MJ. Ultrasound detection of neural tube defects in patients with elevated maternal serum alpha-fetoprotein. Obstet Gynecol 1991; 78:1055–1057.

66. Kyle PM, Harman CR, Evans JA, et al. Life without amniocentesis: Elevated maternal serum alpha-fetoprotein in the Manitoba program 1986–91. Ultrasound Obstet Gynecol 1994; 4:199–204.

67. Sickler GK, Nyberg DA. Neural tube defects: prenatal screening (letter). AJR 1996; 166:466 and Budorick NE, Pretorius D (Reply). AJR 1996; 166:466–467.

68. Candenas M, Villa R, Fernandez-Collar R, et al. Maternal serum alpha-fetoprotein screening for neural tube defects. Report of a program with more than 30 000 screened pregnancies. Acta Obstet Gynecol Scand 1995; 74:266–269.

69. Alembrik Y, Dott B, Roth MP, Stoll C. Prevalence of neural tube defects in northeastern France, 1979–1992; impact of prenatal diagnosis. Ann Genet 1995; 38:49–53.

70. Chan A, Robertson EF, Haan EA, Ranieri E, Keane RJ. The sensitivity of ultrasound and serum alpha-fetoprotein in population based antenatal screening for neural tube defects, South Australia 1986–1991. Br J Obstet Gynaecol 1995; 102:370–376.

71. Northern Region Survey Steering Group. Fetal abnormality: An audit of its recognition and management. Arch Dis Child 1992; 67:770–774.

72. Cuckle HS. Screening for neural tube defects. Ciba Foundation Symposium 1994; 181:253–266; discussion: 266–269.

Spina bifida: prognosis

73. Mapstone TB, Rekate HL, Nulsen FE, et al. Relationship of CSF shunting and IQ in children with myelomeningocele: A retrospective analysis. Childs Brain 1984; 11:112–118.

74. Sutherland RS, Mevorach RA, Baskin LS, Kogan BA. Spinal dysraphism in children: An overview and an approach to prevent complications. Urology 1995; 46:294–304.

Spina bifida: management

75. Grevengood C, Shulman LP, Dungan JS, et al. Severity of abnormality influences decision to terminate pregnancies affected with fetal neural tube defects. Fetal Diagn Ther 1994; 9:273–277.

76. White-Van Mourik MC, Connor JM, Ferguson-Smith MA. Patient care before and after termination of pregnancy for neural tube defects. Prenat Diagn 1990; 10:497–505.

77. Chervenack FA, Duncan C, Ment LR, et al. Perinatal management of meningomyelocele. Obstet Gynecol 1984; 63:376–380.

78. Bensen JT, Dillard RG, Burton BK. Open spina bifida: Does Cesarean section delivery improve prognosis. Obstet Gynecol 1988; 71:532–534.

Spina bifida: variants

79. Kofinas AD, Hatjis CG, Ernest JM, Parker RL. Anterior sacral meningocele in pregnancy. Obstet Gynecol 1987; 69:441–444.

80. Chreston J, Sherman SJ. Sonographic detection of lipomyelomeningocele: A retrospective documentation. JCU 1997; 25:50–51.

Diastematomyelia

81. Williams RA, Barth RA. In utero sonographic recognition of diastematomyelia. AJR 1985; 144:87–88.

82. Winter RK, McKnight L, Byrne RA, Wright CH. Diastematomyelia. Prenatal ultrasonic appearances. Clin Rad 1989; 40:291–294.

83. Caspi B, Gorbacz S, Appelman Z, Elchalal U. Antenatal diagnosis of diastematomyelia. JCU 1990; 18:721–725.

84. Pachi A, Maggi E, Giancotti A, et al. Prenatal sonographic diagnosis of diastematomyelia in a diabetic woman. Prenat Diagn 1992; 12:535–539.

85. Boulot P, Ferran JL, Charlier C, et al. Prenatal diagnosis of diastematomyelia. Pediatr Radiol 1993; 23:67–68.

86. Anderson NG, Jordan S, MacFarlane MR, Lovell-Smith M. Diastematomyelia: Diagnosis by prenatal sonography. AJR 1994; 163:911–914.

87. Yamada S, Mandybur GT, Thompson JR. Dorsal midline proboscis associated with diastematomyelia and tethered cord syndrome. Case report. J Neurosurg 1996; 85:709–712.

Scoliosis: hemivertebrae

88. Harrison LA, Pretorius DH, Budorick NE. Abnormal spinal curvature in the fetus. J Ultrasound Med 1992; 11:473–479.

89. Zelop CM, Pretorius DH, Benacerraf BR. Fetal hemivertebrae: Associated anomalies, significance and outcome. Obstet Gynecol 1993; 81:412–416.

90. McMaster MJ, Ohtuka K. The natural history of congenital scoliosis. J Bone Joint Surg 1982; 64:1128–1147.

91. Connor JM, Connor AN, Connor RAC, Tolmie JL, Yeung B, Goudie D. Genetic aspects of early childhood scoliosis. Am J Med Genet 1987; 27:412–424.

Sacral agenesis and caudal regression syndrome

92. Depraetere M, Dehauwere R, Marien P, Fryns JP. Severe axial mesodermal dysplasia spectrum in the infant of a diabetic mother. Genet Couns 1995; 6:303–307.

93. Goto MP, Goldman AS. Diabetic embryopathy. Curr Opin Paediatr 1994; 6:486–491.

94. Twickler D, Budorick N, Pretorius D, Grafe M, Currarino G. Caudal regression versus sirenomelia: sonographic clues. J Ultrasound Med 1993; 12:323–330.

95. Baxi L, Warren W, Collins MH, Timor-Tritsch IE. Early detection of caudal regression syndrome with transvaginal scanning. Obstet Gynecol 1990; 75:486–489.

96. Adra A, Cordero D, Mejides A, Yasin S, Salman F, O'Sullivan MJ. Caudal regression syndrome: Etiopathogenesis, prenatal diagnosis and perinatal management. Obstet Gynecol Survey 1994; 49:508–516.

97. Muthukumar N. Surgical treatment of non-progressive neurological deficits in children with sacral agenesis. Neurosurgery 1996; 38:1133–1138.

Iniencephaly

98. Scherrer CC, Hammer F, Schinzel A, Briner J. Brainstem and cervical cord dysraphic lesions in iniencephaly. Pediatr Pathol 1992; 12:469–476.

99. Shoham Z, Caspi B, Chemke J, Dgani R, Lancet M. Iniencephaly: prenatal ultrasonographic diagnosis – a case report. J Perinat Med 1988; 16:139–143.

100. Katz VL, Aylsworth AS, Albright SG. Iniencephaly is not uniformly fatal. Prenat Diagn 1989; 9:595–599.

101. Gartman JJ, Melin TE, Lawrence WT, Powers SK. Deformity correction and long term survival in an infant with iniencephaly: Case report. J Neurosurg 1991; 75:126–130.

102. Meizner I, Levi A, Katz M, Maor E. Iniencephaly. A case report. J Reprod Med 1992; 37:885–888.

103. Sherer DM, Hearn-Stebbins B, Harvey W, Metlay LA, Abramowicz JS. Endovaginal sonographic diagnosis of iniencephaly apertus and craniorachischisis at 13 weeks, menstrual age. JCU 1993; 21:124–127.

104. David TJ, Nixon A. Congenital malformations associated with anencephaly and iniencephaly. J Med Genet 1976; 13:263–265.

105. Morocz I, Szeifert GF, Molnar P, Toth Z, Csecsei K, Papp Z. Prenatal diagnosis and pathoanatomy of iniencephaly. Clin Genet 1986; 30:81–86.

Sacrococcygeal teratoma

106. Gross SJ, Benzie RJ, Sermer M, Skidmore MB. Sacrococcygeal teratoma: Prenatal diagnosis and management. Am J Obstet Gynecol 1987; 156:393–396.

107. Altman RP, Randolph JG, Lilly JR. Sacrococcygeal teratoma. American Academy of Pediatrics surgical section survey – 1973. J Pediatr Surg 1974; 9:389–398.

108. Winderl LM, Silverman RK. Prenatal identification of a completely cystic internal sacrococcygeal teratoma (Type IV). Ultrasound Obstet Gynecol 1997; 9:425–428.

109. Flake AW, Harrison MR, Adzick NS. Fetal sacro-coccygeal tumour. J Pediatr Surg 1986; 21:563–566.

110. Holzgreve W, Ming P, Anderson R, Golbus MS. Experience with 8 cases of prenatally diagnosed sacrococcygeal teratomas. Fetal Ther 1987; 2:88–94.

111. Hogge WA, Thiagarajah S, Barber VG. Cystic sacrococcygeal teratoma: Ultrasound diagnosis and perinatal management. J Ultrasound Med 1987; 6:707–709.

112. Sheth S, Nussbaum AR, Sanders RC. Prenatal diagnosis of sacrococcygeal teratoma: Sonographic–pathological correlation. Radiology 1988; 169:131–133.

113. Ein S, Adeyemi SD, Mancer K. Benign sacrococcygeal teratomas in infants and children, a 25 year review. Ann Surg 1980; 191:382–384.

114. Kirkinen P, Partanen K, Merikanto J, Ryyanen M. Ultrasonic and magnetic resonance imaging of fetal sacrococcygeal teratoma. Acta Obstet Gynecol Scand 1997; 76:917–922.

115. Shipp TD, Shamberger RC, Benacerraf BR. Prenatal diagnosis of a Grade IV sacrococcygeal teratoma. J Ultrasound Med 1996; 15:175–177.

116. Warkany J. Congenital malformations. Chicago: Year Book Medical Publishers; 1981.

117. Elcholal U, Benschaehar I, Nadjari M, Gross E. Prenatal diagnosis of acute bladder distension associated with fetal sacrococcygeal teratoma – a case report. Prenat Diagn 1995; 15:1160–1164.

118. Schmidt KG, Silverman NH, Harrison MR, Callen PW. High output cardiac failure in fetuses with large sacrococcygeal teratoma; diagnosis by echo-cardiography and Doppler ultrasound. J Pediatr 1989; 114:1023–1028.

119. Bloechle M, Bollman R, Wit J, Buttenberg S. Neuroectodermal cyst may be a rare differential diagnosis of fetal sacrococcygeal teratoma: first case report of a prenatally observed neuroectodermal cyst. Ultrasound Obstet Gynecol 1996; 7:64–67.

120. Adzick NS, Crombleholme TM, Morgemar M, Quinn TM. A rapidly growing fetal teratoma. Lancet 1997; 349:538.

121. Langer JC, Harrison MR, Schmidt KG, Silverman NH, et al. Fetal hydrops and death from sacrococcygeal teratoma: Rationale for fetal surgery. Am J Obstet Gynecol 1989; 160:1145–1150.

122. Bullard KM, Harrison MR. Before the horse is out of the barn: fetal surgery for hydrops. Semin Perinatol 1995; 19:462–473.

123. Hecker K, Hackeloer BJ. Intrauterine endoscopic laser surgery for fetal sacrococcygeal teratoma. Lancet 1996; 347:470.

CHAPTER 8

Cardiac abnormalities

Gurleen Sharland

Introduction

The earliest experiences with ultrasound examination of the fetal heart were obtained using time-motion and B-mode recording and in the late 1970s advances in the resolution of real time equipment allowed clear visualization of the structure of the moving heart.[1-3] Detailed descriptions of the cross-sectional appearance of the normal human fetal heart were published by several authors in 1980.[4-6] Since the early descriptions, imaging systems have improved and now allow a high degree of diagnostic accuracy in the detection of congenital heart disease from the mid-trimester of pregnancy.[7,8] The addition of pulsed and colour flow Doppler to the study adds further information to the cross-sectional images.[9,10]

Embryology of the human heart

Heart development is first seen in embryos of 18 or 19 days.[11] In the cardiogenic area, aggregation of the splanchnic mesenchymal cells occurs producing two cellular strands, which become canalized to form two, thin-walled, endocardial tubes. These heart tubes gradually approach each other and fuse to form a single heart tube. As the heart tubes fuse, the mesenchyme around them thickens to form a myoepicardial mantle. This will give rise to the myocardium and the epicardium, whereas the inner endocardial tube will become the endocardium. The tubular heart then elongates and develops alternate dilatations and constrictions. The primordia of the bulbus cordis, ventricle and atrium appear first, but the truncus arteriosus and the sinus venosus can soon be recognized. The truncus arteriosus is continuous caudally with the bulbus cordis and cranially it enlarges to form the aortic sac which gives rise to the aortic arches. The sinus venosus receives the umbilical, vitelline and common cardinal veins. As the bulbus cordis and

ventricle grow faster than the other regions, the heart tube bends upon itself forming a loop.

Partitioning of the atrioventricular canal, the atrium and ventricle begins around the 4th week and is complete by the end of the 5th week. During the 4th week, bulges (atrioventricular, endocardial cushions) form on the dorsal and ventral walls of the atrioventricular canal. During the 5th week these grow towards each other and fuse, forming the atrioventricular septum. The primitive atrium is divided into right and left by the formation and subsequent fusion of two septa, the septum primum and the septum secundum. The septum primum also fuses with atrioventricular septum. Division of the primitive ventricle into right and left ventricles is first indicated by a muscular ridge or fold, the interventricular septum and is usually complete by 7 weeks. The method of closure of the interventricular septum links the aorta to the left ventricle and the pulmonary artery to the right. Development of the two great arteries occurs in the 5th week when bulges form in the walls of the bulbus cordis and in the truncus arteriosus. The truncal ridges are continuous with the bulbar ridges and form a spiral aorto-pulmonary septum when they fuse. This septum divides the bulbus cordis and truncus arteriosus into two channels, the aorta and pulmonary trunk. Because of the spiral nature of this septum, the pulmonary trunk twists around the ascending aorta.

Conventional teaching suggests that the heart is formed by the 8th to 10th week of pregnancy. However, some of the conventional ideas about the embryology of congenital heart disease have been disproved by the observations made by fetal echocardiography. It has been observed that obstructive lesions of any of the cardiac valves can be a dynamic and progressive process.[12,13] It therefore seems likely that abnormalities where the connections are inappropriate are related to an early insult, whereas obstructive valve lesions can develop in severity throughout gestation.

Examining the fetal heart

Many of the major cardiac malformations affect the connections of the heart and it is therefore easiest to consider examination of the fetal heart by examining the cardiac connections. Additional cardiac anomalies can be sought once the major connections have been checked.

Essentially there are six connections to consider, three on each side of the heart. These are the veno-atrial connection, the atrio-ventricular connection and the ventriculo-arterial connection. On the right side of the heart, the inferior and superior vena cavae drain to the right atrium, which then connects through the tricuspid valve to the right ventricle, which in turn gives rise to the pulmonary artery. On the left side of the heart, the left atrium receives the pulmonary veins. The left atrium then connects via the mitral valve to the left ventricle which gives rise to the aorta. The method of imaging these connections must be learnt in order to detect major forms of congenital heart disease.

Normal appearance

The 4-chamber view

Pulmonary venous connection and atrioventricular connections

The most easily obtained view of the fetal heart is the 4-chamber view. Examination of this view will demonstrate the pulmonary veins and atria, the atrioventricular connections and the two ventricles. Thus, three of the six connections are seen in this one view alone, and clues to the normality of the great arteries can be identified. Including the recognition of this view in a routine ultrasound examination can lead to the possibility of screening the whole pregnant population for major forms of congenital heart disease.[14-16] Once this section can be reliably obtained, the operator can attempt to recognize the more difficult arterial views.

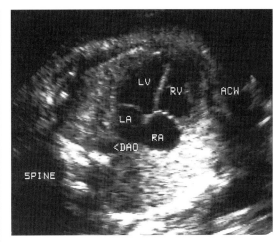

Fig. 8.1 The fetal heart is seen in a 4-chamber projection with the apex nearest to the ultrasound beam. One complete rib is visualized in the section. ACW, anterior chest wall; DAO, descending aorta; LA, left atrium; LV, left ventricle; RA, right atrium; RV, right ventricle.

Obtaining the 4-chamber view

The 4-chamber view (Fig. 8.1) is achieved in a horizontal section of the fetal thorax just above the diaphragm. One complete rib should be seen to ensure that the section is truly transverse. The heart lies mainly in the left chest with the apex pointing out of the left anterior chest wall. The apex is displaced upwards by the large fetal liver so that the right ventricle lies directly anterior to the left.

Different appearances of 4-chamber view

The appearance of the 4-chamber view will vary according to the orientation of the fetus to the ultrasound beam. Figure 8.1 illustrates the image obtained when the apex of the heart is closest to the transducer and in Figure 8.2, the normal forward flow into the ventricles with colour flow mapping is demonstrated in this orientation. In this position, the beam is parallel to the interventricular septum. In Figure 8.3, the fetal spine is more anterior and although the cardiac structures can be obscured by spinal shadowing the structures can still be seen. In Figure 8.4, the ultrasound beam is perpendicular to the interventricular septum. In this projection, the ventricular walls will appear thicker as illustrated in the image.

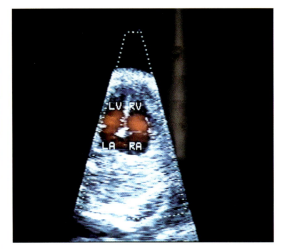

Fig. 8.2 The fetal heart is seen in a 4-chamber projection. Colour Doppler demonstrates flow from the atria to the ventricles. Flow is similar on the two sides of the heart. LA, left atrium; LV, left ventricle; RA, right atrium; RV, right ventricle.

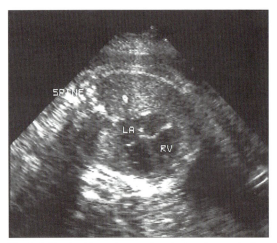

Fig. 8.3 The fetal heart is seen in a 4-chamber projection with the fetal spine nearer to the ultrasound beam. LA, left atrium; RV, right ventricle.

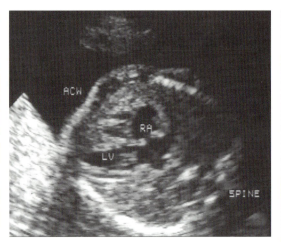

Fig. 8.4 The fetal heart is seen in a 4-chamber projection with the ultrasound beam perpendicular to the interventricular septum. In this projection, the ventricular walls appear thicker. ACW, anterior chest wall; LV, left ventricle; RA, right atrium.

Method of orientation

The same method of orientation is always used in order to identify the cardiac chambers in the normally connected and positioned heart and can be illustrated using Figures 8.1, 8.3 and 8.4. Locate the spine first. Opposite the spine is the anterior chest wall and beneath this is the right ventricle. Returning to the spine, the descending aorta is seen as a circular structure lying anterior to the spine and anterior to this is the left atrium. Once the left atrium and right ventricle have been identified, the right atrium and left ventricle can then also be identified.

If the heart is displaced, for example by a diaphragmatic hernia, the relationship of the aorta to the left atrium is more reliable than that of the right ventricle to the chest wall.

Features to note in a 4-chamber view

Important features of a normal 4-chamber view that should always be noted are:

1. The heart occupies about one-third of the thorax and the apex points out of the left anterior thorax.
2. There are two atria of approximately equal size.
3. There are two ventricles of approximately equal size and thickness. Both show equal contraction in the moving image.
4. The atrial and ventricular septa meet the two atrioventricular valves (mitral and tricuspid) at the crux of the heart forming an offset cross. This offset cross appearance is due to the fact that the septal leaflet of the tricuspid valve inserts slightly lower in the ventricular septum than the mitral valve.
5. The two atrioventricular valves (mitral

and tricuspid) are seen to open equally in the moving image.

6. The interatrial defect, the foramen ovale, is patent in fetal life. It is usually guarded by the foramen ovale flap valve, which can usually be seen flickering in the left atrium.
7. The interventricular septum should appear intact.

It should be noted that all the above features are true of the fetal heart until about 28 weeks' gestation. After this time, the right ventricle may look slightly dilated compared with the left in the normal fetus. Scanning up and down horizontally at the back of the left atrium will allow the pulmonary venous connections to the back of the left atrium to be seen (Figs 8.5 and 8.6).

Ventriculo-arterial connections

The fluid-filled lungs in the fetus allow the two great arteries (aorta and pulmonary artery) to be imaged in a variety of projections.[17] These include both transverse and longitudinal projections. The transverse views are usually the easiest views of the great arteries to obtain following on from a 4-chamber view. The longitudinal views are

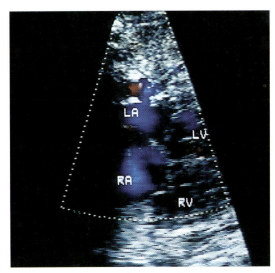

Fig. 8.6 The left upper pulmonary vein can be seen to be draining into the left atrium on colour flow mapping. The blue flow into the left atrium represents the pulmonary vein. LA, left atrium; LV, left ventricle; RA, right atrium; RV, right ventricle.

more easily recognized by those with experience of paediatric echocardiography.

Angling the transducer cranially from the 4-chamber demonstrates the aorta arising in the centre of the chest (Fig. 8.7). Angling further towards the right shoulder shows the aorta arising from the left ventricle and sweeping out into the right thorax. In this long-axis view of the left ventricle, all the left

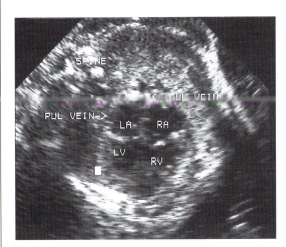

Fig. 8.5 The fetal heart is seen in a 4-chamber projection with the spine nearest to the ultrasound beam. At least two of the four pulmonary veins can be seen to be draining into the back of the left atrium. LA, left atrium; LV, left ventricle; RA, right atrium; RV, right ventricle; PUL VEIN = pulmonary vein.

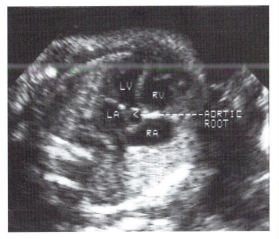

Fig. 8.7 Angling cranially from the 4-chamber view allows visualization of the aortic root in the centre of the heart. LA, left atrium; LV, left ventricle; RA, right atrium; RV, right ventricle.

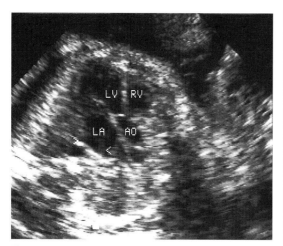

Fig. 8.8 Further angulation from Figure 8.7 towards the right shoulder demonstrates a long-axis view of the left ventricle. In this view, the left heart connections, the pulmonary veins to the left atrium (shown by the two arrows), the mitral valve between the left atrium and left ventricle, and the aorta arising from the left ventricle, can all be identified. AO, aorta; LA, left atrium; LV, left ventricle; RV, right ventricle.

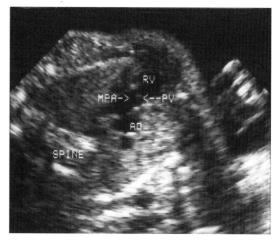

Fig. 8.9 The horizontal section cranial to the plane in Figures 8.7 and 8.8 will demonstrate the pulmonary artery. This artery arises anteriorly, close to the chest wall and is directed straight back towards the spine. The ascending aorta can be seen next to the pulmonary artery in this view. AO, aorta; MPA, main pulmonary artery; PV, pulmonary valve; RV, right ventricle.

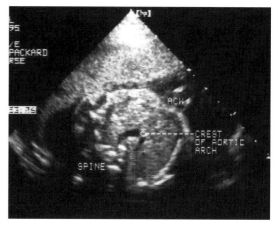

Fig. 8.10 The crest of the arch of the aorta can be seen in a section slightly more cranially than Figure 8.9. ACW, anterior chest wall.

heart connections, the pulmonary vein to left atrium, the mitral valve, between the left atrium and left ventricle, and the aorta arising from the left ventricle, can be identified (Fig. 8.8). The transverse section cranial to this plane will demonstrate the pulmonary artery (Fig. 8.9). This artery arises anteriorly, close to the chest wall and is directed straight back towards the spine. Slightly further cranially, the crest of the arch of the aorta can be seen (Fig. 8.10). Transducer angulation in the other direction from the long-axis view of the left ventricle will allow the right heart connections to be seen (Fig. 8.11). This section of the fetus demonstrates the inferior vena cava entering the right atrium, the tricuspid valve between the right atrium and ventricle, the origin of the pulmonary artery from the right ventricle and its connection to the duct. The aortic arch can also be imaged in a longitudinal section of the fetus (Fig. 8.12). The aorta normally arises in the centre of the thorax and forms a tight, hook shape with the head and neck vessels arising from the crest of the arch. Diagrammatic representation of the sections relative to the intracardiac structures for the above views is shown in Figures 8.13A–C.

Features of the aorta and pulmonary artery

The following are important features of the great arteries and allow major anomalies of the great arteries to be excluded:

1. Two arterial valves should always be seen.
2. The aorta arises from the centre of the chest and is wholly committed to the left ventricle. It gives rise to the aortic arch

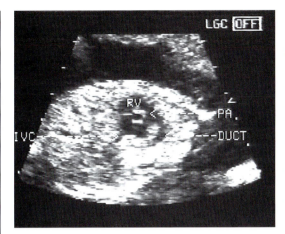

Fig. 8.11 The right heart connections are shown in this section. IVC, inferior vena cava; PA, pulmonary artery; RV, right ventricle.

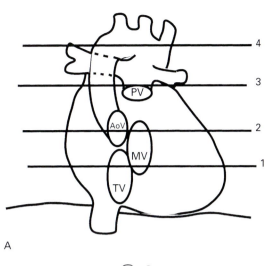

A

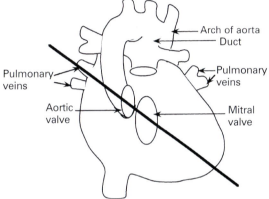

B

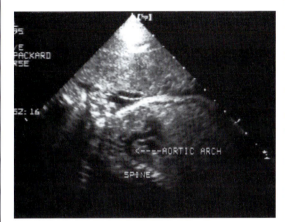

Fig. 8.12 A longitudinal section of the fetus showing the aortic arch. This arch is a tight-hooked arch and the three head and neck vessels can clearly be seen arising from it.

which can be identified by head and neck vessels.

3. The pulmonary artery arises from the right ventricle and is a branching vessel giving rise to the branch pulmonary arteries and the arterial duct.

4. The great arteries are similar in size but the pulmonary artery at the valve ring may be slightly bigger than the aorta.

5. The pulmonary valve is anterior and cranial to the aortic valve.

6. The great arteries cross over each other at their origin.

7. The arch of the aorta is of similar size to the pulmonary artery and duct and is complete.

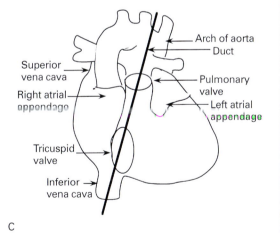

C

Fig. 8.13 Heart diagrams showing sections described in the text. (A) Horizontal sections of heart. 1 = 4-chamber view, 2 = aortic root view, 3 = pulmonary artery and duct view, 4 = crest of aortic arch. (B) Section required to obtain long-axis view of left ventricle. (C) Section required to visualize right ventricular outflow tract structures.

Systemic venous connection and situs

Abdominal situs is examined in the fetus by visualizing the aorta and inferior vena cava in transverse or longitudinal views. The inferior vena cava should lie to the right of the spine and anterior to the aorta, which lies slightly to the left of the spine (Fig. 8.14). The systemic venous connections to the right atrium (inferior and superior vena cavae) are best visualized in a longitudinal section (Fig. 8.15).

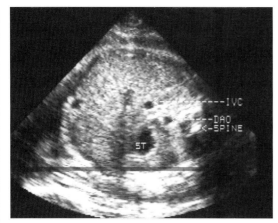

Fig. 8.14 The relationship of the descending aorta and inferior vena cava in the abdomen is shown. The inferior vena cava should lie to the right of the spine and anterior to the aorta, which lies slightly to the left of the spine. DAO, descending aorta; IVC, inferior vena cava; ST, stomach which is in the left of the abdomen.

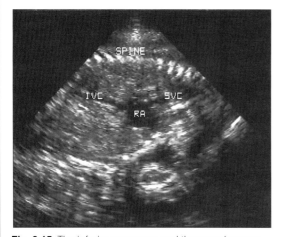

Fig. 8.15 The inferior vena cava and the superior vena cava are shown draining into the right atrium in a longitudinal section. IVC, inferior vena cava; SVC, superior vena cava; RA, right atrium.

Cardiac abnormalities

Segmental examination of the connections of the heart will allow detection of abnormalities at the veno-atrial, atrioventricular and ventriculo-arterial junctions. Additional anomalies can then also be sought.

CONNECTION ABNORMALITIES AT THE VENO-ATRIAL JUNCTION

Anomalous systemic venous connection

Abnormalities of the venous connections to the right side of the heart usually occur in the context of more complex congenital heart disease and the prognosis will be influenced by this.

Anomalous pulmonary venous connection

One or more pulmonary veins can drain anomalously to one or more of three different sites. These are intracardiac to the coronary sinus, supracardiac to the innominate vein or superior vena cava or infracardiac to the hepatic venous system and inferior vena cava. Surgical correction is required for total anomalous pulmonary venous drainage and is usually successful if the newborn is in a good condition for surgery, whereas the infant presenting later may be in severe heart failure owing to obstruction of pulmonary venous return which may develop either within the anomalous channels or at the atrial septum.

Thus, prenatal diagnosis would be expected to improve the survival rate in this malformation. Unfortunately, however, this is a very difficult diagnosis to make in the fetus.[18,19] The signs in the fetus are right atrial and right ventricular dominance, giving an abnormal appearance of the 4-chamber view. There will be no pulmonary veins seen draining to the usual sites in the left atrium and the left atrium will be small (Fig. 8.16). The coronary sinus may appear dilated if the veins are draining anomalously to the

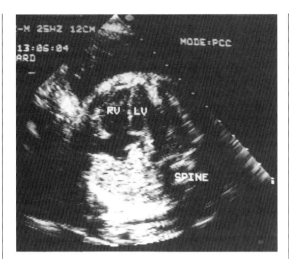

Fig. 8.16 The left ventricle is significantly smaller than the right ventricle and the left atrium appears compressed. The arrowhead indicates the normal position of the left atrium. LV, left ventricle; RV, right ventricle.

coronary sinus. In cases where the drainage is supracardiac, the degree of right ventricular volume overload will depend on the degree of obstruction to drainage and, in some cases, the 4-chamber view in the fetus may appear normal, although the pulmonary veins will not be seen draining to the left atrium. The infracardiac form is usually obstructed and right ventricular volume overload is not a feature.

Partial anomalous pulmonary venous drainage is not usually a fetal or neonatal problem as some of the pulmonary veins drain normally, protecting the fetus or neonate from serious compromise.

CONNECTION ABNORMALITIES AT THE ATRIOVENTRICULAR JUNCTION

Atrioventricular septal defect

Complete

There is a defect in the lower part of the atrial septum and the inlet part of the ventricular septum, at the crux of the heart. A common atrioventricular valve bridges the defect and there is loss of the normal differential insertion of the two atrioventricular valves.

Thus, the echocardiographic appearance is of a single valve opening into both ventricular chambers. An example of a common valve bridging the defect in systole is shown in Figure 8.17. In diastole, both atria communicate with both ventricles as illustrated in Figure 8.18.

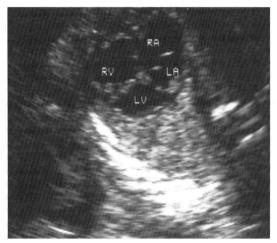

Fig. 8.17 An example of an atrioventricular septal defect with the common valve shown in systole. Note the loss of differential insertion at the crux of the heart. LA, left atrium; LV, left ventricle; RA, right atrium; RV, right ventricle.

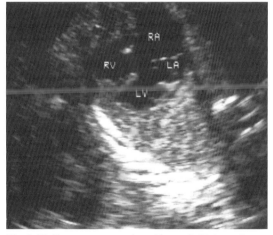

Fig. 8.18 The same example as Figure 8.17 shown in diastole with the valve open. The defect in the atrial and ventricular septa can be seen and both atria communicate with both ventricles. In diastole, both atria communicate with both ventricles. LA, left atrium; LV, left ventricle; RA, right atrium; RV, right ventricle.

Partial

The junction of the lower part of the atrial septum to the atrioventricular valve insertion is not intact. There is a defect in the lower portion of the atrial septum, the primum septum. There is loss of the normal differential insertion of the two atrioventricular valves so that they are equally positioned at the crest of the ventricular septum. An example is shown in Figure 8.19.

When the normal fetal heart is viewed directly from the apex with the atrioventricular septum in line with the ultrasound beam, there may be septal 'dropout' which resembles the appearance of a complete atrioventricular septal defect. It is therefore particularly important to obtain multiple, angled views of this region of the fetal heart.

Atrioventricular septal defects are one of the commonest forms of heart disease seen in prenatal life.[20] This type of defect is commonly associated with chromosomal anomalies, in particular with trisomy 21, although it can occur with other chromosome anomalies.[21] It is also frequently found associated with isomerism of the atrial appendages although it can occur with normal situs in patients with normal chromosomes.

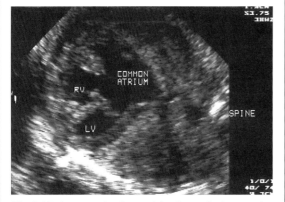

Fig. 8.19 An example of a partial atrioventricular septal defect. There is loss of the normal differential insertion of the two atrioventricular valves. There is a common atrium with no atrial septum seen, but no ventricular component is apparent. LV, left ventricle; RV, right ventricle.

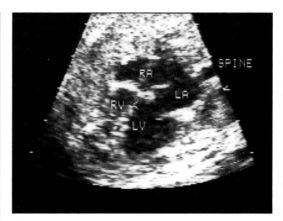

Fig. 8.20 An example of tricuspid atresia where a patent tricuspid valve is not seen and the right ventricular chamber is very small. The arrowhead points to a ventricular septal defect. LA, left atrium; LV, left ventricle; RA, right atrium; RV, right ventricle.

Tricuspid atresia

There is no connection between the right atrium and right ventricle and no opening valve can be seen between these two chambers. The 4-chamber view in the fetus will be abnormal as a patent tricuspid valve is not seen and the right ventricular chamber is small or may even be indiscernible (Fig. 8.20). Typically, there is a ventricular septal defect, which can be of variable size and the size of this will influence the size of the right ventricular cavity. In the majority, the great arteries are normally related, but they may be transposed in about 20% of cases. This is important as it will influence the prognosis. There is no flow detected across the tricuspid valve on pulsed or colour Doppler flow mapping, and there is brightly echogenic 'sulcus tissue' in the area where the tricuspid valve might be expected to be (Fig. 8.21). Tricuspid atresia is rarely associated with extracardiac anomalies.

Mitral atresia

The mitral valve is not patent in this condition and the 4-chamber view will be abnormal as an opening mitral valve is not seen and the left ventricle is small (Fig. 8.22). There is no demonstrable flow across the posterior atrioventricular valve on colour

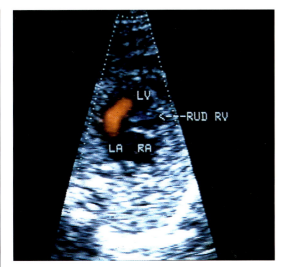

Fig. 8.21 An example of tricuspid atresia. There is no flow detected across the tricuspid valve on colour Doppler flow mapping, whereas flow can be seen from left atrium to left ventricle across the mitral valve. LA, left atrium; LV, left ventricle; RA, right atrium; RUD RV, rudimentary right ventricle.

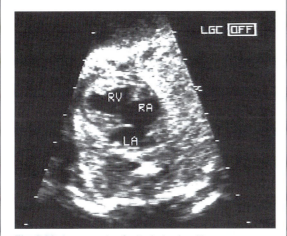

Fig. 0.22 An example of mitral atresia with an indiscernible left ventricle. LA, left atrium; RA, right atrium; RV, right ventricle.

flow mapping (Fig. 8.23). Mitral atresia can occur in three settings. It most commonly occurs in association with aortic atresia in the hypoplastic, left heart syndrome, which is discussed further under aortic atresia. Alternatively, mitral atresia can occur with a ventricular septal defect with either a normally connected but patent aorta or with double outlet right ventricle. An example of mitral atresia, ventricular septal defect and

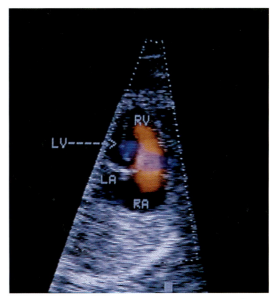

Fig. 8.23 In mitral atresia there is no demonstrable flow across the mitral valve on colour flow mapping. LA, left atrium; LV, left ventricle; RA, right atrium; RV, right ventricle.

double outlet right ventricle is shown in Figures 8.24 and 8.25. In this setting, the aorta is often malpositioned anterior to the pulmonary artery, as shown in these examples.

In fetal life, mitral atresia has a significant association with chromosomal anomalies

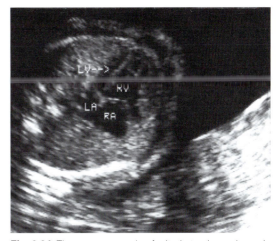

Fig. 8.24 The same example of mitral atresia as shown in Figure 8.23. The left ventricular cavity is more easily seen in this example compared with Figure 8.22. This is due to the associated ventricular septal defect. LA, left atrium; LV, left ventricle; RA, right atrium; RV, right ventricle.

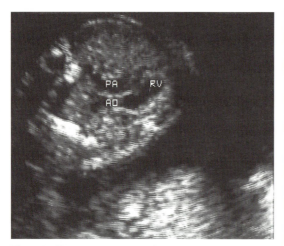

Fig. 8.25 The same example of mitral atresia as illustrated in Figures 8.23 and 8.24, showing a view of the great arteries. Both the great arteries arise from the right ventricle with the aorta being anterior to the pulmonary artery. AO, aorta; PA, pulmonary artery; RV, right ventricle.

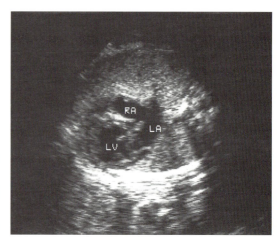

Fig. 8.26 An example of double inlet left ventricle where both the atrioventricular valves drain into the dominant left ventricle and no ventricular septum is seen dividing the ventricular mass equally between the two atrioventricular valves. LA, left atrium; LV, left ventricle; RA, right atrium.

(18%), usually trisomy 18 but 13, 21 and translocation/deletion syndrome are also possible.[20]

Double inlet ventricle

In a double inlet connection, both atrioventricular valves drain predominantly to one ventricle. In most cases there is one dominant ventricle and one rudimentary chamber. The 4-chamber view will be abnormal as no ventricular septum is seen dividing the ventricular mass equally between the two atrioventricular valves (Fig. 8.26). The flow from both atrioventricular valves drains into the same ventricular chamber which is usually of left ventricular morphology (Fig. 8.27). The great arteries are frequently transposed and arise in parallel orientation (Fig. 8.28) with the aorta arising from the rudimentary chamber (usually an anterosuperior morphologically right ventricle) which communicates with the main chamber via a ventricular septal defect.

Double inlet ventricle is rarely associated with extracardiac syndromes.

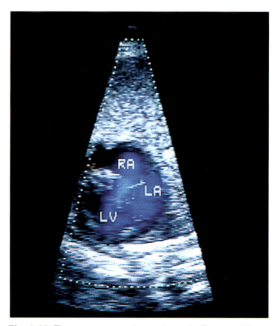

Fig. 8.27 The same example as shown in Figure 8.26. On colour flow mapping, flow can be identified across two separate atrioventricular valves draining into the same ventricular chamber. LA, left atrium; LV, left ventricle; RA, right atrium.

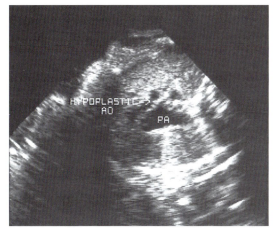

Fig. 8.28 A view of the great arteries in the same example of double inlet left ventricle as illustrated in Figures 8.26 and 8.27. The two arteries are seen arising in parallel orientation and the aorta is significantly hypoplastic in comparison with the pulmonary artery. This baby had an associated coarctation of the aorta. AO, aorta; PA, pulmonary artery.

ADDITIONAL ABNORMALITIES AT THE ATRIOVENTRICULAR JUNCTION

Tricuspid dysplasia

This condition is easily detected in the fetus because of cardiomegaly.[22] The 4-chamber view will be abnormal as a result of the cardiomegaly, which is a result of right atrial and ventricular enlargement. Tricuspid valve thickening and nodularity (Fig. 8.29) can

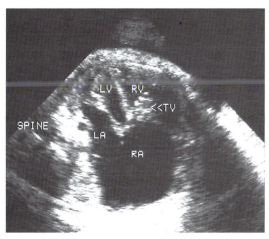

Fig. 8.29 An example of tricuspid valve dysplasia. There is marked cardiomegaly, with the right atrium in particular being enlarged. The tricuspid valve appears thickened and nodular. LA, left atrium; LV, left ventricle; RA, right atrium, RV, right ventricle; TV, tricuspid valve.

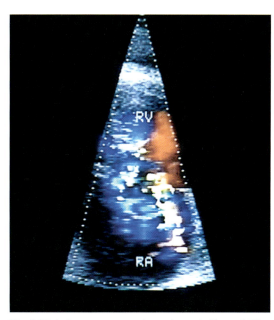

Fig. 8.30 In the same example as shown in Figure 8.29, there is marked tricuspid regurgitation seen on colour flow mapping. RA, right atrium; RV, right ventricle.

often be seen and there is a variable degree of tricuspid regurgitation (Fig. 8.30). Secondary lung hypoplasia as a result of long-standing compression from severe cardiomegaly can be a life-threatening, associated feature.

Obstruction to the right ventricular outflow tract is commonly manifest as pulmonary stenosis or atresia.

Tricuspid dysplasia can be difficult to distinguish from Ebstein's malformation, as the two overlap each other in terms of anatomical findings.[23] The differentiation is not important in fetal life as the prognosis is similar when diagnosed in utero. Tricuspid dysplasia is uncommonly associated with extracardiac lesions but chromosomal anomalies can occur.

Ebstein's malformation

In Ebstein's malformation, the attachment of the septal leaflet of the tricuspid valve is displaced into the right ventricle (Fig. 8.31). The degree of displacement is variable and a displaced tricuspid valve can sometimes be difficult to find in a severe case of Ebstein's malformation. There will be a variable

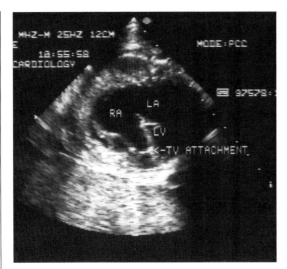

Fig. 8.31 An example of Ebstein's malformation of the tricuspid valve. The attachment of the septal leaflet of the tricuspid valve is displaced into the right ventricle and the right atrium is enlarged. LA, left atrium; LV, left ventricle; RA, right atrium; TV, tricuspid valve.

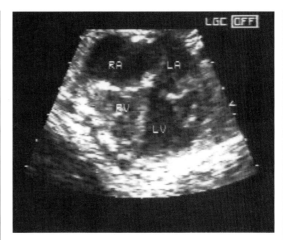

Fig. 8.32 An example of pulmonary atresia with an intact interventricular septum where the right ventricle is hypertrophied. LA, left atrium; LV, left ventricle; RA, right atrium; RV, right ventricle.

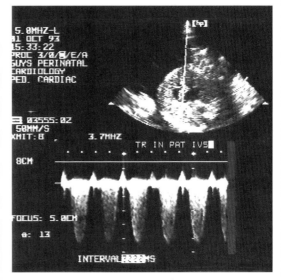

Fig. 8.33 A high velocity jet (4 m.s⁻¹) of tricuspid regurgitation detected in a case of pulmonary atresia with an intact interventricular septum.

degree of tricuspid incompetence and a variable degree of right atrial enlargement, resulting in an increased cardiothoracic ratio. This can result in secondary pulmonary hypoplasia, as in cases with tricuspid valve dysplasia. Obstruction to the right ventricular outflow tract is common. Ebstein's malformation is rarely associated with extracardiac anomalies.

CONNECTION ABNORMALITIES AT THE VENTRICULO-ARTERIAL JUNCTION

Pulmonary atresia with intact ventricular septum

The pulmonary valve is completely atretic so that there is no communication between the right ventricle and the main pulmonary artery. This condition is associated with an abnormal 4-chamber view. Usually the right ventricle is hypertrophied and contracts poorly (Fig. 8.32). The tricuspid valve movement is restricted and there may be a jet of tricuspid regurgitation at high velocity (Fig. 8.33). If the pulmonary valve can be visualized, it will be noted that it does not open. There will be no forward flow

detectable into the pulmonary artery, but reverse flow from the arterial duct is frequently seen, as the branch pulmonary arteries fill retrogradely from the duct. The pulmonary artery may be smaller than normal for the gestational age and is often smaller than the aorta.[24] Pulmonary atresia with an intact interventricular septum in the fetus can also be seen with a dilated right ventricle and tricuspid incompetence. This form is usually associated with either tricuspid valve dysplasia or Ebstein's malformation, which have been discussed above. This condition is not commonly associated with extracardiac malformations.

Aortic atresia (hypoplastic left heart syndrome)

Aortic atresia usually occurs when the aorta is arising from the left ventricle in association with mitral atresia, in the setting of the hypoplastic left heart syndrome. An example of the 4-chamber view of such a case is shown in Figure 8.22. The aortic valve is atretic so that there is no forward flow into the ascending aorta (Fig. 8.34). The left ventricle varies in size from small to slit-like and indiscernible,[25] with usually no detectable flow into the cavity. In cases where the mitral valve is severely restricted but still patent, the left ventricle may be echogenic and poorly contracting (Fig. 8.35).

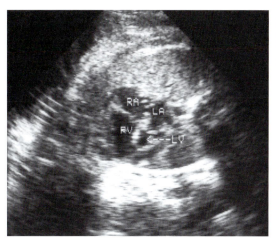

Fig. 8.35 An example of aortic atresia where the mitral valve is severely restricted but still patent. The left ventricle is small, echogenic and poorly contracting on the moving image. LA, left atrium; LV, left ventricle; RA, right atrium; RV, right ventricle.

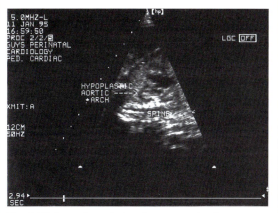

Fig. 8.36 An aortic arch view in an example of hypoplastic left heart syndrome. The ascending aorta and aortic arch are very hypoplastic.

The ascending aorta and aortic arch in this condition are hypoplastic (Fig. 8.36) and there is reversal of flow in the aortic arch (Fig. 8.37) with blood reaching the head and neck branches and the coronary arteries retrogradely from the duct. The foramen ovale may be restrictive or intact.

The hypoplastic left heart syndrome can occasionally be associated with chromosomal anomalies, particularly Turner's syndrome, but also trisomy 18 and 13. Repeated examinations of left ventricular size may therefore be required in borderline cases or where there is a family history.

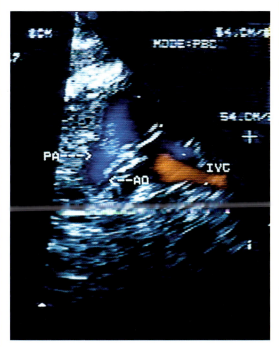

Fig. 8.34 A view of the two great arteries in hypoplastic left heart syndrome. The aorta is tiny compared with the pulmonary artery. There is no forward flow in the ascending aorta, although the normal flow in the pulmonary artery is clearly seen on colour flow mapping. AO, aorta; PA, pulmonary artery; IVC, inferior vena cava.

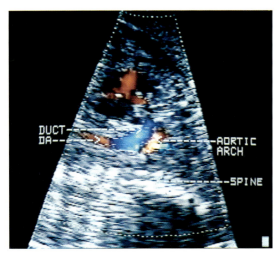

Fig. 8.37 Colour flow mapping in this example of hypoplastic left heart syndrome shows reverse flow in the aortic arch (red), whereas there is normal forward flow (blue) from the pulmonary artery into the duct and descending aorta. DA, descending aorta.

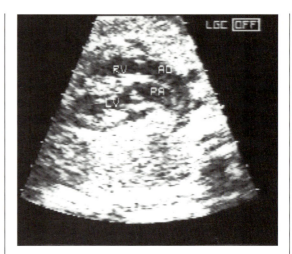

Fig. 8.38 An example of simple transposition with the aorta arising anteriorly from the right ventricle and the pulmonary artery arising from the left ventricle. The two arteries arise in parallel orientation. AO, aorta; LV, left ventricle; PA, pulmonary artery; RV, right ventricle.

Simple transposition of the great arteries

The aorta (artery forming the arch with head and neck vessels) arises from the right ventricle and the pulmonary artery (the branching great artery) from the left ventricle. The relative positions of the two arteries are abnormal as the aorta arises anterior and in parallel orientation to the pulmonary artery. The normal 'cross-over' of the great arteries is therefore not found and the two great arteries arise in parallel orientation (Fig. 8.38). The aortic arch will form a wide-sweeping arch instead of the normal, tight-hooked arch (Fig. 8.39). In simple transposition, the interventricular septum is intact. Simple transposition is rarely associated with extracardiac lesions.

Transposition of the great arteries with ventricular septal defect

The aorta arises from the right ventricle and the pulmonary artery arises from the left ventricle, as above, but there is an associated ventricular septal defect, which can be of variable size (Fig. 8.40). This condition can be associated with either pulmonary stenosis or a coarctation of the aorta. In the former, the

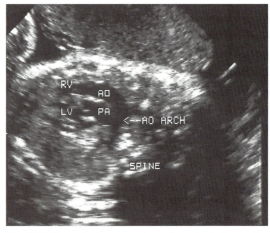

Fig. 8.39 The anterior great artery gives rise to the aortic arch in transposition. AO, aorta; AO ARCH, aortic arch; LV, left ventricle; PA, pulmonary artery; RV, right ventricle.

pulmonary valve may be thickened and the pulmonary artery will be smaller in size than the aorta. Turbulent flow across the pulmonary valve will be seen. This condition can be mistaken for double outlet right ventricle with a subpulmonary ventricular septal defect but the difference is academic rather than of great practical importance. In cases with a coarctation, the aorta is smaller than the pulmonary artery and there may be associated subaortic narrowing.

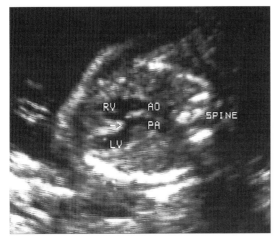

Fig. 8.40 An example of transposition of the great arteries with a ventricular septal defect (arrow). AO, aorta; LV, left ventricle; PA, pulmonary artery; RV, right ventricle.

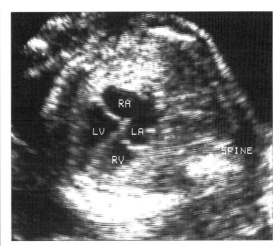

Fig. 8.41 The 4-chamber view in an example of congenitally corrected transposition. The posterior atrioventricular valve is inserted more apically in the septum than the anterior atrioventricular valve, the reverse of normal. LA, left atrium; LV, left ventricle; RA, right atrium; RV, right ventricle.

Discordant atrioventricular connection with discordant ventriculo-arterial connection (corrected transposition)

The right atrium is connected to the left ventricle, which in turn gives rise to the pulmonary artery. The left atrium is connected to the right ventricle, which gives rise to the aorta. Thus, the systemic venous return passes to the pulmonary artery and the pulmonary venous return to the aorta, so that the circulation is anatomically 'corrected' even though the ventricular anatomy is inverted. On the 4-chamber view, the posterior atrioventricular valve will be inserted more apically in the septum than the anterior atrioventricular valve, the reverse from normal. This is illustrated in Figure 8.41.

If these are isolated findings, this condition is compatible with a long and uncomplicated life. However, there may be associated pulmonary stenosis, a ventricular septal defect, complete heart block or Ebstein's malformation. Extracardiac malformations are rarely associated.

Tetralogy of Fallot

This condition is made up of four components: anterior deviation of the aorta, a ventricular septal defect, infundibular

pulmonary stenosis and right ventricular hypertrophy. The 4-chamber view of the fetal heart is usually normal. On long-axis views of the left ventricle the ventricular septal defect and aortic override are seen as illustrated in Figure 8.42. The other features of tetralogy – subpulmonary stenosis and right ventricular hypertrophy – may not be very evident in the fetus. The pulmonary artery is usually smaller than the aorta (Fig. 8.43).

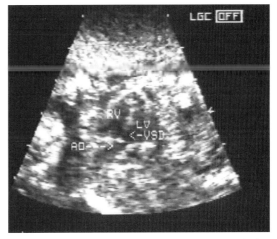

Fig. 8.42 An example of an aorta overriding a ventricular septal defect, where the aorta arises astride the crest of the ventricular septum. AO, aorta; LV, left ventricle; RV, right ventricle; VSD, ventricular septal defect.

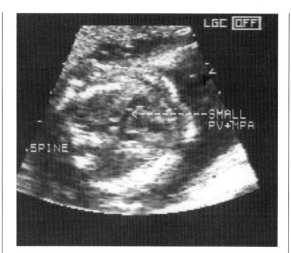

Fig. 8.43 A small pulmonary artery which was detected in association with aortic override (Fig. 8.42) in an example of tetralogy of Fallot. PV, pulmonary valve; MPA, main pulmonary artery.

This type of ventricular septal defect is a malalignment defect and in addition to being a feature of tetralogy of Fallot, it can also be found as an isolated defect or can occur with a common arterial trunk or with pulmonary atresia with a ventricular septal defect (see below).

Tetralogy of Fallot is commonly associated with extracardiac malformations. These include omphalocoele and diaphragmatic hernia in addition to trisomy 21, 13, 18 and additions/deletions,[26] particularly of the short arm of chromosome 22 (DiGeorge and Shprintzen syndromes).

Pulmonary atresia with ventricular septal defect

The pulmonary artery is atretic and there is a ventricular septal defect and anterior displacement of the aorta as in the simpler form of tetralogy. Often there are large collateral vessels arising directly from the aorta supplying the lungs. The 4-chamber view of the fetal heart may be normal. There is a defect in the interventricular outlet septum and the aorta overrides the crest of the ventricular septum. No main pulmonary artery can be identified, although branch pulmonary arteries can sometimes be found. It may be difficult to distinguish tetralogy

from a case with pulmonary atresia if the main pulmonary artery is very small. It may also be difficult to distinguish this condition from a common arterial trunk.

This condition can be associated with chromosomal defects and has been associated with the 22q⁻ phenotypes.

Common arterial trunk

In this condition, a single, great artery arises from the heart astride the crest of the ventricular septum and gives rise to both the aortic arch and the branch pulmonary arteries. The 4-chamber view will usually be normal. There is a malalignment type of ventricular septal defect, as described above. The truncal valve is often thickened and dysplastic (Fig. 8.44). There may be turbulence at the truncal valve and an increase in truncal velocity (Fig. 8.45). There may also be truncal valve regurgitation. The branch pulmonary arteries can be identified arising from the common trunk (Fig. 8.46).[27]

This condition can be associated with chromosomal anomalies and DiGeorge or Shprintzen syndromes.

Double outlet right ventricle

In this condition, both great arteries arise predominantly from the right ventricle

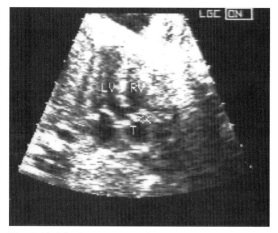

Fig. 8.44 A further example of a vessel overriding a ventricular septal defect. In this example the large vessel is a common arterial trunk (T) and the truncal valve is thickened and dysplastic. LV, left ventricle; RV, right ventricle.

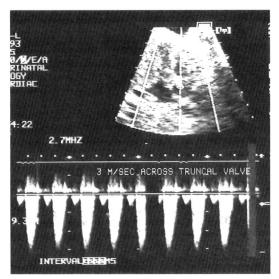

Fig. 8.45 In the same example as shown in Figure 8.44, a high velocity jet of 3 m.s^{-1} is detected across the truncal valve indicating truncal valve stenosis.

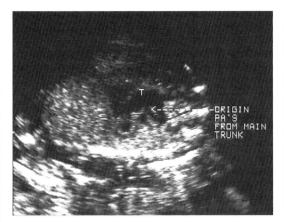

Fig. 8.46 In this example of a common arterial trunk, the branch pulmonary arteries (PAs) can be identified arising from the common trunk.

anterior to the ventricular septum (Figs 8.25 and 8.47). There is an associated ventricular septal defect. Double outlet right ventricle can occur in the setting of more complex heart disease, for example, with an atrioventricular septal defect or mitral atresia. The position of the two great arteries is usually variable and either artery can be obstructed or partially obstructed. The relationship between the site of the ventricular septal defect and the great arteries is important for surgical repair.

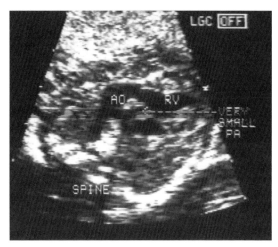

Fig. 8.47 An example of a double outlet right ventricle, with both great arteries arising from the right ventricle. In this example, the aorta is anterior to the pulmonary artery, which is very small as there is associated pulmonary stenosis. AO, aorta; PA, pulmonary artery; RV, right ventricle.

Double outlet right ventricle can be associated with chromosomal defects. This condition can also be associated with DiGeorge and Shprintzen syndromes.

ADDITIONAL ABNORMALITIES AT THE VENTRICULO-ARTERIAL JUNCTION

Pulmonary stenosis

There is obstruction to flow through the pulmonary valve. Pulmonary stenosis can be isolated, or it can be part of a complex of heart malformation which is more common in fetal practice.

The more minor forms of the isolated forms of pulmonary stenosis are not usually detectable during fetal life. The fetal echocardiographic appearance will depend on the severity of the lesion.[24] If pulmonary stenosis is severe, there may be right ventricular hypertrophy and depressed function. However, in some cases, the right ventricle may appear normal (Fig. 8.48). The pulmonary valve may appear thickened and restrictive in motion. An increased velocity may be detectable across the abnormal valve (Fig. 8.49) and the growth of the pulmonary artery may be affected. Pulmonary stenosis

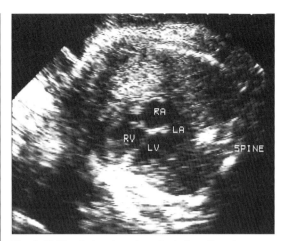

Fig. 8.48 The 4-chamber view of a baby with pulmonary stenosis diagnosed antenatally. The right ventricle in this example appears normal. LA, left atrium; LV, left ventricle; RA, right atrium; RV, right ventricle.

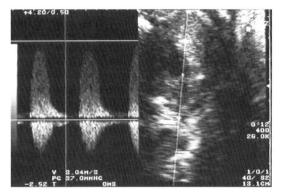

Fig. 8.49 In the same example as shown in Figure 8.48, a high velocity jet (3 m.s⁻¹) was detected with Doppler evaluation across the pulmonary valve, thus confirming the diagnosis of pulmonary stenosis.

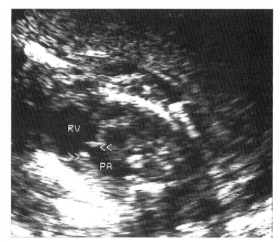

Fig. 8.50 The pulmonary valve, indicated by the arrowheads, is very abnormal in this example of absent pulmonary valve syndrome. PA, pulmonary artery; RV, right ventricle.

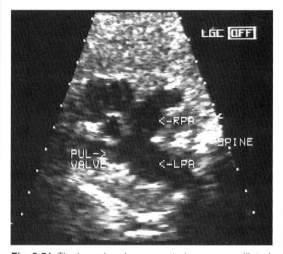

Fig. 8.51 The branch pulmonary arteries are very dilated in this example of absent pulmonary valve syndrome. LPA, left pulmonary artery; RPA, right pulmonary artery; PUL VALVE, pulmonary valve.

may progress to complete atresia of the pulmonary valve before gestation is complete.

Absent pulmonary valve syndrome

This term is a misnomer because there is usually tissue seen in the position of the pulmonary valve both echocardiographically and anatomically. The valve leaflets are very abnormal (Fig. 8.50), resulting in free pulmonary regurgitation and often massive dilatation of the main and branch pulmonary arteries (Fig. 8.51).[28] There is usually an associated ventricular septal defect most often in the outlet septum.

Aortic stenosis

There is obstruction to flow through the aortic valve. As in cases of pulmonary stenosis the stenosis varies in severity, and may progress during fetal life but is usually severe or critical if detected in the fetus.[29] If aortic stenosis is moderate to severe the left ventricle may appear normal or only mildly hypertrophied. The aortic valve may appear thickened (Fig. 8.52) and the aortic Doppler will be normal or increased depending on the degree of left ventricular compromise. If aortic stenosis is critical, there will typically be a dilated, poorly contracting left ventricle with evidence of increased echogenicity of the ventricular walls and papillary muscles of the mitral valve (Fig. 8.53). The mitral

valve will be restricted in opening and there may be mitral regurgitation at high velocity.

Coarctation of aorta and aortic arch anomalies

The aortic arch can be partially obstructed as in coarctation of the aorta, or it may be completely interrupted. Coarctation can occur as an isolated defect or as a component of a complex malformation. In its isolated form in fetal life, the narrowing is preductal and there is usually associated hypoplasia of the isthmus and transverse arch.[30] One of the difficulties with this diagnosis in utero is that the coarctation shelf lesion is not seen and the diagnosis is suspected on other soft signs.[31]

The first clue to the diagnosis is asymmetry of the 4-chamber view, with the right ventricle dilated relative to the left (Fig. 8.54). The pulmonary artery appears dilated compared with the aorta. The aortic arch is narrowed in the transverse views, especially in comparison with the pulmonary artery and arterial duct (Fig. 8.55). Associated cardiac lesions which are common include ventricular septal defect and aortic stenosis. Other causes of right heart dominance should be excluded. An increase in the right

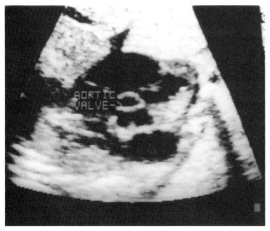

Fig. 8.52 A view of the aortic valve in an example of critical aortic stenosis. The valve leaflets appear dysplastic.

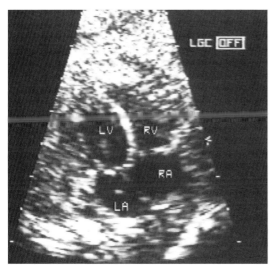

Fig. 8.53 The 4-chamber view of an example of critical aortic stenosis. The left ventricle is dilated with evidence of increased echogenicity of the ventricular walls. LA, left atrium; LV, left ventricle; RA, right atrium; RV, right ventricle.

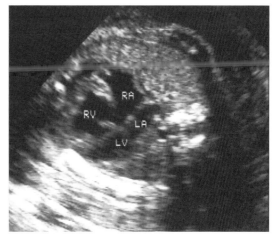

Fig. 8.54 The 4-chamber view of an example of coarctation of the aorta. The right-sided structures appear dilated compared with the left. LA, left atrium; LV, left ventricle; RA, right atrium; RV, right ventricle.

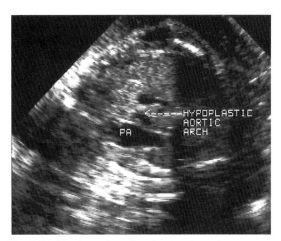

Fig. 8.55 A horizontal section showing the pulmonary artery and aortic arch in an example of coarctation of the aorta. The aortic arch is very hypoplastic in comparison with the pulmonary artery. PA, pulmonary artery.

ventricle/left ventricle ratio can be normal in late gestation, after about 28 weeks. Cardiac causes of an increase in right ventricular size include total anomalous pulmonary venous drainage and tricuspid valve anomalies.

OTHER ANOMALIES

Ventricular septal defect

A defect in the ventricular septum can occur in the outlet, perimembranous inlet or trabecular septum. It is one of the most common forms of congenital heart disease although it is detected much less commonly in the fetus than in postnatal life. A ventricular septal defect can occur in isolation or may be a component of many complex forms of congenital heart disease. A defect in the outlet or perimembranous ventricular septum will be detected in the subaortic position in the long-axis view of the left ventricle (Figs 8.56A–C). A defect in the inlet septum will be seen in the 4-chamber views of the fetal heart and will cause loss of differential insertion of the atrioventricular valves. A trabecular defect can be found in any part of the muscular septum and is usually evident in a 4-chamber view (Fig. 8.57).

Ventricular septal defects are commonly associated with extracardiac malformations and karyotypic anomalies.[20,21]

Tumours

Cardiac tumours are rare heart lesions, but are seen relatively frequently in the fetus.[20,32] The only histological type of intracardiac tumour which has been described in the fetus is a rhabdomyoma. They are usually multiple but can be single. They can cause obstruction to blood flow leading to fetal hydrops or intra-uterine death. They are variable in size and site. They tend to increase in size in fetal life so may only become visible as pregnancy advances. The natural history of rhabdomyomas is to regress spontaneously. Cardiac rhabdomyomas are strongly associated with tuberous sclerosis, particularly when multiple lesions are present. An example of a rhabdomyoma is shown in Figure 8.58.

A teratoma, which is much more rare, is a cystic pericardial tumour which can compress the heart and cause fetal hydrops and intra-uterine death because of its size, although it is histologically benign.

Ectopia cordis

This occurs when the heart in its pericardial sac lies partially or completely outside the chest cavity. It is due to partial or complete absence of the sternum. There may be associated congenital heart malformation. An example of ectopia associated with tetralogy of Fallot is shown in Figure 8.59. On this image, the ventricular septal defect associated with tetralogy is clearly demonstrated. There may or may not be skin covering the defect. If there is no skin cover, the heart appears to float freely in the amniotic fluid. The anterior abdominal wall must be examined for evidence of an associated gut protrusion.

Atrial isomerism

In left atrial isomerism, the inferior vena cava is interrupted and the hepatic veins drain directly to the atrial floor. Both atria have the morphological characteristics of left atria. This is also known as a heterotaxy syndrome, the Ivemark or polysplenia syndrome. It tends to be associated with complex cardiac

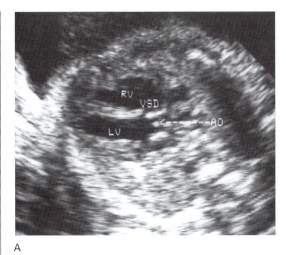

A

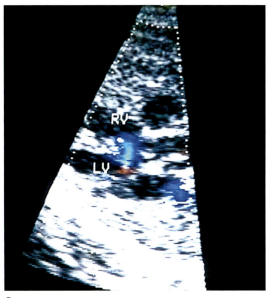

C

Fig. 8.56 An example of a ventricular septal defect in the outlet septum. (A) Colour flow mapping shows bidirectional shunting across the defect (B & C). AO, aorta; LV, left ventricle; RV, right ventricle; VSD, ventricular septal defect.

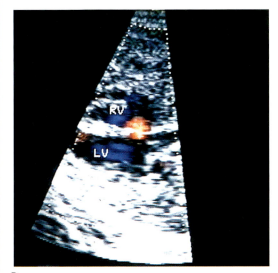

B

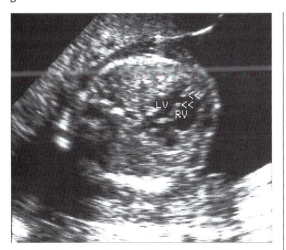

Fig. 8.57 An example of a mid-trabecular ventricular septal defect (shown by arrowheads). LV, left ventricle; RV, right ventricle.

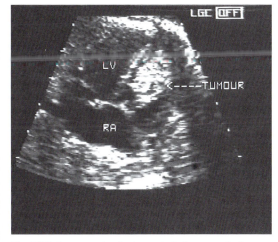

Fig. 8.58 An example of a large rhabdomyoma in the right ventricle. LA, left atrium; LV, left ventricle; RA, right atrium.

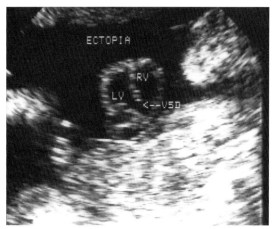

Fig. 8.59 An example of ectopia associated with tetralogy of Fallot is shown. On this view, the ventricular septal defect associated with tetralogy is clearly demonstrated. LV, left ventricle; RV, right ventricle; VSD, ventricular septal defect.

disease, which frequently takes the form of an atrioventricular septal defect, but other lesions also occur.[33] Complete heart block is a common accompanying feature. When the inferior vena cava is interrupted, it cannot be seen in a horizontal section of the upper abdomen in its normal position and a dilated vessel can usually be seen behind the aorta instead. This is the azygous or hemi-azygous vein which carries the venous drainage of the lower body in the absence of the inferior vena cava. The azygous continuation of the inferior vena cava can be clearly seen behind the aorta in the long- or short-axis view of the fetal thorax (Fig. 8.60).

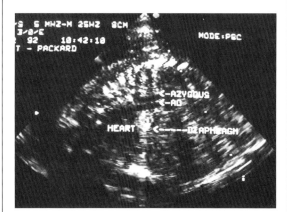

Fig. 8.60 The azygous continuation of the inferior vena cava can be clearly seen behind the aorta in this example of left atrial isomerism. AO, aorta.

In right atrial isomerism, there are two morphologically right atria. There is often asplenia, bilaterally trilobed lungs and bilateral right (short) main bronchi. There is often complex heart disease associated with this syndrome which may take the form of anomalous pulmonary venous drainage, an atrioventricular septal defect, and double outlet right ventricle with pulmonary stenosis or atresia. In the upper abdomen, the relationship of the inferior vena cava to the aorta is abnormal.

AREAS OF CONTROVERSY

Golfballs

These are bright echogenic lesions seen within the right or left ventricular cavities. It is most common to see a single lesion in the left ventricle (Fig. 8.61) but multiple lesions can occur.[34] From a cardiac point of view, these lesions are usually of no consequence, provided that the structure of the heart is normal.[35] A detailed examination of the heart should therefore be performed. Lesions that might correlate with the ultrasound appearance of golfballs have been reported in pathological specimens of fetuses with chromosomal anomalies.[36] This has given reason for concern following detection of

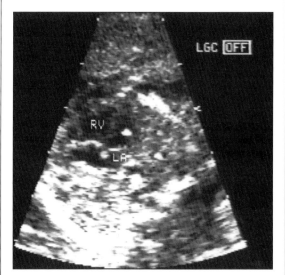

Fig. 8.61 A bright echogenic lesion is seen in the left ventricle. This is an example of a golfball. LA, left atrium; RV, right ventricle.

golfballs. A detailed fetal anomaly scan is therefore recommended in all cases and fetal karyotyping should be discussed with the parents, particularly if any other markers of a karyotypic anomaly are detected. The risk of a karyotypic abnormality in the absence of any other ultrasound marker is low (see Ch. 14).[34]

Pericardial effusions

It is common to see a rim of fluid around the ventricular chambers during fetal life (Fig. 8.62). This should be distinguished from a true pericardial effusion, which usually extends around the atrioventricular groove and measures more than 2 mm (Fig. 8.63). Isolated pericardial effusions can be a marker of chromosomal anomalies, in particular trisomy 21.[37] Fetal karyotyping should therefore be considered in these cases, even in the absence of any other ultrasound markers of a karyotype abnormality.

Organization of fetal echocardiography

Pregnancies at increased risk of congenital heart disease include those with:

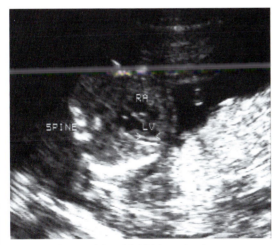

Fig. 8.62 A normal rim of fluid (shown by the arrowheads) can be seen in this example of a normal 4-chamber view. LV, left ventricle; RA, right atrium.

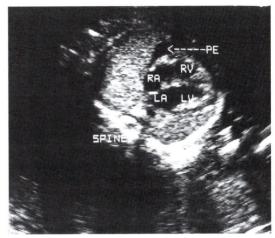

Fig. 8.63 An example of a true pericardial effusion, which extends around the atrioventricular groove. LA, left atrium; LV, left ventricle; RA, right atrium; RV, right ventricle; PE, pericardial effusion.

- maternal factors identified at booking
- fetal high risk factors.

Maternal factors identified at booking:

1. A family history of congenital heart disease (CHD). If one previous child has had CHD, the recurrence risk in any subsequent pregnancy is 2%. Where there have been two affected children, the risk increases to 10%. When a parent is affected, the risk to the next generation is higher if the mother is affected (6%) than if the father is affected (2%).

2. Maternal diabetes is associated with a statistical risk of cardiac malformation of about 2%, but in practice it has been found to be higher (Sharland, unpublished data). Good diabetic control in early pregnancy is thought to diminish this risk.

3. Exposure to teratogens in early pregnancy such as lithium, phenytoin or steroids is reported to be associated with a 2% risk of heart malformation.

Fetal high risk factors:

1. The detection of an extracardiac fetal anomaly on ultrasound should lead to a complete examination of the fetal heart as many types of abnormality, for example exomphalos, are often associated with heart disease.[21,38] Abnormalities in more than one system in the fetus should arouse the suspicion of a chromosome defect.

2. Some fetal arrhythmias are associated with structural heart disease, particularly complete heart block.[39] Evaluation of a fetal arrhythmia must therefore include examination of the cardiac structure.

3. Non-immune fetal hydrops can be due to CHD.[40] Fetal hydrops will have a cardiac cause in up to 25% of cases.

4. A very important high-risk group can now be identified in a low-risk population. This group comprises the 'normal' pregnancies where the obstetrician/ultrasonographer notices an abnormality of the 4-chamber view during a routine obstetric scan. Over 90% of pregnant women have a scan in the UK at the present time. The timing and intensity of the routine scan varies but in those units where a thorough anomaly scan takes place at 18 weeks' gestation or after, potentially the scan can detect severe cardiac anomalies in up to 2 per 1000 studies. The 4-chamber view has been shown to be an effective method of detecting some of the severe forms of cardiac malformation in utero.[15,16] There is no doubt that including examination of the arterial connections of the heart would greatly improve the detection rate of CHD prenatally,[41–43] but the practicality and feasibility of this in the setting of routine obstetric scanning is debatable.

Management and outcome

It has now become widely acknowledged that a different spectrum of disease is seen in prenatal life from that observed in those who survive to infancy.[20,44] Malformations detected are frequently the more severe forms of heart disease and defects which are not commonly seen postnatally are frequently recognized, such as tricuspid dysplasia and cardiac tumours. There is a higher incidence of associated extracardiac lesions compared with postnatal life and, in addition, a significant number of affected pregnancies may result in a spontaneous intra-uterine loss.[45] These factors will

influence the outcome for prenatally diagnosed CHD and must be taken into account at the time of counselling. Additionally, some forms of cardiac lesions are progressive in nature, so that obstructive lesions can change in severity and there may be a reduced rate of growth observed in the chambers or arteries as a result of reduced blood flow.[12,13,25,29,31] Although progression is usually to a more severe form of lesion, rarely it can be to a less severe form.[46]

Following the diagnosis of a cardiac malformation, the clinician should be able to provide the parents with detailed information about the problem. This includes an accurate description of the anomaly, along with information regarding the need for surgical intervention and the type of surgery available for the condition, the number of procedures likely to be required, the mortality and morbidity associated with this, and the overall long-term outlook for the child. Perhaps the most critical anatomical factor influencing cardiac prognosis is whether or not two useful ventricles are present. Long-term survival for almost all forms of 'single ventricle' (e.g. tricuspid atresia, hypoplastic left heart syndrome or double inlet ventricle) is now achievable with a 'Fontan-like' circulation (single systemic ventricular pump, 'passive' systemic venous to pulmonary artery flow). However, at best, this always requires multiple operations and carries significant morbidity and mortality for what will always be only a palliative result. Most lesions with two adequate ventricles will now achieve satisfactory biventricular repair. The parents need to understand all these facts before they can make any decisions about how to proceed. Thus, it is vital to make as accurate a diagnosis as possible and to involve a paediatric cardiologist in the discussion with the parents. It is normal for parents to be extremely distressed at the time of disclosure of an abnormality and further information is likely to be required after the initial explanations. Some parents find it very helpful to talk to others who have been in a similar situation and some will find it beneficial to talk to a paediatric cardiac surgeon before making their final decisions. Since there is a high association with other anomalies, it is prudent to recommend or organize further investigations to exclude any associated lesions. The finding of an associated anomaly may influence the parents' decision about how to proceed.

The major decision the parents face when a severe cardiac defect is diagnosed in early pregnancy is whether they wish to continue with the pregnancy or whether they wish to interrupt it. Termination of pregnancy is an option available before 24 weeks' gestation in the UK, with later termination for critical abnormalities also a possibility, but, as stressed above, the parents should have accurate and adequate information before making their final choice. Should a termination take place, it is vital to try to obtain permission for autopsy in order to confirm the diagnosis and to look for any associated malformations. Ideally this should be performed by a pathologist who is familiar with the examination of congenital heart anomalies.

In continuing pregnancies, appropriate arrangements should be made to re-study the fetal heart in later pregnancy, as some lesions may progress, and some will be at risk of developing non-immune fetal hydrops. The parents can meet the paediatricians, paediatric cardiologists, and paediatric cardiac surgeon likely to be looking after their baby. In some conditions, it may be beneficial for the neonate to be transferred to allow delivery in a unit with paediatric cardiology facilities available. This would be particularly beneficial in lesions that are duct-dependent.

Once the fetus is mature, delivery can be timed to occur when appropriate personnel are available. Vaginal delivery should be possible in most cases as most babies with severe congenital heart defects are unlikely to have problems until after delivery. The advantage of prenatal diagnosis is that it allows immediate cardiac assessment of the neonate and avoids late diagnosis after an infant has become cyanotic or acidotic.

The outcome of 1340 consecutive, structural, cardiac abnormalities diagnosed

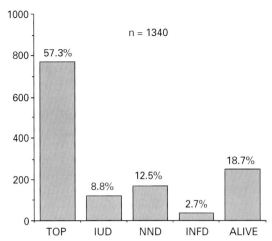

Fig. 8.64 The outcome of 1340 consecutive cases of congenital heart disease diagnosed prenatally at Guy's Hospital from 1980–94. INFD, death in infancy; IUD, spontaneous intra-uterine death; NND, neonatal death; TOP, termination of pregnancy.

at Guy's Hospital between 1980 and 1994 is shown in Figure 8.64. During this time 57% of parents opted to stop the pregnancy following prenatal diagnosis. However, of the 573 continuing pregnancies, only 44% are currently surviving. In 1994 and 1995, the termination rate in our unit fell significantly (Fig. 8.65). There are multiple reasons for this, which include the fact that with increasing ability of ultrasonographers, more correctable lesions are being detected, for

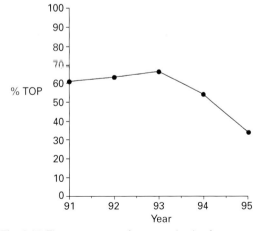

Fig. 8.65 The percentage of parents electing for termination of pregnancy each year from 1991–95, following the prenatal detection of congenital heart disease at Guy's Hospital.

example, simple transposition. Another factor is that detection of all fetal anomalies has improved considerably, so that many chromosomal anomalies are detected before referral for fetal echocardiography, resulting in interruption of pregnancy in some instances before the fetal heart is evaluated. These factors suggest that perhaps the spectrum of cardiac abnormalities being detected in the fetus is starting to change. The fact that more parents are opting to continue with pregnancy will give us the opportunity to re-evaluate the outcome for babies with a prenatal diagnosis of CHD.

References

1. Garrett WJ, Robinson DE. Fetal heart size measures in vivo by ultrasound. Pediatrics 1970; 46:25–27.
2. Egeblad H, Bang J, Northeved A. Ultrasonic identification and examination of fetal heart structures. J Clin Ultrasound 1975; 3:95–105.
3. Baars AM, Merkus JMWM. Fetal echocardiography: a new approach to the study of the dynamics of the fetal heart and its component parts. Eur J Obstet Gynaecol Repro Biol 1977; 7:91–100.
4. Allan LD, Tynan MJ, Campbell S, Wilkinson J, Anderson RH. Echocardiographic and anatomical correlates in the fetus. Br Heart J 1980; 44:444–451.
5. Kleinman CS, Hobbins JC, Jaffe CC, Lynch DC, Talner NS. Echocardiographic studies of the human fetus: prenatal diagnosis of congenital heart disease and cardiac dysrhythmias. Pediatrics 1980; 65:1059–1067.
6. Lange LW, Sahn DJ, Allen HD, Goldberg SJ, Anderson C, Giles H. Qualitative real-time cross-sectional echocardiographic imaging of the human fetus during the second half of pregnancy. Circulation 1980; 62:799–805.
7. Allan LD, Chita SK, Sharland GK, Fagg NLK, Anderson RH, Crawford DC. The accuracy of fetal echocardiography in the diagnosis of congenital heart disease. Int J Cardiol 1989; 25:279–288.
8. Huhta JC, Strasburger JF, Carpenter RJ, Reiter A. Fetal echocardiography: accuracy and limitations in the diagnosis of cardiac disease. J Am Coll Cardiol 1985; 5:387(abstract).
9. Allan LD, Chita SK, Al-Ghazali W, Crawford DC, Tynan MJ. Doppler echocardiographic evaluation of the normal human fetal heart. Br Heart J 1987; 57:528–533.
10. Sharland GK, Chita SK, Allan LD. The use of colour Doppler in fetal echocardiography. Int J Cardiol 1990; 28:229–236.
11. Moore KL, Persaud TVN. The developing human – clinically orientated embryology. Philadelphia: WB Saunders; 1993: 304–353.
12. Allan LD, Sharland GK, Tynan M. Natural history of

13. Hornberger LK, Sanders SP, Sahn DJ, Rice MJ, Spevak PJ, Benacerraf BR. In utero pulmonary artery and aortic growth and potential for progression of pulmonary outflow tract obstruction in tetralogy of Fallot. J Am Coll Cardiol 1995; 25:739–745.
14. Allan LD, Crawford DC, Chita SK, Tynan MJ. Prenatal screening for congenital heart disease. BMJ 1986; 292:1717–1719.
15. Fermont L, De Geeter B, Aubry MC, Kachener J, Sidi D. A close collaboration between obstetricians and cardiologists allows antenatal detection of severe cardiac malformations by 2D echocardiography. In: Paediatric cardiology: Proceedings of the Second World Congress. New York: Springer-Verlag; 1986:34–37.
16. Sharland GK, Allan LD. Screening for congenital heart disease prenatally. Results of a 2½ year study in the South East Thames Region. Br J Obstet Gynaecol 1992; 99:220–225.
17. Allan LD. Manual of fetal echocardiography. Lancaster: MTP Press; 1986.
18. Allan LD, Sharland G, Cook A. Color atlas of fetal cardiology. London: Mosby-Wolfe; 29–31 (Anomalies of venous connection).
19. Yeager SB, Parness IA, Spevak PJ, Hornberger LK, Sanders SP. Prenatal echocardiographic diagnosis of pulmonary and systemic venous anomalies. Am Heart J 1994; 128:397–405.
20. Allan LD, Sharland GK, Milburn A et al. Prospective diagnosis of 1,006 consecutive cases of congenital heart disease in the fetus. J Am Coll Cardiol 1994; 23:1452–1458.
21. Allan LD, Sharland GK, Chita SK, Lockhart S, Maxwell DJ. Chromosomal anomalies in fetal congenital heart disease. Ultrasound Obstet Gynecol 1991; 1:8–11.
22. Sharland GK, Chita SK, Allan LD. Tricuspid valve dysplasia or displacement in intrauterine life. J Am Cardiol 1991; 17:944–949.
23. Lang D, Oberhoffer R, Cook A et al. The pathological spectrum of malformations of the tricuspid valve in prenatal and neonatal life. J Am Coll Cardiol 1991; 17:1161–1167.
24. Hornberger LK, Benacerraf BR, Bromley BS, Spevak PJ, Sanders SP. Prenatal detection of severe right ventricular outflow tract obstruction: pulmonary stenosis and pulmonary atresia. J Ultrasound Med 1994; 13:743–750.
25. Sharland GK. Left heart disease in the fetus. MD thesis. University of London, 1993.
26. Allan LD, Sharland GK. The prognosis in fetal tetralogy of Fallot. Pediatric Cardiol 1992; 13:1–4.
27. de Araujo LM, Schmidt KG, Silverman NH, Finkbeiner WE. Prenatal detection of truncus arteriosus by ultrasound. Pediatr Cardiol 1987; 8:261–263.
28. Ettedgui JA, Sharland GK, Chita SK, Cook A, Fagg N, Allan LD. Absent pulmonary valve syndrome with ventricular septal defect: role of the arterial duct. Am J Cardiol 1990; 66:233–234.
29. Sharland GK, Chita SK, Fagg N et al. Left ventricular

dysfunction in the fetus: relation to aortic valve anomalies and endocardial fibroelastosis. Br Heart J 1991; 66:219–224.

30. Hornberger LK, Sahn DJ, Kleinman CS, Copel J, Silverman NH. Antenatal diagnosis of coarctation of the aorta: a multicenter experience. J Am Coll Cardiol 1994; 23:417–423.

31. Sharland GK, Chan K, Allan LD. Coarctation of the aorta: difficulties in prenatal diagnosis. Br Heart J 1994; 71:70–75.

32. Groves AM, Fagg NLK, Cook AC, Allan LD. Cardiac tumours in intrauterine life. Arch Dis Child 1992; 67:1189–1192.

33. Phoon CK, Neill CA. Asplenia syndrome: insight into embryology through an analysis of cardiac and extracardiac anomalies. Am J Cardiol 1994; 73:581–587.

34. Simpson JM, Rowlands ML, Sharland GK. The significance of echogenic foci ('golfballs') in the fetal heart: a prospective study of 147 cases. (Abstract) BMUS meeting, Torquay; 1995.

35. How HY, Villafane J, Parihus RR, Spinnato JA. Small hyperechogenic foci of the fetal cardiac ventricle: a benign sonographic finding? Ultrasound Obstet Gynecol 1994; 4:205–207.

36. Roberts DJ, Genest D. Cardiac histologic pathology characteristic of trisomies 13 and 21. Hum Path 1992; 23:1130–1140.

37. Sharland GK, Lockhart SM. Isolated pericardial effusion: an indication for fetal karyotyping? Ultrasound Obstet Gynecol 1995; 6:29–32.

38. Copel JA, Pilu G, Kleinman CS. Congenital heart disease and extracardiac anomalies: associations and indications for fetal echocardiography. Am J Obstet Gynecol 1986; 154:1121–1132.

39. Machado MVL, Tynan MJ, Curry PVL, Allan LD. Fetal complete heart block. Br Heart J 1988; 60:512–515.

40. Kleinman CS, Donnerstein RL, DeVore GT et al. Fetal echocardiography for evaluation of in utero congestive cardiac failure. N Engl J Med 1982; 10:568–575.

41. Wigton TR, Sabbagha RE, Tamura RK, Cohen L, Minogue JP, Strasberger JF. Sonographic diagnosis of congenital heart disease: comparison between the four-chamber view and multiple cardiac views. Obstet Gynecol 1993; 82:219–224.

42. Kirk JS, Riggs TW, Comstock CH, Lee W, Yang SS, Weinhouse E. Prenatal screening for cardiac anomalies: the value of routine addition of the aortic root to the four chamber view. Obstet Gynecol 1994; 84:427–431.

43. Bromley B, Estroff JA, Sanders SP et al. Fetal echocardiography: accuracy and limitations in a population at high and low risk for heart defects. Am J Obstet Gynecol 1992; 166:1473–1481.

44. Allan LD, Crawford DC, Anderson RH, Tynan MJ. Spectrum of congenital heart disease detected echocardiographically in prenatal life. Br Heart J 1984; 54:523–526.

45. Sharland GK, Lockhart SM, Chita SK, Allan LD. Factors influencing the outcome of congenital heart disease detected prenatally. Arch Dis Child 1990; 64:284–287.

46. Sharland GK, Qureshi SA. Closure of the ventricular component of an atrioventricular septal defect during fetal life. Cardiol in the Young 1995; 5:272–274.

CHAPTER 9

Diagnosis and treatment of fetal arrhythmias

Frances Bu'Lock
David Pilling

Introduction

Disturbances of fetal cardiac rhythm are reported in up to 7% of pregnancies,[1] with true tachyarrhythmias in 1 in 10–25 000 pregnancies[2] and isolated heart block in 15 per 20 000 live births.[3] It is likely that more occur and go unreported, but the majority of these are benign extrasystoles. However, some rhythm disturbances are more serious and may be associated with fetal haemodynamic compromise, structural cardiac abnormalities, or both. True 'electrical' arrhythmia needs to be differentiated from heart rate changes associated with fetal distress, particularly in the preterm fetus in whom early delivery with an arrhythmia may be both unnecessary and detrimental. Although technically feasible, fetal electrocardiography is cumbersome and unsuitable for routine application, and fetal echocardiography has become the method of choice both for diagnosis and monitoring of fetal arrhythmias.[4–7]

Extrasystoles

Atrial premature beats are probably the commonest cause of referral for fetal arrhythmia assessment. They may present as irregular fetal heartbeat, tachycardia, or bradycardia caused by the compensatory pause after a premature contraction. After echocardiographic assessment to exclude structural cardiac anomalies, the parents can usually be reassured that this is a benign, normal variant which may well resolve in the third trimester, and that no further follow-up is required. However, monitoring to exclude more sustained arrhythmia may be necessary in some cases.

Tachyarrhythmias

The cardiac conducting system forms in parallel with other cardiac structures and pathways differentiate very early in fetal development. However, maturation of the physiological relationships between autonomic and anatomic elements of the conduction system occurs much more slowly.[8] This has particular relevance to the regulation of both atrial and atrioventricular 're-entry' circuits, which underlie the majority of fetal tachyarrhythmias.

Fetal heart rates of > 200 bpm require further investigation. Persistent fetal tachycardias may be associated with non-immune hydrops and intra-uterine death, in addition to polyhydramnios and preterm delivery.[9] Maternal drug therapy may be very successful in controlling fetal arrhythmias and treating fetal heart failure.[10–13] Maximal information on the fetal rhythm may optimize the chances of gaining control, and close co-operation with a paediatric cardiologist is essential. Intermittent fetal tachycardias may also be associated with hydrops and prolonged monitoring may be required.[13]

Cross-sectional echocardiography may show evidence of a structural cardiac malformation predisposing to arrhythmia such as cardiac tumours,[14] aneurysm of the foramen ovale[2,15] (Fig. 9.1) or Ebstein's

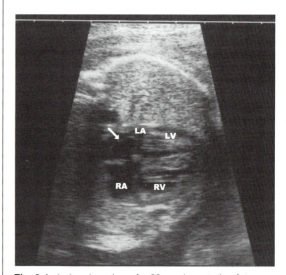

Fig. 9.1 4-chamber view of a 28-week gestation fetus with frequent atrial extrasystoles, showing aneurysmal dilatation (arrow) of the flap valve of the oval foramen of the atrial septum. LA, left atrium; RA, right atrium; LV, left ventricle; RV, right ventricle.

anomaly of the tricuspid valve and permits assessment of cardiothoracic ratio and ventricular function. The presence of oedema or effusions should also be noted. M-mode echocardiography should be performed, usually steered from the cross-sectional image. Depending on the fetal lie, the ventricles and atria may be studied separately but it is frequently possible to obtain a view in which atrial and ventricular wall motion can be examined simultaneously (Fig. 9.2). Atrial and ventricular rate can then be calculated and the presence or absence of atrioventricular synchrony noted[4-7] (Fig. 9.3). Doppler interrogation of the fetal vasculature may also provide helpful information on fetal rhythm as well as haemodynamic state.[16-18]

An irregularly irregular atrial rhythm suggests atrial fibrillation, whereas a regular atrial rate of ≥ 300 bpm suggests atrial flutter. Where the atrial rate exceeds the ventricular rate, any link between the atrial and ventricular contractions (e.g. 2:1 or 3:1) should also be noted and is suggestive of atrial flutter with associated atrioventricular block. One-to-one atrioventricular conduction at lower rates suggests more classical supraventricular (atrioventricular re-entrant tachycardia) such as Wolff–Parkinson–White syndrome (Fig. 9.4).

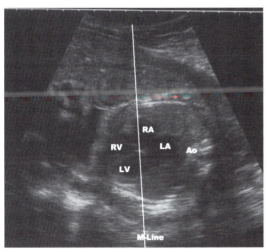

Fig. 9.2 4-chamber view of fetal heart showing potential for positioning of M-line to transect atrial (RA, right atrium; LA, left atrium) and ventricular structures. LV, left ventricle; RV, right ventricle; Ao, aorta.

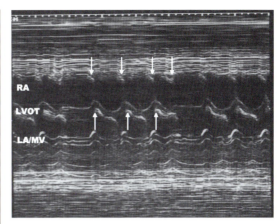

Fig. 9.3 M-mode echocardiogram from same fetus as Figure 9.1, showing frequent non-conducted atrial extrasystoles, with a compensatory pause in ventricular activity. RA, right atrium; LVOT, left ventricular outflow tract; LA/MV, left atrium/mitral valve junction.

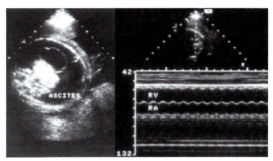

Fig. 9.4 Fetal ultrasound scans from a hydropic fetus with ascites (left). The steered M-mode echocardiogram shows a sustained tachycardia of 240 bpm. There is atrioventricular synchrony, suggesting Wolff–Parkinson–White syndrome. RA, right atrium; RV, right ventricle. (Courtesy of Dr I. Sullivan, Great Ormond Street Hospital, London.)

Atrioventricular dissociation with a rapid ventricular rate suggests either congenital His bundle/junctional ectopic tachycardia or a true ventricular tachycardia but these are rare.

Therapy

Although direct fetal administration of anti-arrhythmic therapy has been reported, it carries significant risks and should be reserved as a 'last resort'.[19] Transplacental treatment of the fetus with maternally administered anti-arrhythmic agents is now well established, although the optimum drug regimen required remain as controversial as those for extra-uterine therapy! The use of verapamil, digoxin, beta-blockers, flecainide and amiodarone have all been reported and advocated.[10–12] Digoxin and flecainide cross the placenta well (40% and 80% respectively) and maternal drug levels can be readily monitored.[11] Ventricular tachycardia should be identified[4] as digoxin and verapamil are contraindicated. All fetuses with evidence of hydrops should receive anti-arrhythmic therapy with maternal hospitalization and close fetomaternal observation until control of the tachycardia is achieved. Resolution of the hydrops may take some time even once ventricular function returns to normal.[11] Although up to 70% of preterm fetuses with a tachyarrhythmia have been reported to develop hydrops,[2] this may be an overestimate, and since all anti-arrhythmic agents have side effects, the role of treatment for the asymptomatic fetus remains controversial.[2,4,11] Lower gestational age at presentation and the presence of sustained tachycardias are significant risk factors for the development of hydrops, whereas ventricular rate and precise mechanism of tachycardia are not.[20] In all cases, frequent fetal echocardiography and assessment of fetal wellbeing are required, and preterm delivery should be avoided.[9,11]

Bradyarrhythmias

Normal variation in fetal heart rate with autonomic tone is common, but persistent fetal bradycardia (< 80 bpm) is almost always due to fetal heart block and requires further investigation. Regular atrial ectopic beats may mimic a sinus bradycardia owing to the ventricular compensatory pauses[7,21] (Fig. 9.5) and congenital long QT syndromes may rarely present in utero with moderate fetal bradycardia.[22] As with fetal tachycardias, differentiation of heart block from end-stage fetal distress is vital in avoiding unnecessary preterm delivery, and careful assessment of fetal wellbeing is mandatory.

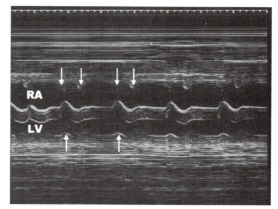

Fig. 9.5 Fetal M-mode echocardiogram across right atrium (RA) and left ventricle (LV) showing atrial bigemini. The second atrial beat is not conducted to the ventricle and the regular compensatory pauses produce an apparent bradycardia. The arrhythmia is generally benign.

The diagnosis of fetal heart block requires either M-mode (Fig. 9.6) or Doppler sampling (Fig. 9.7) of both atrial and ventricular structures (e.g. M-mode of aorta or right ventricle (depending on orientation) with left atrial free wall); preferably simultaneously in order to assess atrioventricular synchrony as well as rate.[23–25] The presence of chamber dilatation, reduced ventricular function, atrioventricular valve

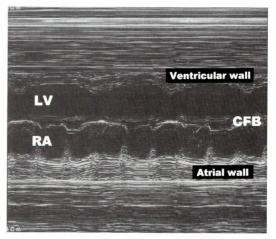

Fig. 9.6 M-mode fetal echocardiogram showing complete dissociation of left ventricular (LV) activity from the atrial rhythm (RA, right atrium; CFB, central fibrous body). The ventricular rate is around 60 bpm whereas the atrial rate is 150 bpm. The mother had both anti-Rho and anti-La auto-antibodies but no clinical evidence of a lupus syndrome.

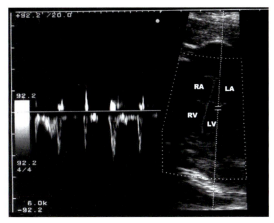

Fig. 9.7 Transmitral Doppler signal from a fetus with complete heart block. Note the variable peak velocities and duration of transmitral flow as a result of variable atrioventricular synchronicity. RA, right atrium; LA, left atrium; RV, right ventricle; LV, left ventricle.

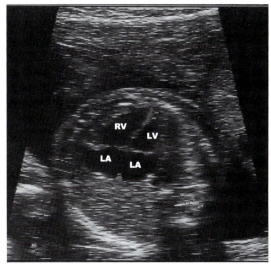

Fig. 9.8 4-chamber view of a fetus with left atrial isomerism, complex complete atrioventricular septal defect and complete heart block. The prognosis for this combination of lesions is very poor. LA, left atrium; RV, right ventricle; LV, left ventricle.

regurgitation and evidence of fetal heart failure (oedema, ascites, pleural or pericardial effusions) should also be noted.

As in postnatal life, fetal heart block may be complete (i.e. with total dissociation of atrial and ventricular contraction), or with lesser degrees of block. First degree heart block, i.e. with delayed atrioventricular conduction but retention of 1:1 conduction, does not cause bradycardia and is unlikely to be recognized in utero. Second degree heart block, with either regular or irregular intermittent conduction (e.g. 2:1 or 3:1), may be recognized, but differentiation from complete heart block may be difficult, especially when the ventricular rate is well preserved.

Interruption of the fetal atrioventricular conducting system may be anatomic, in association with congenital heart disease, or functional, usually related to maternal autoimmune disease,[23,24] but is occasionally idiopathic or related to viral infections.[26] The prognosis for congenital heart disease with in utero heart block is extremely poor, whereas that for auto-immune heart block is better although there is still a significant risk of the development of fetal hydrops and intra-uterine death.[23,27,28] The first aim of fetal echocardiography in this situation is therefore to identify any associated fetal cardiac malformations. In the complex, isomeric conditions, there is usually an atrioventricular septal defect with variable additional abnormalities (Fig. 9.8). In so-called 'congenitally corrected transposition', the heart may look normal other than reversal of the usual atrioventricular valve offsetting, with a left-sided right ventricle identifiable by its moderator band. Early consultation with a paediatric cardiologist is highly desirable in such cases.

In the fetus with an apparently structurally normal heart, maternal screening for auto-antibodies is positive in the vast majority, although many of the mothers will be completely asymptomatic. Identification of maternal auto-immune status is important as around 25% of future pregnancies may also be affected.[29] In addition, the mother may develop symptomatic connective tissue disease at a later date.[23,30]

Once the likely underlying pathology has been determined, repeated fetal echocardiography is important both to monitor for any progression in the heart block itself and for the assessment of fetal wellbeing at least on a weekly basis. Although lower heart rates (< 55 bpm) early in pregnancy appear to be associated with a poorer outcome, the relationship is not absolute[5,27,28] and falling fetal heart rate (decrease > 5 bpm) is also a poor prognostic indicator. The development of fetal hydrops is an ominous sign and carries a mortality rate of 80 to 100%.[27,28] Since some success with in utero supportive therapy has been reported,[31–35] close collaboration with both obstetric and paediatric cardiac colleagues is essential. The cardiac size and ventricular rate should be monitored and early identification of fetal oedema and effusions or reduced ventricular function is important.

Therapy

In utero cardiac pacing has been reported but with very limited success at present.[36,37] The use of maternal plasmapheresis or steroid administration (dexamethasone has good transplacental passage) has been reported to reverse hydrops or modify the progression of heart block in some cases.[31,32] Steroids may also suppress any associated fetal myocarditis[33] and have the additional advantage of enhancing pulmonary maturation in the preterm fetus. Beta sympathomimetics such as ritodrine and salbutamol have also been used with reports of increase in fetal heart rate and resolution of hydrops.[34,35] Close liaison with obstetric and paediatric cardiac colleagues for optimum perinatal management is also required.

References

1. Elkayman U, Gleicher N. Cardiac problems in pregnancy. In: Elkayman U, Gleicher N, eds. Diagnosis and management of maternal and fetal disease. New York: Alan R. Liss; 1982:535–565.
2. Wladmiroff J, Stewart P. Treatment of fetal cardiac arrhythmias. Br J Hosp Med 1985; 34:134–140.
3. Cobbe SM. Congenital complete heart block. BMJ 1983; 286:1769–1770.
4. Allan LD, Anderson RH, Sullivan ID, et al. Evaluation of fetal arrhythmias by echocardiography. Br Heart J 1983; 50:240–245.
5. Kleinman CS, Donnerstein RJ, Jaffe CC, et al. Fetal echocardiography for the evaluation of in utero cardiac arrhythmias and the monitoring of in utero

6. Silverman NH, Enderlain MA, Stranger P, et al. Recognition of fetal arrhythmias by echocardiography. J Clin Ultrasound 1985; 13:255–263.
7. Steinfeld L, Rappaport HL, Rossbach HC, Martinez E. Diagnosis of fetal arrhythmias using echocardiographic and Doppler techniques. J Am Coll Cardiol 1986; 8:1425–1433.
8. Janse MK, Anderson RH, van Capelle FJ, Durrer D. A combined electrophysiological and anatomic study of the human fetal heart. Am Heart J 1976; 91:556–562.
9. Maxwell D, Crawford D, Curry P, Tynan M, Allan L. Obstetric importance, diagnosis and management of fetal tachycardias. BMJ 1988; 297:107–110.
10. Rey E, Duperron L, Gauthier R, et al. Trans-placental treatment of tachycardia induced fetal heart failure with verapamil and amiodarone: A case report. Am J Obstet Gynecol; 1985:311–312.
11. Allan L, Chita S, Maxwell D, Priestley K, Sharland G. Use of flecainide in fetal atrial tachycardia. Br Heart J 1991; 65:46–48.
12. Arnoux P, Seyral P, Llurens M, et al. Amiodarone and digoxin for refractory fetal tachycardia. Am J Cardiol 1987; 59:166–167.
13. Smoleniec JS, Martin R, James DK. Intermittent fetal tachycardia and hydrops. Arch Dis Child 1991; 66:1160–1161.
14. Birnbaum SE, McGahan JP, Janos GG, Meyers M. Fetal tachycardia and intramyocardial tumours. J Am Coll Cardiol 1985; 6:1358–1361.
15. Rice MJ, McDonal RW, Reller MD. Fetal atrial septal aneurysm: a cause of fetal atrial arrhythmias. J Am Coll Cardiol 1988; 12:1292–1297.
16. Chan FY, Woo SK, Ghosh A, Tang M, Lam C. Prenatal diagnosis of congenital fetal arrhythmias by simultaneous pulsed Doppler velocimetry of the fetal abdominal aorta and inferior vena cava. Obstet Gynecol 1990; 76:200–205.
17. DeVore GR, Horenstein J. Simultaneous Doppler recording of the pulmonary artery and vein: a new technique for the evaluation of a fetal arrhythmia. J Ultrasound Med 1993; 12:669–671.
18. Tonge H, Wladmiroff J, Noordam M, Stewart P. Fetal cardiac arrhythmias and their effect on volume blood flow in descending aorta of human fetus. J Clin Ultrasound 1986; 14:607–612.
19. Weiner P, Thompson M. Direct treatment of fetal supraventricular tachycardia after failed transplacental therapy. Am J Obstet Gynecol 1988; 158:570–573.
20. Naheed ZJ, Strasburger JF, Deal BJ, Benson DW, Gidding SS. Fetal tachycardia: Mechanisms and predictors of hydrops fetalis. J Am Coll Cardiol 1996; 27:1736–1740.
21. Crawford D, Chapman A, Allan L. The assessment of persistent bradycardia in fetal life. Br J Obst Gynaecol, 1985; 92:941–944.
22. Vigliani M. Romano–Ward syndrome diagnosed as

moderate fetal bradycardia. A case report. J Reprod Med 1995; 40:725–728.

23. Machado MVL, Tynan MJ, Curry PVL, Allan LD. Fetal complete heart block. Br Heart J 1988; 60:512–515.

24. Gembruch U, Hanasmann M, Redel DA, Bald R, Knopfle G. Fetal complete heart block: antenatal diagnosis, significance and management. Eur J Obst Gynecol 1989; 31:9–22.

25. Chan FY, Ghosh A, Tang M, Lam C. Simultaneous pulsed Doppler velocimetry of fetal aorta and inferior vena cava. Diagnosis of fetal congenital complete heart block; two case reports. Eur J Obstet Gynecol Reprod Biol 1990; 35:89–95.

26. Lewis PE, Cefalo RC, Zaritsky AL. Fetal heart block caused by cytomegalovirus. Am J Obstet Gynecol 1980; 136:967–968.

27. Schmidt KG, Ulmer HE, Silverman NH, Kleinman CS, Copel JA. Perinatal outcome of fetal complete atrioventricular block: a multicenter experience. J Am Coll Cardiol 1991; 17:1360–1366.

28. Groves AMM, Allan LD, Rosenthal E. Outcome of isolated congenital complete heart block diagnosed in utero. Heart 1996; 75:190–194.

29. Scott JS, Maddison PJ, Taylor PV, et al. Connective tissue disease, antibodies to ribonucleoprotein and congenital complete heart block. N Engl J Med 1985; 312:98–100.

30. Buyon J, Roubey R, Swersky S, et al. Complete congenital heart block: risk of recurrence and therapeutic approach to prevention. J Rheumatol 1988; 15:1104–1108.

31. Barclay CS, French MH, Ross LD, Sokol RJ. Successful pregnancy following steroid therapy and plasma exchange in a woman with anti-Rho (SS-A) antibodies: case report. Br J Obstet Gynecol 1987; 94:369–371.

32. Copel JA, Buyon JP, Kleinman CS. Successful in utero therapy of fetal heart block. Am J Obstet Gynecol 1995; 173:1384–1390.

33. Horsfall AC, Venables PJW, Taylor PV, Maini RM. Ro and LA antigens and maternal autoantibody idiotype on the surface of myocardial fibres in congenital complete heart block. J Autoimmun 1991; 4:165–176.

34. Groves AMM, Allan LD, Rosenthal E. Therapeutic trial of sympathomimetics in three cases of complete heart block in the fetus. Circulation 1995; 92:3394–3396.

35. Koike T, Minakami H, Shiraishi H, Sato I. Fetal ventricular rate in case of congenital complete heart block is increased by ritodrine. Case report. J Perinat Med 1997; 25:216–218.

36. Carpenter RJ, Strasburger JF, Garson A, Smith RT, Deter RL, Engelhart HT. Fetal ventricular pacing for hydrops secondary to complete atrioventricular block. J Am Coll Cardiol 1986; 8:1434–1436.

37. Walkinshaw SA, Welch CR, McCormack J, Walsh K. In utero pacing for fetal congenital heart block. Fetal Diagn Ther 1994; 9:183–185.

CHAPTER 10

Pulmonary abnormalities

David Pilling

Introduction

With the exception of cardiac abnormalities (see Ch. 8), abnormalities of the chest are quite unusual. Abnormalities of shape and size are diagnostically usually quite obvious and associated with other system abnormalities on many occasions. Isolated lung abnormalities are uncommon, but when present are easily detected either by texture change in the lung parenchyma or by the effect they have on the adjacent heart or both.

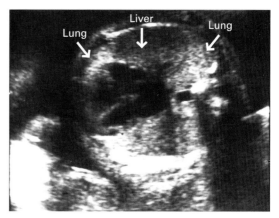

Fig. 10.1 Axial section of normal chest, showing the normal echodensity of the lungs is slightly greater than the liver.

Normal appearances excluding the first trimester

The chest is most easily assessed in the axial section in continuum with the abdomen inferiorly and the neck superiorly. The normal shape of the chest is almost circular, tending to an ellipse in axial section. The size of the chest can be assessed by obtaining an axial section and measuring the chest circumference at the level of the 4-chamber view. The accuracy of this section because of the relative lack of specificity of the exact landmarks is not as good as the abdominal circumference, but has been used to confirm or exclude reductions in thoracic size.[1] The relative circumferences of the thorax and heart are almost unchanged in the second and third trimesters.[1] The orientation and position of the heart are very important in assessing the chest. The heart lies with its axis (the interventricular septum) at about 45° to the midline on the axial section. Most of the heart lies in the anterior left quadrant of the chest with its apex touching the left anterior chest wall. The axial view can be supplemented with coronal or sagittal views depending on fetal position. An appreciation of the overall shape of the chest is best seen from the coronal view with the diaphragm in particular being well seen on the sagittal view. Full assessment of the normal chest includes assessment of the shape of the ribs

and the integrity of the thoracic spine (see Ch. 7)

The overall echogenicity of the normal lungs is slightly increased compared to the liver, but the texture differs slightly. Minor changes in echogenicity with gestational age (and from patient to patient) do not seem to have any clinical significance[2,3] (Figs 10.1 and 10.2).

Pitfalls and artefacts

It is sometimes impossible to obtain a good thoracic circumference measurement, particularly in the context of oligohydramnios when a true axial section may be very difficult to obtain because of a relatively fixed fetal position and lack of liquor causing loss of the normal fluid/soft tissue interface. Assessing lung volume can be difficult on a series of axial sections, but obtaining a coronal section of the chest, except in very early pregnancy to complement the axial sections, is extremely difficult and the typical, 'bell-shaped' chest seen postnatally with reduced lung volume cannot always be appreciated antenatally. In later pregnancy, sequestrated lung segments can be very difficult to demonstrate when closely applied to the spine as they may be lost by the shadow caused by the spine and it can be impossible to manoeuvre the probe

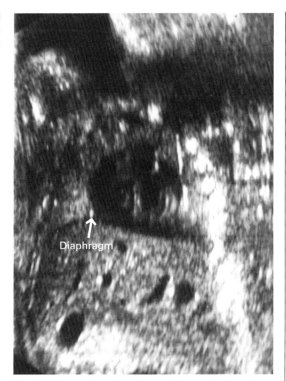

Fig. 10.2 Coronal section of normal chest, showing the normal diaphragm as echolucency below the heart and lungs.

into such a position that all areas of both lungs have been covered. The apices of the lungs can be also difficult to demonstrate because of the shoulders in later pregnancy, but this is rarely a practical problem as there are very few isolated apical lung lesions occurring antenatally. The diaphragm can only be demonstrated well in the sagittal and coronal views and this is often restricted in later pregnancy. The diaphragm is seen as a thin line of low echogenicity compared with the adjacent organs. Small defects can easily be missed when it is only possible to examine the structure completely in one plane.

Abnormal appearances

Lungs

Pulmonary hypoplasia

The definition of pulmonary hypoplasia is an absolute decrease in lung volume and weight for gestation age.[4]

In unilateral hypoplasia, one lung is either completely absent or considerably reduced in volume. In the case of the right lung, this is relatively easy to demonstrate, but in the left lung it is often more difficult to appreciate. Rotation and displacement of the heart are the two most easily demonstrated ultrasound features. In the case of the right lung being reduced in volume, the heart is shifted towards the right, but its axis is usually maintained, the apex pointing towards the left anteriorly. In the case of left lung hypoplasia, the changes are more subtle with rotation of the heart and the interventricular septum being more in the coronal plane than usual. There can sometimes be more obvious cardiac displacement if the lung is entirely absent.

In bilateral pulmonary hypoplasia, the chest volume is usually considerably reduced with the heart appearing relatively enlarged. Measurement of thoracic circumference and cardiac diameters will help to differentiate reduced chest volume from increased cardiac size.[1] There is, however, an association between growth retardation, with pulmonary hypoplasia, oligohydramnios and apparent cardiac enlargement which adds to the difficulties of diagnosis. Whilst pulmonary hypoplasia can be suggested by measuring fetal lung length[5] and by comparing the thoracic circumference with other body parameters such as abdominal circumference, biparietal diameter and femur length, the ultimate diagnosis of pulmonary hypoplasia can only be made at post-mortem when the lungs can be weighed and thus only the most severe degrees of bilateral pulmonary hypoplasia are going to be diagnosed by antenatal ultrasound and be confirmed postnatally. Many of the ratios used have drawbacks, especially in the growth-retarded fetus. More subtle degrees may be suspected and not confirmed and some cases will only be evident postnatally.

In summary, antenatal diagnosis of moderate or mild degrees of pulmonary hypoplasia is not good.[6,7] The accompanying features of oligohydramnios and growth retardation will increase the suspicion of pulmonary hypoplasia antenatally. Bilateral

Table 10.1
Causes of bilateral pulmonary hypoplasia

Feature	Related condition

Oligohydramnios	Result of premature rupture of membranes
	• Growth retardation
	• Renal abnormality
	    agenesis
	    dysplasia
	    bladder outlet obstruction
	    polycystic disease
	    (autosomal recessive)

Intrathoracic mass	• Pleural effusions • Diaphragmatic hernia • Cystic adenomatoid malformation
Cardiac	• Cardiomyopathy
Neuromuscular	• Myopathy • Skeletal dysplasia
Chromosomal	• Trisomies 13, 18, 21
Idiopathic	

pulmonary hypoplasia as well as being associated with all causes of oligohydramnios is also a feature of a number of other conditions (see Table 10.1). Unilateral pulmonary hypoplasia is associated with any lesion which compresses the lung and many of these lesions are described in the following paragraphs.

The degree of pulmonary hypoplasia and its effects are determined by the histological appearances of the lungs which in turn are determined by the gestational age at the onset of the insult. Early onset such as in renal agenesis will usually produce more severe hypoplasia than late onset whatever the underlying cause.[8] However, the amniotic fluid volume early in the second trimester in renal agenesis is usually normal so that oligohydramnios per se cannot explain the histological changes of pulmonary hypoplasia and other features such as pulmonary fluid dynamics must contribute. The prognosis of pulmonary hypoplasia is very varied, depending on the underlying causes. Mortality in the neonatal period can be as high as 80%.

Echogenic lung – bilateral

Uniform increased echogenicity of both lungs is caused by any condition which prevents the normal circulation of lung fluid. This is a rare condition and often associated with tracheal or laryngeal atresia. The lung volume in these circumstances is considerably enlarged with the diaphragms being pushed downwards so that the chest volume is considerably greater and abdominal volume is reduced. This condition is sometimes associated with renal agenesis and microphthalmia as part of Fraser's syndrome (Fig. 10.3). It is important to make this diagnosis as this is an autosomal recessive condition with a 1 in 4 risk of recurrence. Bilateral cystic adenomatoid malformations have been described as causing the same appearances, but are very uncommon and it would be very unusual for uniformity of echogenicity to be equal bilaterally in this condition. In addition the demonstration of a dilated trachea may be seen in laryngeal atresia.

Echogenic lungs – unilateral

Uniform echogenicity of a single lung with increase in volume can be caused by bronchial atresia.[9] The mechanism is similar to that of tracheal atresia, but only one lung is affected. The mediastinum may be displaced and the contralateral lung somewhat compressed by this condition. This is a very rare condition, but is compatible with life if early neonatal surgery is undertaken to remove the non-functioning lung.

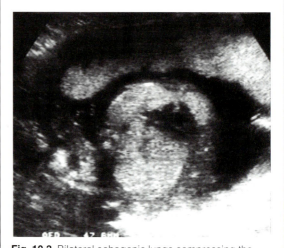

Fig. 10.3 Bilateral echogenic lungs compressing the heart. The fetus had other features of Fraser syndrome also.

Bronchopulmonary sequestration

Bronchopulmonary sequestration is a condition where part of the lung has ceased during development to be connected to the bronchial tree. A vascular aetiology has been suggested. In this condition, there is a uniform increased echogenicity of part of one of the lungs. This more commonly affects the lower lobes. It can sometimes be difficult to differentiate between this and bronchial atresia if the normal part of the lung is compressed. A bright section of lung can be demonstrated from 18 weeks onwards.[10] Many of these lung abnormalities become less marked in the late second trimester and some cannot be demonstrated after delivery by any imaging means (Fig. 10.4). It is thought that the mechanism of production of these abnormalities is a bronchial atresia, occurring during the later development of the lung with retention of lung fluid caused by the bronchial occlusion. The reason for the reduction in size of many of these in later pregnancy is uncertain, but it has been suggested that transient bronchial occlusion as a result of 'plugging' may account for those cases where no postnatal pulmonary abnormality is detected. Because the blood supply of these lesions is usually systemic from the aorta, it is sometimes possible to demonstrate a large vessel entering the lesion from the aorta. The postnatal outlook can be good, particularly if the lesion shows evidence of reduction in size in utero as often happens in the third trimester. If hydrops develops, the outlook is more guarded.[11] Infradiaphragmatic pulmonary sequestrations have been described and diagnosed antenatally.[12] These tend to grow slowly with the fetus and most require postnatal removal although a more conservative approach has been advocated by some authors recently.

Cystic adenomatoid malformation

This is a rare condition of the lung presenting with a varied appearance. This ranges from bright lung as seen in sequestration to a cystic lesion causing space occupation which can sometimes be difficult to differentiate from a diaphragmatic hernia. Traditionally

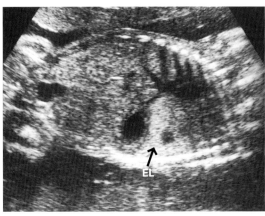

A

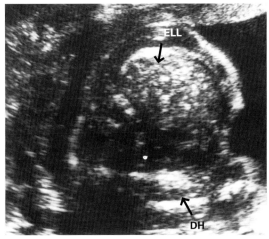

B

Fig. 10.4 (A) Coronal image of echogenic lung with small, echo-poor area. EL, echogenic lung. (B) Echogenic lung on axial section causing cardiac displacement. This lesion showed complete antenatal resolution. DH, displaced heart; ELL, echogenic left lung.

three types of congenital cystic adenomatoid malformation of the lung (CCAM) have been recognized.[13] Type 1 is predominantly macrocystic and is the type sometimes confused with diaphragmatic hernia; type 2 is mixed; and type 3 is microcystic which appears predominantly echogenic antenatally and may cause confusion with bronchopulmonary sequestration (Figs 10.5 and 10.6). Lesions may change in character during pregnancy and have even been known to resolve. The underlying cause is again thought to be a local bronchial atresia or bronchial occlusion,[14] occurring at an earlier stage in pregnancy than that which

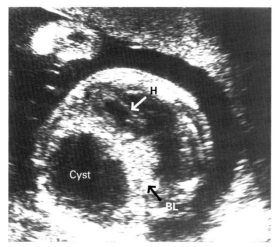

Fig. 10.5 Axial section of the fetal chest, showing left lower lobe lesion displacing the heart to the right. The lesion is largely cystic and histologically proved to be a congenital cystic adenomatoid malformation. BL, bright lung; H, heart.

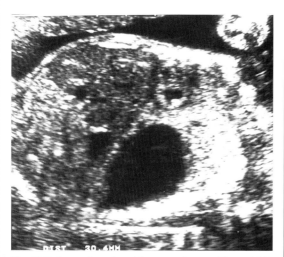

Fig. 10.6 Coronal section of the same fetus as Figure 10.5.

causes sequestration. Prognosis is affected if associated trisomy 21 or hydrops fetalis is present although early diagnosis and mediastinal shift are not indicators of poor prognosis.[15] In up to 30% of cases where there is hydrops, this will resolve.[15] If hydrops is not present at diagnosis, there is only a small chance that it will develop. Many cases have been seen to resolve during pregnancy although histological proof of the diagnosis is lacking in many such cases.[14] Diagnosis in utero by lung biopsy has been undertaken.

Lobar emphysema has been demonstrated in pregnancy either as a uniformly echogenic lesion which does not reduce in size or occasionally as a cystic lesion. Cases related to cytomegalovirus infection or respiratory syncytial virus infection have been described. It is thought these viruses cause inflammation of the bronchus and occlusion in utero, the mechanism being very similar to that seen with the bronchial atresia causing cystic adenomatoid malformation or sequestration.

It can be very difficult to differentiate between bronchopulmonary sequestration and CCAM antenatally. Cases of sequestration with large cystic elements have been described mimicking CCAM and cases of type 3 CCAM, which appear uniformly bright mimicking bronchopulmonary sequestration, have likewise been seen. A definitive prenatal diagnosis is probably not necessary to determine prognosis.

Bronchogenic cyst

These lesions have been diagnosed in utero as cystic chest lesions arising near the midline.[17]

Cystic hygromas

These appear as transonic lesions in the chest and may extend into the neck. Antenatally diagnosed, chest, cystic hygromas are very much rarer than neck hygromas.[18]

Pleural abnormalities

Virtually the only pleural abnormality seen on ultrasound antenatally is a pleural effusion. This appears as a transonic area surrounding one or both lungs. Large effusions cause depression of the diaphragm and mediastinal shift. The very earliest pleural effusions are seen as small collections around the lung bases on a coronal view (Figs 10.7 and 10.8). When slightly larger, these are seen on the axial view as a rim around the lung. Effusions can be unilateral or bilateral. Unilateral effusions can be transudates or chyle.

Unilateral chylothorax is the commonest cause of an isolated pleural effusion. It can be seen from 19 weeks onwards. Postnatally no cause for it is usually found and in most

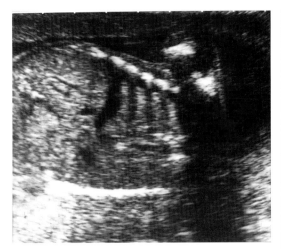

Fig. 10.7 Coronal section shows small pleural effusion predominantly between the lung base and the lung.

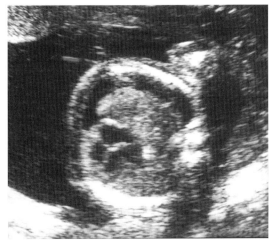

Fig. 10.8 Axial section, showing moderate right pleural effusion.

circumstances the condition is self-limiting with the effusion resolving following drainage or repeated aspiration over a period of days or weeks. The chylous nature of the effusion can be determined postnatally by the typical 'milky' appearance of the fluid, but this only happens when the baby has been fed a milk diet.

Chylothoraces have been described with other lymphatic abnormalities, including Turner's syndrome and trisomy 21 and, rarely, congenital pulmonary lymphangiectasia.[19–22] Whilst there may be significant lung compression by a unilateral pleural effusion, the timing on onset

determines the long-term effect of this. Significant pulmonary compression between 17 and 24 weeks' gestation can cause pulmonary hypoplasia with subsequent respiratory difficulties postnatally.

Transudate pleural effusions are also seen as unilateral transonic appearances. These may also be seen in isolation and can vary in size; spontaneous disappearance has been described. An isolated pleural effusion is an indication for karyotyping and trisomy 21 is the underlying cause in a significant number of cases.

Bilateral pleural effusions can be of the same underlying causes. They may also be seen as part of the spectrum of features of hydrops fetalis with other effusions and soft tissue oedema (see Ch. 17). Aspiration of the fluid for diagnostic reasons to exclude chromosome abnormalities by lymphocyte culture is often used. It can also be therapeutic with complete resolution of the effusion following a single aspiration. Recurrences, however, are common and shunting of the fluid into the amniotic cavity using a percutaneously inserted pigtail catheter is often required. Aspiration reduces lung compression, enables a more comprehensive cardiac assessment and improves cardiac venous return which in turn improves cardiac function. The outlook for fetuses with pleural effusions is very varied. It is worse if bilateral or associated with hydrops fetalis.[23] It is also worse if occurring early in pregnancy, if a cause can be defined, e.g. chromosomal abnormality or cardiac anomaly, or if it causes chronic pulmonary compression and consequent pulmonary hypoplasia.

Chest wall

The commonest deviation of chest shape is the so-called 'bell-shaped' chest. This is often seen in pulmonary hypoplasia as a secondary phenomenon.

In many skeletal dysplasias such as thanatophoric dysplasia, osteogenesis imperfecta, achondrogenesis, several syndromes associated with short rib polydactyly syndrome and Ellis–van-Creveld syndrome, the chest shape is abnormal. As well as the lung volume and chest volume being reduced, short ribs can be demonstrated in some cases and in osteogenesis imperfecta, the unusual shape of the ribs ('violin shape') or healing fractures can be demonstrated (see Ch. 12).

Chest wall tumours

Hamartomas of the chest wall presenting as echogenic masses have been described. It can be difficult to exclude a thoracic neuroblastoma involving the chest wall and to differentiate this from a primary chest wall lesion involving the thorax. Lymphangiomas and haemangiomas of the chest wall appear as mixed echo lesions. The latter may be associated with limb haemangiomas and the Klippel–Trenaunay–Weber syndrome.

Diaphragmatic hernias

There are a number of sites for potential hernia formation through the diaphragm. The commonest are the pleuroperitoneal canals, the site of foramen of Bochdalek hernias and, most uncommonly, the foramen of Morgagni more anteriorly.

Posterior diaphragmatic hernias (Bochdalek type)

Posteriorly situated hernias of the Bochdalek type are most commonly seen on the left side (75%).[24] Diagnosis can be made from about 18 weeks onwards.[25] Cardiac displacement from left to right is usually the most obvious and earliest sign to suggest such an abnormality. Whilst the apex of the heart is usually unaffected, in orientation it is displaced from the left to right by the herniated abdominal contents. If these include the stomach, then a transonic area adjacent to the heart is clearly seen with absence of the normal stomach in its usual position in the abdomen. It is usually very difficult at around 20 weeks to see the compressed left lung separate from the herniated bowel so that direct assessment of lung volume on the affected side is very difficult (Fig. 10.9). The right lung in left-sided hernias can usually be identified and seen in its compressed state.

With right-sided, diaphragmatic hernias, the liver is usually the primary organ herniating although small bowel may also form part of the hernial contents. Such hernias are more difficult to diagnose because of the relatively subtle changes in echo appearances in the right side of the chest, as the right lung, liver and small bowel all have very similar echodensities. Although the texture of the three organs is somewhat different, such differences are not easily

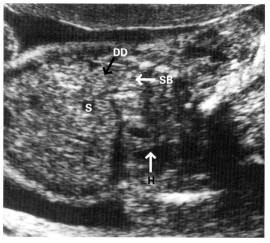

A

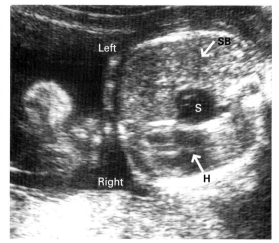

B

Fig. 10.9 (A) Coronal section, showing defect in the left diaphragm with a diaphragmatic hernia. DD, defect in diaphragm; H, heart; S, stomach; SB, small bowel in chest. (B) Axial section of left diaphragmatic hernia, showing stomach and small bowel in the left chest with heart displaced to the right. H, heart; S, stomach; SB, small bowel.

appreciated even with high resolution equipment, especially if the mother is somewhat obese. Right-sided hernias should be suspected if the heart is displaced more to the left than would be usual and, in particular, if the axis of the interventricular septum is more coronally placed than the usual oblique positioning. In later pregnancy, it is often possible to differentiate the small bowel from the lung and liver to confirm the diagnosis.

A further indirect sign of diaphragmatic hernia is a rotatory movement of the thoracic and abdominal contents with fetal breathing movements. This is due to upward movement into the chest of the abdominal contents on the affected side with normal downward movement on the unaffected side.

Identifying a defect in the diaphragm can sometimes be extremely difficult and, indeed, even with good image quality, moderate-sized diaphragmatic defects sometimes go undetected although the secondary effects of the herniation are usually well seen. An apparently intact diaphragm does not exclude a diaphragmatic hernia.

The time of occurrence of Bochdalek hernias is very variable, the earliest being seen at 15 to 16 weeks' gestation, but there is evidence that some hernias occur well into the third trimester and indeed it is well recognized that some hernias do not manifest themselves until later in postnatal life. Right-sided hernias are more prone to late diagnosis than left-sided ones. A late complication of diaphragmatic hernia is polyhydramnios, but this usually only develops in the third trimester.[26,27] Associated abnormalities are common, especially chromosomal abnormalities and those affecting the cardiovascular, genitourinary, musculoskeletal and central nervous systems. An associated abnormality raises the mortality to between 80 and 90%.[27,28] The differential diagnosis includes cystic adenomatoid malformation, bronchopulmonary sequestration, bronchogenic and enteric cysts and mediastinal teratomas.[29]

The suspicion of a diaphragmatic hernia is ample justification for karyotyping.

Diaphragmatic hernias are commonly seen with trisomy 21, trisomy 18 and deletion of the short arm of chromosome 12 (Pallister–Killian syndrome). Caution should be exercised in the tissue being karyotyped as the Pallister–Killian syndrome cannot be excluded on fetal blood sampling and trisomy 18 can occasionally go undetected on placental biopsy.

One recent large series has pointed out that whilst the accuracy of antenatal diagnosis has increased from 6% in 1985 to 41% in 1991, survival has not improved. Associated abnormalities are seen in 29% of cases.

Morgagni hernia

These are rare and often have no sac to contain the contents. They are anteriorly situated and frequently contain liver and large bowel. Associated ascites, pericardial or pleural effusions have been described.[30] Associated structural abnormalities, especially cardiovascular and chromosomal defects, have been described.

Prognosis of diaphragmatic hernia

There are a number of factors which influence the prognosis of diaphragmatic hernias. The survival rate for isolated diaphragmatic hernias diagnosed antenatally is at best 34%. The prognosis is considerably reduced in the presence of other abnormalities. The commonest of these are chromosomal anomalies and cardiac lesions. Poor prognostic signs include diagnosis prior to 24 weeks, polyhydramnios, hydrops fetalis and concomitant intra-uterine growth retardation.[29] The immediate outlook for survival is determined by the degree of pulmonary hypoplasia which is at its most profound in those lesions which have caused compression between 17 and 24 weeks and in those which have the greatest mediastinal shifts. Anterior Morgagni hernias are much less common and have rarely been described antenatally. They tend to be centrally situated and cause cardiac compression and rotation. They usually contain large and/or small bowel and rarely cause significant pulmonary compression.

Hiatus hernias are very unusual in the neonate but have been described in fetal life.[31]

References

Normal appearances

1. De Vore GR, Hovenstein J, Platt LD. Fetal echocardiography: Assessment of cardiothoracic disproportion – A new technique for the diagnosis of thoracic hypoplasia. Am J Obstet Gynecol 1986; 155:1066–1071.
2. Carson PL, Meter CR, Bowrman RA. Prediction of fetal lung maturity at various stages of intrauterine life. Thorax 1961; 16:207–218.
3. Fried AM, Loh FK, Umer MA, et al. Echogenicity of fetal lungs: Relation to fetal age and maturity. AJR 1985; 145:591–594.

Pulmonary hypoplasia

4. Schnizel A, Savodelli G, Briner J, et al. Prenatal sonographic diagnosis of Jeune syndrome. Radiology 1985; 154:777–778.
5. Robert AB, Mitchell J. Pulmonary hypoplasia and fetal breathing in preterm premature rupture of membranes. Early Hum Dev 1995; 41:27–37.
6. Harstad TW, Twickler DM, Leveno KJ, Brown CE. Antepartum prediction of pulmonary hypoplasia: An elusive goal? Am J Perinatol 1993; 10(1):8–11.
7. Ohlsson A, Fong K, Rose T, et al. Prenatal ultrasonic prediction of autopsy proven pulmonary hypoplasia. Am J Perinatol 1992; 9(5–6):334–337.
8. Chamberlain D, Hislop A, Hey E, et al. Pulmonary hypoplasia in babies with severe rhesus isoimmunization: A quantitative study. J Pathol 1977; 122:43–52.

Echogenic lung

9. King SJ, Pilling DW, Walkinshaw S. Fetal echogenic lung lesions: prenatal ultrasound diagnosis and outcome. Pediatr Radiol 1995; 25(3):208–210.

Bronchopulmonary sequestration

10. Romero R, Chervenak FA, Kotzen J, et al. Antenatal sonographic findings of extralobar pulmonary sequestration. J Ultrasound Med 1982; 1:131–132.
11. Thomas CS, Leopold GR, Hilton S, et al. Fetal hydrops associated with extralobar pulmonary sequestration. J Ultrasound Med 1986; 5:668–671.
12. Davies RP, Ford WDA, Lequesne GW, et al. Ultrasonic detection of subdiaphragmatic pulmonary sequestration in utero and postnatal diagnosis by fine needle aspiration biopsy. J Ultrasound Med 1989; 8:47–49.

Cystic adenomatoid malformation

13. Stocker JT, Madewell JE, Drake RM. Congenital cystic adenomatoid malformation of the lung. Hum Pathol 1977; 8:155–171.
14. Achiron R, Strauss S, Seidman DS, Lipitz S, Mashiach S, Goldman B. Fetal lung hyperechogenicity: prenatal ultrasonographic diagnosis, natural history and neonatal outcome. Ultrasound Obstet Gynecol 1995; 6(1):40–42.
15. Barret J, Chitayat D, Sermer M, et al. The prognostic factors in the prenatal diagnosis of the echogenic fetal lung. Prenat Diagn 1995; 15(9):849–853.
16. McCullagh M, MacConnachie I, Garvie D, Dykes E. Accuracy of prenatal diagnosis of congenital cystic adenomatoid malformation. Arch Dis Child 1994; 71(2):F111–F113.

Bronchogenic cyst

17. Hoeffel JC, Didier F, Marx D, et al. Imaging of bronchogenic cysts in children. Ann Radiol Paris 1994; 37(6):417–423.

Cystic hygroma

18. Zalel Y, Shalev E, Ben-Ami M, Mogilner G, Weiner E. Ultrasonic diagnosis of mediastinal cystic hygroma. Prenat Diagn 1992; 12(6):541–544.

Pleural abnormalities

19. Castillo RA, Devoe LD, Falls G, et al. Pleural effusions and pulmonary hypoplasia. Am J Obstet Gynecol 1987; 157:1252–1255.
20. Samuel N, Sirotta L, Bar-Ziv J, et al. The ultrasonic appearance of common pulmonary vein atresia in utero. J Ultrasound Med 1988; 7:25–28.
21. Jaffe R, DiSegni E, Altaras M, et al. Ultrasonic real time diagnosis of transitory fetal pleural and pericardial effusion. Diagn Imag Clin Med 1986; 55L:373–375.
22. Wilson RHJ, Duncan A, Hume R, et al. Prenatal pleural effusion associated with congenital pulmonary lymphangiectasia. Prenat Diagn 1985; 5:73–76.
23. Rodeck CH, Fisk NM, Fraser DI, et al. Longterm in utero drainage of fetal hydrothorax. N Engl J Med 1988; 319:1135–1138.

Posterior diaphragmatic hernia

24. Adzick NS, Harrison MR, Glick PL, et al. Diaphragmatic hernia in the fetus: Prenatal diagnosis and outcome in 94 cases. J Pediatr Surg 1985; 20:357–361.
25. Benacerraf BR, Juul S, Siebert JR. Fetal diaphragmatic hernia: Ultrasound diagnosis and clinical outcome in 19 cases. Am J Obstet Gynecol 1987; 156:573–576.
26. Chinn DH, Filly RA, Callen PW, et al. Congenital diaphragmatic hernia diagnosed prenatally by ultrasound. Radiology 1983; 148:119–123.
27. Constock CH. The antenatal diagnosis of diaphragmatic anomalies. J Ultrasound Med 1986; 5:391–396.
28. Constock CH. The antenatal diagnosis of diaphragmatic anomalies. J Ultrasound Med 1986; 5:391–396.
29. David TJ, Illinsworth CA. Diaphragmatic hernia in the southwest of England. J Med Genet 1976; 13:253–262.
30. Adzick NS, Harrison MR, Glick PL, et al. Diaphragmatic hernia in the fetus: Prenatal diagnosis and outcome in 94 cases. J Pediatr Surg 1985; 20:357–361.

Morgagnia hernia

31. Whittle MJ, Gilmore DH, McNay MB, et al. Diaphragmatic hernia presenting in utero as a unilateral hydrothorax. Prenat Diag 1989; 9:115–118.

Hiatal hernia

32. Bahado-Singh RO, Romero R, Vecchio M, Hobbins J. Prenatal diagnosis of congenital hiatal hernia. J Ultrasound Med 1992; 11:297–300.

CHAPTER 11

Abdominal and abdominal wall abnormalities

David Pilling

Introduction

Abdominal wall abnormalities are one of the commoner fetal abnormalities demonstrated by ultrasound. They were recognized early in the development of fetal ultrasound because disturbance of the abdominal wall contour in the region of the cord insertion was demonstrated even by static B-mode scanning before real time was available. Since many of these abnormalities cause a rise in the serum alphafetoprotein, a specific search for abdominal wall abnormalities as a cause for this has been undertaken in virtually all ultrasound departments using routine serum alphafetoprotein screening. Even though the primary aim of this screening was to exclude neural tube defects, anterior abdominal wall defects as a group are the second commonest anatomical cause for raised serum alphafetoprotein. The spectrum of anterior abdominal wall defects extends from the very minor exomphalos with bowel herniating into the base of the cord to the most major defects, including the pentalogy of Cantrell and body stalk defect or early amnion rupture sequence.

Normal appearances

The anterior abdominal wall is best demonstrated in axial section. The anterior abdominal wall is clearly outlined by amniotic fluid on its external surface with the site of the cord insertion being clearly demonstrated. The lowest part of the anterior abdominal wall is sometimes obscured by the flexed legs with assessment of the anterior abdominal wall below the cord insertion sometimes being extremely difficult, whatever approach is utilized. A midline, sagittal view of the fetus will sometimes give better views of this area but this is not always feasible. The internal aspect of the anterior abdominal wall can be difficult to see clearly because of the similar echodensities of the anterior abdominal wall and adjacent liver and bowel. This becomes

more clearly identified as the pregnancy advances.

Normal variants, pitfalls and artefacts

By 12 weeks' gestation, the bowel has returned to the abdomen so that any herniated abdominal contents are abnormal after this time. The exclusion of abnormality of the anterior abdominal wall is difficult in certain circumstances, particularly where the anterior abdominal wall of the fetus lies adjacent to the maternal uterus or placenta. This is not a major difficulty with adequate amounts of liquor in the first and second trimesters since the fetus will usually turn given time so that the anterior abdominal wall can be checked. With severe oligohydramnios and anhydramnios and, in particular, with the reduced mobility of the fetus in the third trimester, exclusion of an anterior abdominal wall defect can be very difficult. With extreme oligohydramnios, the distortion of the anterior abdominal wall can often mimic a moderate-sized, anterior abdominal wall defect. Defects in the infra-umbilical portion of the abdominal wall are difficult to exclude with flexion of the fetal femora. Since many of these defects are associated with bladder abnormalities, presence of a normal bladder, even in the absence of clear demonstration of the anterior abdominal wall, excludes cloacal exstrophy and thus suggests an intact lower abdominal wall but will not exclude exomphalos or gastroschisis.

Anterior abdominal wall appearances

List of conditions

- Exomphalos
- Gastroschisis
- Limb–body wall complex/early amnion rupture sequence

- Ectopia cordis (including pentalogy of Cantrell)
- Cloacal and bladder exstrophy.

Exomphalos

Exomphalos occurs in about 0.1 to 0.03% of pregnancies,[1,2] the incidence increasing with maternal age.

Exomphalos is an incomplete return of the abdominal contents to the abdominal cavity in early pregnancy. In its minor form this can consist of herniation of a small loop of bowel into the base of the cord and can be extremely difficult to diagnose. Any transonic area at the base of the cord which is not a blood vessel is almost certainly a small loop of bowel in a minor exomphalos. The umbilical vein is seen coursing through the sac and its contents in contradistinction to gastroschisis. The most major exomphalos may indeed be larger in cross-sectional area than the abdomen. The sac of an exomphalos which consists of peritoneum and amnion may contain any of the abdominal organs although bowel is most commonly present, but the stomach, liver and spleen may be partially or entirely present within the exomphalos. Exomphalos containing only bowel are in the minority (10 to 25%).[3,4,5] The relatively thick sac wall restricts the 'leakage' of alphafetoprotein and levels are not as raised as in gastroschisis.[6] There is frequently some free fluid within the larger exomphalos which obviously communicates freely with the peritoneal cavity (Fig. 11.1). As the bowel is contained within a sac, it does not become exposed to amniotic fluid and thus does not become thickened. The relatively wide neck to the sac (Fig. 11.2) seen in exomphalos also contributes to the reduced incidence of bowel atresias compared with gastroschisis.

Other abnormalities are frequently associated with exomphalos. Cardiac malformations are seen in up to 50%, limb abnormalities in about 30% and chromosome abnormalities in 28 to 36%, mainly trisomies 13 and 18.[7] Some authors quote a chromosome abnormality rate of 61% at 11 to 14 weeks' gestation.[2] Chromosome abnormalities are more frequently associated

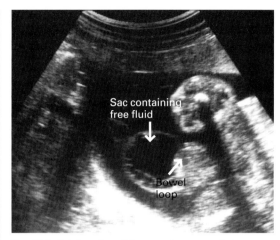

Fig. 11.1 Axial section of the sac of an exomphalos, containing liver, a loop of bowel and some free fluid.

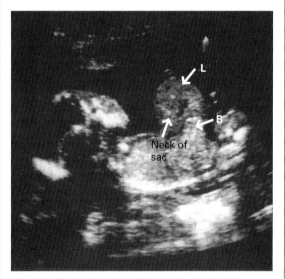

Fig. 11.2 Sagittal section of fetus with exomphalos, showing the wide neck of the sac containing liver and some loops of bowel. B, bowel; L, liver.

with small exomphalos containing only bowel (67% compared with 16% if liver is also present).[1] It is important to differentiate a large exomphalos from limb–body wall complex (see below). Exomphalos is a feature of the Beckwith–Wiedemann syndrome and is seen in 10% of cases. Other features include macroglossia, gigantism and cystic kidneys. Any fetus with exomphalos should be thoroughly examined for other abnormalities, particularly cardiac malformations. With larger exomphalos, the heart is often difficult to examine comprehensively. This is due to the tendency of the heart to rotate, as much of the abdominal contents lie outside the normal abdomen. The fetus also tends to lie on its side which makes an anterior approach to the heart quite difficult. The exomphalos itself may also impede the view of the heart to some extent. Umbilical cord cysts are sometimes associated with exomphalos and in such cases there is a very high risk (44%) of trisomy 18.[8]

Ultrasound diagnosed exomphalos in 66 to 75% of cases[7,9] in two large British series from the late 1980s to early 1990s, but accuracy has increased in later years. Misdiagnosis of exomphalos as gastroschisis occurred in 5%.[7] In view of the high risk of chromosome abnormalities all patients carrying a fetus with exomphalos should be offered karyotyping.

Polyhydramnios has been demonstrated in 30% of fetuses with exomphalos[10] but the cause, whilst sometimes related to other abnormalities, is not always clear.

The fetus with exomphalos should be examined at intervals throughout the pregnancy although complications such as bowel atresia are quite uncommon. Rupture of the sac in utero is rare.[5,11,12] There is no evidence of improved outcome if the fetus is delivered by caesarean section[13,14] and this should be reserved for those pregnancies with obstetric indications for such delivery.

In the absence of other abnormalities, the outcome for a fetus with exomphalos is good, with surgical repair being feasible in most cases although sometimes complex, staged, abdominal wall repairs are required. The survival in exomphalos is strongly related to the incidence of associated anomalies and this has to a large extent prevented an improvement in survival in recent years. In the presence of a major associated anomaly, the survival can be as low as 20%. Interestingly, whilst large size is associated with a poorer prognosis, this is not a major factor.

Although in most cases the relative size of the exomphalos compared to the abdominal cross-section remains unchanged, relative increase in size has been observed in some cases. Relative decrease in size of the exomphalos has also been demonstrated in other cases (Fig. 11.3).

As there is usually an intact sac covering exomphalos at birth, immediate surgery within hours is not always necessary and, indeed, with small exomphalos, delayed repair is often feasible.

Gastroschisis

This condition, which has no known genetic associations, is a herniation of abdominal

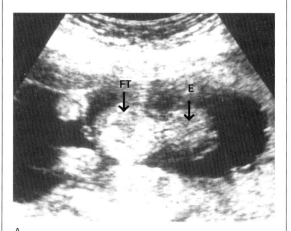

A

B

Fig. 11.3 (A) Axial section of fetus, showing fetal trunk (FT) with exomphalos (E). Note that the exomphalos is almost the same size as the fetal trunk. (B) Same fetus 4 weeks later, showing relative decrease in the size of the exomphalos (E). At birth, the exomphalos was very small and repair was delayed until 3 months of age. Note the umbilical cord (UC) entering the apex of the sac, a diagnostic feature of exomphalos. FT, fetal trunk.

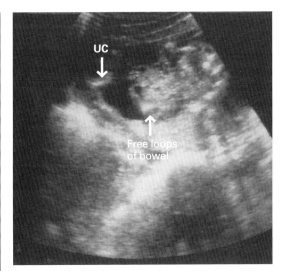

Fig. 11.4 Gastroschisis containing free loops of bowel. Umbilical cord (UC) seen to the right of the loops of bowel, differentiating this from an exomphalos.

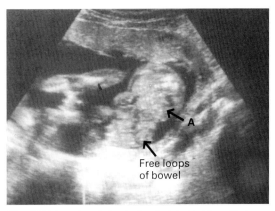

Fig. 11.5 Anterior abdominal wall defect with multiple loops of small bowel free floating in the amniotic fluid – gastroschisis. A, abdomen.

contents usually to the right of the cord insertion (Fig. 11.4). There is some dispute as to the underlying cause, some authorities suggesting that this is due to rupture of an exomphalos, and others suggesting that it is a developmental defect of the abdominal wall with herniation of the contents as a consequence of this. De Vries[16] suggests that it is due to abnormal involution of the right umbilical vein.[17] A gastroschisis never has a surrounding membrane and usually contains only bowel, predominantly small bowel (Fig. 11.5). As the bowel is in direct contact with the amniotic fluid, both serum and amniotic fluid alphafetoprotein levels are elevated more than in exomphalos.[6] The stomach, large bowel and bladder do occasionally herniate from the abdomen, but this is less common. It is unusual for liver, spleen or bladder to herniate. In early pregnancy, the multiple loops of bowel can be seen outlined by the amniotic fluid, with bowel wall thickness and lumen dimensions being normal. In later pregnancy, complications such as bowel wall thickening, shortening and bowel dilatation may supervene. The thickening is thought to be a chemical peritonitis related to the exposure of the bowel to fetal urine in the amniotic fluid.[18] By definition the bowel of

gastroschisis is non-rotated. Intestinal atresias or stenosis secondary to intestinal ischaemia are reported in up to 30%.[19,20] Bowel lumen diameter of greater than 17 mm is very suspicious of significant bowel dilatation.[17] Babcock et al[15] showed that a maximum small bowel diameter of more than 11 mm was related to postnatal bowel complications, but operator variation in measurement makes utilization of this figure in practice difficult. Abnormal ultrasound appearance of bowel is associated with more difficult repair and higher incidence of overall complications.[21] Gastroschisis is not usually associated with other abnormalities although every fetus with gastroschisis should be examined by ultrasound to exclude other abnormalities. Karyotypic abnormalities are extremely uncommon and most centres would not recommend karyotyping for gastroschisis. In the absence of additional abnormalities, the antenatal outlook for fetuses with gastroschisis is good. The antenatal detection rate of gastroschisis in two series has been quoted as 71.6%[22] and 70%.[9]

About 48% of fetuses with gastroschisis will be small for dates.[23] Difficulties in management occur because ultrasound abdominal circumference measurements are not usually valid in this group and as this is the cornerstone of assessment of fetal size in utero, accurate assessment becomes difficult. Cardiotocograph monitoring is also affected

ABDOMINAL AND ABDOMINAL WALL ABNORMALITIES

by the bowel in the amniotic cavity, possibly mediated through tension on the vagus nerve. Whilst caesarean section is not usually considered advantageous over vaginal delivery in this condition,[21] many fetuses with gastroschisis are delivered by caesarean section for obstetric reasons related to the difficulty in monitoring both fetal size and fetal wellbeing.

Misdiagnosis of gastroschisis as exomphalos occurred in 14.7% of cases in one series from the late 1980s to early 1990s.[22] Confusion with limb–body wall complex can be avoided by identifying the other abnormalities usually seen in the latter condition (see below).

Outcome is not affected by delivery in a tertiary obstetric centre as compared with a district general hospital,[7,24] although delivery within easy reach of a neonatal surgery centre is advisable. Postnatal management requires immediate enclosure of the bowel in 'clingfilm' to retain the moisture followed by early transfer to the neonatal surgical unit for early closure. This can almost always be achieved, but sometimes requires complex staging procedures. Because of bowel wall thickening and the incidence of atresias, lengthy intravenous feeding is often required and an overall, neonatal mortality rate of 10% is a combination of the early neonatal deaths caused by bowel ischaemia and later problems relating to short bowel and the complications of intravenous feeding. The majority of survivors will be on full feeding within 4 weeks of delivery, but some may require many months of intravenous feeding. Bowel dilatation in utero of 18 mm or more is associated with significant delay in establishing oral feeding.[25] It is extremely difficult to predict when bowel is at risk in utero. Colour flow Doppler, whilst helpful, has not answered all the questions and the balance between preterm delivery with all its problems and the risks of bowel ischaemia, the symptoms and signs of which in utero are very non-specific, is a difficult one to achieve.

Spontaneous resolution of gastroschisis and closure of the anterior abdominal wall defect has been described.[26]

Limb–body wall complex

This is a very rare condition also known as body stalk anomaly. Some authors consider this to be a variant of early amnion rupture. The cord is shortened and a very large, anterior abdominal wall defect is seen, usually affecting the left side. There is often an associated, extensive, lower spine neural tube defect. Other primary features are exencephaly or encephalocoele, facial cleft and limb defects. All such pregnancies have failure of fusion between the amnion and the chorion. The outcome is uniformly fatal.

Pathogenesis is uncertain, and theories of causation include body stalk dysmorphogenesis and early amnion rupture owing to vascular disruption. Some consider it to be an extreme form of the amniotic band syndrome. Ultrasound findings are of extensive facial, thoracic and abdominal abnormalities entangled with the membranes. The umbilical cord is short. Spinal dysraphism is common and association of anterior abdominal wall defect with scoliosis and spinal defect should suggest the diagnosis. Karyotypic abnormalities have not been described. The condition has been linked with cocaine abuse.[27]

Ectopia cordis

This is a rare, body wall abnormality where the heart has herniated through a defect in the chest or thoraco-abdominal wall. When there is an abdominal element, this is often known as the pentalogy of Cantrell (ectopia cordis, diaphragmatic defect, exomphalos, pericardial defect and intracardiac abnormality).[28,29] The defect is thought to be due to lack of fusion of the lateral body folds. Ectopia cordis is easy to demonstrate by ultrasound as the pulsating heart is clearly identified outside the confines of the chest. The diagnosis can be difficult if amniotic fluid volume is reduced.

The rotation and occasional displacement of the heart seen with a large exomphalos should not be confused with pentalogy of Cantrell.

Cloacal and bladder exstrophy

In cloacal exstrophy as well as an exomphalos, there is a cloacal abnormality which opens on to the anterior abdominal wall. This can sometimes be a very difficult condition to diagnose, but should be suspected in any abdominal wall defect where a normal urinary bladder is not demonstrated within the fetal abdomen (Fig. 11.6). Associated hydronephrosis is a common finding. Less commonly, gastrointestinal, central nervous system and cardiac anomalies are seen. The thorax is usually narrow and there is a large sacral meningomyelocoele.[27,30] Bilateral club-feet are a common association.[31] This is a very serious condition requiring multiple surgical procedures postnatally with complicated urinary bowel and genital implications. Long-term outcome is not good with a 55% mortality.[32]

Bladder exstrophy is a less severe condition which, because the lower abdominal wall is often partially obscured by the femora, is more difficult to demonstrate. The outcome following surgery for bladder exstrophy is very good.

Abdominal abnormalities

Normal anatomy

The normal intra-abdominal anatomy is

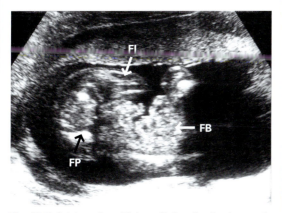

Fig. 11.6 Axial section of fetus with free floating loops of bowel. The section of the lower fetal abdomen does not demonstrate the fetal bladder. At post-mortem following termination of pregnancy, cloacal exstrophy was confirmed. FB, fetal bowel; FL, fetal leg; FP, fetal pelvis, no bladder seen.

dominated by the liver. This fills the upper abdomen and has a uniform echodensity. It contains a number of transonic structures, most notably hepatic veins, the intrahepatic portion of the umbilical vein as it joins the portal vein, and the gall bladder. The inferior vena cava is closely related to the posterior aspect of the liver. The spleen is of the same density as the liver, but is often difficult to differentiate from it. The normal fetal stomach can usually be recognized from early second trimester onwards although not always on a single examination as its size varies with time. Repeat scanning usually enables it to be identified over a period of hours or on separate days. The kidneys are easily recognized by their position and slightly brighter cortex compared to the renal medulla and adjacent liver. The bowel has a slightly increased echodensity compared to the liver and a 'coarser' texture.

Some small fluid-filled loops of small bowel can often be identified in the second and third trimester. The large bowel in the third trimester often has a relatively transonic appearance and is recognized by its haustral appearance and its position in the abdomen. This should not be mistaken for dilated loops of small bowel which would be pathological. The normal calibre of the fetal large bowel is up to 5 mm at 20 weeks and up to 20 mm at term.[33] The pelvic colon can be mistaken for a pelvic mass or ovarian pathology. The fetal bladder is of variable size and transonic in appearance. Its position in the pelvis confirms its nature. Fetal ureters are not identified in utero when normal. The fetal adrenal glands can be clearly identified in many cases in the second and third trimesters. Their position above the kidneys and differentiation between the more echodense medulla and less echodense cortex is typical.

Intra-abdominal abnormalities

Liver

Echo bright areas in the liver, either solitary or multiple, are recognized. In many of these,

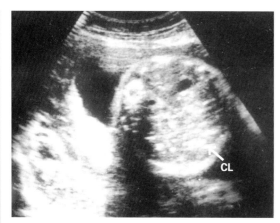

Fig. 11.7 Axial section of fetal abdomen with multiple, small, calcific lesions (CL) within the liver. These were related to fetal varicella.

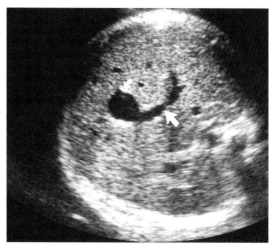

Fig. 11.8 Transverse section through the liver, showing a varix of the umbilical vein (curved arrow) as it joins the portal vein (straight arrow).

the underlying cause is not determined. If they are uncalcified, they may well represent small haemangiomas. Calcified lesions suggest the possibility of previous viral infection, particularly cytomegalovirus, toxoplasmosis or varicella (Fig. 11.7). In the absence of infection, isolated calcified foci in the liver have a good outcome.[34]

Liver tumours, particularly large haemangiomas and hepatoblastomas, have been demonstrated in utero. These manifest themselves as liver enlargement with mixed echogenicity. Large haemangiomas may be the cause of extensive arteriovenous shunting and developing hydrops, but are very rare. Whilst these are benign lesions, the outlook is poor if hydrops is present. Liver cysts, often lymphangiomas, have been described antenatally[35] and if unilocular, they must be differentiated from choledochal cysts and a normal gall bladder. Some are multilocular and they must be differentiated from a duplication cyst or mesenteric cyst. One further differential diagnosis of a cystic mass within the liver is a varix of the intra-abdominal portion of the umbilical vein. This can usually be diagnosed as it communicates with the umbilical or portal vein and shows venous flow on Doppler or colour flow (Fig. 11.8).[36]

Gall bladder

The fetal gall bladder is very variable in size

and whilst absence of the gall bladder can be associated with polysplenia syndromes and biliary atresia, such diagnoses are rarely made antenatally. A subjectively enlarged gall bladder has been reported in association with chromosomal disease.[37] Calcific foci in the fetal gall bladder are well recognized.[38,39] These are due to small gallstones and are usually incidental findings (Fig. 11.9). Most of these have no postnatal implications.

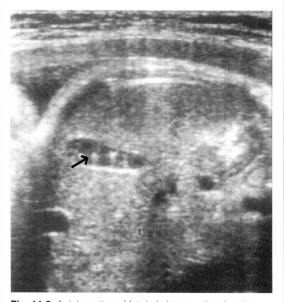

Fig. 11.9 Axial section of fetal abdomen, showing the gall bladder containing several calculi (arrow). No symptoms or signs in the neonatal period.

Choledochal cysts

Transonic areas in the portahepatis or subhepatic area separate from the gall bladder are rare. Such an abnormality should be considered to be a choledochal cyst when a separate gall bladder can be identified and the duodenum is seen separately from this mass.[40] Renal tract abnormalities and adrenal cysts rarely cause confusion. A duplication cyst of the duodenum can give similar appearances as can a simple, hepatic cyst. Some choledochal cysts, however, will be seen communicating with the branching biliary structures and this further confirms the diagnosis. All cases so far diagnosed antenatally have been female[41] and have been diagnosed between 15 and 37 weeks. In 56% of cases, the cyst was seen to grow in utero.

Spleen

In utero splenic abnormalities are very unusual, but transonic splenic cysts have been described as isolated findings, and normally have a good outcome.

Intra-abdominal cysts (Table 11.1)

Cystic abdominal lesions in the fetus are quite common. When such an abnormality is suspected, confirmation of normality of organ systems is essential. This includes normality of the gall bladder, kidneys, bladder, stomach, duodenum and large

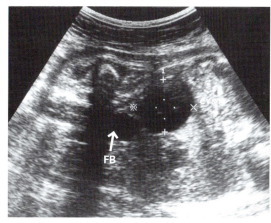

Fig. 11.10 Oblique section of fetal abdomen in the third trimester, showing a cyst adjacent to the fetal bladder (FB). Postnatal follow-up confirmed this to be a follicular ovarian cyst.

bowel if possible. Determination of gender also helps. In females, the commonest cause of a transonic abdominal mass with thin walls is an ovarian cyst (Fig. 11.10). These are usually seen in the third trimester. They can occur in any site within the abdomen and be up to 10 cm in diameter. Such cysts are almost always follicular and are related to hormonal stimulus from the pregnancy.[42–44] Unless very large, these do not usually require in utero management although in utero aspiration has been described. This should be considered if the cyst is thought likely to cause obstruction to delivery or be causing diaphragmatic elevation and subsequent pulmonary compromise. The vast majority of these, however, cause no difficulty in pregnancy or delivery. Postnatally the majority will resolve although this may take up to 6 months. If they are large and thought to be causing compression, then postnatal aspiration may be appropriate with postnatal ultrasound follow-up to check for resolution. Any recurrence or enlargement in size should raise the possibility of an alternative cause. Aspirate should be clear and straw-coloured in an uncomplicated cyst. Some authorities would advise early surgical removal of these cysts to preserve fertility,[45] but other authorities would suggest that this is unlikely to affect the long-term outlook for ovarian function in later life. Auto-

Table 11.1
Intra-abdominal cysts (excluding renal tract)

Liver	Simple cyst/lymphangioma Choledochal cyst (exclude large gall bladder) Varix of umbilical vein
Adrenal	Simple cyst Haemorrhage (evolving) Neuroblastoma
Bowel	Duplication cyst Mesenteric cyst/lymphangioma Meconium peritonitis (exclude dilated bowel loops)
Ovarian	Follicular cyst
Uterus/vagina	Hydrometrocolpos

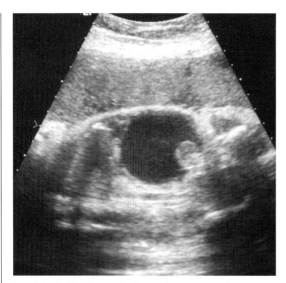

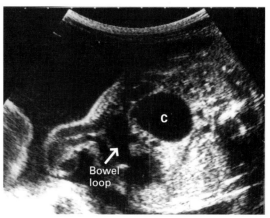

Fig. 11.13 Axial section of fetal abdomen, showing a cyst (C). At surgery postnatally, this was a duplication cyst of the ileum. The adjacent loop of bowel was a transient finding.

Fig. 11.11 Ovarian cyst with a solid component – representing clot retraction – which suggests torsion.

amputated cysts have been described.[46] Cysts larger than 50 mm may be candidates for postnatal aspiration[47] or removal.[48] Ovarian cysts that show solid areas (Fig. 11.11) or debris (Fig. 11.12) usually indicate torsion or haemorrhage and should be removed postnatally.[48–50] Polyhydramnios occurs in some pregnancies.[48]

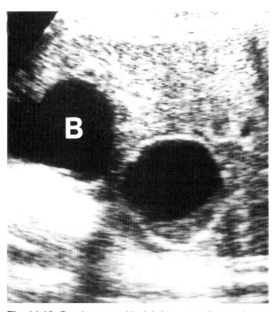

Fig. 11.12 Ovarian cyst with debris suggesting torsion. B, bladder.

The second commonest cause (Fig. 11.13) is a duplication cyst.[51,52] This is usually unilocular and, with high resolution, it is occasionally possible to demonstrate a multilayered wall. These cysts may be up to several centimetres in diameter and may be recognized in the second or third trimester. As they are closely related to bowel, they may sometimes cause compression of bowel in the postnatal period. They do not require intervention in utero, and, ex utero, if they are not causing symptoms, urgent surgery is not usually required. Interestingly, since many of these cysts are relatively flaccid, they may well not be palpable in the neonatal period.[53,54]

Mesenteric cysts which are usually lymphangiomas may also be seen in utero as transonic lesions, but are usually multilocular and not usually confused with the two former diagnoses (Fig. 11.14). These cysts frequently require operation after delivery and cannot always be entirely removed.

A pseudo-cyst related to meconium peritonitis can sometimes be diagnosed[55,56] but additional features including dilated bowel, peritoneal or bowel calcification and ascites often help to differentiate the cause (Fig. 11.15).

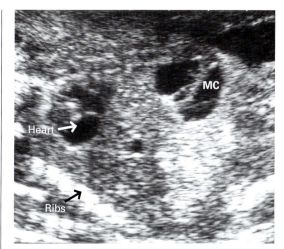

Fig. 11.14 Oblique section of the chest and abdomen. The multiloculated cyst was shown postnatally to be a mesenteric cyst (MC).

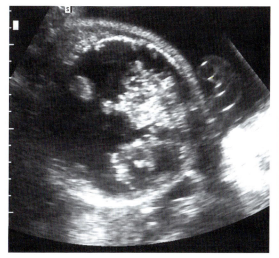

Fig. 11.15 Meconium pseudocyst – large abdominal cyst with calcification in its wall and containing debris. At surgery, there was a sigmoid perforation.

Posterior abdominal wall tumour

Masses arising from the tissues of the posterior abdominal wall are extremely rare, but may arise from striated muscle or fibrous tissue. The appearances are those of a soft tissue mass of slightly different density to the liver and spleen, usually extending into the abdomen, but sometimes seen extending outwards and distorting the abdominal circumference. They can be suspected by excluding other organs of origin such as adrenal, kidney or bowel as the source of origin of the mass, but the ultimate diagnosis usually can only be confirmed postnatally, especially if the mass extends into the abdominal cavity.

There is no established routine of management of these lesions. The ultimate diagnosis is usually only made after delivery although termination of a lesion occurring earlier in pregnancy is feasible.

As most of these lesions are aggressive in character, the long-term outlook is poor, particularly if adjacent structures such as the spine are involved. Cystic enteric duplication cysts have been described as a cause of retroperitoneal mass.[57]

Adrenal masses

The normal adrenal gland in the fetus is relatively larger than the adrenal gland in the older child and adult. The glands are relatively inconspicuous with normal tissue density slightly higher than the adjacent liver, spleen or kidney. The density of the medulla is usually higher than the density of the cortex, and the glands are most easily recognized in the transverse section. The typical Y-shaped appearance of the adrenal gland in longitudinal section is best appreciated in cases of renal agenesis where the adrenal gland may fill the renal fossa and be mistaken for renal tissue. Appreciation of the similarity in appearances is usually sufficient to enable differentiation of a normal adrenal gland in cases of suspected renal agenesis.

Adrenal haemorrhage

Haemorrhage into the left adrenal gland in particular is an uncommon event seen in the second or third trimester.[55,58] It is sometimes associated with fetal distress and growth retardation. Adrenal haemorrhage presents as a mass above the kidney, distorting the normal adrenal anatomy. The mass is usually hypoechoic, but can be mixed in character and will usually change in appearance over a period of time. The echogenicity varies with time and the size usually reduces. The condition has been described in association with renal vein thrombosis, particularly on the left side, and close examination of the kidneys is necessary. The condition usually has a benign outcome with the mass resolving in utero or early neonatal life without any long-term sequelae if the haemorrhage is isolated. Occasionally, a calcified residual lesion is seen. Adrenal function is not usually affected. Haemorrhagic cysts of the adrenal cortex are described in Beckwith–Wiedemann syndrome.[59]

Neuroblastoma

The other, well-described adrenal mass is a neuroblastoma. It is usually only seen in the third trimester. The appearance is variable, but it should be suspected in a suprarenal mass which is increasing in size with time. Evidence of spinal involvement should be sought, but is difficult to exclude. Secondary deposits in the liver, whilst subtle and often of density only slightly more than the surrounding liver, should be sought. Antenatally diagnosed neuroblastomas, as neonatal ones, have a good long-term prognosis, but the diagnosis, which may be suspected antenatally, cannot be confirmed until the postnatal period. Unless the mass is enlarging rapidly, early delivery is probably not justified. Some neuroblastomas will have a cystic component and can entirely mimic an adrenal haemorrhage in utero.[60] The diagnosis can only be confirmed biochemically and histologically after delivery.[60] Other neuroblastomas will be solid isoechoic or complex.[61] Whilst some tumours do well, others do not. The DNA index may be the most important predictor.[62] Hydrops is a complication seen in the more advanced stages of the disease (Stages IV and IVS).[63] Accurate antenatal staging is impossible. Metastases to the umbilical cord and placenta are described.[63] Masses can become so large that dystocia results (Fig. 11.16).

Extralobar pulmonary sequestration

Intrathoracic pulmonary sequestrated segments are easily recognized. Intra-

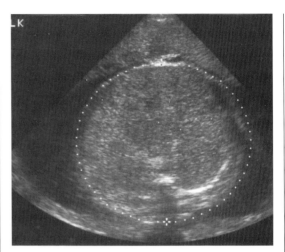

Fig. 11.16 Neuroblastoma – extensive abdominal mass in a 34-week fetus. Following delivery, a diagnosis of neuroblastoma was made.

abdominal sequestrated lung is a more difficult diagnosis to make, presenting usually as a solid suprarenal mass most often on the left side (Fig. 11.17). It is impossible to differentiate from an adrenal lesion in utero. The relative lack of change in size with time makes haemorrhage unlikely although the differential diagnosis from neuroblastoma cannot be made with certainty in utero.[64] Most of these lesions are hypoechoic,[61] but some are mixed. These lesions are usually left-sided and have been described in association with diaphragmatic hernia.[65]

Uterus and vagina

The normal uterus and vagina, like the ovary, are not visible in utero because of similarity of echotexture to the surrounding structure. Vaginal atresia or an imperforate hymen may present in utero as a cystic pelvic mass (hydrometrocolpos). This is a unilocular cyst arising from the pelvis.[66–68] On high-quality scans it is sometimes possible to determine that the echogenicity of the fluid is greater than that of urine in the adjacent bladder. Frequently, because of the size of the mass, the adjacent bladder is compressed and differentiation of this mass from a distended bladder or other causes of pelvic

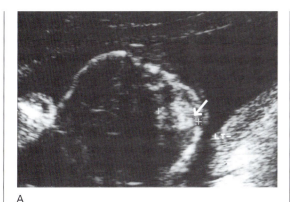

A

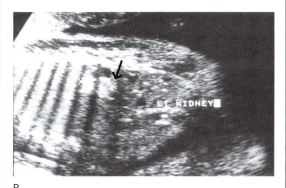

B

Fig. 11.17 (A) Axial section, showing echogenic suprarenal lesion which proved histologically postnatally to be an extrapulmonary sequestration (arrow). (B) Longitudinal section, showing the suprarenal position of the extrapulmonary sequestration (arrow).

mass such as an ovarian cyst can be difficult. There is frequently dilatation of the ureters and pelvicalyceal systems with this condition which is unusual with an ovarian cyst, but this does not differentiate this condition (hydrometrocolpos) from a dilated obstructed or neurogenic bladder. Associated anomalies have been described, including anorectal atresia, other bowel atresias and polycystic kidneys. It is impossible to determine antenatally whether the cause of the abnormality is a simple, imperforate hymen which would require only a minor surgical procedure or vaginal atresia requiring major reconstructive surgery in later life. Amniotic fluid volume in hydrometrocolpos is usually normal, but can be reduced, sometimes critically so.[69]

Bowel abnormalities

Oesophageal atresia

The normal oesophagus can occasionally be demonstrated in utero with high-resolution equipment (Fig. 11.18). Oesophageal atresia

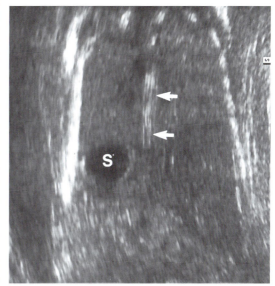

A

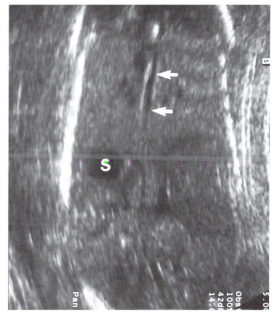

B

Fig. 11.18 Normal oesophagus. Coronal scan through thorax of 20-week fetus. (A) Collapsed oesophagus (arrows). (B) Swallowing with fluid in oesophagus (arrows). S, stomach.

may be suspected if the fetal stomach is either small or not easily demonstrated on more than one occasion in utero in the second trimester. Caution must be exercised, however, in attributing this to oesophageal atresia as a number of other conditions with poor swallowing can cause the same appearance and primary microgastria (small stomach) can also give this same appearance. A small stomach is the hallmark of oesophageal atresia without a tracheo-oesophageal fistula (Type A).[70–74] Some cases of oesophageal atresia with fistula will also have a small stomach, but many cases of oesophageal atresia with a tracheo-oesophageal fistula will have normal ultrasound appearances in the second trimester, because fluid can pass into the stomach via the trachea and distal tracheo-oesophageal fistula. Polyhydramnios developing in the third trimester may raise the possibility of this diagnosis again even when the second trimester scan was normal. About two-thirds of cases of tracheo-oesophageal fistula and oesophageal atresia will have polyhydramnios and one-third will have a small, fetal stomach. Confident diagnosis of oesophageal atresia with a fistula at 20 weeks is virtually unheard of. Differential diagnosis of polyhydramnios with absent stomach in the third trimester includes craniofacial anomalies, neuromuscular abnormalities and misplaced stomach, e.g. diaphragmatic hernia or situs inversus. Associated abnormalities are common including the VATER association (see Table 11.2). Cardiac, skeletal, genitourinary and other gastrointestinal abnormalities, central nervous system anomalies and facial anomalies have been described.

Chromosome anomalies, especially trisomies 18 and 21, are also associated. The prognosis in the absence of other anomalies is good with a mortality rate of less than 10% for liveborn infants.[75] Much of the mortality is related to complications of polyhydramnios and prematurity.

Stomach

The normal stomach can usually be demonstrated on a mid-trimester scan. Its

Table 11.2 Features of VATER association	
V	Vertebral anomalies
A	Anorectal anomalies
T E	Tracheo-oEsophageal anomalies
R	Renal anomalies Radial anomalies

Cardiac abnormalities are also a common associated feature. (Smith DW. The VATER association. Am J Dis Child 1974; 128:767–770.)

size is variable from time to time and patient to patient, but it is an easily identified transonic structure to the left of the midline in the upper abdomen. Other surrounding structures such as the left kidney and the liver should be identified to exclude the possibility of a renal cyst, hydronephrosis or a large gall bladder in situs inversus as a cause of a cystic structure in the left upper abdomen. Other uncommon causes of cysts in the left upper quadrant include duplication cysts, mesenteric cysts and ovarian cysts. In situs inversus, the stomach will be on the right side, but the heart will also in the complete form be on that side. In partial situs inversus, the abdominal situs and cardiac situs will be different and this is commonly associated with complex isomeric cardiac malformations.

A small stomach can be an isolated finding (microgastria)[76] or associated with other malformations such as oesophageal atresia, tracheo-oesophageal cleft or any cause of diminished or absent fetal swallowing such as major neuromuscular disorders.

Duodenal atresia

The normal duodenum can only occasionally be demonstrated in the second and third trimester. Dilatation of the duodenum which can be as large as or larger than the stomach in its most marked forms suggests a diagnosis of duodenal atresia or stenosis (Fig. 11.19). The typical appearance is of a 'double bubble' with the stomach and duodenum each forming similarly sized,

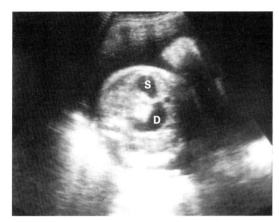

Fig. 11.19 Axial section of second trimester fetus. Dilated stomach (S) and duodenum. Note the duodenum (D) is often as large as the stomach. Polyhydramnios is present. Fetus is shown to have associated trisomy 21.

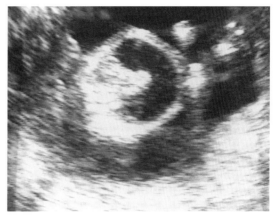

Fig. 11.20 Duodenal and oesophageal atresia. Coronal scan through abdomen of 16-week fetus, showing typical 'C'-shaped cystic mass.

fluid-filled structures. Duodenal peristalsis with variation in size of the two bubbles relative to one another can sometimes be seen. It is important not to mistake a normal gall bladder for a slightly enlarged duodenum. Continuity between the two bubbles in duodenal obstruction prevents this mistake being made.

This diagnosis is rarely made before the latest part of the second trimester and when made in the third trimester is often associated with polyhydramnios. An isolated diagnosis of the condition in the first trimester has been made.[77]

Duodenal atresia can be an isolated abnormality or part of the VATER association. 30% of duodenal atresias occur in fetuses with Down's syndrome.

Duodenal obstruction is usually caused either by complete obliteration of the duodenal lumen or by a web in the lumen of the duodenum. It is impossible to determine the cause antenatally. The postnatal association of Ladd's bands and malrotation of the bowel also cannot be identified antenatally. Apart from the association with Down's syndrome and the VATER association, other concurrent isolated abnormalities have been described in all systems. About 50% of duodenal atresia fetuses have other abnormalities. In the absence of other abnormalities the postnatal outlook is excellent.[78]

Duodenal atresia will occasionally be associated with oesophageal atresia to produce a characteristic 'C'-shaped cystic mass within the upper abdomen (Fig. 11.20).[79,80]

Jejunal and ileal atresia

Separate loops of normal jejunum and ileum are not visible on antenatal scanning although with modern, high-resolution scanners, the loops of bowel can be clearly differentiated from the other abdominal organs. If multiple, fluid-filled, bowel loops are demonstrated persistently on antenatal scanning, a small bowel atresia must be suspected. Small bowel atresias are rare (probably less than 1 in 5000 deliveries). Atresias of the jejunum (Fig. 11.21) are almost twice as common as those of the ileum[81] (Fig. 11.22). The exact site and cause of the atresia cannot be determined, but, in general terms, the more loops of bowel present and the more dilated they are, the more distal the atresia is likely to be. Multiple atresias are well described. Association with malrotation cannot be determined antenatally. Associated abnormalities of the bowel are described (malrotation, gastroschisis, duplication, meconium ileus) but outside the gastrointestinal tract abnormalities are uncommon. The gastrointestinal tract associations in many situations are thought

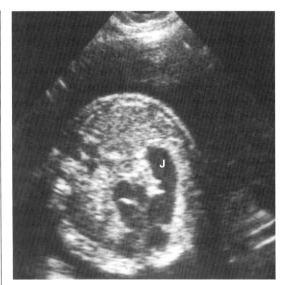

Fig. 11.21 Axial section of fetal abdomen. Several dilated loops of small bowel (arrow). Postnatally, this was shown to be jejunal atresia. Note polyhydramnios. J, dilated jejunum.

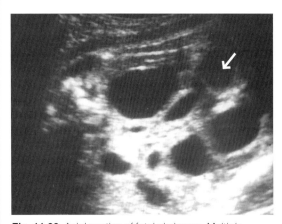

Fig. 11.22 Axial section of fetal abdomen. Multiple dilated loops of small bowel. Postnatally, ileal atresia was confirmed.

to be the cause of the atresia rather than the effect. In the absence of other abnormalities, the outlook for small bowel atresias is excellent, ileal atresias slightly better than jejunal because of the association of polyhydramnios and prematurity with some jejunal atresia. Differentiation from ureteric dilatation is essential. Differentiation from large bowel dilatation is usually possible by considering the position of the bowel loops. This diagnosis is rarely made before the late second trimester and more usually in the third trimester.[82] Associated polyhydramnios is common. As well as atresia of the small bowel, associated conditions such as meconium ileus should also be considered.

Meconium ileus

Meconium ileus is a common manifestation of cystic fibrosis in the fetal and neonatal period. The condition is one in which the bowel content becomes extremely thick and tenacious causing occlusion of the bowel that typically starts in the terminal ileum. Dilatation of the bowel proximal to the occlusion usually occurs. Complications such as volvulus and atresia are well recognized. The condition is, however, not often suspected antenatally, but should be suspected if the bowel is 'bright as bone' and particularly if this bright bowel is associated with dilatation or abdominal calcification. The brightness in the bowel is due to increased reflectivity of the inspissated meconium in the terminal ileum.[83–86] The diagnosis can be confirmed by genotyping the parents and if both have one of the cystic fibrosis genes (most commonly Delta F 508), then the diagnosis is confirmed. About 80% of cases of cystic fibrosis presenting as meconium ileus can be diagnosed by parental genotyping. The condition is inherited in an autosomal recessive manner, each succeeding pregnancy having a 1 in 4 risk. The prognosis for neonates with meconium ileus is good, but the long-term prognosis for the individual is related to the outlook for cystic fibrosis which, whilst improving, causes significant morbidity with increasing mortality from the late teens onwards.

Meconium peritonitis

This condition occurs when perforation of the bowel occurs in utero. It is manifested by calcification in the peritoneum typically peripherally arranged in the abdomen or associated with an intra-abdominal cyst or ascites or meconium calcification. (Fig. 11.15). It can be associated with meconium ileus (10%),[87] but other causes of perforation are more common. The calcification is caused by a chemical reaction between the peritoneum and irritant meconium. The prognosis depends on the underlying cause, but, in the absence of cystic fibrosis, is generally good.[88–91] Cases have been described in association with cocaine abuse[92] and in the rubella syndrome[93] and associated with cytomegalovirus infection[94] but most are associated with volvulus, atresia or meconium ileus.[95]

Large bowel pathology

The normal large bowel is not always clearly identified in the second trimester. In the third trimester, the appearances are very varied and frequently the meconium is of low echogenicity so that the colon stands out from the other abdominal contents and can be mistaken for dilated small bowel or ureters. The typical haustral pattern and peripheral position of the bowel in the abdomen almost always enables the normal large bowel to be differentiated from dilated small bowel. Dilatation of the large bowel has been described in imperforate anus,[96–98] but this condition is more frequently diagnosed postnatally following a normal antenatal scan.

Intraluminal, large bowel calcification has been described antenatally and postnatally with imperforate anus with communication between the large bowel and the urinary tract. The reaction between urine and meconium causes the calcification of meconium.[99,100] Imperforate anus is often associated with the other anomalies of the VATER association (Table 11.2), the renal and sacral abnormalities being the most frequent.

Persistent cloaca

This results from lack of development of the cloacal septum, so that the genital, gastrointestinal and urinary tracts all open into a single structure. Several cases have been reported antenatally,[101–103] usually presenting as a septated pelvic mass with oligohydramnios and poor fetal growth. Associated anomalies are common.

Prognosis is good in the absence of life-threatening, associated anomalies.

Hirschsprung's disease

This has only occasionally been diagnosed in utero with variable appearances suggesting both large and small bowel dilatation.[104–106] Differentiating this from other causes of bowel dilatation is virtually impossible. Colon atresia has not yet been described antenatally.

Bright bowel

The observation of increased echogenicity of the bowel above the normal is a non-specific finding. The standard is that the bowel should be as 'bright as bone' to be considered abnormal (Fig. 11.23). This appearance is associated in some cases with Down's syndrome, intra-uterine growth retardation, cystic fibrosis, swallowed blood and viral infections[107–109] but in the majority of cases no underlying cause is found.[110] If this appearance is seen in the second trimester, some would consider invasive testing for karyotype to be advisable together with testing to exclude cystic fibrosis. Long-term follow-up to exclude intra-uterine growth retardation would also be considered appropriate.

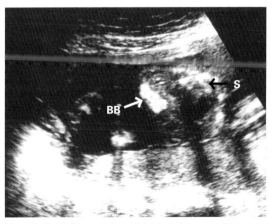

Fig. 11.23 Oblique section of fetal abdomen at 20 weeks. Echogenic bowel 'bright as bone'. This fetus developed intra-uterine growth retardation in the third trimester which is a well-recognized association. BB, bright bowel; S, spine.

Megacystis microcolon intestinal hypoperistalsis syndrome (MMIH)

This rare condition can be suspected in utero if the fetal bladder is particularly large and there is hydronephrosis.[111–113] Dilated bowel may also be seen in this circumstance, but is not usually a predominant feature. It is an important condition to consider as a differential diagnosis of posterior urethral valves because invasive management with drainage of the bladder in this condition is futile as the long-term outlook for affected babies is extremely poor. Differential diagnosis is helped by the fact that the vast majority of fetuses with this condition are female whereas posterior urethral valves are an entirely male condition. Recent evidence suggests an autosomal recessive mode of inheritance in some cases.[114,115]

Sacrococcygeal teratomas

Whilst the majority of these lesions arising from the coccyx produce a mass at the lower end of the spine or in the buttock, the intrapelvic form of these lesions can appear isolated and should be considered with any mixed solid and cystic mass arising in the pelvis.

According to the accepted classification,[116] these are type IV tumours. An intra-abdominal component has been seen in 40% of cases[117] but rarely has the tumour been entirely intrapelvic or intra-abdominal. The masses can be entirely cystic and difficult to differentiate from hydrometrocolpos, a dilated urinary bladder or an anterior meningocoele. Polyhydramnios is a common feature, especially in later diagnosed cases and hydrops occurs in some as a result of high output cardiac failure secondary to the vascular nature of some of these tumours. Associated musculoskeletal abnormalities have been described.[101,118] The outlook for these cases must be guarded since a confident diagnosis of type IV tumour is unlikely in utero and an entirely intra-abdominal or intrapelvic tumour has a greater risk of malignancy than the commoner lesions presenting as external masses. Overall mortality of 32% for the

lesion relates to the complications of polyhydramnios and hydrops as much as to the lesion itself.[116,119] As these tumours produce alphafetoprotein maternal serum, alphafetoprotein should be elevated although only occasionally is this a cause of raised alphafetoprotein assay in the second trimester.

Ascites

Any fluid seen surrounding the bowel is abnormal. A very thin, black line around the inner aspect of the abdomen is, however, a normal appearance and should not be confused with small amounts of ascites. Small amounts of ascites can be sometimes identified adjacent to the right lobe of the liver. Isolated ascites is a frequent, early manifestation of hydrops fetalis and the causes of this should be sought both by ultrasound, excluding cardiac lesions and other fetal abnormalities, and by appropriate invasive testing to exclude the other causes although persistent isolated ascites is most commonly associated with intra-abdominal pathology. Ascites caused by intra-abdominal pathology is quite uncommon. However, the two most frequent associations are urinary ascites secondary to obstructive uropathy and meconium peritonitis. Rare associations are with liver disease and certain metabolic storage diseases.

Intra-abdominal calcification

Calcification within the fetal abdomen is rare

Table 11.3
Intra-abdominal calcification

Liver	Viral infection • varicella • cytomegalovirus Tumoural • haemangioma • hepatoblastoma
Gall bladder	Stones
Peritoneum	Meconium peritonitis
Bowel	Intraluminal • meconium ileus • anorectal atresia and urinary fistula
Tumoural	Teratoma

and has many individual causes. If the organ of origin can be determined, then the cause of calcification can often be determined (see Table 11.3).

References

Exomphalos

1. Snijders RJM, Nicolaides KH. Ultrasound markers. In: Snijders RJM, Nicolaides KH, eds. Ultrasound markers for chromosomal defects. Frontiers in Fetal Medicine series. London: Parthenon; 1994:95.
2. Snijders RJM, Sebire NJ, Souka A, Santiago C, Nicolaides KH. Fetal exomphalos and chromosomal defects: relationship to maternal age and gestation. Ultrasound Obstet Gynecol 1995; 6:250–255.
3. Bair JH, Russ PD, Pretorius DH, et al. Fetal omphalocele and gastroschisis: A review of 24 cases. AJR 1986; 147:1047–1051.
4. Brown BSJ. The prenatal ultrasonographic features of omphalocele: A study of 10 patients. J Can Assoc Radiol 1985; 36:312–316.
5. Redford DH, McNay MB, Whittle MJ. Gastroschisis and exomphalos: Precise diagnosis by mid-pregnancy ultrasound. Br J Obstet Gynaecol 1985; 92:54–59.
6. Palomaki GE, Hill LE, Knight GJ, et al. Second-trimester maternal serum alpha-fetoprotein levels in pregnancies associated with gastroschisis and omphalocele. Obstet Gynecol 1988; 71:906–909.
7. Dillon E, Renwick M. The antenatal diagnosis and management of abdominal wall defects: the Northern Region experience. Clin Radiol 1995; 50:855–859.
8. Chen CP, Jan SW, Liu FF, et al. Prenatal diagnosis of omphalocele associated with umbilical cord cyst. Acta Obstet Gynecol Scand 1995; 74:832–835.
9. Morrow RJ, Whittle MJ, McNay MB, et al. Prenatal diagnosis and management of anterior abdominal wall defects in the west of Scotland. Prenat Diagn 1993; 13:111–115.
10. Hughes MD, Nyberg DA, Mack LA, Pretorius DH. Fetal omphalocele: Prenatal detection of concurrent anomalies and other predictors of outcome. Radiology 1989; 173:371–376.
11. Martin LW, Torres AM. Omphalocele and gastroschisis. Symposium on pediatric surgery. Surg Clin North Am 1985; 65:1235–1244.
12. Schwaitzenberg SD, Pokorny WJ, McGill CW, et al. Gastroschisis and omphalocele. Am J Surg 1982; 144:650–654.
13. Hasan S, Hermansen. The prenatal diagnosis of ventral abdominal wall defects. Am J Obstet Gynaecol 1986; 155:842–845.
14. Kirk EP, Wah R. Obstetric management of the fetus with omphalocele or gastroschisis: A review and report of one hundred and twelve cases. Am J Obstet Gynecol 1983; 146:512–518.

Gastroschisis

15. Babcock CJ, Hedrick MH, Goldstein RB, et al. Gastroschisis: Can sonography of the fetal bowel accurately predict postnatal outcome? J Ultrasound Med 1994; 13:701–706.
16. De Vries PA. The pathogenesis of gastroschisis and omphalocele. J Pediatr Surg 1980; 15:245–251.
17. Pryde PG, Bardicef M, Treadwell MC, et al. Gastroschisis: Can antenatal ultrasound predict infant outcomes? Obstet Gynecol 1994; 84:505–510.
18. Kluck P, Tibboel D, Van Der Kamp AWM, et al. The effect of fetal urine on the development of bowel in gastroschisis. J Pediatr Surg 1983; 18:47–50.
19. Luck SR, Sherman J, Raffensperger JG, et al. Gastroschisis in 106 consecutive newborn infants. Surgery 1985; 98:677–683.
20. Mabogunje OOA, Mahour GH. Omphalocele and gastroschisis: Trends in survival across two decades. Am J Surg 1984; 148:679–686.
21. Adra AM, Landy HJ, Nahmias J, Gomez-Marin O. The fetus with gastroschisis: Impact of route of delivery and prenatal ultrasonography. Am J Obstet Gynecol 1996; 174:540–546.
22. Walkinshaw SA, Renwick M, Hebisch G, Hey EN. How good is ultrasound in the detection and evaluation of anterior abdominal wall defects? Br J Radiol 1993; 65:298–301.
23. Fries MH, Filly RA, Callen PW, et al. Growth retardation in prenatally diagnosed cases of gastroschisis. J Ultrasound Med 1993; 12:583–588.
24. Nicholls G, Upadhyaya V, Gornall P, Buick RG, Corkery JJ. Is specialist centre delivery of gastroschisis beneficial? Arch Dis Child 1993; 69:71–73.
25. Langer JC, Khanna J, Caco C, Dykes EH, Nicolaides KH. Prenatal diagnosis of gastroschisis: development of objective sonographic criteria for predicting outcome. Obstet Gynecol 1993; 81:53–56.
26. Pinette MG, Pan Y, Pinette SG, et al. Gastroschisis followed by absorption of the small bowel and closure of the abdominal wall defect. J Ultrasound Med 1994; 13:719–721.

Limb/body wall complex

27. Viscarello RR, Ferguson DD, Nores J, Hobbins JC. Limb–body wall complex associated with cocaine abuse: Further evidence of cocaine's teratogenicity. Obstet Gynecol 1992; 80:523–526.
28. Ravitch MM. Cantrell's pentalogy and notes on diverticulum of the left ventricle. In: Congenital deformities of the chest wall and their operative corrections. Philadelphia: WB Saunders; 1977:53–57.
29. Toyama WM. Combined congenital defects of the anterior abdominal wall, sternum, diaphragm, pericardium, and heart: A case report and review of the literature. Pediatr 1972; 50:778–792.

Cloacal and bladder exstrophy

30. Meglin AJ, Balotin RJ, Jelinek JS, et al. Cloacal exstrophy radiologic findings in 13 patients. AJR 1990; 155:1267–1272.
31. Meizner I, Levy A, Barnhard Y. Cloacal exstrophy sequence: an exceptional ultrasound diagnosis. Obstet Gynecol 1995; 86:446–450.

32. Howell C, Caldamone A, Snyder H, et al. Optimal management of cloacal exstrophy. J Pediatr Surg 1983; 18:365–369.

Normal anatomy

33. Walkinshaw SA, Renwick M, Hebisch G, Hey EN. How good is ultrasound in the detection and evaluation of anterior abdominal wall defects? Br J Radiol; 1992; 65:298–301.

Liver

34. Carroll SG, Maxwell DJ. The significance of echogenic areas in the fetal abdomen. Ultrasound Obstet Gynecol 1996; 7:295–298.

35. Chung WM. Antenatal detection of hepatic cyst. J Clin Ultrasound 1986; 14:217–219.

36. Estroff JA, Benacerraf B. Fetal umbilical vein varix: sonographic appearance and postnatal outcome. J Ultrasound Med 1992; 11:69–73.

Gall bladder

37. Sepulveda W, Nicolaidis P, Hollingsworth, Fisk N. Fetal cholecystomegaly. A prenatal marker of aneuploidy. Prenat Diagn 1995; 15:193–197.

38. Beretsky I, Lanken DH. Diagnosis of fetal cholelithiasis using real-time high-resolution imaging employing digital detection. J Ultrasound Med 1983; 2:381–383.

39. Klingensmith WC III, Ragan-Cioffi DT. Fetal gallstones. Radiology 1988; 167:143–144.

Choledochal cysts

40. Rha SY, Stovroff MC, Glick PL, Allen JE, Ricketts RR. Choledochal cysts: a ten year experience. Am Surg 1996; 62:30–34.

41. Lugo-Vicente HL. Prenatally diagnosed choledochal cysts: observation or early surgery? J Pediatr Surg 1995; 30:1288–1290.

Intra-abdominal cysts

42. Bower R, Dehner LP, Tenberg JL. Bilateral ovarian cysts in the newborn. Am J Dis Child 1974; 128:731–733.

43. Carlson DH, Griscom NT. Ovarian cysts in the newborn. AJR 1972; 116:664–672.

44. Desa DJ. Follicular ovarian cysts in stillbirths and neonates. Arch Dis Child 1975; 50:24–50.

45. Yokoyama Y, Kagiya A, Ozaki T, et al. Two cases of twisted fetal ovarian cysts. J Obstet Gynecol 1996; 22:85–88.

46. Aslam A, Wong C, Haworth JM, Noblett HR. Autoamputation of ovarian cyst in an infant. J Pediatr Surg 1995; 30:1609–1610.

47. Sapin E, Bargy F, Lewin F, et al. Management of ovarian cyst detected by prenatal ultrasound. Eur J Pediatr Surg 1994; 4:137–140.

48. Brandt ML, Luks FI, Filiatrault D, et al. Surgical indications in antenatally diagnosed ovarian cysts. J Pediatr Surg 1991; 26:276–281.

49. Sakala EP, Leon ZA, Rouse GA. Management of antenatally diagnosed fetal ovarian cysts. Obstet Gynecol Surv 1991; 46:407–414.

50. Meizner I, Levy A, Katz M, Maresh AJ, Giezerman M. Fetal ovarian cysts: prenatal ultrasonographic detection and postnatal evaluation and treatment. Am J Obstet Gynecol 1991; 164:874–878.

51. Bidwell JK, Nelson A. Prenatal ultrasonic diagnosis of congenital duplication of the stomach. J Ultrasound Med 1986; 5:589–591.

52. van Dam LJ, de Groot CJ, Hazeborek FW, et al. Intra uterine demonstration of bowel duplication by ultrasound. Eur J Obstet Gynecol Reprod Biol 1984; 18:229.

53. Degani S, Mogilner JG, Shapiro I. In utero sonographic appearance of intestinal duplication cysts. Ultrasound Obstet Gynecol 1995; 5:415–418.

54. Goyert GL, Blitz D, Gibson P, et al. Prenatal diagnosis of duplication cyst of the pylorus. Prenat Diagn 1991; 11:483–486.

55. Suda H, Matsuda I, Chida S, Maete H. Neonatal adrenal hemorrhage detected antenatally. Acta Pediatr Jpn 1992; 34:606–610.

56. Lin MH, Jeng CJ, Wang KG, Yang YC. Prenatal diagnosis of meconium peritonitis: a case report with literature review. Chung Hua I Hsueh Tsa Chih Taipei 1992; 49:48–52.

Posterior abdominal wall tumours

57. Duncan BW, Adzick NS, Eraklis A. Retroperitoneal alimentary tract duplication detected in utero. J Pediatr Surg 1992; 27:1231–1233.

Adrenal masses

58. Burbidge KA. Prenatal adrenal hemorrhage confirmed by postnatal surgery. J Urol 1993; 150:1867–1869.

59. McCaulet RG, Beckwith JB, Elias ER, et al. Benign hemorrhagic adrenocortical macrocysts in Beckwith Wiedemann syndrome. AJR 1991; 157:549–552.

60. Dreyfus M, Neuhart D, Baldauf JJ, et al. Prenatal diagnosis of cystic neuroblastoma. Fetal Diagn Ther 1994; 9:269–272.

61. Rubenstein SC, Benacerraf BR, Retik AB, Mandell J. Fetal suprarenal masses: sonographic appearance and differential diagnosis. Ultrasound Obstet Gynecol 1995; 5:164–167.

62. Saylors RL III, Cohn SL, Morgan ER, Broduer GM. Prenatal detection of neuroblastoma by fetal ultrasonography. Am J Pediatr Haematol Oncol 1994; 16:356–360.

63. Jennings RW, LaQuaglia MP, Leong K, Hendren WH, Adzick NS. Fetal neuroblastoma prenatal diagnosis and natural history. J Pediatr Surg 1993; 28:1168–1174.

Extra-lobar pulmonary sequestration

64. Plattner V, Haustein B, Llanas B, et al. Extra-lobar pulmonary sequestration with prenatal diagnosis. A report of 5 cases and review of the literature. Eur J Pediatr Surg 1995; 5:235–237.

65. White J, Chan YF, Neuberger S, Wilson T. Prenatal sonographic detection of intra-abdominal extralobar pulmonary sequestration: report of three cases and literature review. Prenat Diagn 1994; 14:653–658.

Uterus and vagina

66. Dacis GH, Wapner R, Kurtz AB, et al. Antenatal diagnosis of hydrometrocolpos by ultrasound examination. J Ultrasound Med 1984; 3:371–374.
67. Valenti C, Kassner EG, Yermakow V, et al. Antenatal diagnosis of a fetal ovarian cyst. Am J Gynecol 1975; 123:216–219.
68. Russ PD, Zavitz WR, Pretorius DH, et al. Hydrometrocolpos, uterus didelphys and septate vagina: An antenatal sonographic diagnosis. J Ultrasound Med 1986; 5:211–213.
69. Shimada K, Hosokawa S, Sakaue K, Kishima Y. Fetal genitourinary abnormalities associated with oligohydramnios. Nippon Hinyokika Gakkai Zasshi 1994; 84:990–995.

Oesophageal atresia

70. Farrant P. The antenatal diagnosis of oesophageal atresia by ultrasound. Br J Radiol 1980; 53:1202–1203.
71. Hobbins JC, Grannum PAT, Berkowitz RI, et al. Ultrasound in the diagnosis of congenital anomalies. Am J Obstet Gynecol 1979; 134:331–334.
72. Pretorius DH, Meier PR, Johnson ML. Diagnosis of esophageal atresia in utero. J Ultrasound Med 1983; 2:475.
73. Pretorius DH, Drose JA, Dennis MA, et al. Tracheoesophageal fistula in utero. J Ultrasound Med 1987; 6:509–513.
74. Loveday BJ, Barr JA, Aitken J. The intra-uterine demonstration of duodenal atresia by ultrasound. Br J Radiol 1975; 48:1031–1032.
75. Bishop PJ, Klein MD, Phillipart AL, et al. Transpleural repair of esophageal atresia without a primary gastrotomy. 240 patients treated between 1951 and 1983. J Pediatr Surg 1985; 20:823–828.

Stomach

76. Tanaka K, Tschuida Y, Hashizume K, Kawarasaki H, Sugiyama M. Microgastria – case report and a review of the literature. Eur J Pediatr Surg 1993; 3:290–292.

Duodenal atresia

77. Tsukerman GL, Krapiva GP, Kirillova IA. First trimester diagnosis of duodenal stenosis associated with oesophageal atresia. Prenat Diagn 1993; 13:371–376.
78. Grosfeld JL, Rescorlla FJ. Duodenal atresia and stenosis: Reassessment of treatment and outcome cased on antenatal diagnosis, pathological variance and long-term follow up. World J Surg 1993; 17:301–309.
79. Chitty LS, Goodman J, Seller M, Maxwell D. Oesophageal and duodenal atresia in a fetus with Down's syndrome. Ultrasound Obstet Gynaecol 1996; 7:430–432.
80. Estroff JA, Parad RB, Share JC, Benacerraf B. Second trimester prenatal findings in duodenal and oesophageal atresia without tracheoesophageal fistula. J Ultrasound Med 1994; 13:375–379.

Jejunal and ileal atresia

81. De Lorimier AA, Fonkalsrud EW, Hays DM. Congenital atresia and stenosis of the jejunum and ileum. Surgery 1969; 65:819–827.
82. Weissman A, Goldstein I. Prenatal sonographic diagnosis and clinical management of small bowel obstruction. Am J Perinatol 1993; 10:215–216.

Meconium ileus

83. Benacerraf B, Chaudhury AK. Echogenic fetal bowel in the third trimester associated with meconium ileus secondary to cystic fibrosis. J Reprod Med 1989; 34:299–300.
84. Gilbert F, Kwei-Lan T, Mendoza A, et al. Prenatal diagnostic options in cystic fibrosis. Am J Obstet Gynecol 1988; 158:947–952.
85. Muller F, Frot JC, Aubry J, et al. Meconium ileus in cystic fibrosis fetuses. Lancet 1984; ii:223.
86. Muller F, Aubry MC, Gasser B, et al. Prenatal diagnosis of cystic fibrosis. Prenat Diagn 1986; 5:109–117.

Meconium peritonitis

87. Foster MA, Nyberg DA, Mahony BS, et al. Meconium peritonitis: Prenatal sonographic findings and clinical significance. Radiology 1987; 165:661–665.
88. Estroff JA, Bromley B, Benacerraf BR. Fetal meconium peritonitis without sequelae. Pediatr Radiol 1992; 22:277–278.
89. Paulson EK, Hertzberg BS. Hyperechoic meconium in the third trimester fetus: an uncommon normal variant. J Ultrasound Med 1991; 10:677–680.
90. Dirkes K, Crombleholme TM, Craigo SD, et al. The natural history of meconium peritonitis diagnosed in utero. J Pediatr Surg 1995; 30:979–982.
91. Wang YJ, Chen HC, Chi CS. Meconium peritonitis in neonates. Chung hua I Hsueh Rsa Chih Taipei 1994; 53:49–53.
92. Hume RF Jr, Gingras JL, Martin LS, et al. Ultrasound diagnosis of fetal anomalies associated with in utero cocaine exposure: further support for cocaine-induced vascular disruption teratogenesis. Fetal Diagn Ther 1994; 9:239–245.
93. Radner M, Vergesslich KA, Woninger M, et al. Meconium peritonitis: a new finding in rubella syndrome. J Clin Ultrasound 1993; 21:346–349.
94. Pletcher BA, Williams MK, Mulivor RA, Barth D, Linder C, Rawlinson K. Intrauterine cytomegalovirus infection presenting as fetal meconium peritonitis. Obstet Gynecol 1991; 78:903–905.
95. Forouhar F. Meconium peritonitis: Pathology, evolution, and diagnosis. Am J Clin Pathol 1982; 78:208–213.

Large bowel pathology

96. Barss VA, Benacerraf BR, Firgolotto FD. Antenatal sonographic diagnosis of fetal gastrointestinal malformation. Pediatrics 1985; 76:445–449.
97. Bean WJ, Calonge MA, Aprill CN, et al. Anal atresia: A prenatal ultrasound diagnosis. J Clin Ultrasound 1978; 6:111–112.

98. Harris RD, Nyberg DA, Mack LA, et al. Anorectal atresia: Prenatal sonographic diagnosis. AJR 1987; 149:395–400.
99. Berdon WE, Baker DH, Wigges HJ, et al. Calcified intraluminal meconium in newborn males with imperforate anus. AJR 1975; 125:449–455.
100. Shalev E, Weiner E, Zuzherman H. Prenatal ultrasound diagnosis of intestinal calcifications with imperforate anus. Acta Obstet Gynecol Scand 1983; 62:95–96.

Persistent cloaca

101. Holzgreve W. Brief diagnosis of persistent common cloaca with prune belly and anencephaly in the second trimester. Am J Med Genet 1985; 20:729–732.
102. Lande IM, Hamilton EF. The antenatal sonographic visualisation of cloacal dysgenesis. J Ultrasound Med 1986; 5:275–278.
103. Shalev E, Feldman E, Weiner E, et al. Prenatal sonographic appearance of persistent cloaca. Acta Obstet Gynecol Scand 1986; 66:517–518.

Hirschsprung's disease

104. Jarmas AL, Weaver DD, Padilla AM, et al. Hirschsprung's disease: Etiologic implications of unsuccessful prenatal diagnosis. Am J Med Genet 1983; 16:163–167.
105. Vermish M, Mayden KI, Confino E, et al. Prenatal sonographic diagnosis of Hirschsprung's disease. J Ultrasound Med 1986; 5:37–39.
106. Wrobleski D, Wesselhoeft C. Ultrasound diagnosis of prenatal intestinal obstruction. J Pediatr Surg 1979; 14:598–600.

Bright bowel

107. Fakhry J, Reiser M, Shapiro LR, et al. Increased echogenicity in the lower fetal abdomen: A common normal variant in the second trimester. J Ultrasound Med 1986; 5:489–492.
108. Lince DM, Pretorius DH, Manco-Johnson ML, et al. The clinical significance of increased echogenicity in the fetal abdomen. AJR 1985; 145:683–685.
109. Manco LG, Nunan FA Jr, Sohnen H, et al. Fetal small bowel simulating an abdominal mass at sonography. J Clin Ultrasound 1986; 14:404–407.

110. Sipes SL, Weiner CP, Wenstrom KD, et al. Fetal echogenic bowel on ultrasound – is there clinical significance? Fetal Diagn Ther 1994; 9:38–43.

Megacystis microcolon intestinal hypoperistalsis syndrome

111. Manco LG, Osterdahl P. The antenatal sonographic features of megacystis–microcolon–intestinal hypoperistalsis syndrome. J Clin Ultrasound 1984; 12:595–598.
112. Vezina WC, Morin FR, Winsberg F. Megacystis–microcolon–intestinal hypoperistalsis syndrome: Antenatal ultrasound appearance. AJR 1979; 133:749–750.
113. Vintzileos AM, Eisenfeld LI, Herson VC, et al. Megacystis–microcolon–intestinal hypoperistalsis syndrome: Antenatal sonographic findings and review of the literature. Am J Perinatol 1986; 3:297–302.
114. McNamara HM, Onwude JL, Thornton JG. Megacystis microcolon intestinal hypoperistalsis syndrome: a case report supporting autosomal recessive inheritance. Prenat Diagn 1994; 14:153–154.
115. Carlsson SA, Hokegard KH, Mattson LA. Megacystis microcolon intestinal hypoperistalsis syndrome. Antenatal appearance in two cases. Acta Obset Gynecol Scand 1992; 71:645–648.

Sacrococcygeal teratoma

116. Altman RP, Randolph JG, Lilly JR. Sacrococcygeal teratoma. American Academy of Pediatrics Surgical section Survey 1973; 9:389–398.
117. Tank ES. The urological complications of imperforate anus and cloacal dysgensis. In: Harrison JH, Gittes RF, Perimuuter AD, et al, eds. Campbell's Urology. 4th ed. Philadelphia: WB Saunders; 1979:1889–1900.
118. Puri P, Lake BD, Gorman F, et al. Megacystis–microcolon–intestinal hypoperistalsis syndrome: a visceral myopathy. J Pediatr Surg 1983; 18:64–69.
119. Heloury Y, Vergnes P, Classe JM, et al. Prenatal diagnosis of sacrococcygeal teratoma. Chir Pediatr 1990; 31:202–206.

CHAPTER 12

Skeletal abnormalities

Josephine M. McHugo

Introduction

Skeletal abnormalities are relatively common congenital abnormalities which have heterogeneous aetiology and include the following groups:

- Abnormalities associated with **syndromes** or **chromosomal** abnormalities
- Isolated bony abnormalities – the malformations which represent failure of development or disruption of previously normal bone structures, e.g. amniotic bands
- Abnormalities reflecting a generalized disorder of bone formation – the **bone dysplasias**.

This chapter aims to provide a systematic approach to the antenatal diagnosis and assessment of this heterogeneous group.

Abnormalities of the skeletal system are not uncommon with an incidence of 1:500 births. However, true skeletal dysplasias are less common.

The international nomenclature for skeletal dysplasia is broadly divided into five groups:

1. Dysostosis (malformation of bones either singly or in combinations)
2. Osteochondrodystrophies (abnormalities of cartilage and bone)
3. Osteolysis (disorders associated with multifocal resorption of bone)
4. Skeletal abnormalities associated with chromosomal disorders
5. Primary metabolic disorders.

The nomenclature for limb abnormalities is given in Table 12.1.

In view of the complex development of limbs that occurs between 4 and 8 weeks of gestation, this is the time of highest susceptibility to damage either from environmental or mechanical effects.

Abnormalities in cellular and molecular interactions can also occur from gene mutations and chromosomal defects.[1,2] Limb defects can also arise from trauma once formed, e.g. constriction from amniotic bands, resulting in amputations and slash defects. The polydactylies and syndactylies

Table 12.1
Nomenclature for limb abnormalities

Achiria	Absence of hands
Achiropody	Absence of hands and feet
Acromelia	Shortening of the distal segments (hands and feet)
Adactyly (ectrodactyly)	Absence of fingers and toes
Amelia (ectomelia)	Absence of an extremity
Apodia	Absence of the foot
Brachydactyly	Abnormally short fingers
Camptomelia	Bent limb
Clinodactyly	In-turning of the finger
Diastrophic	Distorted
Ectrodactyly	Split hand
Equinus	Extension of the foot
Hemimelia	Absence (partial or complete) of the distal portion of the limb below the elbow or knee
Mesomelia	Shortening of the middle segment of the limbs
Micromelia	Shortening of all the long bones
Oligodactyly	Partial loss of the fingers
Phocomelia	Deficient development of the middle segments with normal development of the proximal and distal segments
Polydactyly	Extra digits
Pre-axial	Extra digit on radial or tibial side
Post-axial	Extra digit on ulnar or fibular side
Rhizomelia	Shortening of the proximal segment (femur–humerus)
Syndactyly	Fused digits
Talipes	Club-foot
Valgus	Bent outwards
Varus	Bent inwards

are usually inherited autosomally. Limb defects are not infrequently associated with other structural abnormalities, particularly of cardiac, renal, facial and skin development.

Skeletal chondrodysplasias are defined as abnormalities of the formation of cartilage, bone growth and development. They are, however, uncommon abnormalities – the commonest apparent at birth is thanatophoric dysplasia with an incidence of 1:30 000 births. Although rare, these abnormalities are amenable to antenatal diagnosis as bone is an excellent reflector of ultrasound, and abnormalities of bone are therefore well imaged with ultrasound. The skeletal dysplasias represent a heterogeneous group that to date have been defined by the specific skeletal radiological abnormalities, clinical features, genetic inheritance and histological features of the growth plate. However, increasingly, the gene locus and the specific mutations that cause these disorders are being defined. Those now defined are given in Table 12.2. Advances in the genetics of the human chondrodysplasias have resulted in greater understanding of this group of disorders, e.g. mutations of the fibroblast growth factor receptor number 3 are involved in the group of abnormalities which has similar phenotypes to achondroplasia, thanatophoric dysplasia and hypochondroplasia. Osteogenesis imperfecta is due to at least 100 different mutations of the collagen 1 chain genes.

Embryology

The fetal skeleton forms in two distinct ways:

- Membranous ossification that occurs in the clavicle and mandible
- Intracartilaginous (enchondral) when ossification occurs from pre-existing cartilage.

Intracartilaginous is the more common type of ossification.

Normal bone nomenclature is given in Figure 12.1. This is important as accurate descriptive terms will aid the differential diagnosis.

The fetal limbs

Both the upper and lower limbs form from the lateral plate mesoderm. The beginning of the upper limb buds are apparent by 26 days

Table 12.2
Human chondrodysplasias in which mutations are known

Disorder	Inheritance	Gene locus	Chromosome
Achondrogenesis type II	AD	COL2A1	12q13.11
Hypochondrogenesis	AD	COL2A1	12q13.11
SED congenita	AD	COL2A1	12q13.11
Kneist dysplasia	AD	COL2A1	12q13.11
Late onset SED	AD	COL2A1	12q13.11
Stickler's dysplasia	AD	COL2A1	12q13.11
Stickler-like dysplasia	AD, AR	COL11A2	6p21.3
Schmid metaphyseal chondrodysplasia	AD	COL10A1	6q21–q22
Jansen metaphyseal dysplasia	AD	PTHrPR	3p21–p22
Thanatophoric dysplasia	AD	FGFR3	4p16.3
Achondroplasia	AD	FGFR3	4p16.3
Pseudoachondroplasia	AD	COMP	19p13.1
MED Faifbanks	AD	COMP	19p13.1
Diastrophic dysplasia	AR	DTDST	5q31–q34
Chondrodysplasia punctata	XLR	ARSE	Xp22.3
Camptomelic dysplasia	AD	SOX9	17q24.1–q25.1

Reproduced with permission from Horton WA. Advances in the genetics of human chondrodysplasia. Paediatr Radiol 1997: 27:5, 419–421 Copyright Springer-Verlag
AD, autosomal dominant; AR, autosomal recessive; XLR, X-linked recessive; SED, spondyloepiphyseal dysplasia; MED, metaphyseal epiphyseal dysplasia

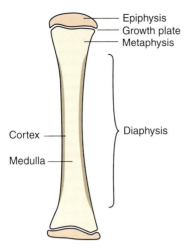

Epiphysis
Growth plate
Metaphysis

Cortex

Medulla

Diaphysis

Fig. 12.1 Normal bone nomenclature.

Table 12.3
Fetal ossification centre

Structure	Gestation (weeks)
Clavicle	8
Mandible/palate	9
Vertebral bodies	9
Neural arches	9
Frontal bones	10–11
Long bones	11

Table 12.4
Bones assessed on a routine 18- to 20-week ultrasound examination

Cranial vault	Biparietal diameter/head circumference measurements
Ribs	Imaged on the 4-chamber view of the heart
Femur	Morphology and length assessed while obtaining an image to measure femoral length

post-fertilization. The lower limb buds develop 1 to 2 days later. These buds consist of mesochyme covered by an epithelium. This thickens to form the apical ectodermal ridge. This region is important in the normal development of the limbs. By 32 to 34 days post-fertilization, the rudimentary hand has formed. Condensation of the central mesochyme results in the area where the fetal cartilaginous elements form. Chondrogenesis is apparent by the 5th week. By the 6th week, all skeletal structures are cartilaginous and the digital rays are present.

Osteogenesis begins and the interdigital tissue is broken by programmed cell death. By the end of the 8th week, the limbs are formed but not yet ossified.

Fetal ossification (membranous) starts in the clavicle at 8 weeks.

Enchondral ossification occurs in the primary ossification centres in the diaphysis of the long bones and extends towards the epiphysis. Epiphyseal secondary centres of ossification mainly appear after birth. However, the distal femoral epiphysis is usually present from 32 weeks gestation in the normal fetus; this can be used as an assessment of maturity in later pregnancy.[4] The proximal tibial secondary centre is present soon after and the proximal humeral head may appear by 40 weeks gestation. Table 12.3 lists the timing of fetal ossification in the skeleton.

Normal ultrasound appearances

A structured approach to the routine 18 to 20-week anomaly scan includes a careful survey of many bony structures which are listed in Table 12.4. In the screening anomaly scan, routine measurements of the femur length and biparietal diameter and head circumference should aid diagnosis. Shortening of the long bones in a known-gestation-age fetus below 2 standard deviations should promote a full assessment of all the bones. Bone lengths should always be plotted on the appropriate normograms (see Appendix).

The long bone should be appropriately modelled – straight and in proportion; the proximal bones (humeri and femora) should be slightly longer than the distal bones (radius and ulna; tibia and fibula). An abnormality of bone morphology or length on this screening survey should always promote a more extensive survey of the fetal skeleton with measurement of all long bones as outlined in Table 12.5. Ossification of the bone can be assessed by posterior acoustic shadowing (Fig. 12.2), and by reference to the fetal falx and intracranial structures; in the

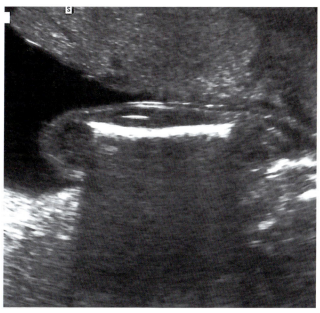

Fig. 12.2 Normal straight femur showing posterior acoustic shadowing which is an indicator of normal ossification.

Table 12.5
Extended ultrasound examination following a suspicion of a skeletal abnormality

Image and measure all the long bones	Length Width Structure Texture Ossification? Fractures?
Cranium Facial profile Ribs	Vault bones Length Shape Fractures?
Spine Hands Feet	
Associated abnormalities	Cardiac Facial clefting Renal

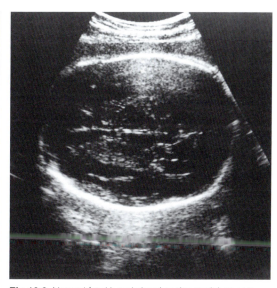

Fig 12.3 Normal fetal head showing the vault bones to be slightly more echogenic than the falx, indicating normal ossification.

normally ossified vault, the bones are more reflective than the falx and midline structures (Fig. 12.3). This relationship is lost or reversed when ossification is deficient.

As with any structural abnormality detected by ultrasound, a systematic survey of the fetal anatomy is appropriate as certain syndromes and dysplasias have common associated structural abnormalities. If present, the type of associated abnormalities will aid a definitive or differential diagnosis.

For many structural bone abnormalities, antenatal detection results in a differential or working diagnosis prior to the delivery, the precise diagnosis only being apparent at birth with the aid of postnatal radiographs and at post-mortem. This makes accurate prenatal counselling very difficult. It is often only possible to predict outcome by a multidisciplinary approach involving the following groups: antenatal imagers, geneticists, neonatologists, orthopaedic surgeons and skeletal radiologists. More recently, some of the inherited single gene disorders have been identified and some of these are now available for prenatal diagnosis from DNA.[5]

The majority of skeletal abnormalities occur in the low-risk population and it is a careful and structured approach that allows the antenatal diagnosis by a routine scan. Where recessive disorders have resulted in a known, previously affected fetus, the ultrasound examination can be more tailored and the scan carried out at a more appropriate time. It must be remembered that the majority of lethal, short limb dysplasias will show marked shortening by 18 to 20 weeks but the non-lethal, short limb dysplasias apparent at birth essentially show normal ultrasound appearances at this gestation (20 weeks). Therefore, if there is a known recurrence risk, a further scan at a later gestation is appropriate. Severe intra-uterine growth restriction can result in short femoral length. It is however usually associated with other features of growth restriction such as oligohydramnios, abnormal head-to-abdomen ratio and abnormal Doppler velocimetry.[6]

The common skeletal dysplasias with the incidence are given in Table 12.6.

The structured ultrasound should assess the following:

Bone length

If the bone length is apparently short, the type of shortening must be assessed. The appropriate nomenclature is given in Figure 12.4.

Micromelia occurs when the shortening affects both the proximal and distal bones equally. It is often of practical importance to divide this group further into severe or mild shortening.

Rhizomelia is where the limb shortening affects the proximal bones more than the distal bones.

Mesomelia is where the shortening affects the distal bones most. Appropriate plotting

Table 12.6
Common skeletal dysplasias with birth prevalence rates per 10 000

	Source			
	1	2	3	4
Thanatophoric dysplasia	0.60	0.24	0.09	0.28
Achondroplasia	0.37	—	0.46	0.64
Achondrogenesis	0.23	0.09	0.03	0.28
Osteogenesis imperfecta	0.18	0.18	0.43	0.64
Asphyxiating thoracic dysplasia	0.14	—	—	0.09
Chondrodysplasia punctata	0.09	0.12	0.06	0.18
Diastrophic dysplasia	—	—	0.03	0.09
Camptomelic dysplasia	0.05	0.09	0.09	0.09
Chondroectodermal dysplasia	0.05	—	—	—
Larsen syndrome	0.05	—	—	—
Mesomelic dysplasia (Langer)	0.05	—	—	—
Others	0.46	—	—	—
Total skeletal dysplasia	2.44	1.10	2.29	3.22

Sources
1 Camera G and Mastoiacovo P.[8]
2 Connor JM, Connor RAC, Sweet EM, et al. Lethal neonatal chondrodysplasias in the West of Scotland, 1970–1983 with a description of a thanatophoric, dysplasia-like autosomal recessive disorder. Am J Med Genet 1985; 22:243.
3 Orioli I et al.[9]
4 Stoll C, Dott B, Roth MP, et al. Birth prevalence rates of skeletal dysplasias. Clin Genet 1989; 35:88.
Reproduced with permission from Fleischer et al sonography in obstetrics and gynaecology. Practice and principles, 5th ed. New York: Appleton and Lange; 1996:448.

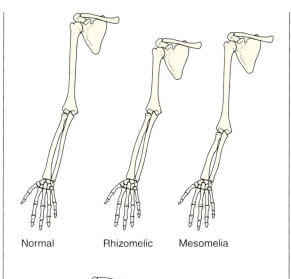

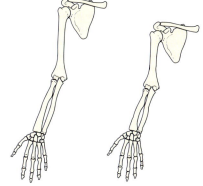

Fig. 12.4 Types of limb shortening.

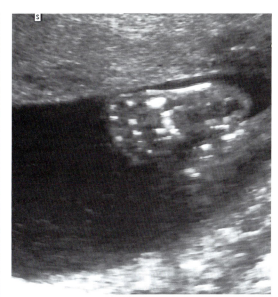

Fig. 12.5 Normal foot length.

on normograms is only possible if the gestation is known accurately, preferably by early ultrasound scan.

When there is uncertainty of the gestation in the presence of limb shortening, the femoral length cannot be used for estimating the gestational age. In this situation, the foot length is more appropriate (Fig. 12.5). This measurement is obtained by imaging the length of the foot and measuring the maximum length. The foot is usually uninvolved in skeletal dysplasias apart from positional deformities and polydactyly. Normograms should be used for plotting the foot length (see Appendix).

If there is doubt about the normality or otherwise of the bones, an assessment of bone growth is appropriate after an interval of time (minimum 2 weeks). Bone dysplasias do not show normal growth. Other disorders of growth that are not true bone dysplasias will also show abnormally slow incremental growth. This can range from placental causes of growth restriction to syndromic abnormalities, e.g. Russell–Silverman syndrome.

As stated previously, a structured approach must be undertaken to assess the ultrasound abnormalities in order that a differential diagnosis can be reached and the appropriate management options discussed and planned. As many of the bone dysplasias are first detected on a screening anomaly scan, this approach for the practical assessment of the fetal skeleton and associated abnormalities will first be discussed followed by detailed text on the specific dysplasias apparent at birth. Being apparent at birth, they are potentially amenable to antenatal diagnosis. It must be stressed, however, that frequently only a differential diagnosis can be achieved before birth. Marked femoral shortening at 18 to 20 weeks has a very poor outcome as this defines the lethal dysplasias.[7]

Morphology

The following important questions need to be addressed.

Long Bones: are the long bones as assessed by ultrasound normal or abnormal?

If abnormal, are they:

Broad?

Bent?

Fractured?

Which bones are involved?

Is the bone mineralization normal?

Ribs: Are the ribs involved?

If so, are they short or fractured?

Is the thorax narrow?

Cranial vault

Is the ossification normal?

Is the **facial profile**, including the contour of the frontal bone and mandible, normal or abnormal?

Having assessed all the skeleton in this systematic way, other anomalies must be searched for.

Is there an associated **facial cleft?** If present, is this midline or lateral?

Table 12.7
Classification of skeletal dysplasias

Ultrasound diagnosis	Pathological diagnosis	Comments
Short limbs		
Severe micromelia	Achondrogenesis types I, II, III	Hypomineralized. Rib fractures only type I. Autosomal recessive
Mild micromelia but marked bowing	Camptomelic dysplasia	Scapulae hypoplastic/absent, scoliosis from vertebral anomalies. Often autosomal recessive
Marked rhizomelia hypertelorism	Rhizomelic chondrodysplasia punctata	Similar syndrome follows warfarin therapy. Autosomal recessive
Mild micromelia talipes, facial clefting. Hitch-hiker thumb	Diastrophic dysplasia	Autosomal recessive
Mild rhizomelia. Often normal at 20 weeks, apparent by 27/28 weeks. Distal long bones normal	Heterozygous achondroplasia	Autosomal dominant. 80% new mutations
Thoracic deformity		
Multiple vertebral/spinal rib abnormalities	Spondylothoracic dysostosis (Jarcho–Levin syndrome)	Autosomal recessive. Lethal
Thoracic/spinal deformity		
Profound micromelia. Camptomelia of long bones. Narrow thorax – short ribs. Polyhydramnios	Thanatophoric dysplasia	Commonest lethal dysplasia (1 in 30 000). Sporadic but recurrences have been seen if associated with clover-leaf skull
Mild micromelia. Marked thoracic hypoplasia. Polydactyly may be present	Asphyxiating thoracic dysplasia (Jeune's)	Often lethal but survivors exist. Autosomal recessive
As for Jeune's but with renal and cardiac anomalies	Chondroectodermal dysplasia (Ellis van Creveld)	Autosomal recessive
Short ribs, polydactyly. Narrow thorax. Cardiac and renal malformations. Short or absent tibias	Type I Saldino–Noonan Type II Majewski Type III Naumoff	All autosomal recessive and lethal
Mineralization defects		
Severe hypomineralization without fractures	Hypophosphatasia	Autosomal recessive. Absent or low alkaline phosphatase. Lethal
Hypomineralization. Severe micromelia owing to multiple fractures. Bones appear broad. Rib fractures	Osteogenesis imperfecta IIa	Lethal. Recurrence risk non-consanguineous parents 3%. About 90% autosomal dominant new mutations, 10% autosomal recessive
As for osteogenesis imperfecta IIa. Less extensive fractures	Osteogenesis imperfecta III	Autosomal recessive. Non-lethal but progressive.

Reproduced with permission from Whittle M, Connor JM, eds. Prenatal diagnosis in obstetric practice. Oxford: Blackwell Science; 1995:179.

If lateral, does this involve one or both sides?

Is the **mandible** of normal size or small?

The assessment of the **fetal spine** should include the vertebral bodies and the appendages.

Although the neonatal spine shows striking X-ray abnormalities in skeletal dysplasias, these features often are difficult to assess antenatally.

> Are the **hands** and **feet** normal in position? If abnormal, is there talipes or positional abnormalities of the digits?
> Is there associated **polydactyly** and if so, is this pre- or post-axial?
> Are there other associated structural abnormalities? In particular, is the **renal tract** and **heart normal** as assessed by ultrasound?

Having assessed the above features, it is then possible to provide a differential diagnosis. Syndromic data may be available from a dysmorphology database. If not, a systematic approach is outlined in Table 12.7.

Dysplasias associated with a narrow thorax are given in Table 12.8.

Normograms are available for thoracic length which is measured from the apex of the thorax to the diaphragm (Fig. 12.6) and

Table 12.8
Dysplasia associated with a narrow thorax

Thanatophoric dysplasia
Achondrogenesis
Hypochondrogenesis
Asphyxiating thoracic dystrophy
Chondroectodermal dysplasia
Short rib polydactyly syndrome
    Type I Saldino–Noonan syndrome
    Type II Majewski syndrome
    Type III Naumoff syndrome
    Type IV Beemer–Langer syndrome
Camptomelic dysplasia

for the thoracic circumference which is measured at the level of the 4-chamber view to the heart (Fig. 12.7).

Clearly gestational age must be known for an accurate assessment and therefore some age-independent ratios have been used, e.g. the thoracic-to-abdominal circumference ratio (normal value 0.77–1.01).

The evaluation of the thoracic dimensions is an important part of the assessment of the fetus with skeletal dysplasias as in the lethal dysplasias, it is pulmonary hypoplasia that is the cause of death in the majority of cases.

This structured approach is most appropriate in the practical scanning situation and once a working differential diagnosis is reached, the more precise, abnormal ultrasound findings of the specific

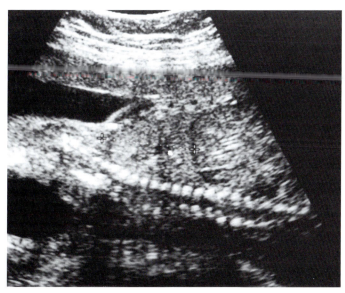

Fig. 12.6 Normal thoracic length on a longitudinal scan.

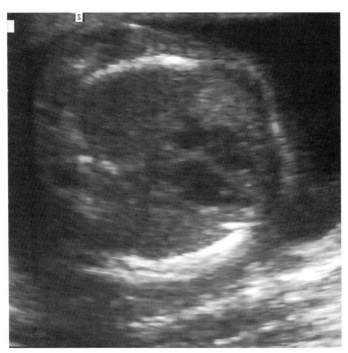

Fig. 12.7 Normal thoracic circumference at the level of the heart showing that the normal ribs extend two-thirds around the thorax.

bone dysplasia can be assessed. Bone abnormalities are rare and for best and safe practice, referral to a tertiary centre is appropriate.

Having defined the type of bone shortening – micromelia, rhizomelia or mesomelia and the degree of shortening – the group of micromelias can be further subdivided into those with mild or

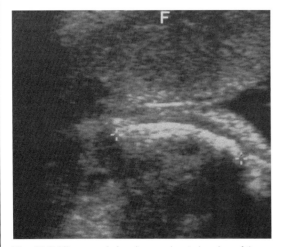

Fig. 12.8 Ultrasound showing moderate bowing of the femur.

moderate-to-severe shortening and the presence or absence of bowing (Fig. 12.8).

This structured approach to the abnormalities of the skeleton and the presence of other associated abnormalities should result in a differential diagnosis that can be assessed in relationship to the published data on specific conditions at specific gestations.

There follows a description of the abnormal ultrasound features of the commoner skeletal dysplasias.

The reporting of the antenatal findings of specific diagnoses is ongoing but the current list available is given in Table 12.9.

Dysplasias associated with abnormal thoracic dimensions

Lethal

Thanatophoric dysplasia

This is the commonest of the lethal skeletal dysplasias seen prenatally with an incidence of 1:4000–30 000.[8,9,10]

Table 12.9
Skeletal dysplasias detected prenatally

Achondrogenesis type I
Achondrogenesis type II
Achondroplasia
Amelia
Apert syndrome
Arthrogryposis multiplex congenita
Asphyxiating thoracic dysplasia
Atelosteogenesis type I
Atelosteogenesis type II
Camptomelic dysplasia
Carpenter's syndrome
Caudal regression syndrome
Chondrodysplasia punctata (rhizomelic type)
Chondrodysplasia punctata (non-rhizomelic)
Chondroectodermal dysplasia
Cleidocranial dysplasia
Diastrophic dysplasia
Dyssegmental dysplasia
Ectrodactyly–ectodermal dysplasia
Fanconi anaemia
Femur–fibula–ulna syndrome
Fibula aplasia
Fraser syndrome
Greenberg dysplasia
Hemivertebrae
Holt–Oram syndrome
Hypochondrodysplasia
Jarcho–Levin syndrome
Larsen's syndrome
Mandibulofacial dysostosis
Mesomelic dysplasia
Osteogenesis imperfecta type I
Osteogenesis imperfecta type II
Osteogenesis imperfecta type III
Proximal focal femoral deficiency
Radial ray aplasia
Roberts syndrome
Short rib polydactyly type I
Short rib polydactyly type II
Short rib polydactyly type III
Sirenomelia
TAR syndrome
Thanatophoric dysplasia
VACTERL syndrome

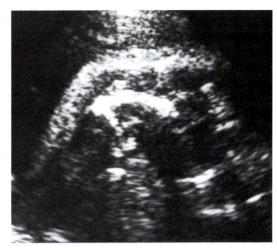

Fig. 12.9 Short and bent femur in thanatophoric dysplasia.

The main features are of profound limb shortening with bowing associated with a narrow, shortened thorax with short ribs. The abdomen by comparison is protuberant and the head is large with a prominent forehead. There is associated poly-hydramnios in 70% of cases and this clinical sign of large-for-gestational age is the presenting feature in those who have not had a screening anomaly scan.

There are two sub-groups which depend on the appearances of the head:

- **Type I** with typical short, bent ('telephone receiver') femora without a clover-leaf skull.
  This type is seen in approximately 85% of cases (Fig. 12.9).
- **Type II** shows clover-leaf skull with less long bone shortening or abnormal curvature and is seen in less than 20% of cases (Fig. 12.10). Approximately 25% of these cases will have agenesis of the corpus callosum.

The extreme shortening of the long bones is easily apparent and is well demonstrated by 18 weeks' gestation.

The differential diagnosis includes homozygous achondroplasia but, in this case, the fact that both parents have heterozygous achondroplasia will readily be apparent. Other very rare conditions have been described with similar appearances. All carry a very poor prognosis and the final diagnosis is often not possible prenatally. These include atelosteogenesis, fibrochondro-genesis, San Diego dysplasia, Schneckenbecken dysplasia and Torrance dysplasia.

Outcome. This is a uniformly lethal abnormality and neonatal death from respiratory failure is the norm for those that survive to term.

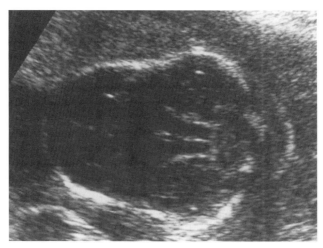

Fig. 12.10 Clover-leaf deformity in thanatophoric dysplasia.

Homozygous achondroplasia

The antenatal ultrasound findings are of marked micromelia and narrow thorax secondary to the rib shortening. The long bones are broad and bent. These features are similar to thanatophoric dysplasia.

This condition clearly only occurs when both parents have heterozygous achondroplasia, therefore the diagnosis is relatively easy to make as both parents will have the classical appearances of heterozygous achondroplasia (Fig. 12.11).

Short rib polydactyly

This group is characterized by severe micromelia, short horizontal ribs, postaxial polydactyly and frequently cardiac and renal abnormalities. These disorders are probably inherited as autosomal recessive disorders. They are very rare and the distinguishing features between the groups are the presence of facial clefting, tibial length and metaphyseal morphology.[11]

There are now four groups of short rib polydactyly:

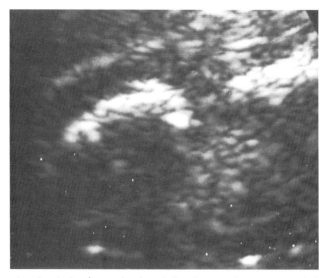

Fig. 12.11 Homozygous achondroplasia – femur showing similar ultrasound appearances to thanatophoric dysplasia.

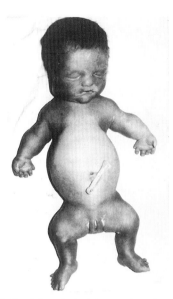

Fig. 12.12 Short rib polydactyly – post-mortem external appearances.

- **Type 1 Saldino–Noonan** – is characterized by short horizontal ribs and polydactyly with severe micromelia. The metaphyses in this condition are narrow (Fig. 12.12).
- **Type 2 Majewski** – has additional facial clefting and marked shortening of the tibia.[13]
- **Type 3 Naumoff** – has wide metaphyses with spurs in addition to the severe micromelia, short ribs and polydactyly.[14]
- **Type 4 Beemer–Langer** – is characterized by a median facial cleft, small thorax owing to very short ribs and protuberant abdomen and omphalocoele. The genitalia may be ambiguous in 46 XY fetuses. The iliac wings are small.[15]

In practical terms, the exact type of short rib polydactyly dysplasia is unimportant for prenatal counselling as all groups are lethal. This knowledge allows parents informed choices relating to interruption of the pregnancy.

Outcome. The outcome for all groups of short rib polydactyly is lethal.

Achondrogenesis

This is characterized by severe micromelia, a short narrow thorax and a large head. There may be associated hydrocephalus, facial clefting and heart and renal abnormalities. The incidence is approximately 1:40 000 births.

The pathophysiology of this condition is defective cartilage formation, resulting in poor ossification. There may be associated polyhydramnios seen in approximately 50% of cases and hydrops may develop (30%).

Two distinct types are recognized:

- Achondrogenesis type I (Parenti–Fraccora) In type I, there is severe limb shortening with almost complete lack of ossification in the skull vault, spine and pelvis with multiple rib fractures (Fig. 12.13). This is an autosomal recessive inheritance.
- Achondrogenesis type II (Langer–Saldino) In type II, there is more calcification in the bones of the vault, spine and pelvis and there are no rib fractures. These cases are thought to be the result of spontaneous, new, dominant mutations.[16]

Hypochondrogenesis is now considered by some to be the same entity as achondrogenesis type II but with variable penetrance, resulting in a less severe phenotype and with better mineralization of bone.

Fibrochondrogenesis

This has similar manifestations to thanatophoric dysplasia with severe limb shortening. However, there is vertebral body clefting and metaphyseal clefting which are not seen in thanatophoric dysplasia. This feature is not apparent on antenatal ultrasound and the precise diagnosis can only be confirmed by postnatal investigations, particularly X-rays. It is inherited in an autosomal pattern and is lethal.[17]

Atelosteogenesis

This lethal dysplasia has severe micromelia but with hypoplasia of the distal humerus and femur, a narrow thorax, marked bowing of the long bones with dislocation at the elbow and knee and the mandible is small. Talipes is often present. There is coronal clefting of the vertebral bodies. Polyhydramnios has been described.[18] Two sub-groups are recognized.[19–22]

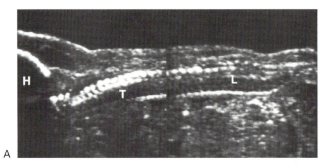

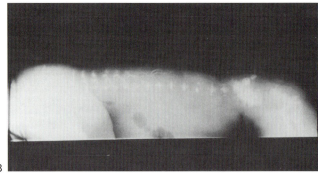

Fig. 12.13 (A) Prenatal ultrasound appearances. H, head; T, thoracic spine; L, lumbar spine. (B) Lateral spine in achondrogenesis, showing marked lack of ossification.

- Type I   a sporadic condition
- Type II   autosomal recessive inheritance.

Hypophosphatasia

This disorder is characterized by lack of mineralization in bones and is associated with low serum and cellular alkaline phosphatase. It has an autosomal recessive inheritance pattern.

Four clinical groups are described, depending on the time of presentation:

- Neonatal
- Juvenile
- Adult
- Latent.

The antenatal diagnosis is possible for the neonatal type when the ultrasound features and/or chorionic villus sampling for tissue alkaline phosphatase levels can be performed. The ultrasound features of this disease are of undermineralization of bone although there are fewer fractures than seen in osteogenesis imperfecta type IIa.

Osteogenesis imperfecta

This is a heterogeneous group of disorders, characterized by abnormalities of type I collagen which interferes with the normal process of ossification of the bones.[23] The most popular classification is that of Sillence and is outlined in Table 12.10.[24] This classification results in four groups, types I to IV. Types I and IV have repeated fractures

Table 12.10 Sillence classification of osteogenesis imperfecta	
Type I	Blue sclera Presenile conduction deafness Sub-group A: normal dentition Sub-group B: abnormal dentition Sub-group C: blue sclera 　　　　　　　wormian bones 　　　　　　　abnormal dentition
Type II	
	Sub-group A: short and fractured long bones 　　　　　　　beaded ribs from multiple 　　　　　　　fractures
	Sub-group B: short and fractured long bones 　　　　　　　no rib fractures
	Sub-group C: thin and fractured long bones 　　　　　　　thin ribs
Type III	Normal sclera Variable fractures
Type IV	Normal sclera Severe deformities of the long bones

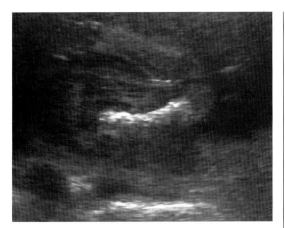

Fig. 12.14 Broad and fractured femur in osteogenesis imperfecta type IIa.

but with survival; these groups are further subdivided by the appearance of the dentition and sclera. Type II is lethal in utero or early in the neonatal period for most cases.

Type II, the perinatal group, will be considered in detail here as this is the type most commonly seen in the antenatal department. Type II is divided into three further sub-groups on the basis of the morphology of the ribs and the presence of rib fractures.

Type IIa is characterized by multiple fractures which result in profound limb shortening as the bones telescope from the fractures (Fig. 12.15). The incidence is approximately 1:60 000 births. Most cases are new mutations but an autosomal recessive inheritance has also been described. The bone shortening is apparent by 18 to 20 weeks and has been described as early as 13 weeks.[25,26]

The ultrasound features are of broad, bent, fractured and very shortened long bones. The thorax shows an abnormal contour on the transverse scan (Fig. 12.15) secondary to the multiple rib fractures.[27] The lack of ossification in the skull vault bones results in particular clarity of the brain when the head is examined with ultrasound. The normal relationship of the echogenicity of the bones to the falx is lost. The falx in this condition is a stronger reflector than bone, the reverse of the normal relationship.

This lack of mineralization of the vault results in very soft bone so that gentle pressure from the ultrasound transducer on the fetal head while scanning will result in the distortion of the vault bones (Fig. 12.16). Polyhydramnios has been described.

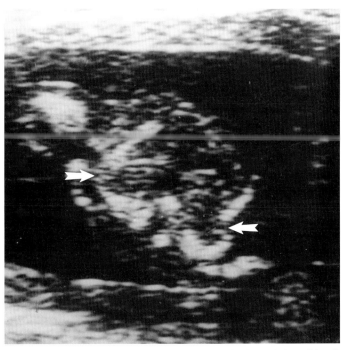

Fig. 12.15 Fractured ribs on a transverse scan of the thorax showing marked angulation of the ribs (arrows).

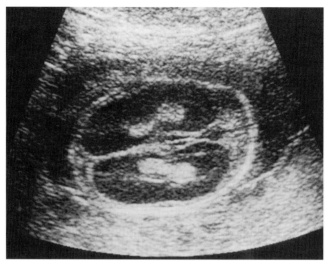

Fig. 12.16 Fetal head in osteogenesis imperfecta where the lack of ossification in the vault bones results in the falx being a stronger reflector than the abnormal bone.

Outcome. This condition is lethal.

Type IIb shows moderately shortened femurs and discrete fractures are seen in the long bones. The ribs are not fractured (Figs 12.17 and 12.18).

Outcome. This condition is not invariably lethal but results in severe disease postnatally.

Type IIc shows shortening of all limbs but discrete fractures may not be apparent.

Type I (**non-lethal**) is late in onset and, by comparison to type II, and is mild. This makes antenatal diagnosis often difficult. The ultrasound examination at 20 weeks would be expected to be normal in this condition. The incidence is 1:30 000 births with a dominant inheritance.

Spontaneous mutation is relatively rare and therefore there will be a positive family history. Only 5% or fewer show fractures at birth and therefore, if present, there will be

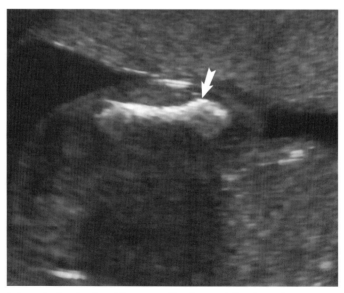

Fig. 12.17 Osteogenesis imperfecta – fractured femur resulting in angulation (arrow).

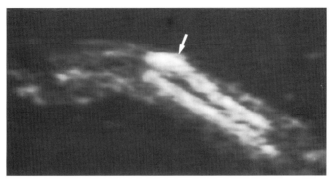

Fig. 12.18 Osteogenesis imperfecta – a subtle fracture of the distal radius (arrow).

the ultrasound signs of a fracture – the exact ultrasound findings will depend on the age of the fracture. There will be a distinct break in the normal contour of the involved bone with some angulation if recent. As callous forms, the bone demonstrates broadening and bowing. Rarely, there may be bowing of the fractured long bones but for many affected babies the antenatal ultrasound remains normal. This is an important fact to remember when counselling the couple when one partner is known to have osteogenesis imperfecta with a dominant inheritance.

Type III: this condition has variable expression and variable postnatal progression of the disease although the majority of those affected are in wheelchairs by early adulthood. The main antenatal ultrasound feature is of shortening of the long bones that have fractured. This may not be apparent in the early second trimester. The shortening only becomes apparent after 24 weeks. Therefore women with at-risk pregnancies should have a detailed examination at this gestation.

Camptomelic dysplasia

This condition is characterized by mild shortening or normal length but with marked bowing of the long bones of the lower limbs, particularly the femora and tibia. This bowing occurs in the anteroposterior plane of the bone and therefore careful scanning in this plane is essential to assess the degree of abnormal bowing. There is hypoplasia of the scapulae and the thorax may be bell-shaped. The pedicles of the thoracic vertebra are undermineralized and the iliac bones are more vertical than normal and narrowed. There is often associated hip dislocation. These features of the thoracic vertebra and iliac wings are unique to this condition but these signs are difficult to elicit antenatally (Fig. 12.19).[28,29]

Associated ultrasound structural abnormalities include:

- heart – ventricular septal defect, atrial septal defect, Fallot tetralogy and aortic stenosis
- renal tract –hydronephrosis
- facial clefts
- talipes.

50% of cases are phenotypically female although the chromosomes indicate 46 XY and testes are present.[30–30a]

There are two broad types in this heterogeneous group:[31]

- Type I – slightly short limb length with anterior bowing of the femora and tibia. The bones are of normal width. The upper limbs are not involved.
- Type II – short bent bones which are widened. There may be associated craniostenosis.

The ultrasound appearances are apparent at 18 to 20 weeks in the published cases and the most striking features are of the anterior

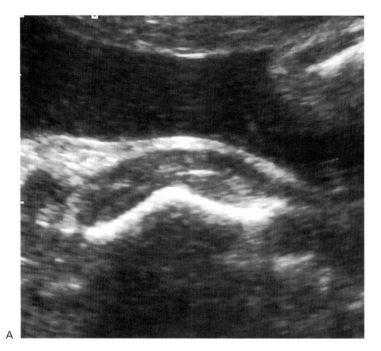

A

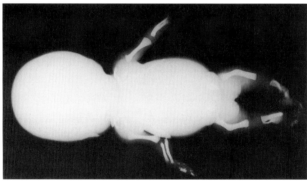

B

Fig. 12.19 (A) Ultrasound of angulated femur. (B) X-ray of camptomelic dysplasia.

bowing of the femur and tibia with hypoplasia of the fibula.[32] The scapula is hypoplastic and the scapular length can be plotted against published normograms[33,34] (see Appendix).

Outcome. This is lethal in most, but not all, cases, secondary to respiratory failure, which is the result of the tracheobronchial malacia; deficiency of the cartilage of the trachea and main bronchi.

Dyssegmental dysplasia

There is severe micromelia associated with a disordered spine from multiple vertebral body abnormalities. In addition, there is

frequently an associated occipital encephalocoele.

Outcome. The outcome is lethal.[35,36]

Non-lethal or variable outcome

Asphyxiating thoracic dysplasia (Jeune's syndrome)

This is an autosomal recessive disorder but with a variable phenotypic expression. This condition is characterized by a long and narrow thorax caused by short and horizontal ribs. This is a rare disorder with an approximate incidence of 1:70 000 births (Fig. 12.20). The long bones show only mild

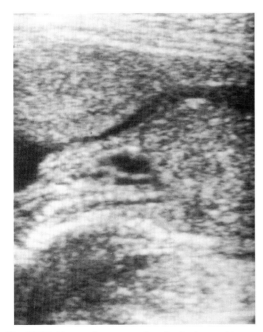

Fig. 12.20 Narrow thorax on a longitudinal scan in asphyxiating thoracic dysplasia (Jeune's syndrome).

shortening or may be normal in length. The shortening is rhizomelic (proximal). The long bone lengths may be normal at 18 to 20 weeks and the shortening becomes apparent in later pregnancy, e.g. after 24 to 26 weeks. This is similar to most non-lethal, short limb dysplasias where the impaired long bone growth is not apparent until a later gestation compared with the lethal disorders.

The following are associated features:

— facial cleft lip and palate which may occur together or separately
— polydactyly – seen in approximately 14%[37,39]
— renal cystic dysplasia – the cystic changes are progressive and not usually apparent before birth although cases have been described associated with oligo-hydramnios, presumably the result of the renal dysplasia
— polyhydramnios may be apparent in those without renal impairment.

Outcome. Those that survive the neonatal period usually have progressively less thoracic constriction with growth but progressive renal impairment owing to the cystic renal dysplasia which results in renal failure for many. Early neonatal or infantile deaths are the result of respiratory failure from pulmonary hypoplasia.[38,39]

Chondroectodermal dysplasia (Ellis van Creveld)

This is an autosomal recessive condition with an incidence of 1:200 000. The abnormal gene is common in the Amish communities. It is characterized by shortening of the limb bones and shows similar appearances in the thorax as asphyxiating thoracic dysplasias, i.e., a narrow thorax. There is usually polydactyly (postaxial) which distinguishes this condition from asphyxiating thoracic dysplasia. Approximately 50% of cases have an associated cardiac defect, usually an atrial septal defect.

The ultrasound features are less severe than the lethal, short rib polydactly syndromes and this should allow differentiation from these disorders.[40]

Outcome. There is survival with normal intelligence.

Diastrophic dysplasia

This autosomal recessive disorder shows variable phenotypic expression which ranges from the mild to the severe. The location of the gene has been mapped to the long arm of chromosome 5.[41,42] DNA analysis from chorionic villus sampling allows early diagnosis in affected at-risk pregnancies. This dysplasia results in generalized disorder of cartilage and a destructive process in the cartilage matrix. This destructive process results in scar formation with fibrous and osseous tissue formation. It is this process that is responsible for the contractures.

The typical features are of micromelia with flexion limitations at the elbows, hips and finger joints, resulting in the classical hitchhiker thumb owing to fixed lateral position of this digit. There is a progressive scoliosis which may be apparent before birth. Other features include talipes, cleft palate and micrognathia. Less common findings are anterior chamber disorders of the eye, facial haemangioma, craniostenosis, stenosis of the larynx and trachea, and cardiac defects, most commonly atrial septal defect, ventricular septal defect and patent ductus arteriosus.

The ultrasound findings in the severe cases have been apparent by 20 weeks with severe micromelia but these cases were in known at-risk pregnancies for this disorder.[43]

Outcome. This is variable. For the less severe expression of this disease, survival past infancy results in good survival with normal intelligence.

Metatrophic dysplasia

This condition is very rare with an incidence of 1:100 000 and appears to be a hetero-geneous group. There is a variable mode of inheritance with both autosomal dominant and recessive forms being described.

The features prenatally consist of a narrow thorax with moderate shortening of the long bones. The appearances prenatally are similar to asphyxiating dysplasia; therefore a differential diagnosis only can be reached. The bone shortening as in most non-lethal dysplasia is not apparent until after 22 weeks when normal, incremental bone growth decreases and the absolute limb length measurements fall below the 3rd centile by 27 to 28 weeks.

Outcome. Death may occur in infancy secondary to respiratory failure. After this period, survival is the norm but with progressive spinal deformities. The intelligence is normal.

Jarcho–Levin syndrome

This is characterized by disorders of the segmentation of the spine resulting in hemi- and fused vertebra. This affects all parts of the spine: cervical, thoracic and lumbar. The features seen on ultrasound are of a profoundly abnormal spine with distortion of the thorax as a result of the multiple vertebral anomalies and the associated rib malformations (Fig. 12.21).

Two sub-types are recognized postnatally:

- Spondylothoracic dysostosis is an autosomal recessive condition where the ribs show marked flaring.
- Spondylocostal dysostosis has more marked rib abnormalities and has been described as an autosomal recessive or dominant inheritance.

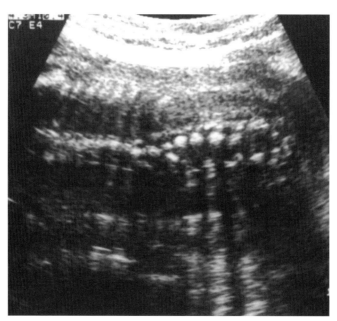

Fig. 12.21 Spine disorder in Jarcho–Levin syndrome.

These abnormalities have been described from 20 to 22 weeks.[44,45]

Cleidocranial dysplasia

This is an autosomal dominant disorder which shows a wide variation in expression but usually complete penetrance. It is characterized by abnormalities of bone formed in cartilage. The clavicles are hypoplastic or absent and the base of the skull abnormal. Prenatally, the cases have been described as showing a small thorax owing to rib shortening.[46] There are normograms available for clavicular length that allow measurement of the case under suspicion to be assessed in comparison to the normal fetus[47] (see Appendix).

Outcome is good.

Metatrophic dysplasia type II (Kneist syndrome)

This condition is an autosomal dominant condition, showing mild-to-moderate micromelia. It is extremely rare with an incidence of 0.1:1 000 000. There is a shortened thorax which may be broad owing to the kyphoscoliosis which is usually progressive (Fig. 12.22). The long bones show widening towards the metaphysis.

Outcome. There is survival but with marked shortening of the bones resulting in very short stature.

Otopalatalodigital syndrome type II

This is a rare disorder with an incidence of 0.1:1 000 000 and is most likely an X-linked recessive disorder. The features consist of polydactyly, syndactyly, and talipes associated with facial clefting. The long bones show moderate micromelia.

Outcome. 50% have impaired intellect. There is progressive conductive deafness.

De la Chappelle dysplasia

This is a rare condition characterized by severe micromelia, and on post-mortem X-rays, classical triangular appearances to the ulna and fibula. Talipes and facial clefting also occur. The thorax is narrow and there are multiple vertebral anomalies. It is most likely to be an autosomal recessive condition.

Outcome. The outcome is neonatal death from respiratory failure.[48]

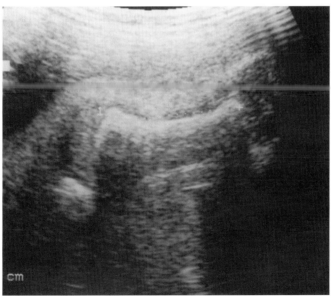

Fig. 12.22 Kneist syndrome (metatrophic dysplasia). Femur showing widened metaphysis.

Other conditions not associated with a markedly abnormal thorax

Lethal

Boomerang dysplasia

This rare condition has short broad and bowed long bones with absence of the radii and fibulae. The long bones have a characteristic 'boomerang' configuration. There is abnormal ossification of the lower spine and the iliac wings are small.[49]

Chondrodysplasia punctata (rhizomelic form)

This is a group of disorders that all show disordered mineralization, resulting in typical stippling seen on postnatal radiographs (Fig. 12.23). The severe and lethal form shows proximal shortening of the limbs that is apparent by 20 weeks.[50–52]

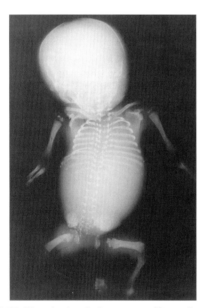

Fig. 12.23 Chondrodysplasia punctata (Conradi–Hunermann syndrome). Post-mortem X-ray shows stippled epiphyses.

Non-lethal

Heterozygous achondroplasia

This condition has an incidence of approximately 1:30 000 births and most cases (80%) occur as new mutations. It is an autosomal dominant disorder. Therefore there is a 50% chance of recurrence with an affected parent. The homozygous condition is lethal and resembles thanatophoric dysplasia.

The main features consist of rhizomelic shortening that is not apparent until 22 weeks and the absolute limb lengths only become less than the 3rd centile by 24 to 26 weeks. Therefore in at-risk pregnancies, it is insufficient to scan only at 20 weeks. Further growth scans are essential after 24 weeks (Fig. 12.24). The reduced growth profile of the abnormal limbs will be apparent.

The skull vault is relatively large compared to the base. There is frontal bossing and a depressed nasal bridge, resulting in a saddle nose deformity (Fig. 12.25). The hands are broad with shortening of the bones – brachydactyly.[53]

Outcome. The child has short stature but will have normal intelligence and life-span.

Chondrodysplasia punctata (Conradi–Hunermann syndrome)

The sonographic findings are of early ossification of the epiphysis of the proximal humerus and femora.[54,55]

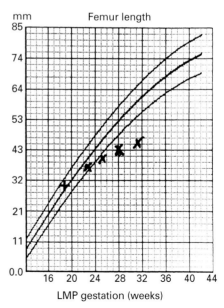

Fig. 12.24 Growth profile in heterozygous achondroplasia.

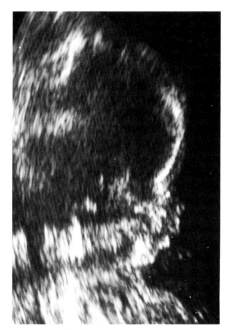

Fig. 12.25 Facial profile in heterozygous achondroplasia.

Acromesomelic dysplasia

This is an autosomal recessive disorder with mesomelic shortening; the bones show flaring of the metaphysis.

Outcome. The child has short stature but will have normal intelligence.

Larsen syndrome

This condition has multiple joint dislocations, talipes, abnormal broad thumbs and short metacarpals. Vertebral abnormalities consisting of hemi- and butterfly vertebrae are seen. There is an association with facial clefting and cardiac defect. This condition has been diagnosed in at-risk pregnancies at 20 weeks.[56,57]

Mesomelic dysplasia

This is a heterogeneous group of disorders where the limb shortening is most marked in the middle segment. Mesomelic dysplasia is subdivided into the following groups with mesomelic shortening in both the arms and legs:[58]

- Langer – autosomal recessive
- Neivergelt – autosomal dominant
- Reinhart–Pfeiffer – autosomal dominant

- Robinow – autosomal dominant. This condition is associated with typical facies and genital anomalies, consisting of hypoplasia of the penis or clitoris. The degree of bone shortening tends to be more marked in the radius and ulna compared to the tibia and fibula
- Werner – autosomal dominant. In this condition, there are dysplastic or absent tibia; there may be dislocation at the knees and the hands. Although the hand has five digits, there is no normal thumb. Polydactyly of the feet may be present.

The precise diagnosis is only possible postnatally unless there is a known antenatal diagnosis of the specific condition in a previous pregnancy.[59]

Limb deficiencies and amputations

These abnormalities have an incidence of 1:20 000 births. Approximately one-half of these result from amputations secondary to amniotic bands. In these cases, there is a transverse defect with no other associated abnormalities (Fig. 12.26). In the remainder there are multiple defects and internal or craniofacial abnormalities.[60] The majority of reductions of the upper limbs are isolated events but those involving the lower limbs are often part of more complex anomalies or syndromes.

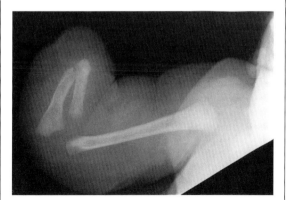

Fig. 12.26 Amputation of the distal portion of the ulna and radius secondary to an amniotic band.

Isolated amputations are due to the following:

> Amniotic band
> Vascular compromise
> Teratogens
> Limb reduction following chorion villous sampling prior to 66 days' gestation are reported.[61–65]

Limb reductions as part of syndromes include:

> Aglossia–adactyly syndrome
> Oromandibular limb hypogenesis syndrome
> Mobius syndrome
> Congenital hemidysplasia with ichthyosiform erythroderma and limb defects (child syndrome)

Fibula aplasia–complex brachydactyly syndrome
Roberts syndrome
Grebe syndrome.

Sirenomelia

This condition is a lethal disorder that shows fusion of the lower limbs (Fig. 12.27). It has three sub-groups, depending on the bones present in the lower limb:

— Absent feet and a single tibia and femur
— Single foot and two femora and two tibiae and two fibulae
— Two feet with fused legs.

In all conditions there are usually multiple, internal, structural abnormalities, particularly in the renal tract.[66–70]

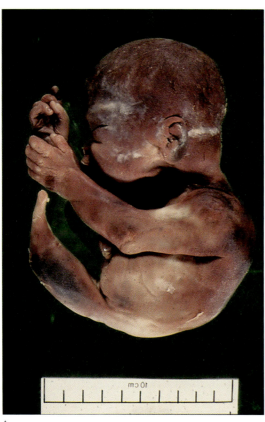
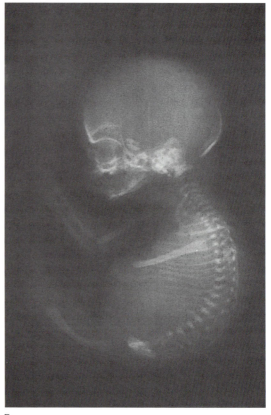

A   B

Fig. 12.27 Sirenomelia. (A) Post-mortem photograph. (B) X-ray of 20-week fetus with sirenomelia.

Ectrodactyly lobster claw deformity; split hand and foot

This is a rare condition and is subdivided into two groups:

- Those where there is absence of the digits and metacarpal/metatarsal bones, resulting in a central, V-shaped loss in the centre of the hands and feet resulting in a distinct radial/ulnar or tibial/fibular component (Fig. 12.28). This type has an incidence of 1:90 000 births and is inherited usually as an autosomal dominant condition.
- The less common type consists of a wider central loss with only a small digit remaining on the ulnar side. This occurs in 1:150 000 births.

The ectrodactyly deformity may occur in isolation but more commonly occurs as part of a syndrome, e.g. split hand and foot and absent bones syndrome – this may be an autosomal dominant or an X-linked recessive inheritance pattern. In this condition, the abnormalities of the hands and feet are associated with aplasia of the ulna. Other bones may be involved, e.g. the femur, fibula or clavicle.

Ectrodactyly-ectodermal dysplasia cleft palate syndrome

In this syndrome the upper limbs are more severely affected than the lower and there is variable expression.[71]

Club-hand

This is divided into abnormalities of either radial or ulnar deformities.

Radial club-hand. The abnormalities range from hypoplasia to absence of the thumb

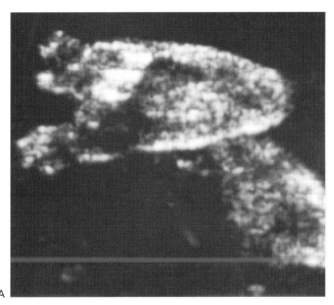

A

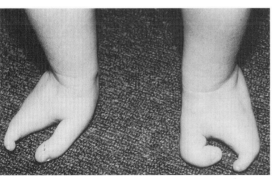

B

Fig. 12.28 (A) Ultrasound, showing the appearance of a lobster claw deformity of the foot with (B) clinical photograph for comparison.

Table 12.11
Radial ray abnormalities

Isolated non-syndromic
Syndromes with blood disorders
   Fanconi anaemia
   TAR syndrome (thrombocytopenia and absent radii)
   Aase syndrome
Syndromes with heart defects, e.g.
   Holt–Oram syndrome
Syndromes with craniofacial abnormalities, e.g.
   Nager acrofacial dysostosis
   Radial club-hand and cleft lip syndrome
Syndromes with vertebral anomalies, e.g.
   VACTERL syndrome
   Goldenhar syndrome
Radial abnormalities associated with chromosomal
abnormalities, e.g.
   trisomy 18
   Turner's syndrome
Syndromes with mental retardation, e.g.
   Seckel's syndrome

Adapted and reproduced with permission from Goldberg MD. The dysmorphic child: An orthopaedic perspective. New York: Raven Press; 1987.

with deformities of the associated metacarpals and absence of the radius. The differential diagnosis of radial ray abnormalities is outlined in Table 12.11.

Clearly in this situation, once the abnormal position of the fetal hand has been diagnosed, a careful search for associated ultrasound structural defects is mandatory. In particular, the fetal heart should be examined carefully. Fetal blood sampling for karyotype and fetal blood count with platelet estimation are essential to diagnose Fanconi's pancytopenia, TAR (Thrombocytopenia and Absent Radii) syndrome and Aase syndrome. In the Holt–Oram syndrome, congenital abnormalities of the heart are present.

Ulnar club-hand. This abnormality is less common than the radial abnormalities and ranges from ulnar deviation of the hand to absence of the ulna. It is usually an isolated abnormality.

TAR syndrome. This syndrome consists of thrombocytopenia and bilateral absent radii. It is a recessive condition. 30% of cases have cardiac defects, most commonly ventricular septal defect or Fallot tetralogy. Antenatal

platelet transfusions have been given to reduce the risk of antepartum intracranial haemorrhage.[72,73]

Fanconi anaemia. This is an autosomal recessive disorder with pancytopenia from bone marrow failure with radial hypoplasia, radial club-hand and absent thumbs.[74]

Aase syndrome. This autosomal recessive disorder differs from Fanconi anaemia in that the thumb is tripharangeal. This abnormality is also seen in the Holt–Oram and Nager syndromes but in these the blood picture is normal whereas in Aase syndrome there is a hypoplastic anaemia.

Holt–Oram syndrome. This is an autosomal dominant disorder with variable expression but 100% penetrance. It consists of congenital heart disease, usually ventricular septal defect and secundum atrial septal defect and upper limb abnormalities.[75] The abnormalities are asymmetric. There may be abnormalities of the thumbs including hypoplasia, tripharangeal, clinodactyly, syndactyly, or absent first metacarpal. The fifth finger may have a short middle phalanx or clinodactyly. The carpal bones may show modelling abnormalities or have extracarpal bones. The radius may be absent or hypoplastic. The shoulder may have an abnormal scapula, an abnormal humeral head or abnormal clavicle.

Radial club-hand is also seen in the following syndromes connected with VACTERL association:

Vertebral segmentation abnormalities (70%)
Anal atresia (80%)
Congenital cardiac abnormality (50%)
Tracheo-oesophageal atresia (65%)
Radial abnormalities (53%)
Renal (53%)
Single umbilical artery (35%)
Limb abnormality.

The radial club-hand-type abnormality has been demonstrated in trisomies 18 and 21. Deletions of the long arm of 13 and ring formation of chromosome 4 have been described.[76]

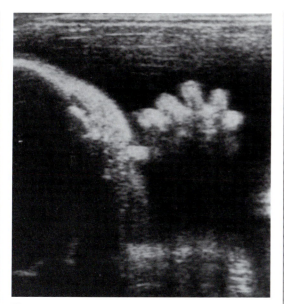

Fig. 12.29 Polydactyly of hand.

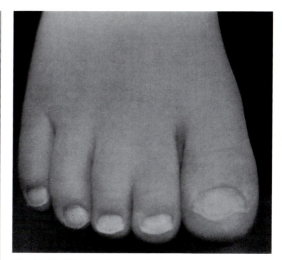

Fig. 12.30 Clinical photograph showing syndactyly between the second and third toes.

Polydactyly

This is the condition of extra digits which can range from small, extra, soft tissue structures to a complete digit with controlled flexion and extension. Polydactyly is divided into:

- **Pre-axial** when the extra digit is on the radial side of the hand and the tibial side of the foot
- **Postaxial** when the extra digit is on the ulnar side of the hand and the fibular side of the foot.

The ultrasound features are best demonstrated with the fingers extended but may be difficult to demonstrate and are often missed because of the limitations of ultrasound examination (Fig. 12.29).

Most cases of polydactyly are isolated with a dominant inheritance but many are part of defined syndromes. The commoner conditions are given in Table 12.12. A complete list of the known associated syndromes will be available from a dysmorphology database.

Syndactyly

This occurs when there is webbing of the fingers (Fig. 12.30). It is difficult to detect antenatally but is best seen when the fingers are extended but not separated. It has an association with many syndromes (Table 12.13) but may be an isolated finding with an autosomal dominant inheritance.

Fetal akinesia sequence

Although not a skeletal abnormality per se, it presents as a positional abnormality of the limbs related to the lack of normal movement. There is frequently poly-

Table 12.12
Skeletal dysplasia associated with polydactyly

Pre-axial polydactyly
  Short rib polydactyly type II
  Chondroectodermal dysplasia
  Carpenter's syndrome

Postaxial polydactyly
  Short rib polydactyly types I and II
  Chondroectodermal dysplasia
  Asphyxiating thoracic dysplasia
  Mesomelic dysplasia
  Otopalatal digital syndrome

Table 12.13
Skeletal dysplasia associated with syndactyly

Carpenter's syndrome
Alpert's syndrome
Otopalatal digital syndrome type II
Mesomelic dysplasia
TAR syndrome
Roberts syndrome
Jarcho–Levin syndrome
Poland syndrome

hydramnios in the third trimester. This has also been termed arthrogryposis congenita when there are multiple joint contractures present at birth. However, any cause of limited joint movement can result in contractures and it is therefore considered here for completeness.

Fetal akinesia should be considered as a group of disorders that results in decrease in movement of the skeleton. The aetiology includes pathology occurring anywhere in the pathway from the cerebral cortex, spinal connections, anterior horn cells, peripheral nerves, nerve muscle interface and, finally, muscle.[77,78]

Ultrasound findings. These are variable but the fixed flexion at the elbows with lack of movement, often associated with positional abnormalities of the feet, are the most common ultrasound findings.

Craniostenosis (see cranial abnormalities)

Spinal abnormalities

These are divided into abnormalities of formation resulting in hemivertebrae if unilateral, anterior central defects, resulting in butterfly vertebrae and abnormalities of segmentation, resulting in block vertebrae.

Hemivertebrae can result in scoliosis whereas block vertebrae can result in scoliosis, kyphosis or lordosis. Vertebral abnormalities are frequently seen as part of syndromes and therefore a careful search for associated structural abnormalities that may be apparent on ultrasound is mandatory.

Ultrasound findings. There is loss of the normal curvature and alignment of the fetal spine (Fig. 12.31). When the abnormality is seen antenatally, there are usually several abnormal vertebrae. There will be associated rib abnormalities if the thoracic vertebrae are involved.

Associated abnormalities include limb–body wall complex (see Ch. 11) and those affecting the gastrointestinal, renal and central nervous systems.

Prognosis. This depends on the aetiology, the extent of the vertebral abnormalities and the associated structural abnormalities.[79]

Isolated hemivertebrae are of no clinical consequence. More extensive vertebral involvement usually results in progressive curvature deformities requiring surgery. Syndromic and multiple structure abnormalities result in an outcome relating to all of the abnormalities which is usually poor.[80]

Caudal regression/sacral agenesis

This consists of agenesis of the lower lumbar

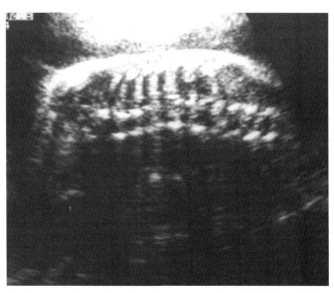

Fig. 12.31 Ultrasound, showing scoliosis resulting from abnormal vertebral body in the mid-thoracic region.

spine and sacrum with hypoplasia of the lower limbs. This abnormality is seen in insulin-dependent diabetes. It is diagnosed at the routine anomaly scan by a failure to visualize the normal, lower lumbar and sacral segments of the normal spine. These can easily be visualized in the normal fetus on the transverse section of the fetus at the level of the iliac wings, a view that is needed to examine the lower spine and bladder. This normal arrangement is lost in sacral agenesis (Fig. 12.32).[81]

Summary

A structured approach to the routine screening ultrasound at 18 to 20 weeks will allow the detection of many skeletal abnormalities. As in any screening tests it is important to define the aims and acknowledge the limitations of the test. If a skeletal abnormality is detected, then a thorough examination of the fetus should be undertaken. The skeletal dysplasias are rare conditions and in order to allow informed choices to be made by the parents of the unborn child, referral to a tertiary centre where a multidisciplinary team is available is appropriate. It should be remembered that often a precise diagnosis is not possible before birth.

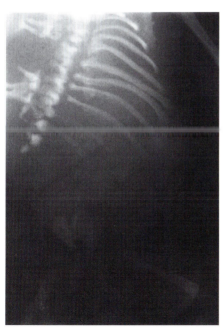

Fig. 12.32 Sacral agenesis with absence of the sacral segments.

References

1. Winter RM. Recent molecular advances in dysmorphology. Human Molecular genetics, vol. 4. 1995:1699–1704.
2. Jacenko O, Otsen BR, Warman ML. Of mice and man: Heritable skeletal disorder. Am J Hum Genet 1994; 54:163–168.
3. Horton WA. Advances in the genetics of human chondrodysplasias. Paediatr Radiol 1997; 27:419–421.
4. Goldstein I, Lockwood C, Belanger K, et al. Ultrasonographic assessment of gestational age with the distal femoral and proximal tibial ossification centers in the third trimester. Am J Obstet Gynecol 1988; 158:127.
5. Wilkie AOM, Amberger JS, McKusick VA. A gene map of congenital malformations. J Med Genet 1994; 31:507–517.
6. Pattarelli P, Pretorius DH, Edwards DK. Intrauterine growth retardation mimicking skeletal dysplasia on antenatal sonography. J Ultrasound Med 1990; 9:7376
7. Kurt AB, Goldberg BB, Wapner RJ. Predictive value of the short femur in the detection of in utero skeletal dysplasias. Radiology 1989; 173:40.
8. Camera G, Mastoiacovo P. Birth prevalence of skeletal dysplasias in the Italian multicenteric monitoring system for birth defects. In: Papadatos CJ, Bartsocas CS, eds. Skeletal dysplasia. New York: Alan R Liss; 1982:441–449.
9. Orioli IM, Castilla EE, Barbosa JG. Birth prevalence of skeletal dysplasias. J Med Genet 1986; 23:328.
10. Saunders RC, Blahemore K. Lethal fetal anomalies. Sonographic demonstration. Radiology 1989; 172:1–6.
11. Beighton P, Giedion ZA, Gorlin R, et al. An international classification of osteochondro-dysplasias. International working group on constitutional disease of bone. Am J Med Genet 1992; 44:223.
12. Meizner I, Bar Ziv J. Prenatal ultrasonic of short rib polydactyly type 1: a case report. J Reprod Med 1989; 34:668.
13. Benacerraf BR. Prenatal sonographic diagnosis of short rib polydactyly syndrome type II. Majewski type. J Ultrasound Med 1993; 12:552.
14. Meizner I, Bar Ziv J, Prenatal ultrasonic diagnosis of short rib polydactyly (SRPS) type III: A case report and a proposed approach to the diagnosis of SRPS and related conditions. J Clin Ultrasound 1985; 13:284.
15. Sharma AK, Phade SR, Agarwall SS. Short rib (polydactyly) syndrome Type IV: Beemer–Langer syndrome. Am J Med Genet 1993; 46:345.

16. van de Harten JJ, Brons JTJ, Dijkstra PF, et al. Achondrogenesis, hypochondrogenesis, the spectrum of chondrogenesis imperfecta: A radiographic, ultrasonographic and histopathologic study of 13 cases. Paediatr Pathol 1988; 8:571.

17. Whitley CB, Langer LO, Ophoven J, et al. Fibrochondrogenesis: Lethal autosomal recessive chondrodysplasia with distinctive cartilage histopathology. Am J Med Genet 1988; 19:265.

18. Chervenak FA, Isacson G, Rosenberg JC, et al. Antenatal diagnosis of frontal cephalocoele in a fetus with atelosteogenesis. J Ultrasound Med 1986; 5:111.

19. den Hollander NS, Stewart PA, Brandenburg H, et al. Atelosteogenesis, type I. The Fetus 1993; 3:7562. 23–26.

20. Nores JA, Rotmensch S, Romero R, et al. Atelosteogenesis type II: Sonographic and radiological correlation. Prenat Diagn 1992; 12:741.

21. Hunter AGW, Carpenter BF. Atelosteogensis I and boomerang dysplasia: A question of nosology. Clin Genet 1991; 39:471.

22. Greally MT, Jewett T, Smith WL, et al. Lethal bone dysplasia in a fetus with the manifestations of ateleogenesis type I and boomerang dysplasia. Am J Med Genet 1993; 47:1086.

23. Marion MJ, Gannon FH, Fallon MD, et al. Skeletal dysplasia in perinatal osteogenesis imperfecta. Clin Orthop 1993; 293:327.

24. Sillence DO, Senn A, Danks DM. Genetic heterogeneity in osteogenesis imperfecta. J Med Genet 1979; 16:101–116.

25. Dimaro MS, Barth R, Koprivinkar KE, et al. First trimester diagnosis of osteogenesis imperfecta type II by DNA analysis and sonography. Prenat Diagn 1993; 13:589.

26. Bronstein M, Weiner Z. Anencephaly in a fetus with osteogenesis imperfecta: Early diagnosis by transvaginal sonography. Prenat Diagn 1992; 12:831.

27. Constantine G, McCormick J, McHugo J, et al. Prenatal diagnosis of severe osteogenesis imperfecta. Prenat Diagn 1991; 11:103.

28. Hall BD, Springer JW. Camptomelic dysplasia. Further elucidation of a distinct entity. Am J Dis Child 1980; 134:289.

29. Balcar I, Beiber FR. Sonographic and radiological findings in camptomelia dysplasia. AJR 1983; 141:481.

30. Winter R, Rosenkranz W, Hofmann H, et al. Prenat Diagn 1995; 5:132.

30a. Beluffi G, Fraccaro M. Genetical and clinical aspects of camptomelic dysplasia. Prog Clin Biol Res 1982; 104:5333.

31. Khajavi A, Lachman R, Rimoin D, et al. Heterogeneity in the camptomelic syndromes: Long- and short-bone varieties. Radiology 1976; 120:641.

32. Valcammonico A, Jeanty P. Camptomelic dysplasia. The Fetus 1992; 2:7544–7551.

33. Cordone M, Lituania M, Zampatti C, et al. In utero ultrasound features of camptomelic dysplasia. Prenat Diagn 1989; 9:745.

34. Sherer DM, Allen TA, Plessinger MA. Fetal scapular length in the ultrasound assessment of fetal age. J Ultrasound Med 1994; 13:52337.

35. Anderson PE, Hauge M, Bang J, et al. Dyssegmental dysplasia in sibling. Prenatal ultrasonic diagnosis. Skeletal Radiol 1988; 17:29.

36. Izquierdo LA, Kushnir O, Asse J, et al. Antenatal ultrasonic diagnosis of dyssegmental dysplasia: A case report. Prenat Diagn 1990; 10:587.

37. Lipson M, Waskey J, Rice J, et al. Prenatal diagnosis of asphyxiating thoracic dysplasia. Am J Med Genet 1984; 8:273.

38. Skiptunas SM, Weiner S. Early prenatal diagnosis of asphyxiating thoracic dysplasia (Jeune's syndrome). Value of in fetal thoracic measurements. J Ultrasound Med 1987; 6:41.

39. Kozlowski K, Masel J. Asphyxiating thoracic dystrophy without respiratory distress. A report of 2 cases of the latent form. Pediatr Radiol 1976; 5:30.

40. Qureshi F, Jacques SM, Evans MI, et el. Skeletal histopathology in fetuses with chondroectodermal dysplasia (Ellis van Creveld syndrome). Am J Med Genet 1993; 45:471.

41. Hastabacka J, De la Chappelle A, Mahtani MM, et al. The diastrophic dysplasia gene encodes a novel sulphate transporter: Positional cloning by fine structure linkage disequilibrium mapping. Cell 1994; 78:1073–1087.

42. Babcosk C, Filly RA. Diastrophic dysplasia. The Fetus 1993; 3:7564. 19–22.

43. Horton WA, Rimoin DL, Lachman RS, et al. The phenotypic variability of diastrophic dysplasia. J Paedr 1978; 93:609.

44. Karmes PS, Day D, Berry SA, et al. Jarcho–Levin syndrome: four new cases and classification of subtypes. Am J Med Genet 1991; 40:264.

45. Romero R, Ghidini A, Eswara MS, et al. Prenatal findings in a case of spondylocostal dysplasia type I (Jarcho–Levin syndrome). Obstet Gynecol 1988; 71:988.

46. Hammer LH, Fabbri EL, Browne PC. Prenatal diagnosis of cleido cranial dysostosis. Obstet Gynecol 1994; 83:856.

47. Yarkoni S, Schmidt W, Jeanty P, et al. Clavicle measurements; A new biometric parameter for fetal evaluation. J Ultrasound Med 1985; 4:467.

48. Whitley CB, Burke BA, Granroth G, Gorlin RJ. De la Chappelle dysplasia. Am J Med Genet 1986; 25:29–39.

49. Kozlowski K, Sillence D, Cortis-Jones R. Osborn boomerang dysplasia. Br J Radiol 1989; 58:369–371.

50. Duff P, Harlass FE, Milligan DA. Prenatal diagnosis of chondrodysplasia punctata by sonography. Obstet Gynecol 1990; 76:497.

51. Sastrowijoto SH, Vandenberghe K, Moerman P, et al. Prenatal ultrasound diagnosis of rhizomelic chondrodysplasia punctata in a primigravida. Prenat Diagn 1994; 14:770–776.

52. Gendall PW, Baird CE, Beecroft DMO. Rhizomelic chondrodysplasia punctata: Early recognition with antenatal ultrasonography. J Clin Ultrasound 1994; 22:271.

53. Cordone M, Lituania M, Bocchino G, et al. Ultrasonographic features in a case of heterozygous achondroplasia at 25 weeks' gestation. Prenat Diagn 1993; 13:395.

54. Pryde PG, Bawle E, Brandt F, et al. Prenatal diagnosis of non-rhizomelic chondrodysplasia punctata (Conradi Hunerman). Am J Med Genet 1993; 47:426.

55. Sherer DM, Glatz JC, Allen TA, et al. Prenatal sonographic diagnosis of non rhizomelic chondrodysplasia punctata. Obstet Gynecol 1994; 83:858.

56. Mostello D, Heochstetter L, Bendon RW, et al. Prenatal diagnosis of recurrent Larsen syndrome: Further definition of a lethal variant. Prenat Diagn 1991; 11:215.

57. Rochelson B, Petrikovsky B, Shmoys S. Prenatal diagnosis and obstetric management of Larsen syndrome. Obstet Gynecol 199; 81:845.

58. Evans MI, Zador IE, Qureshi F, et al. UItrasonographic prenatal diagnosis and fetal pathology of Langer mesomelic dwarfism. Am J Med Genet 1988; 31:915.

59. Spirt BA, Oliphant M, Gottlieb R, et al. Prenatal sonographic evaluation of short limb dysplasia: an algorithmic approach. Radiographics 1990; 10(2):217–236.

60. Firth HV, Boyd PA, Chamberlain P, et al. Severe limb abnormalities after chorionic villus sampling at 56–66 days gestation. Lancet 1991; 377:762.

61. Mastroiacovo P, Cavalcanti L. Limb reduction defects and chorionic villus sampling. Lancet 1991; 337:1091.

62. Shepard TH, Kapur RP, Fantel AG. Limb reduction defects and chorionic villus sampling. Lancet 1991; 337:1092.

63. Hsieh FH, Chen D, Tseng LH, et al. Limb reduction defects and chorionic villus sampling. Lancet 1991; 337:1091–2.

64. Burton BK, Schultz CJ, Burd LI. Limb anomalies associated with chorionic villus sampling. Obstet Gynecol 1992; 79:726.

65. Firth HV, Chamberlain PF, MacKenzie, et al. Analysis of limb reduction defects in babies exposed to chorionic villus sampling. Lancet 1994; 343:1069.

66. Dordoni D, Freeman PC. Sirenomelia sequence. The Fetus 1991; 1:7553. 1–3.

67. Honda N, Shimokawa H, Yamaguchi Y, et al. Antenatal diagnosis of sirenomelia (sympus apus). J Clin Ultrasound 1988; 16:675.

68. Chenoweth CK, Kellog SSJ, Abu-Yosef MM. Antenatal sonography diagnosis of sirenomelia. J Clin Ultrasound 1991; 19:167.

69. Sirtori M, Gidini A, Romero R, et al. Prenatal diagnosis of sirenomelia. J Ultrasound Med 1989; 8:83.

70. Sepulveda W, Romero R, Pryde PG, et al. Prenatal diagnosis of sirenomelus with colour Doppler ultrasonography. Am J Obstet Gynecol 1994; 170:1377.

71. Rodini ES, Richieri-Costa A. EEC syndrome: Report of 20 new patients, clinical and genetic considerations. Am J Med Genet 1989; 37:42.

72. Luthy DA, Hall JG, Graham CB, et al. Prenatal diagnosis of thrombocytopaenia with absent radii. Clin Genet 1979; 15:495.

73. Filkins K, Russo J, Bilinki I, et al. Prenatal diagnosis of thrombocytopaenia absent radius syndrome using ultrasound and fetoscopy. Prenat Diagn 1984; 4:139.

74. Auerbach AD, Sagi M, Adler B. Fanconi anaemia; Prenatal diagnosis in 30 fetuses at risk. Pediatrics 1985; 76:794.

75. Helton K, Goncalves L, Jeanty P. Heart–hand syndrome type I. The Fetus 1993; 3:7552: 125.

76. Meizner I, Bar Ziv J, Barki Y, et al. Prenatal ultrasonic diagnosis of radial-ray aplasia and renal anomaly. Prenat Diagn 1986; 6:223.

77. Banker BQ. Neuropathologic aspects of an arthrogryposis multiplex congenita. Clin Orthop 1985; 194:30.

78. Baty BJ, Cubberley D, Morris C, et al. Prenatal diagnosis of distal arthrogryposis. Am J Med Genet 1988; 29:501.

79. Benacerraf BR, Greene MF, Barass VA. Prenatal sonographic diagnosis of congenital hemivertebrae. J Ultrasound Med 1986; 5:257–259.

80. Zelop CM, Pretorius DH, Benacerraf BR. Fetal hemivertebrae: Associated anomalies, significance, and outcome. Obstet Gynecol 1993; 81:412.

81. Twickler D, Budorik N, Pretorius D, et al. Caudal regression versus sirenomelia: sonographic clues. J Ultrasound Med 1993; 12:323.

CHAPTER 13

Urinary tract abnormalities

Peter Twining

Introduction

Abnormalities of the urinary tract are relatively common, accounting for approximately 20% of all fetal malformations[1]. The exact incidence of prenatally detected urinary tract anomalies is difficult to determine and varies from centre to centre and with the timing of the ultrasound examination.[2-11] Table 13.1

Table 13.1
Incidence of prenatally detected uropathies

Reference	Year	Centre	Incidence
2	1984	Lund, Sweden	1:1200
3	1986	Malmo, Sweden	1:330
4	1988	Nottingham, UK	1:935
5	1989	Leeds, UK	1:600
6	*1989	Stoke-on-Trent, UK	1:154
7	1990	Hameenlinna, Finland	1:208
8	1993	Northern Region, UK	1:333
9	1994	Westmead, Australia	1:200
10	*1995	Auckland, New Zealand	1:70
11	1998	Nottingham, UK	1:364

*Studies based on ultrasound scanning at 28 weeks' gestation.
Reproduced with permission from Thomas DFM. Prenatally detected uropathies: Epidemiological considerations. Br J Urol 1998;81:Supplement 2, 8–12.

outlines the incidence of prenatally detected urinary tract anomalies from various series. Early series reported relatively low incidences of urinary tract anomalies (approximately 1 in 1000 live births)[2,4,5] but this figure has increased in the early 1990s to approximately 1 in 200 to 300 live births. This is explained partly by an improvement in resolution of ultrasound medicines and also by the introduction of routine screening at 18 to 20 weeks' gestation.[7,9,11] It is also seen that scanning in the third trimester detects a higher incidence of urinary tract abnormalities.[6,10]

Although advances in ultrasound machine technology has meant that the diagnosis of renal disease is more accurate,[12,13] there remains a significant false-positive rate which ranges between 39 and 52%.[6,8,14,15] This high false-positive rate is mainly due to the detection of mild hydronephrosis which is subsequently found to be normal after birth.[8,14,15] This problem is still unresolved and to date there is no consensus on the degree of dilatation on the antenatal ultrasound that should prompt full postnatal investigation.[11]

The majority of renal abnormalities are not life threatening. However, severe bilateral renal abnormalities account for 10%

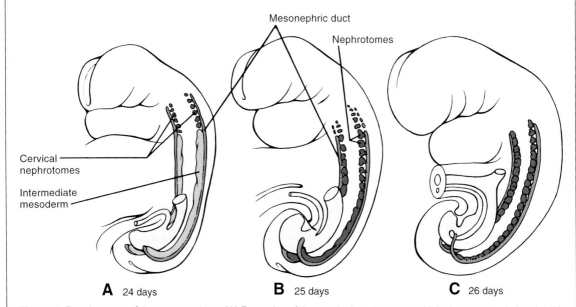

Fig. 13.1 Development of the mesonephros. (A) Formation of the cervical nephrotones which degenerate during the 4th week. (B) Mesonephros forms in cranial coronal sequence. (C) The mesonephros is fully formed by approximately 6 weeks. (Reproduced from Larsen[20] with permission.)

of all terminations for lethal fetal abnormalities.[8]

The assessment and management of bilateral renal abnormalities such as bilateral hydronephrosis secondary to posterior urethral valves have provoked considerable debate within the literature,[5,16,17] and the place of intra-uterine intervention has still to be completely clarified.[18,19]

The detection and management of prenatally detected urinary tract anomalies are therefore still open to discussion and it is the increasing move towards a multidisciplinary approach with obstetricians, radiologists and paediatricians in close communication which will improve the management of such fetuses.[4]

Embryology

The urinary and genital tracts arise from the intermediate mesoderm on either side of the dorsal body wall. This intermediate mesoderm forms three successive structures of increasingly advanced design – the pronephros, mesonephros and metanephros.[20] The pronephros is made up of transitory, non-functional tissue in the cervical region which regresses during the 4th week. As the pronephros regresses the mesonephros forms as two elongated swellings located on either side of the vertebral column extending from the upper thoracic region to the lumbar region. The mesonephros forms rudimentary renal tissue and mesonephric ducts connect this mesonephros to the cloaca (Fig. 13.1). The mesonephros produces small amounts of urine between about 6 and 10 weeks and then regresses.[20]

The definitive kidneys arise from the metanephros which is induced to form from the intermediate mesoderm in the sacral region by the ureteric bud which grows out from the distal mesonephric duct at the end of the 4th week (Fig. 13.2).[21] The metanephros forms the nephrons, whilst the ureteric bud forms the collecting tubules, calyces, renal pelvis and ureter. During the 10th week the

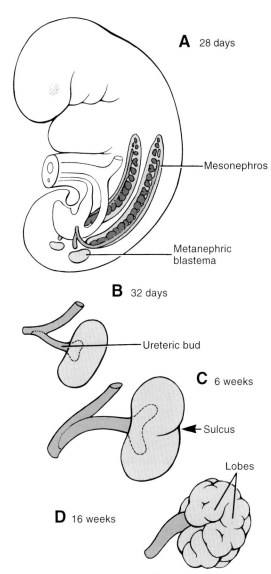

Fig. 13.2 Formation of the definitive kidney. (A) The metanephric blastema develops on each side of the body early in the 5th week. (B) The ureteric bud grows out to the metanephric blastema. (C) The ureteric bud bifurcates to produce superior and inferior lobes in the metanephros. (D) Additional lobules form during the next 10 weeks in response to further bifurcation of the ureteric buds. (Reproduced from Larsen[20] with permission.)

nephrons connect to the collecting ducts and the metanephros becomes functional.[20] Lack of communication between the nephrons and collecting ducts results in cystic renal disease. Between the 6th and 9th weeks the kidneys ascend to the lumbar region

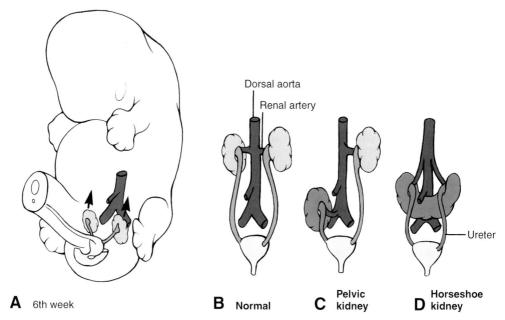

A 6th week   **B** Normal   **C** Pelvic kidney   **D** Horseshoe kidney

Fig. 13.3 Normal and abnormal ascent of the kidneys. (A) The metanephros ascends from the sacral region to the definitive lumbar position between the 6th and 9th weeks. (B) Normal. (C) A kidney may fail to ascend resulting in a pelvic kidney. (D) If the inferior poles make contact and fuse, the result is a horseshoe kidney. (Reproduced from Larsen[20] with permission.)

(Fig. 13.3). Failure of the kidney to ascend results in a pelvic kidney and fusion of the inferior poles of the metanephros produces a horseshoe kidney (Fig. 13.3).

The bladder forms from the anterior part of the cloaca which is separated from the posterior rectum by the urorectal septum (Fig. 13.4). Inferior to the definitive bladder is the urogenital sinus. In males the urogenital sinus becomes the penile urethra and in females the vestibule of the vagina (Fig. 13.4). Between the 4th and 6th week the ureters connect to the trigone of the bladder.

The genital system arises from the genital ridges which are situated just medial to the developing mesonephros.[20] These genital ridges are formed from primordial germ cells which migrate from the yolk sac during the 4th week. During the 6th week the primitive gonads start to develop (Fig. 13.5) and it is during the 8th week that male-female differentiation occurs. In the male the primitive gonads form the testes and the mesonephric duct the vas deferens. In the female the primitive gonad forms the ovary and the mesonephric duct regresses. A

paramesonephric duct forms which gives rise to the fallopian tubes, uterus and superior part of the vagina.

The early development of the external genitalia is similar in males and females. In the 5th week a pair of swellings called the cloacal folds develop on either side of the cloacal membrane. These folds meet anteriorly to form the genital tubercle. During the 7th week the cloacal folds meet posteriorly to form the urogenital fold anteriorly and the anal fold posteriorly.[20] The urogenital membrane breaks down late in the 7th week and this will become the vestibule of the vagina in the female and the urethra in the male (Fig. 13.6). The appearance of the external genitalia is similar up to the 12th week. After this time, in males the urogenital fold and genital tubercle lengthen to form the penis and there is fusion of the urogenital membrane to form the urethra. In females the genital tubercle bends inferiorly to form the clitoris and the urogenital sinus becomes the vestibule of the vagina.[21]

Therefore, by the end of the 10th week the

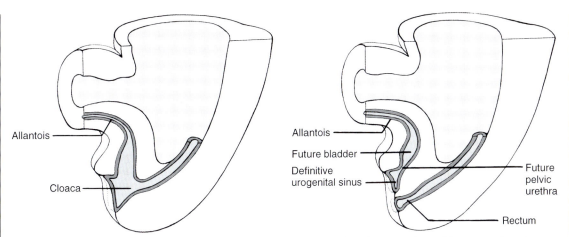

Fig. 13.4 Formation of the bladder and rectum. The bladder and rectum form from the cloaca. The urorectal septum separates the bladder from the rectum. The urogenital sinus becomes the penile urethra in the male and the vestibule of the vagina in the female. (Reproduced from Larsen[20] with permission.)

kidneys and bladder have formed and urine production has commenced. In addition, sex differentiation has occurred but formation of the external genitalia is not complete until after the 14th week.

Normal appearances and variants

The fetal kidneys and bladder can be detected as early as 9 weeks' gestation using transvaginal sonography.[22] At 12 weeks gestation the kidneys appear as bilateral hyperechoic structures in the paravertebral regions (Fig. 13.7). The renal pelves can often be seen as central echo poor regions medially. The bladder is situated in the pelvis as a well defined rounded echo free area (Fig. 13.8). Its position can be confirmed by using colour flow Doppler to demonstrate both umbilical arteries separating around the bladder (Fig. 13.9).

At 18 to 20 weeks' gestation and scanning in the coronal or sagittal plane the kidneys can be clearly seen as oval masses lateral to the psoas muscles and inferior to the adrenal glands. The adrenal glands characteristically appear as triangular hypoechoic shadows which outline the upper poles of the kidneys

(Figs 13.10, 13.11). Scanning in the transverse plane reveals the kidneys as rounded paravertebral structures and the renal pelves as echo free structures situated medial to the kidney (Fig. 13.12). Measurements of the renal pelvis are best carried out in the anteroposterior direction with the fetus either spine up or spine lowermost (Fig. 13.13). The upper limit of normal is 4 mm up to 33 weeks' gestation and 7 mm from 33 weeks' gestation to term.[23] Normal ranges for renal size have also been reported. These include renal length, anteroposterior diameters and renal circumference measurements.

Using high resolution scanners the renal pyramids are often visualized as hypoechoic areas within the renal cortex (Fig. 13.14). These should not be mistaken for renal cysts.

The ureters are not normally visualized and so demonstration of the ureters should raise the possibility of renal obstruction or reflux.

As in the first trimester the bladder is demonstrated as a rounded echo free structure within the pelvis and the rectum may be seen posteriorly (Fig. 13.15). The bladder wall can often be seen distinct from the surrounding bowel; however, measurements of bladder wall thickness are best made at the level of the umbilical artery

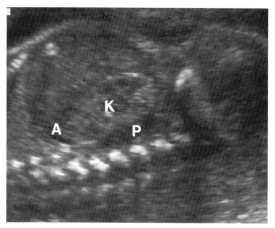

Fig. 13.11 Sagittal scan of the normal kidney. (A – adrenal, K – kidney, P – psoas muscle).

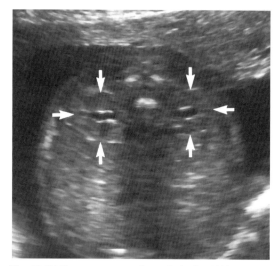

Fig. 13.12 Transverse scan through the fetal kidneys. Both kidneys are seen in a paravertebral location and are outlined by the arrows. Both renal pelves are seen centrally.

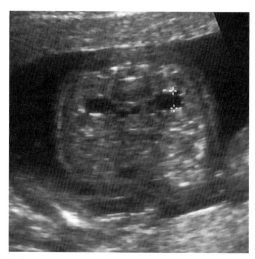

Fig. 13.13 Renal pelvic diameter measurement. The anteroposterior diameter of the renal pelves are best measured with the spine uppermost. The measurement is made as shown by the callipers.

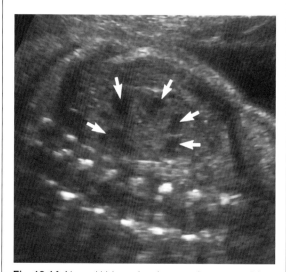

Fig. 13.14 Normal kidney showing prominent pyramids (arrows point to pyramids).

search for the kidney in an ectopic position such as the fetal pelvis. When no other kidney is seen a diagnosis of unilateral renal agenesis should be considered. Bilateral renal agenesis is usually associated with severe oligohydramnios, particularly after 17 weeks' gestation. In the situation where a renal abnormality is seen then it is also essential that the contralateral kidney is examined to confirm or exclude bilateral renal disease.

The size and echogenicity of both kidneys should be assessed.

Kidneys that show increased echogenicity may be normal but also raise the possibility of cystic renal disease, particularly if the kidneys are enlarged.

The presence of macroscopic cysts usually indicates a multicystic kidney; however, care should always be taken to ensure that the cysts do not communicate, as occasionally a multicystic kidney with a large central cyst and smaller peripheral cysts can be mistaken for hydronephrosis. Cysts may also be single

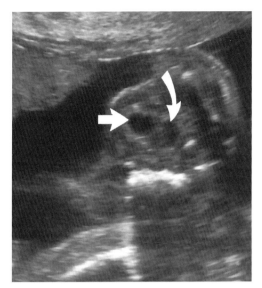

Fig. 13.15 Normal bladder. Transverse scan through the fetal pelvis showing bladder and rectum. (Straight arrow – bladder, curved arrow – rectum).

and as such should be considered simple renal cysts.

The collecting systems of both kidneys should be assessed not only for size but also for number. The presence of two distinct collecting systems should always raise the possibility of a duplex kidney and prompt an examination of the fetal bladder looking for a ureterocoele.

Dilatation of the collecting system should always raise the possibility of an obstruction to the kidney. The level of the obstruction can usually be suggested by the degree of dilatation of renal pelvis, ureter and bladder. Assessment of the echogenicity of renal cortex and the presence or absence of renal cysts should also be carried out when there is dilatation of the collecting system in order to assess the possibility of secondary renal dysplasia.

The bladder

Examination of the fetal bladder includes assessment of bladder size and, if enlarged, visualization of the posterior urethra which, if dilated, suggests a bladder outlet obstruction. Bladder wall thickness can be assessed at the level of the umbilical artery

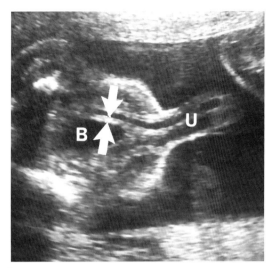

A

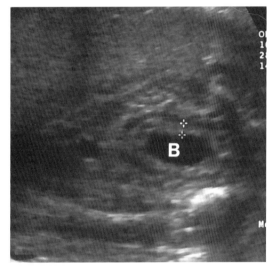

B

Fig. 13.16 Measurement of bladder wall thickness. (A) Transverse scan through fetal pelvis showing the level at which the bladder wall is measured. Bladder wall is best measured at the point where the umbilical artery separates around the bladder. (B – bladder, arrows show bladder wall thickness, U – umbilical cord). (B) A thick-walled bladder. The measurement of the bladder wall thickness was 2.7 mm. The upper limit of normal is 2 mm.

(Fig. 13.16). The presence or absence of ureterocoeles should also be established, particularly in the presence of a duplex kidney. Bladder filling and emptying can normally be demonstrated over a period of 30 to 40 minutes.

Liquor volume

Liquor volume can be assessed in a number of ways. Most workers initially use a subjective assessment and then move on to more objective criteria if there appears to be too much or too little liquor. The best technique would appear to be the amniotic fluid index whereby measurements are made in the four quadrants of the uterus and the mean value obtained.[24] The normal range is demonstrated in Figure 13.17. Severe oligohydramnios in the second trimester usually has a poor outcome and in the absence of ruptured membranes and severe growth retardation usually indicates severe bilateral renal disease.

Abnormalities of the urinary tract

RENAL AGENESIS

Unilateral renal agenesis has an incidence of 1 in 1000 live births[25] and bilateral renal agenesis 1 in 4000.[26] Most cases of renal agenesis are sporadic; however, a number of familial cases have been reported so that various patterns of inheritance have been postulated including autosomal recessive,

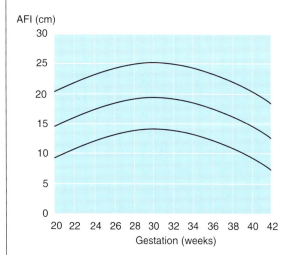

Fig. 13.17 Graph showing the normal range for amniotic fluid index. (Reproduced with permission from Ninosu[24].)

autosomal dominant and X-linked recessive.[27–29]

Bilateral renal agenesis is always associated with severe oligohydramnios producing the typical Potter's syndrome of low set ears, wide set eyes, micrognathia, limb contractures, talipes and pulmonary hypoplasia.[30] The outcome is uniformly lethal secondary to the severe pulmonary hypoplasia. Unilateral renal agenesis has a good outcome with compensatory hypertrophy of the opposite kidney.

Renal agenesis is probably caused by absence of inductive signals from the ureteric bud so that the metanephros fails to develop and so the definitive kidney does not form.[20] (See Embryology section).

Sonographic appearances

Bilateral renal agenesis is associated with oligohydramnios after 17 weeks' gestation. However, prior to this the liquor volume may be normal.[26] It should be noted therefore that normal liquor volume prior to 17 weeks' gestation does not exclude renal agenesis.

The diagnosis rests on demonstration of absence of both kidneys and the bladder. This can be difficult in the setting of severe oligohydramnios as the fetus is often curled up deep in the pelvis.

When the fetus is in a cephalic presentation it is often possible to demonstrate the renal fossae using transabdominal scanning. In this way the psoas muscles are visualized and the adrenal glands flatten to fill in the space left by the absent kidneys, the so-called 'lying down' adrenal sign[31] (Fig. 13.18). This can be confirmed using colour flow Doppler which demonstrates absence of both renal arteries[32] (Fig. 13.19). Colour flow Doppler is also of value in localizing the bladder and demonstrating its absence in renal agenesis (Fig. 13.20).

When the fetus is in a breech presentation the lower abdomen usually lies deep within the maternal pelvis. In this situation transvaginal scanning is extremely useful as the higher frequency transducer and close proximity to the fetus compensate for the lack of liquor and difficult fetal position.[33,34]

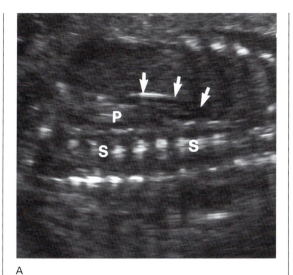

A

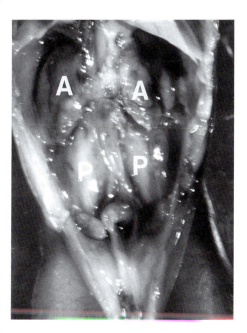

B

Fig. 13.18 Renal agenesis. (A) Coronal scan through a renal fossa showing absence of the kidney and adrenal gland flattened onto the psoas muscle (S – spine, P – psoas muscle, arrows outline flattened adrenal gland). (B) Post-mortem photograph of a fetus with renal agenesis (A – adrenal glands, P – psoas muscles).

Other techniques that have been employed to assess and diagnose renal agenesis include intra-amniotic infusion of fluid[35] and also intraperitoneal fluid infusion.[36] In addition, umbilical artery Doppler studies can be useful to exclude severe intra-uterine growth retardation.[37]

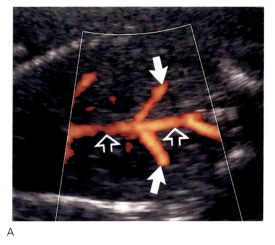

A

B

Fig. 13.19 Colour flow Doppler assessment of renal agenesis. (A) Normal appearances. Open arrows outline aorta, closed arrows point to both renal arteries. (B) Renal agenesis. There is absence of the renal arteries on colour flow Doppler.

Unilateral renal agenesis can be easy to miss unless a very careful assessment is made of each kidney at routine scanning. When an absent kidney is diagnosed a careful assessment should be made of the fetal pelvis to exclude a pelvic kidney and also crossed renal ectopia.[38] Colour flow can also be used to confirm absence of the affected renal artery (Fig. 13.21).

Differential diagnosis

Bilateral renal agenesis presents as severe second trimester oligohydramnios and so the

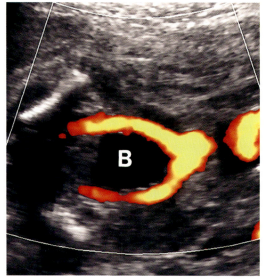

A

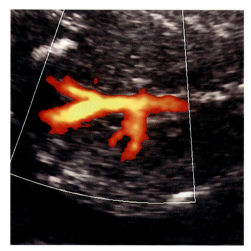

Fig. 13.21 Unilateral renal agenesis. Colour flow Doppler image showing a single renal artery indicating unilateral renal agenesis.

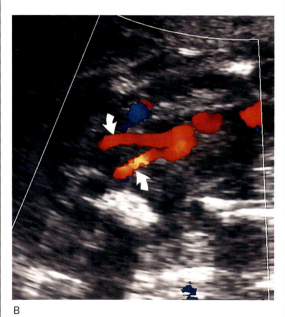

B

Fig. 13.20 Colour flow Doppler assessment of bladder position. (A) Normal appearances. Both umbilical arteries separate around the bladder (B). (B) Renal agenesis. Both umbilical arteries are seen to separate; however, there is absence of the bladder (curved arrows point to umbilical arteries).

differential diagnosis includes other causes of severe bilateral renal disease such as severe bladder outlet obstruction and severe cystic renal disease such as multicystic kidneys or infantile polycystic kidneys. The other two main possibilities are severe early growth retardation which may be secondary to uteroplacental insufficiency or chromosomal disease such as triploidy and spontaneous rupture of the membranes.

Meticulous scanning using both transabdominal and transvaginal scanning will usually confirm absence of the kidneys in renal agenesis and demonstrate a dilated bladder and kidneys in bladder outlet obstruction. Similarly, cystic renal disease can normally be clearly demonstrated by a careful scanning technique. Both kidneys are present in severe growth retardation and small abdominal measurements together with abnormal umbilical artery Doppler waveforms should help to make the diagnosis. The presence of abnormalities should always raise the possibility of chromosomal disease, particularly triploidy.

In spontaneous premature rupture of the membranes there is usually a clinical history; however, occasionally it can be relatively silent and require specific questioning. In addition, both kidneys and the bladder should be demonstrated on scan.

Associated abnormalities

There are a number of syndromes associated with bilateral renal disease and these are outlined in Table 13.2.

Associated abnormalities are seen in over

Table 13.2
Syndromes associated with renal malformations

	Clinical findings
Renal agenesis	
Fraser syndrome	Cryptophthalmos, syndactyly fingers and toes, large hyperechogenic lungs
Cystic renal disease	
Meckel–Gruber syndrome	Large echogenic kidneys, polydactyly encephalocoele
Pataus syndrome (trisomy 13)	Large echogenic kidneys, polydactyly holoprosencephaly, facial clefting
Beckwith–Wiedemann syndrome	Large echogenic kidneys, macrosomia hepatosplenomegaly, macroglossia, omphalocoele
Jeune's syndrome	Echogenic kidneys, dwarfism, small thorax
Short rib polydactyly syndrome (Majewski type)	Large echogenic kidneys, dwarfism, polydactyly, small thorax
Lawrence–Moon–Biedl syndrome (Bardet–Biedl syndrome)	Renal cysts, retinal dystrophy, polydactyly, mental deficiency, hypogonadism
Zellweger syndrome	Cystic kidneys, hypotonicity, limb contractures, congenital cataracts, hypoplastic corpus callosum, heterotopias

50% of cases and the commonest are cardiac and musculoskeletal. Cardiac anomalies occur in 14% of fetuses and include ventricular septal defects, Fallot tetralogy, hypoplastic left heart, transposition of the great vessels and coarctation of the aorta.[29] The musculoskeletal anomalies include sirenomelia (Fig. 13.22), sacral agenesis, radial aplasia and digital anomalies. Neural tube defects, hydrocephalus, microcephaly, holoprosencephaly and gastrointestinal anomalies such as anal atresia, duodenal atresia and omphalocoele may also be seen.[29] Occasionally diaphragmatic hernia and facial clefting are also associated.[30]

Outcome

In bilateral renal agenesis the outcome is uniformly fatal with most babies succumbing in the neonatal period from severe pulmonary hypoplasia. Unilateral renal agenesis has a good outcome with normal life expectancy.

Recurrence risk

The overall recurrence risk is approximately 3%;[28] however, in familial cases the risk is much higher and the author has seen one couple with four consecutive fetuses with bilateral renal agenesis.

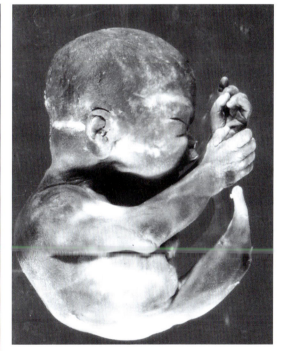

Fig. 13.22 Sirenomelia. There is renal agenesis, gastrointestinal abnormalities and fusion of the lower limbs to produce a single lower limb.

CYSTIC RENAL DISEASE

Cystic renal disease covers a wide range of conditions with differing antenatal appearances and modes of inheritance. The

Table 13.3
Potter classification of cystic renal disease

Type I	Autosomal recessive (infantile) polycystic renal disease
Type II	Multicystic renal dysplasia
Type III	Autosomal dominant (adult) polycystic renal disease
Type IV	Obstructive cystic dysplasia

Table 13.4
Manifestations of autosomal recessive infantile polycystic renal disease according to the subclassification of Blythe and Ockenden

Type	Proportion of dilated renal tubules (%)	Extent of portal fibrosis	Lifespan
Perinatal	90	Minimal	Hours
Neonatal	60	Mild	Months
Infantile	20	Moderate	10 years
Juvenile	<10	Gross	50 years

Reproduced from Deget F, Rudnik-Schoneborn, Zerres K. Course of autosomal recessive polycystic kidney disease in siblings: a clinical comparison of twenty sibships. Clin Genet 1995;47:248–253.

Potter classification, although incomplete, does cover the most important conditions (Table 13.3) and will be used to describe cystic renal disease in this chapter.

Autosomal recessive (infantile) polycystic renal disease (Potter type I cystic disease)

Infantile polycystic renal disease is an autosomal recessive condition which has an incidence of approximately 1 in 40 to 50 000 live births.[39,40] The condition presents as symmetrically enlarged kidneys. Pathologically the renal enlargement is produced by cystic dilatations of the collecting tubules which are arranged in a radial manner throughout the renal parenchyma (Fig. 13.23). Associated with the renal cystic change is a degree of hepatic portal and interlobular fibrosis and also biliary duct hyperplasia.[39,41]

Clinically the disease can be divided into four different subtypes distinguished by

clinical symptoms and pathological findings[42] (Table 13.4). In general, the more severe the renal cystic disease appears the less severe is the hepatic fibrosis, but the prognosis is poor. The best survival occurs when the renal disease is minimal and the hepatic fibrosis severe. In practice, it is the most severe perinatal form that is detected antenatally.

Recent genetic studies have revealed that the gene for infantile polycystic renal disease is located on chromosome 6p.[43]

Sonographic appearances

The classical sonographic appearances are those of enlarged kidneys which show increased echogenicity associated with oligohydramnios[44,45] (Fig. 13.24). These sonographic appearances, however, may not be demonstrable until 24 weeks' gestation and a number of cases have been described where the ultrasound appearances were normal at 16 to 19 weeks' gestation.[46–48] In view of this it is probably true to say that the condition cannot be excluded at 18 to 20 weeks' gestation even if the fetal kidneys appear normal. The parents therefore should be carefully counselled as to the possible risks of the condition appearing later in pregnancy and further follow-up scans arranged.

Although prenatal diagnosis has certain pitfalls in this condition careful attention to detail can provide clues to the diagnosis. There will almost certainly be a family

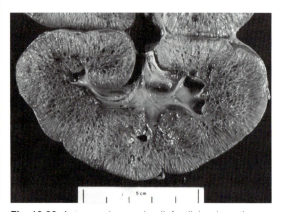

Fig. 13.23 Autosomal recessive (infantile) polycystic kidney disease. Section through an affected kidney showing cystic dilatations of the collecting tubules arranged in a radial manner throughout the renal parenchyma.

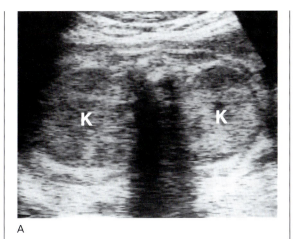

A

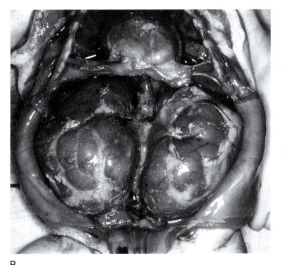

B

Fig. 13.24 Autosomal recessive (infantile) polycystic kidney disease. (A) Transverse scan through the fetal abdomen showing enlarged echogenic kidneys. There is associated oligohydramnios (K – kidney). (B) Post-mortem photograph of same fetus showing massively enlarged kidneys.

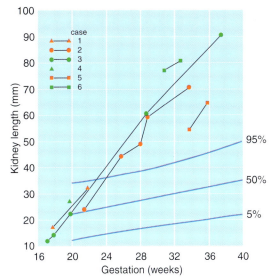

Fig. 13.25 Renal length versus gestational age in six cases of autosomal recessive polycystic kidney disease. Early in gestation renal size may be normal, but the kidneys typically become enlarged later in gestation. (Adapted from Zerres[48].)

history of the condition and so a high index of suspicion. In addition, accurate measurement of anteroposterior, transverse and longitudinal diameters are essential as although in some cases measurements may be normal prior to 24 weeks (Fig. 13.25), increased measurements have been reported as early as 12 weeks' gestation.[49] The other clue to the diagnosis which may be visible as early as 12 weeks' gestation is hyperechogenicity or 'too good looking kidneys' as described by Bronshtein et al,[49] where the kidneys are too easy to see using transvaginal scanning in the first trimester of pregnancy. In the situation where either of these signs are present repeat scanning after 2 weeks may well reveal a significant increase in renal size as the growth profile of affected kidneys is significantly greater than that of normal kidneys (Fig. 13.25).

Although most affected kidneys are bilaterally symmetrically enlarged there have been case reports where one affected kidney is of normal size and the contralateral kidney markedly enlarged.[50]

Differential diagnosis

Adult polycystic renal disease is the main differential diagnosis which can have similar appearances. Other conditions where cystic renal disease is a feature include Meckel–Gruber syndrome, Lawrence–Moon–Biedl syndrome, Jeune's syndrome, Beckwith–Wiedemann syndrome and occasionally chromosomal disease, particularly trisomy 13 (Table 13.5). Careful attention to associated anomalies detectable by ultrasound should raise the possibility of

Table 13.5
Echogenic kidneys – antenatal ultrasound appearances and clinical findings

Condition	Renal size	Cysts present	Hydro-nephrosis	Liquor volume	Cysts in parents' kidneys	Family history	Associated findings
Infantile polycystic kidneys	Large	No	No	Reduced	No	Yes in sibling	Hepatic fibrosis in later life
Adult polycystic kidney disease	Large	Sometimes	No	Normal	Yes >20 years age	Yes in parent	Occasionally cysts in parents' liver, spleen
Obstructive cystic dysplasia	Small	Often	Yes	Depends on degree of renal obstruction	No	No	Hydronephrosis usually urethral obstruction
Finnish type nephrotic syndrome	Large	No	No	Normal	No	Yes in sibling	Raised serum AFP
Beckwith–Wiedemann syndrome	Large	No	No	Normal or increased	No	Occasionally	Macrosomia, large liver, large spleen, macroglossia, omphalocoele
Meckel–Gruber syndrome	Large	Sometimes	No	Reduced	No	Yes in sibling	Polydactyly, encephalocoele
Trisomy 13	Large	Sometimes	No	Normal	No	No	Facial clefting, holoprosencephaly, cardiac defects, polydactyly
Cytomegalovirus infection	Large	No	No	Normal	No	No	Microcephaly, hydrocephaly, intracranial calcification, large liver and spleen, hydrops
Renal vein thrombosis	Large – usually unilateral	No	No	Normal	No	No	Maternal diabetes, maternal pyelonephritis
Normal	Normal	No	No	Normal	No	No	

these conditions. However, this may be very difficult in the presence of severe oligohydramnios. Other much rarer conditions which should also be considered are congenital nephrotic syndrome, renal vein thrombosis and infection with cytomegalovirus (see Echogenic kidneys).

Associated abnormalities

The main associated abnormality is hepatic fibrosis and the severity of the fibrosis is inversely related to the severity of the renal disease (Table 13.4).

Outcome

The outcome depends on the severity of the renal disease with the poorest outcome seen in the perinatal type where most babies die in the neonatal period. With decreasing severity of renal involvement the outcome is progressively better (Table 13.4). Long term complications include hypertension, urinary tract infection and portal hypertension.[39]

Recurrence risk

The autosomal recessive inheritance indicates a 25% risk of recurrence.

Multicystic renal dysplasia (Potter type II)

Multicystic renal dysplasia was first diagnosed antenatally using ultrasound in 1970.[51] It is the commonest form of cystic disease of the kidney in childhood[52] with an incidence of 1 in 3000 live births.[53] It is

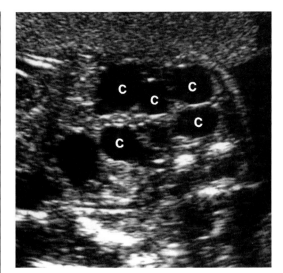

Fig. 13.26 Multicystic dysplastic kidney. Transverse scan through a multicystic dysplastic kidney showing multiple cysts (C – cyst).

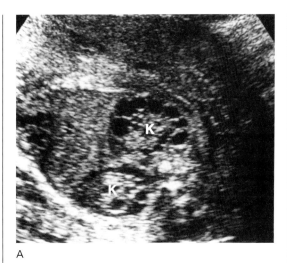

A

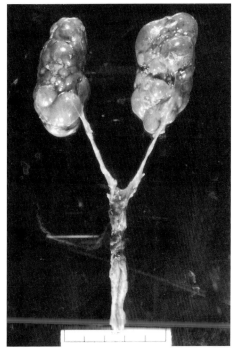

B

Fig. 13.27 Bilateral multicystic dysplastic kidneys. (A) Coronal scan through a fetus with bilateral multicystic kidneys. Both kidneys show multiple peripheral cysts with a dense central stroma. Note severe oligohydramnios (K – kidneys). (B) Post-mortem specimen showing bilateral multicystic kidneys. There are multiple cysts of varying sizes.

commoner in boys[53,54] and is usually unilateral, but may be bilateral in up to 23% of cases. It is quoted as the commonest cause of a urological abdominal mass in a neonate but in practice may only be palpable clinically in 37% of babies.[53]

The abnormality is thought to arise from failed co-ordination and development of the metanephros and the branching ureteric bud. The result is the development of multiple smooth non-functioning, non-communicating cysts of variable size and number (Fig. 13.26). This is associated with atresia of the ureter and renal pelvis and the renal artery is either very small or absent.[55] The pathological process is therefore obstruction to the kidney at a very early stage of development. The condition is usually sporadic.

Sonographic appearances

The affected kidney appears as a paraspinal mass containing multiple cysts of variable size. There is often a dense stroma within the kidney but no normal renal tissue. When the condition is bilateral, there is associated oligohydramnios and absence of urine within the bladder[56,57] (Fig. 13.27).

The diagnosis has been made as early as 12 weeks' gestation; however, the condition is easily demonstrated at 18 to 20 weeks.[22] Careful attention should always be paid to assessment of the contralateral kidney as associated abnormalities can be seen in up to 39% of cases.[58] The most common finding is vesico-ureteric reflux but more severe anomalies have also been documented, such as renal agenesis, renal hypoplasia and pelvi-ureteric junction obstructions.[53,58,59] A search should also be made for non-renal associated anomalies.

Follow-up scans are suggested in later pregnancy to assess the multicystic kidney which can increase in size,[57] and also to re-evaluate the contralateral kidney.

Although multicystic dysplasia usually affects the whole of a kidney, occasionally the condition may affect only part of the kidney (Fig. 13.28), particularly the upper

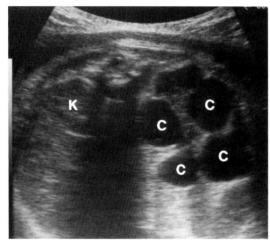

A

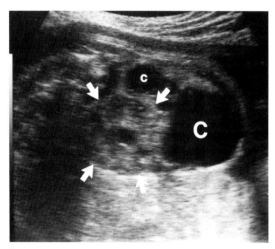

B

Fig. 13.28 Multicystic dysplastic kidney affecting only part of a kidney. (A) Multicystic kidney showing multiple cysts (C – cysts, K – normal contralateral kidney). (B) Same fetus showing a portion of normal renal tissue in the lower pole of the kidney (C – cyst, arrows outline normal renal tissue).

pole of a duplex kidney.[60] Cases have also been reported in association with crossed fused renal ectopia.[61]

Differential diagnosis

The differential diagnosis includes hydronephrosis, particularly where the multicystic kidney has a large central cyst in association with smaller peripheral cysts. High resolution scanning should resolve the problem and lack of communication between the cysts is a useful sign. In the case of bilateral disease the differential includes renal agenesis and infantile polycystic renal disease; however, the presence of well defined cysts of varying sizes should establish the diagnosis. Transvaginal scanning may be of value in this situation.[33]

The presence of associated abnormalities with bilateral disease should raise the possibility of syndromes such as Lawrence–Moon–Biedl syndrome and Zellweger syndrome (Table 13.2).

Associated anomalies

As mentioned in the previous section, associated anomalies occur in the contralateral kidney in up to 39% of cases.[58] Contralateral anomalies include renal agenesis, renal hypoplasia, pelvi-ureteric junction obstruction and vesico-ureteric reflux. Non-renal associated anomalies are commonly cardiac and gastrointestinal; however, central nervous system anomalies, cleft palate and limb anomalies may also be seen.

Outcome

When the condition is unilateral the outcome is good provided the contralateral kidney is normal. When there is a contralateral abnormality the outcome depends on the severity of the associated renal anomaly, the presence of non-renal anomalies also worsens the prognosis. Bilateral disease has a poor outcome with prolonged oligohydramnios producing severe pulmonary hypoplasia and neonatal death.

Postnatal investigations should include a neonatal renal scan. A micturating cystourethrogram with antibiotic cover can usually be carried out within the first month and a dimercaptosuccinic acid (DMSA) scan within the first 3 months.[53] Follow-up examinations should be carried out every 3 months for the first year and then every 6 months up to 3 years and then annually thereafter.

Long term follow-up of infants with unilateral disease reveals that 18% will disappear in the first year of life, 13% during the next 2 years and a further 23% during the following 2 years up to the age of 5 years.[62] Fifty-four percent of multicystic kidneys will therefore remain unchanged after 5 years and it has been estimated that it may take up to 20 years for all cases to resolve.[62]

Complications such as sepsis, hypertension and malignancy have been reported[63–65] but most large series show a low incidence of such complications.[62] Indeed only 12 cases of malignant transformation have been reported and only 6 of these were in infants or children. In all 6 cases the malignancy was a Wilms' tumour.[65,66] In view of this a conservative approach has been adopted to the management of multicystic dysplastic kidney; however, long term follow-up is indicated.[62,67]

Recurrence risk

As most cases are sporadic there is no increased risk of recurrence.

Autosomal dominant (adult) polycystic renal disease (Potter type III)

Adult polycystic renal disease is inherited as an autosomal dominant condition and has an incidence of approximately 1 in 1000 live births.[68] The condition is often asymptomatic and usually presents in the fifth decade with hypertension and end-stage renal failure.[68] It accounts for 10 to 15% of all patients requiring renal dialysis or transplantation.[55] The condition is characterized by cystic dilatation of the nephrons and in the established adult disease the kidneys are enlarged and contain multiple cysts of varying sizes.[69]

The condition does display genetic heterogenicity; however, 90% of cases are linked to the PKD1 gene on the short arm of chromosome 16.[70] A further 1 to 4% are linked to the PKD2 gene on chromosome 4[71] and as yet the PKD3 gene locus remains unmapped.[72] Prenatal diagnosis is therefore possible by gene probes from chorion sampling.[72]

Sonographic appearances

To date only 83 cases of adult type polycystic renal disease have been reported in utero or presenting in the first few months of life.[72] The typical ultrasound appearances are of enlarged echogenic kidneys similar to infantile polycystic renal disease.[73–77] (Fig. 13.29). Some authors have stressed the importance of accentuation of the cortico-medullary junction,[75] whereas others have described disappearance of the differentiation between cortex and medulla.[78] Occasionally macroscopic cysts may be seen within the echogenic kidneys as seen in the adult.[72,73,79] As in infantile polycystic renal disease the fetal kidneys may appear normal in the early second trimester and so follow-up scans are essential in the high risk group.[72,75,79] In addition a number of cases have been reported where the condition is unilateral.[80,81]

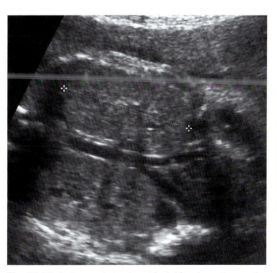

Fig. 13.29 Autosomal dominant (adult) polycystic renal disease. Coronal scan through a 24-week fetus showing bilaterally enlarged echogenic kidneys.

Liquor volume may be normal but when it is reduced the outlook is poorer with the risk of associated pulmonary hypoplasia.

Differential diagnosis

The main differential diagnosis is infantile polycystic renal disease, however this condition is much rarer. In addition, scanning the parents' kidneys is likely to reveal cysts in the case of adult polycystic renal disease[82] whereas there should be a family history in patients having a fetus with infantile polycystic renal disease. In the adult the presence of at least two renal cysts (unilateral or bilateral) in individuals at risk and younger than 30 years may be regarded as sufficient to establish the diagnosis. In older patients the presence of at least two cysts in each kidney may be required.[82]

Other much rarer causes of enlarged echogenic kidneys are infection with cytomegalovirus,[83] congenital nephrotic syndrome of the Finnish type[84] and renal vein thrombosis.[85] Also included in the differential are syndromes where cystic kidneys are a feature (Table 13.2) (see Echogenic kidneys).

Associated abnormalities

Adult patients have cysts in the liver, pancreas and spleen; however these have not been reported in the fetus. Other associations include cardiac disease (mainly mitral valve prolapse),[55] skeletal abnormalities,[74,78] pyloric stenosis[86] and intracranial aneurysms.

Outcome

The outcome for prenatally diagnosed cases is difficult to determine as reported cases are relatively few and the best data have come from family studies. It has been estimated that in prenatal cases 43% die within the first year and 67% of survivors develop hypertension. Approximately 3% will develop end-stage renal failure by the age of 3 years.[72] If a previous child is affected the outcome for the current pregnancy is often similar.[72] Many adult patients are asymptomatic until the fifth decade when hypertension and renal failure may become apparent.

Recurrence risk

As the condition is autosomal dominant the recurrence risk is 50%.

Obstructive cystic dysplasia (Potter type IV)

Obstructive cystic dysplasia is produced by obstruction to the kidney in the first or early second trimester[87] unlike multicystic dysplasia where the obstruction occurs much earlier in renal development.

It is usually produced by urethral obstruction and so may affect both kidneys or can be unilateral when caused by a pelvi-ureteric junction obstruction or lower ureteric obstruction.[87]

Pathologically there is disorganized epithelial tissue surrounded by fibrous tissue and multiple cortical cysts.[88]

Sonographic appearances

The typical sonographic appearance is of a small echogenic kidney which may contain peripheral cortical cysts (Fig. 13.30). The presence of the cortical cysts is an important sign as when associated with obstruction it invariably signifies dysplasia[88] (Fig. 13.31). In addition, although the presence of increased echogenicity is very suggestive of dysplasia a normal renal echodensity does not exclude renal dysplasia.[87]

Occasionally renal obstruction produces calyceal rupture and a perinephric collection and these kidneys often progress to a severe dysplasia[89,90] (Fig. 13.32). Rarely, the dysplasia may affect one segment of a kidney as in the case of obstruction to one part of a duplex kidney, usually the upper moiety.[87,91]

Outcome

The outcome for overall renal function depends on the severity of dysplasia; the presence of oligohydramnios with bilateral echodense hydronephrotic kidneys carries an ominous prognosis (Fig. 13.30). Less severe dysplasia with normal liquor or unilateral dysplasia has a better outcome.

Interventional techniques to aspirate fetal urine and assess fetal renal function will be discussed in the section on renal obstruction.

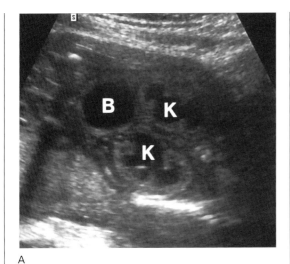

A

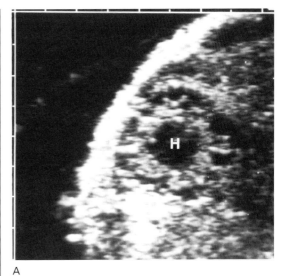

A

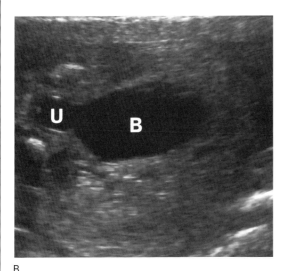

B

Fig. 13.30 Obstructive cystic dysplasia. (A) Coronal section through a fetus with posterior urethral valves. Note the thick-walled bladder – B, Bilateral hydronephrosis – K, and the echogenic cortex. There is severe oligohydramnios. (B) There is a distended bladder – B with dilatation of the posterior urethra – U.

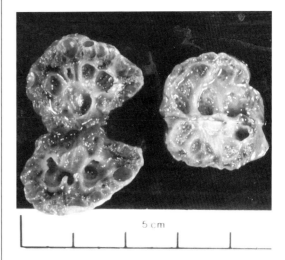

B

Fig. 13.31 Obstructive cystic dysplasia. (A) Transverse scan through the fetal kidney showing a moderate hydronephrosis (H) and multiple cysts throughout the echogenic cortex. (B) Post-mortem specimen of the kidneys showing moderate hydronephrosis and multiple cysts within the cortex.

ECHOGENIC KIDNEYS

The previous sections have discussed the various types of cystic renal disease; however, clinically one is rarely presented with textbook descriptions and classic family histories. The common finding on antenatal ultrasound is echogenic kidneys and so a differential diagnosis and clinical assessment is required.[92]

Table 13.5 outlines the main causes of echogenic kidneys. It can be seen that infantile polycystic renal disease and adult polycystic renal disease can have very similar appearances. The presence of normal liquor volume and the demonstration of cysts in one of the parents' kidneys should favour adult polycystic renal disease. In infantile polycystic renal disease there may be a family history of a previously affected child.

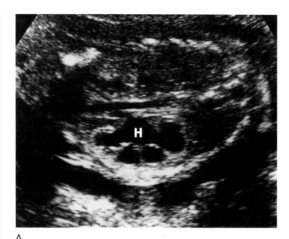

A

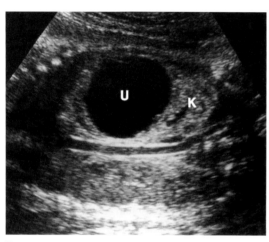

B

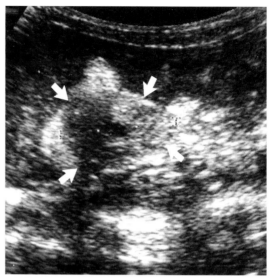

C

Fig. 13.32 Renal dysplasia. (A) Coronal scan at 20 weeks showing a moderate hydronephrosis (H). (B) Same fetus at 26 weeks' gestation showing a large urinoma (U). The kidney (K) is compressed by the urinoma. (C) Follow-up scan in the neonatal period shows a small dysplastic kidney (kidney is outlined by the straight arrows).

Obstructive cystic dysplasia should be fairly easy to diagnose as there is usually hydronephrosis present and cysts may be present in up to 44% of affected kidneys.[88] Finnish type nephrotic syndrome may be difficult to differentiate from infantile and adult polycystic disease; however, the maternal serum alphafetoprotein is often markedly elevated in this condition.[84] Liquor volume is normal and there may be a previous history in a sibling as the condition is autosomal recessive.

The Beckwith–Wiedeman syndrome presents with macrosomia, hepatosplenomegaly, macroglossia, omphalocoele and normal or increased liquor volume and so should not prove to be too difficult a diagnostic dilemma.[93] The

Meckel–Gruber syndrome and trisomy 13 have similar patterns of associated abnormalities; however, oligohydramnios is commoner in the Meckel–Gruber syndrome which is also an autosomal recessive condition and so there may be a previously affected sibling. In addition, midline facial clefting, holoprosencephaly and cardiac anomalies favour trisomy 13, whereas encephalocoele is more in keeping with Meckel–Gruber syndrome.[94]

Cytomegalovirus infection is an uncommon cause of echogenic kidneys; however, the associated features of hydrocephalus, periventricular calcification and microcephaly should raise the possibility of such infection. Additional features include hepatosplenomegaly and hydrops.[83] Renal vein thrombosis, although rare, is often unilateral and liquor volume is normal. Maternal predisposing factors that have been reported include diabetes and pyelonephritis.[85]

Finally, it should not be forgotten that echogenic kidneys can be entirely normal,

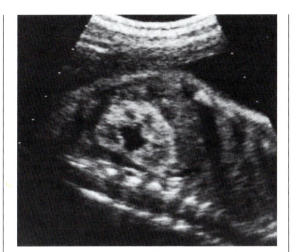

Fig. 13.33 Echogenic kidney. This fetus showed echogenic kidneys which were of normal size throughout pregnancy with normal liquor volume. Follow-up to 5 years shows normal renal function.

Table 13.6
Causes of hydronephrosis

Bilateral hydronephrosis
Bilateral pelvi-ureteric junction obstruction
Bilateral vesico-ureteric junction obstruction
Bilateral vesico-ureteric reflux
Megacystis megaureter syndrome
Posterior urethral valves
Urethral atresia
Obstructing ureterocoele
Megacystis microcolon syndrome
Congenital megalourethra
Persistent cloaca
Hydrometrocolpos

Unilateral hydronephrosis
Pelvi-ureteric junction obstruction
Vesico-ureteric junction obstruction
Duplex kidney with ureterocoele
Normal kidney with ureterocoele
Megaureter

Table 13.7
The final urological diagnosis in infants with significant prenatally detected uropathy

Diagnosis	Percentage
Pelvi-ureteric junction obstruction	35
Vesico-ureteric reflux	20
Multicystic dysplastic kidney	15
Vesico-ureteric junction obstruction	10
Posterior urethral valves	9
Duplex systems	8
Renal agenesis	3

Reproduced with permission from Thomas DFM. Prenatally detected uropathies: epidemiological considerations. B J Urol 1998;81: Supplement 2, 8–12.

particularly if the kidneys are of normal size (Fig. 13.33). Careful follow-up, however, is indicated in fetuses with echogenic kidneys, particularly in the neonatal period and early childhood.

RENAL OBSTRUCTION

Fetal hydronephrosis may be caused by a number of different structural abnormalities producing obstruction to the urinary tract and also due to non-obstructing conditions such as vesicoureteric reflux and prune belly syndrome (Table 13.6). It is clear, however, that the common causes of hydronephrosis are pelvi-ureteric function obstruction, vesico-ureteric reflux, vesico-ureteric junction obstruction, posterior urethral valves and obstruction in duplex kidneys (Table 13.7).

The exact incidence of fetal hydronephrosis is difficult to determine; it has been estimated that dilatations of the urinary tract may be seen in up to 1 in 100 pregnancies. However, follow-up studies reveal significant renal pathology in only 1 in 500.[95] The main cause for this discrepancy is transient or mild hydronephrosis which often resolves after delivery.[11] Indeed individual reported series record false-positive rates for fetal hydronephrosis in a range of 37 to 81% (Table 13.8). Overall sensitivity of antenatal ultrasound in the detection of fetal hydronephrosis, however, is high, with rates ranging between 69 and 100%.[8,23,96–98]

In order to refine the diagnosis of fetal hydronephrosis many workers have proposed different cut-off values for the anteroposterior diameter of the renal pelvis. Values vary between 4 and 10 mm in the second trimester and 7 and 10 mm in the third trimester (Table 13.9). The use of differing cut-off values, however, does not appear to improve sensitivities or the mean false-positive values calculated for each cut-off value.

The degree of renal pelvic dilatation does appear to have some correlation with

Table 13.8
Detection rates and final diagnosis in fetuses with antenatal diagnosis of hydronephrosis

Author	Total population scanned	Number abnormal on scan	Number (%) with significant renal disease	Pelvi-ureteric junction obstruction	Vesico-ureteric junction obstruction	Posterior urethral valves	Duplex kidney	Vesico-ureteric reflux
				Final diagnosis				
Arger et al 1985	3530	30	6 (20)	2	1	2	–	–
Grignon et al 1986	34 592	92	47 (51)	29	8	4	–	3
Livera et al 1989	6292	79	29 (37)	12	4	2	2	2
Mandell et al 1991	–	154	87 (56)	45	6	2	3	8
Corteville et al 1991	–	63	45 (71)	23	3	1	1	–
Johnson et al 1992	7500	47	17 (36)	7	1	1	–	3
Tam et al 1994		105	63 (60)	43	7	3	8	13
Anderson et al 1995	12 100	257	24 (9)	23	3	1	1	–
Adra et al 1995		84	30 (36)	11	2	–	2	10
Ouzouncan et al 1996	–	84	48 (57)	–	–	–	–	–
Dudley et al 1997	18 766	100	21 (21)	3	3	–	1	6
James et al 1998	105 542	154	97 (63)	52	16	3	12	14

Table 13.9
Cut-off values for anteroposterior diameters of the renal pelvis in different studies

Author	Cut-off values
Arger et al 1985	> 5 mm (16 weeks to term)
Grignon et al 1986	> 10 mm (16 weeks to term)
Scott et al 1988	> 5 mm (16 weeks to term)
Livera et al 1989	> 10 mm (28 weeks to term)
Mandell et al 1991	> 5 mm (16 weeks to 20 weeks)
	> 8 mm (20 weeks to 30 weeks)
	> 10 mm (30 weeks to term)
Corteville et al 1991	> 4 mm (16 weeks to 33 weeks)
	> 7 mm (33 weeks to term)
Johnson et al 1992	> 10 mm (16 weeks to term)
Lam et al 1993	> 10 mm (16 weeks to term)
Tam et al 1994	> 4 mm (16 weeks to term)
Anderson et al 1995	> 4 mm (16 weeks to 23 weeks)
	> 6 mm (23 weeks to 30 weeks)
	> 8 mm (30 weeks to term)
Adra et al 1995	> 8 mm (28 weeks to term)
Barker et al 1995	> 5 mm (16 weeks to term)
Ouzouncan et al 1996	> 5 mm (16 weeks to term)
Dudley et al 1997	> 5 mm (16 weeks to term)
James et al 1998	> 5 mm (16 weeks to 28 weeks)
	> 7 mm (28 weeks to term)

Table 13.10
The mean differential function shown for each grade of early prenatal anteroposterior renal pelvic dilatation

Dilatation at median of 19 weeks in mm	Mean differential function %
Normal < 4	48.2
Mild 5–9	42.7
Moderate 10–15	37.3
Severe > 15	26.6

Reproduced with permission from Barker AP, Case MM, Thomas DSM et al. Pelviureteric junction obstruction: predictors of outcome. Br J Urol 1995;76:649–652.

outcome and most authors would agree that renal pelvic diameters of greater than 15 mm are highly predictive of significant renal pathology with a high incidence of postnatal surgery[14,15,99–101]. In addition, when prenatal renal pelvic diameters are compared with postnatal differential renal function it is seen that diameters greater than 15 mm have a mean differential function of only 27% (Table 13.10).

Renal pelvic diameters between 10 and 15 mm also have a high incidence of significant renal pathology[9,11,14,15,23,101,102] and most authors suggest follow-up and investigation in the neonatal period.

The main difficulty arises in the case of mild renal pelvic dilatation when measurements are between 4 and 10 mm. Reference to Table 13.10 reveals only a small drop in mean differential function which is not statistically significant.[101] More important, however, is the link with vesico-ureteric reflux and a number of studies have shown that significant reflux in the neonatal period was associated with mild renal pelvic dilatation of 4 to 10 mm at 18 to 20 weeks' gestation.[9,100,103–105]

In addition, further follow-up studies have shown that mild renal pelvic dilatation can progress in utero to produce significant renal pathology in up to 4% of cases.[106]

Interestingly, in a recent study, Anderson et al found that most kidneys with hydronephrosis in later pregnancy and the neonatal period had renal pelvic diameters of less than 10 mm before 23 weeks' gestation. The study also showed that by plotting renal pelvic diameters for obstructed and normal kidneys the measurements were very similar for both groups until 22 weeks, after which time they began to diverge (Fig.13.34).[96] The study demonstrated that before 23 weeks a renal pelvic diameter cut-off of 5 mm had a sensitivity of 53% for detecting hydronephrosis, whereas a cut-off of 4 mm had a 76% sensitivity.[96] These figures were associated with false-positive rates in the region of 90%. However, the reason for such high false-positive rates is unclear as other studies using a 4 mm cut-off for renal pelvic diameter had much lower false-positive rates in the region of 45 to 56%.[23,103,106]

It would seem therefore that before 23 weeks renal pelvic diameters between 4 and 10 mm can be associated with significant renal pathology including pelvi-ureteric junction obstruction and reflux, and that

follow-up scans are required at around 28 weeks' gestation to determine whether the pelvic dilatation has progressed. In addition it would certainly be prudent to follow these babies up with ultrasound in the neonatal period and probably once more at 3 to 6 months to look for further signs of obstruction or reflux.

The other important finding in fetal hydronephrosis is the demonstration of caliectasis. Grignon et al reported that the presence of caliectasis doubled the rates of surgery to hydronephrotic kidneys[15] and Corteville reported similar findings.[23] Newell et al found that the presence of caliectasis was more likely to indicate a significant hydronephrosis.[107] These findings suggest that caliectasis may be a further marker for more severe disease than if renal pelvic dilatation alone is seen.

A number of papers have reported the association of hydronephrosis with chromosomal disease.[108–111] In most cases there are multiple abnormalities present and the risk of chromosomal disease is then approximately 30%. However, even when hydronephrosis is isolated the risk of chromosomal disease is about 3%.[108] In addition there has been considerable debate as to the association of mild renal pelvic dilatation and trisomy 21;[109–113] however, when age-specific risks are taken into consideration the risk of trisomy 21 is not increased[109,114] (See Ch. 14).

The prenatal diagnosis of hydronephrosis does pose some difficulties; however, some clear guidelines are emerging. Most cases of renal pelvic dilatation less than 4 mm diameter are likely to be normal. Renal pelvic diameters of 5 to 10 mm need follow-up later in pregnancy and also into the neonatal period with a final scan at 3 to 6 months. Renal pelvic diameters greater than 1 cm are likely to have significant renal disease and require investigations including a micturating cystourethrogram to look for reflux and a DMSA scan to assess renal function.

Prenatal diagnosis of hydronephrosis is important for a number of reasons. The clinical diagnosis of renal abnormalities is

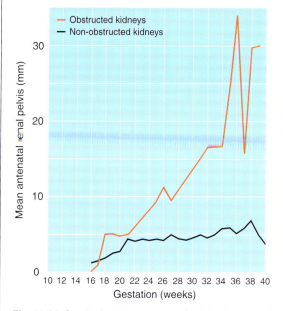

Fig. 13.34 Graph showing mean renal pelvic diameter of obstructed and non-obstructed fetal kidneys in relation to gestational age. The curves overlap at 16 to 21 weeks' gestational age before beginning to diverge. (Published with permission from Anderson et al[96].)

poor with only 15 to 27% detected by abdominal examination[11,115–117] so potentially the majority of renal abnormalities could be missed using clinical examination alone. In this respect prenatal diagnosis has been found to be of definite value in up to 26% and of probable value in 50% of cases.[12] In addition prenatal detection may improve outcome by allowing the site of delivery to be changed to tertiary care setting for early postnatal intervention. In rare cases intervention in utero may be indicated to prevent fatal consequences of obstructive uropathy.[95]

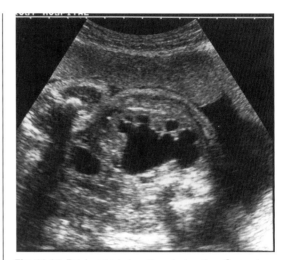

Fig. 13.35 Pelvi-ureteric junction obstruction. Coronal section showing moderate dilatation of the collecting system and renal pelvis. The condition was unilateral, note the normal liquor volume.

PELVI-URETERIC JUNCTION OBSTRUCTION

Pelvi-ureteric junction obstruction is the commonest cause of hydronephrosis (Table 13.7) and has an incidence of approximately 1 in 2000 live births.[11] The condition is more common in boys and is unilateral in 90% of cases.[118] The aetiology is unclear as a true narrowing is seldom demonstrated; it is likely the problem is of a functional nature.[119]

Sonographic appearances

Pelvi-ureteric junction obstruction typically shows dilatation of the renal pelvis and calyces without ureteric dilatation, and a normal bladder (Fig. 13.35). When obstruction is severe the collecting system becomes effaced with thinning of the renal cortex (Fig. 13.36). The degree of renal pelvic dilatation does correlate with the postnatal function of the kidney, with increasing renal pelvic diameter indicating a poorer differential renal function in the neonate (Table 13.10).[101] (See Renal obstruction section).

Liquor volume is usually normal and may be increased, even with bilateral obstruction.[118,119] The reason for this is unclear, but one hypothesis is that obstruction impairs renal concentrating ability and results in a state of high urine output.[118]

Severe obstruction can result in calyceal rupture and the development of a perinephric urinoma (Fig. 13.32). This

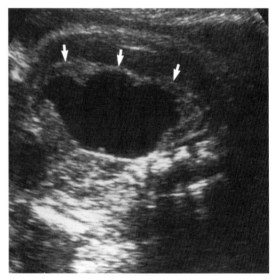

Fig. 13.36 Pelvi-ureteric junction obstruction. Coronal scan through the kidney showing hydronephrosis with thinning of the cortex (arrows).

invariably has a very poor outlook for the affected kidney with a high incidence of renal dysplasia.[89,90,118] Very rarely the dilated renal pelvis can enlarge to massive proportions and mimic an abdominal cyst.[120]

The affected kidney should also be assessed for increased echogenicity and/or cortical cysts which may suggest a degree of renal dysplasia. In addition the contralateral kidney should be evaluated for associated renal abnormalities. The fetal ureters and bladder should also be assessed to exclude lower obstructions such as vesico-ureteric or bladder outlet obstruction.

Differential diagnosis

The differential diagnosis includes multicystic renal dysplasia and also other forms of renal obstruction such as vesico-ureteric junction obstruction and bladder outlet obstruction. Occasionally renal cysts or perinephric urinomas can mimic a pelvi-ureteric junction obstruction.

Associated abnormalities

Associated renal abnormalities occur in approximately 25% of cases and include renal agenesis, multicystic renal dysplasia and vesico-ureteric reflux.[121] Extrarenal abnormalities are seen in 12% but have no specific pattern unless associated with a particular chromosomal abnormality.[119]

Outcome

Outcome in both unilateral and bilateral disease is usually good.[1,118,119] However, the degree of dilatation seen antenatally does correlate with postnatal renal function (Table 13.10) so that the greater the degree of dilatation seen in utero, the poorer the renal function seen in the neonate. Follow-up scans are indicated later in pregnancy to monitor the renal dilatation. If the condition is bilateral then careful monitoring is required, particularly to evaluate liquor volume. The development of oligohydramnios would tend to worsen the prognosis indicating increasing renal compromise.

Postnatal evaluation includes renal ultrasound, and a DMSA scan to assess differential renal function.[11] The surgical management of pelvi-ureteric junction obstruction has become more conservative in recent years with surgery only contemplated in the situation of increasing hydronephrosis and poor differential renal function.[122–125] Indeed, conservative management has revealed remarkable spontaneous improvements even in relatively poorly functioning kidneys.[126]

Recurrent risk

As most cases are sporadic the recurrence risk is low. A few familial cases, however, have been reported.[127,128]

VESICO-URETERIC JUNCTION OBSTRUCTION (NON-REFLUXING MEGAURETER)

Vesico-ureteric junction obstruction accounts for about 10% of causes of fetal hydronephrosis and has an approximate incidence of 1 in 6500 live births.[11] This condition should be diagnosed where there is no evidence of reflux or bladder outlet obstruction. It is thought that the cause of the obstruction is a localized region of dysfunction or physiological obstruction in the distal ureter, which is often narrowed.[129] The condition is commoner in boys with a male to female ratio of 2:1.[130]

Sonographic appearances

There is dilatation of the ureter and usually of the renal pelvis. The bladder should appear normal and liquor volume is usually normal. The condition may be bilateral in up to 25% of cases.[130,131] The dilated ureter is often seen as a serpiginous echo free tubular structure in the paraspinal region and communicates with the renal pelvis (Fig. 13.37). The ureter can usually be differentiated from bowel as bowel contains

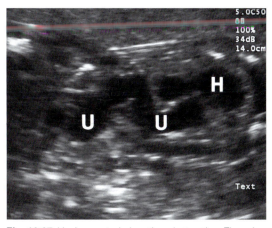

Fig. 13.37 Vesico-ureteric junction obstruction. There is hydronephrosis with dilatation of the ureter (U).

low level echoes from meconium whereas the ureter is relatively echo free.

A careful search should always be made for anomalies in the contralateral kidney and follow-up scans carried out to assess renal dilatation and liquor volume.

Differential diagnosis

The differential diagnosis includes unilateral vesico-ureteric reflux from which it is impossible to distinguish in the antenatal period.[130] Occasionally bladder outlet obstruction will produce asymmetry of the upper tracts with marked hydro-ureter and hydronephrosis in one kidney and relatively normal appearances in the other. This usually indicates the presence of vesico-ureteric reflux dysplasia (VURD) in which one kidney has been essentially destroyed by massive reflux yet the other is relatively well preserved due to the 'pop off' of pressure into the refluxing system.[132] The other main cause for a dilated ureter is ureteric obstruction secondary to a ureterocoele usually associated with a duplex kidney. The presence of the ureterocoele within the bladder can often be demonstrated (Fig. 13.40).

Associated anomalies

Associated renal abnormalities occur in approximately 16% and include pelvi-ureteric junction obstruction, multicystic renal dysplasia, pelvic kidney, renal agenesis and vesico-ureteric reflux.[131]

Outcome

The overall outcome for the condition is good and up to 40% of cases will resolve spontaneously without any intervention. Prenatal studies have found that ureteric diameters of less than 6 mm have a good outcome with a low incidence of surgery. Ureters greater than 10 mm, however, have a poorer outcome with a high incidence of surgical correction.[130] Babies with this condition need to be followed-up into the neonatal period and have a micturating cystourethrogram to exclude reflux and a DMSA scan to assess differential renal function. Those with a poor differential function are usually candidates for surgery and reimplantation of the ureter.

OBSTRUCTION SECONDARY TO URETEROCOELE AND ECTOPIC URETER

Ureterocoeles are cystic dilatations of the intravesical segment of the distal ureter.[133] The ureterocoele balloons into the bladder and consists of bladder and ureteral epithelium separated by varying amounts of connective tissue and smooth muscle. These lesions are most often associated with duplex kidneys and the ureterocoele usually drains the upper pole moiety[134] (Fig. 13.38). In 10 to 20% of cases the ureterocoele arises from a solitary renal pelvis.[135] Ureterocoeles associated with a duplex kidney are more common in girls. However, in boys with a ureterocoele 40% drain a single collecting system. Ureterocoeles and ectopic ureters are bilateral in 10 to 15% of cases.[1]

Ectopic ureters may insert into the urethra, bladder neck or in the trigone inferomedial to the normal location. In males the ureters may also insert in the seminal vesicle, vas deferens or ejaculatory ducts, and in females the vestibule, vagina or uterus.[135] Ectopic ureters and ureters associated with ureterocoeles are almost

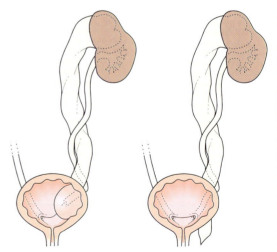

Fig. 13.38 Diagram of two duplex kidneys. Both have hydronephrosis of the upper pole; one with and one without an ectopic ureterocoele. (Printed with permission from Winters[137].)

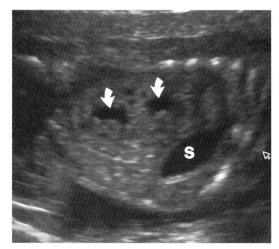

Fig. 13.39 Duplex kidney. Sagittal scan through a duplex kidney showing two collecting systems (curved arrows point to two separate collecting systems, S – stomach).

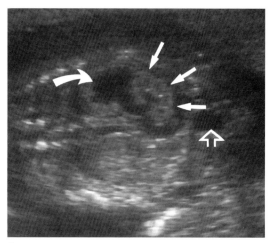

A

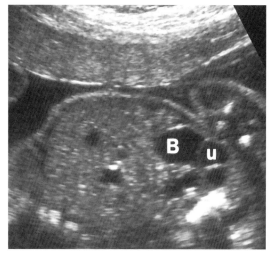

B

Fig. 13.40 Duplex kidney with hydronephrosis in the upper pole moiety secondary to a ureterocoele. (A) Coronal scan through the duplex kidney showing hydronephrosis of the upper pole moiety (curved arrow). The lower pole (outlined by the straight arrows) is normal. Open arrow points to the bladder. (B) Same fetus showing a ureterocoele (U) within the bladder (B).

always dilated and so are amenable to prenatal diagnosis.

The incidence of ectopic ureters and ureterocoeles is difficult to determine but is probably in the order of 1 in 9000 live births.[11]

Sonographic appearances

Duplex kidneys can be difficult to diagnose prenatally if hydronephrosis is not present. However, clues to the diagnosis include a slightly large kidney, which with careful evaluation, may show two collecting systems (Fig. 13.39). Hydronephrosis usually affects the upper pole moiety (Fig. 13.40) and on occasion can be quite marked. A dilated ureter may be visible and a ureterocoele can often be demonstrated within the bladder (Fig. 13.40). An ectopic ureter should be suspected if there is upper pole hydronephrosis in a duplex kidney, a dilated ureter which appears to insert below the bladder base and absence of a ureterocoele within the bladder.[135]

Ureterocoeles can be large and obstruct the contralateral kidney or can herniate into the urethra producing bladder outlet obstruction and bilateral obstruction.[136] Ureterocoeles may also be bilateral.[134]

In one series prenatal diagnosis was only possible in 39% of cases and this may be due to a number of factors.[137] The upper pole hydronephrosis may be quite marked,

compressing the lower pole calyces and making the diagnosis of the duplex system difficult. The ureterocoele may also be difficult to demonstrate because if the bladder is empty it may be mistaken for the bladder, and if the bladder is full this can result in effacement of the ureterocoele.[137,138] In addition severe upper pole hydronephrosis can lead onto renal dysplasia and subsequent poor renal function. In this situation the upper pole may not excrete sufficient urine to continuously distend the ureterocoele,[133] and so the ureterocoele may be missed.

Differential diagnosis

The differential diagnosis includes vesico-ureteric junction obstruction and reflux. A ureterocoele obstructing the urethra can produce similar appearances to posterior urethral valves. The fetal gender is a useful differentiating factor, as urethral valves occur in males and ureterocoeles are much more common in females.

Associated anomalies

Vesico-ureteric reflux is often seen in the lower pole moiety, and is present in up to 50% of fetuses that have a ureterocoele affecting the upper pole.[137] There is no increased incidence of other abnormalities.

Outcome

The outcome is improved with prenatal diagnosis as only 35% of babies have clinical signs or symptoms of ureterocoele or ectopic ureter.[137] Outcome for the affected kidney depends on the degree of renal function present in the upper pole moiety. Postnatal investigations should include a neonatal renal scan, a micturating cystourethrogram and a DMSA scan. When there is good function of the upper pole the ureterocoele can be punctured via the transurethral route.[139] This procedure, however, does increase the risk of reflux into the upper pole moiety. Non-functioning upper poles are usually surgically resected.[1]

POSTERIOR URETHRAL VALVES

Posterior urethral valves are the most common cause of severe obstructive uropathy in children and account for about 9% of all causes of fetal urinary obstruction (Table 13.7).[1] The incidence is approximately 1 in 5000 to 1 in 8000 boys.[95] The condition is caused by tissue leaflets which fan distally from the prostatic urethra to the external urinary sphincter. Typically the leaflets are separated by a slit-like opening.[1] It is the

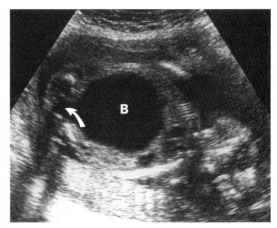

Fig. 13.41 Posterior urethral valves. Sagittal section through the fetal abdomen showing a distended bladder (B). Curved arrow points to the dilated posterior urethra.

underlying cause of end-stage renal disease in almost one-third of boys under the age of 4 years.[132] The condition only affects males.

Sonographic appearances

The typical appearances are a dilated thick-walled bladder with a dilated posterior urethra (Figs 13.30, 13.41). This is usually associated with dilated ureters and bilateral hydronephrosis[140,141] (Fig. 13.42). Liquor volume is variable and there may be oligohydramnios which carries a very poor prognosis. The obstruction may be so severe

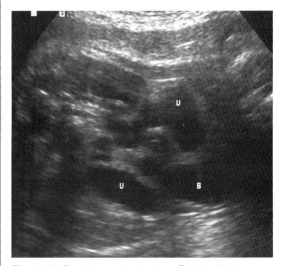

Fig. 13.42 Posterior urethral valves. The bladder is distended (B) and there is dilatation of both ureters (U). Note associated oligohydramnios.

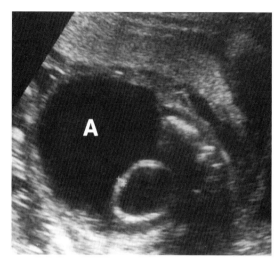

Fig. 13.43 Urinary ascites. A thick-walled bladder is noted, surrounded by the urinary ascites. Note associated oligohydramnios (A – ascites).

as to cause bladder rupture and urinary ascites[141,142] (Fig. 13.43). This, however, is considered a good prognostic sign as the kidneys are decompressed.[1] Similarly, in the kidneys calyceal rupture can occur producing perinephric urinomas (Fig. 13.32). This finding in the kidney is usually associated with severe renal dysplasia.[89,90,118] The presence of echogenic kidneys with or without cortical cysts also indicates renal dysplasia and is often associated with oligohydramnios (Fig. 13.30). The hydronephrosis is occasionally asymmetrical and is thought to represent massive reflux into one kidney which is essentially destroyed with relative sparing of the other kidney due to the 'pop off' of pressure into the refluxing system.[100] This is recognised as vesico-ureteric reflux dysplasia (VURD), and is thought to be a good prognostic sign as the non-refluxing kidney is protected to a certain extent from the back pressure effects of the bladder outlet obstruction.[1]

Differential diagnosis

The most important differential diagnosis is severe bilateral vesico-ureteric reflux producing the megacystis megaureter association.[132] It is often very difficult to differentiate severe reflux from urethral valves; however, in reflux the bladder is usually thin-walled and liquor volume is usually normal.[143] Urethral atresia usually presents with massive bladder distension, bilateral hydronephrosis and severe oligohydramnios and so may be difficult to differentiate from severe urethral valves. The distinction, however, is really academic as the outlook is very poor for either condition. Congenital megalourethra can display similar appearances; however, in addition to bladder distension there will also be dilatation of the penile urethra producing a cyst-like structure between the fetal legs.[144] Persistent cloaca, a condition only occurring in females, may also produce bilateral hydronephrosis and scanning the pelvis one may see a midline cystic mass between the bladder and rectum which represents part of the cloacal complex (see section on cloacal malformations). A hydrometrocolpos can produce bladder outlet obstruction by direct compression of the bladder. It may have similar appearances to persistent cloaca. Megacystis microcolon syndrome can also produce a dilated bladder and bilateral hydronephrosis; however, the clue to this diagnosis is that the stomach is also markedly dilated and the condition is autosomal recessive.[145]

Associated abnormalities

Associated abnormalities are seen in 43% of fetuses[140,146] and include cardiac anomalies, bowel rotation, imperforate anus and vesicorectal fistula. Chromosomal disease can be seen in up to 8% of fetuses; however, there is no specific syndrome.[147]

Pulmonary hypoplasia is commonly seen when there is severe oligohydramnios from the early part of pregnancy. In addition, the typical findings of Potter's syndrome will also be present and include low set ears, wide set eyes, micrognathia, limb contractures and talipes.

The prune belly syndrome describes the distended abdomen due to abdominal muscle laxity associated with any form of urethral obstruction and also severe cases of bilateral vesico-ureteric reflux. There may be urinary ascites[148] and there is also cryptorchidism.

Outcome

The overall mortality rate can be as high as 63%[95] and of the survivors 30% will develop end-stage renal failure.[149] One important prognostic factor is the gestational age at detection. Cases diagnosed before 24 weeks have a poor outcome with a 53% risk of perinatal mortality or chronic/end-stage renal failure. Those cases diagnosed after 24 weeks have a much better prognosis with a 7% risk of poor outcome.[150]

It is well established that cases presenting in the second trimester with severe oligohydramnios and hydronephrotic kidneys that show echogenic cortex have a poor outlook with almost 100% perinatal mortality. Conversely, normal liquor throughout pregnancy with static hydronephrosis has a good outlook.

The difficult group of fetuses are those where the hydronephrosis is getting worse and/or the liquor volume is reducing. It is in this group that fetal intervention has been proposed in order to improve survival and hopefully prevent the development of renal dysplasia.[1,95,132] Experimental work on animals has shown that the relief of urinary obstruction at the appropriate time can prevent the development of renal dysplasia[151] and it is this work that has provided the rationale for urinary decompression in the fetus. The best assessment of prognosis appears to be the assessment of the urinary electrolytes by aspirating fetal urine from the bladder.[18,19,152,153] Table 13.11 outlines the prognostic indicators for sonography and urinary electrolytes. The most appropriate technique appears to be serial urine aspirations over a period of 2 to 3 days in order that fresh urine from the kidneys is sampled rather than stagnant urine within the bladder.[19,95] In this way serial measurements are made and the final values are used to designate the fetus into either a good or poor prognostic group. A fetal karyotype is also carried out to exclude a chromosomal abnormality. It is suggested that fetuses in the poor prognostic group would not benefit from fetal intervention. Those in the good prognostic group could

Table 13.11
Prognostic factors in fetuses with posterior urethral valves

Good prognostic indicators		Poor prognostic indicators
Sonographic signs		
Normal liquor		Oligohydramnios
Diagnosis after 24 weeks		Diagnosis before 24 weeks
Asymmetrical hydronephrosis		Echogenic kidneys with cysts
Urinary ascites		Perinephric urinoma
Isolated		Associated abnormalities
Urine biochemistry		
Sodium	< 100 mEq/l	> 100 mEq/l
Chlorine	< 90 mEq/l	> 90 mEq/l
Osmolality	< 210 mOsm/l	> 210 mOsm/l
Calcium	< 2 mmol/l	> 2 mmol/l
Phosphate	< 2 mmol/l	> 2 mmol/l
B$_2$ Microglobulin	< 2 mg/l	> 2 mg/l

undergo placement of a vesico-amniotic shunt to decompress the urinary tract, if detected before 32 weeks' gestation. After 32 weeks, early delivery with immediate postnatal decompression is the more appropriate management strategy.[95] Placement of vesico-amniotic shunts is not without complications with chorio-amnionitis, anterior abdominal wall defects, shunt malplacement and fetal death.[95] Newer innovations include direct vision endoscopic valve resection using a transabdomino-uretofetal abdominal puncture;[154] however, this is in the experimental stage at present.

The exact place of fetal intervention in bladder outlet obstruction is still controversial;[1,5,17] however, improvements in techniques and refinements in urinary biochemical analysis have meant the prediction of outcome is more accurate. Further studies on affected fetuses are required before the place of fetal intervention is clearly defined.

URETHRAL ATRESIA

In this condition there is complete urethral obstruction so the bladder is usually massively dilated, completely filling the ureterine cavity. There is anhydramnios and the thorax and other structures are so compressed that they are often difficult to visualize. The prognosis is uniformly poor with a lethal outcome.

MEGACYSTIS-MICROCOLON-INTESTINAL HYPOPERISTALSIS SYNDROME

This condition is thought to be due to a degenerative disease of smooth muscle and comprises small intestinal obstruction, microcolon and megacystis. Sonographically the characteristic appearances are of a dilated bladder with bilateral hydonephrosis and a distended fluid-filled stomach.[145] Liquor volume may be normal or increased. The outcome is poor as the syndrome is uniformly lethal.

CONGENITAL MEGALOURETHRA

This condition which only affects boys is caused by partial or complete absence of the corpus spongiosum and the corpora cavernosa. This produces dilatation of the penile urethra which may be massive, presenting as a cystic mass between the fetal legs associated with a dilated bladder and bilateral hydronephrosis.[144] The disorder is often associated with other anomalies including imperforate anus, heart defects and renal anomalies such as renal agenesis or hypoplasia.

VESICO-URETERIC REFLUX

Vesico-ureteric reflux is more common in females with a female to male ratio of 4:1, and it is usually diagnosed following one or more urinary tract infections.[155] It has been established that vesico-ureteric reflux may account for up to 10% of cases of fetal hydronephrosis. However, 80% of this prenatally diagnosed group are boys.[156] The reason for this is unclear but could be related to the high voiding pressures seen in some neonates which in utero could distort the fetal ureterovesical junction resulting in reflux.[156] Another possibility is the development of a transient urethral valve-like obstruction which resolves before

birth.[157] The reflux is bilateral in up to 66% of babies and scarring may be seen in 40% of neonates even before the development of infections.[155,156,158] This suggests that the renal scarring and damage may well occur in utero. Interestingly, up to 35% of cases of reflux resolve spontaneously within 2 years.[159]

Sonographic appearances

Prenatal reports are scanty; however, the common appearance is fetal hydronephrosis which may appear as renal pelvic dilatation only.[160] In severe cases there may be bilateral hydronephrosis, hydro-ureters and a dilated thin-walled bladder – the so-called megacystis megaureter association – and this can mimic posterior urethral valves.[143] However, liquor volume is usually normal in vesico-ureteric reflux.

Differential diagnosis

The differential diagnosis includes virtually any cause of unilateral or bilateral hydronephrosis in the fetus, and includes pelvi-ureteric junction obstructions, vesico-ureteric junction obstruction and, when severe, posterior urethral valves and other causes of bladder outlet obstruction. (See differential diagnosis for posterior urethral valves.) A definitive diagnosis of reflux cannot be made until a micturating cystourethrogram is carried out in the neonatal period.

Associated abnormalities

Vesico-ureteric reflux can be associated with many other renal abnormalities and in particular ureterocoele in a duplex kidney, pelvi-ureteric junction obstruction, multicystic renal dysplasia and unilateral renal agenesis.[104] Non-renal abnormalities are rare.

Outcome

Up to 35% of prenatally detected vesico-ureteric reflux will resolve by 2 years of age.[159] However, all babies require prophylactic antibiotic treatment. Severe reflux is usually treated surgically with reimplantation of the ureter, but there

contain low level echoes. There is often hydronephrosis and in severe cases cystic renal dysplasia with oligohydramnios.[166] The cystic mass may be large, almost filling the abdomen.

Differential diagnosis

The main differential diagnoses are severe posterior urethral valves and the cloacal malformation.

Associated abnormalities

Associated anomalies include renal agenesis and intersex phenotype, i.e. ambiguous genitalia.

Outcome

The presence of renal dysplasia and oligohydramnios has a poor outcome with high perinatal mortality rates. Long term outcome is reasonably good following reconstructive surgery.

CLOACAL EXSTROPHY

This rare condition has an incidence of approximately 1 in 250 000 live births and may occur more frequently in twins.[168] The condition is also referred to as OEIS complex (Omphalocoele, vesical exstrophy, Imperforate anus, Spinal abnormalities). The condition is more common in males and is thought to represent maldevelopment of the cloacal membrane and defective sub-umbilical abdominal wall development.[169] The neonate presents with exstrophy of the bladder, epispadias and a short, hypoplastic externalized hindgut that separates and displaces laterally the two lateral halves of the exstrophied bladder. There is anal atresia and there may also be an omphalocoele.

Sonographic appearances

Sonographically there is a low anterior abdominal wall defect which occurs below the level of the umbilical cord which itself may have a low insertion (Fig. 13.46). In addition there will be absence of the bladder within the pelvis. There is usually normal liquor volume. There are many associated abnormalities but the most important is a lumbar-sacral meningocoele which may be seen in up to 70% of cases.[168]

Differential diagnosis

The differential diagnosis includes other anterior abdominal wall defects such as gastroschisis and omphalocoele. In these two conditions the defect is higher, at the level of the cord insertion, and the bladder will always be present. Bladder exstrophy may have identical sonographic appearances but has a low incidence of associated anomalies and spina bifida is not normally a feature. Amniotic band syndrome would conceivably produce a low anterior abdominal wall defect but there are many other abnormalities present such as scoliosis, facial clefting and amputation defects of the limbs.[170]

Associated abnormalities

Cloacal exstrophy has a number of associated anomalies including omphalocoele, oesophageal atresia, cardiac defects, duodenal atresia and spina bifida. There may also be a double vagina in females.[169]

Outcome

Cloacal exstrophy is a severe condition and if left untreated is fatal.[171] With improved surgical techniques survival rates are now in the range of 70 to 90%.[172] Multiple surgical procedures are required to create a colostomy and close the exstrophied bladder and bring together the pubic symphysis which is often widely separated. After a variety of bladder reconstruction and urethral and bladder neck continence procedures, urinary continence may be possible, although intermittent catheterization is required.[170] Due to the difficulties in creating functioning male genitalia it is usually recommended that genetic males should have gender reassignment and be brought up as females.

Recurrence risk

The condition is sporadic.

BLADDER EXSTROPHY

Bladder exstrophy has an incidence of approximately 1 in 25 to 40 000 live births

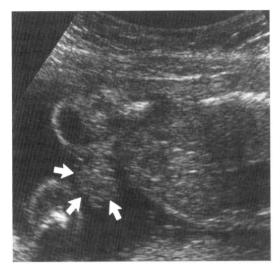

A

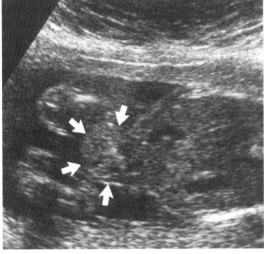

B

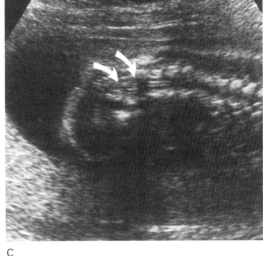

C

Fig. 13.46 Cloacal exstrophy. (A) Sagittal scan through the fetal abdomen showing a low anterior abdominal wall defect (arrows). This represents the everted bladder and short externalized hind gut. (B) Transverse section through the lower abdomen demonstrating the low cloacal defect (outlined by arrows). (C) Coronal section through the lower spine demonstrating a closed neural tube defect (curved arrows point to the defect).

and has a male to female ratio of 2·1.[173] The major clinical finding is a ventral defect in the infra-umbilical abdominal wall with exposure of the bladder. The pubic symphysis is widened and the umbilicus is low set.[174] The bladder wall is usually everted and may protrude outwards from the lower abdominal wall. Unlike cloacal exstrophy the anus is present but is anteriorly situated.[169] In addition, in bladder exstrophy associated abnormalities are less common than in cloacal exstrophy.

Sonographic appearances

The sonographic diagnosis is based on non-visualization of the fetal bladder in the presence of normal liquor and normal kidneys.[174] The umbilical cord is low set and there may be a lower abdominal wall defect which represents the everted bladder.[173] Extended scanning may be required to confirm the absence of the bladder.

Differential diagnosis

Differential diagnosis includes cloacal exstrophy; however, there are often associated anomalies, particularly spina bifida.[168] Other forms of anterior abdominal wall defects need to be considered; however, these defects are usually higher at the level of the cord insertion.

Associated abnormalities

Associated anomalies are uncommon but include renal agenesis, horseshoe kidney and hydronephrosis.[171]

Outcome

Major reconstructive surgery is required following initial bladder closure and although complications are common, long term follow-up suggests that overall outcome is relatively good with expected normal urinary and genital function in many patients.[169]

Recurrence risk

The condition is sporadic and has not occurred in children of mothers with bladder exstrophy.[174]

HORSESHOE KIDNEY, PELVIC KIDNEY AND CROSSED RENAL ECTOPIA

Horseshoe kidney

Horseshoe kidney is usually a result of fusion of the lower poles of both kidneys. In 10% of cases the upper poles are fused. Horseshoe kidney is a common abnormality and has an incidence of 1 in 400 live births, it is more common in boys and 90% of patients with a horseshoe kidney are asymptomatic.[175] The most common presenting symptom in children is urinary tract infection; however, most cases are discovered incidentally.

Sonographic appearances

Sonographically the horseshoe kidney is best demonstrated on a transverse section where at the inferior poles of the kidneys renal tissue will be seen to cross the midline joining both kidneys.[176] The bridge of renal tissue crosses anterior to the aorta and may also be demonstrated on coronal views.[177]

Associated abnormalities

Horseshoe kidney is frequently associated with other anomalies including urogenital, central nervous system, cardiovascular, gastrointestinal, musculoskeletal and chromosomal abnormalities.[178] Vesico-ureteric reflux can be seen in up to 50% of patients. The commonest chromosomal abnormalities associated are trisomy 18 and Turner's syndrome.[175]

Outcome

Outcome is generally good provided there are no other abnormalities. There is, however, an increased incidence of renal calculi, chronic urinary tract infections and hydronephrosis.[177]

Pelvic kidney

An ectopic kidney lies outside its normal position in the renal fossa. Ectopic kidneys are pelvic in 55%, crossed fused ectopic in 27%, lumbar in 12% and non-fused ectopic in 5%. Rarely the kidney may be thoracic.[175] Ectopic kidney has an incidence of 1 in 1200 live births.[179]

Sonographic appearances

The affected renal fossa is empty (Fig. 13.47) and the kidney is seen within the pelvis superior to the bladder.[179]

Outcome

Although long term outcome is good, there is an increased incidence of urinary tract infection.

Crossed renal ectopia

This condition occurs when one kidney is seen on the opposite side of the body. The kidney may be fused with the other kidney

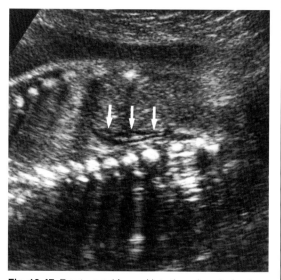

Fig. 13.47 Empty renal fossa. Note the adrenal gland lying horizontally within the renal fossa (arrows) and absence of the kidney.

usually at its lower pole or may be unfused.[175] It is more common in boys and the left kidney crosses over to the right more frequently than the right crossing to the left.

Sonographic appearances

As in pelvic kidney one renal fossa, usually the left, will be empty (Fig. 13.47) and an enlarged, usually bilobed, kidney is seen in the right lower abdomen. In addition two collecting systems may be seen.[180]

Associated abnormalities

The commonest anomalies seen are vertebral, especially spina bifida and sacral agenesis, and anal atresia.[175]

Outcome

Most patients are asymptomatic but there is a higher incidence of urinary tract infections.

RENAL TUMOURS

Fetal renal tumours are rare and the incidence of all renal tumours in childhood is 1 in 125 000 live births.[181] The commonest fetal renal tumour is mesoblastic nephroma which is a benign tumour. Pathologically the features are similar to a hamartoma with a well defined capsule and elongated spindle-shaped mesenchymal cells.

Sonographic appearances

The tumour presents as a fairly homogeneous mass in the renal area (Fig. 13.48). The mass may be large and compress the other intra-abdominal organs.[182,183] Polyhydramnios is seen in up to 70% of cases and is thought to be related to hypercalcaemia with resulting fetal polyuria.[184]

Outcome

The outcome is good as the tumour is benign and surgical removal is usually curative.[182–186] Rupture of the tumour in the neonatal period has been described but this is a rare complication.[183]

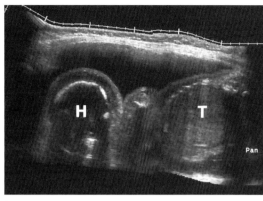

A

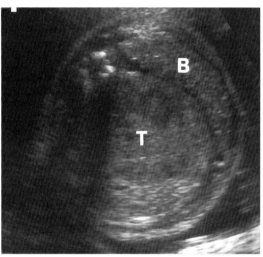

B

Fig. 13.48 Renal tumour. (A) Extended field of view scan showing a hydropic fetus with a renal tumour (H – head, T – tumour). (B) Transverse scan through the fetal abdomen showing a massive renal tumour (T) compressing the bowel (B).

FETAL GENDER

Accurate determination of the fetal gender is possible at or after 20 weeks' gestation in 94 to 100% of cases.[187,188] In the female positive identification of the labia is as essential to the diagnosis as demonstration of the scrotum and penis is in the male (Fig. 13.49).

Demonstration of the fetal sex is of particular importance in X-linked genetic conditions where a female fetus will not be affected by the condition but may still be a carrier.

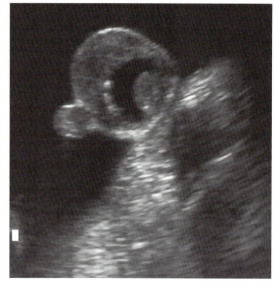

A

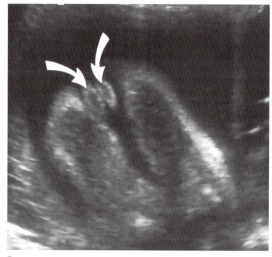

B

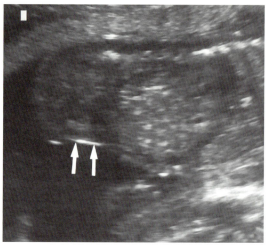

C

Fig. 13.49 Fetal gender. (A) Male fetus. Sagittal scan showing scrotum and penis. There is also a small hydrocoele outlining the testes. Fetal hydrocoeles are not uncommon and are of no clinical significance.· (B) Female fetus. Coronal scan showing both labial folds (curved arrows). (C) Female fetus, sagittal scan showing labial folds (arrows).

References

General

1. Elder J S. Antenatal hydronephrosis fetal and neonatal management. Pediatr Clin North Am 1997;44:1299–1321.
2. Kullendorf C M, Larson L T, Jorgenson C. The advantage of antenatal diagnosis of intestinal and urinary tract malformation. Br J Obstet Gynaecol 1984;91:144–147.
3. Helen I, Personn P H. Prenatal diagnosis of urinary tract abnormalities by ultrasound. Paediatrics 1986;78:879–883.
4. Watson A R, Readett D, Nelson C S. Dilemmas associated with antenatally detected urinary tract abnormalities. Arch Dis Child 1988;63:719–722.
5. Arthur R J, Irving M C, Thomas D F M. Bilateral fetal uropathy: what is the outlook. BMJ 1989; 298:1419–1420.
6. Livera L N, Brookfield D S K, Egginton J A, Hawnaur J M. Antenatal ultrasonography to detect fetal renal abnormalities, a prospective screening programme. BMJ 1989;298:1421–1423.
7. Rosendahl H. Ultrasound screening for fetal urinary tract malformations. A prospective study in the general population. Eur J Obstet Gynecol Reprod Biol 1990;36:27–33.
8. Scott J E, Renwick M. Urological anomalies in the Northern Region Fetal Abnormality Survey. Arch Dis Child 1993;68:22–26.
9. Tam J C, Hodson E M, Choong K L, Cass D T, Cohen R C. Postnatal diagnosis and outcome of urinary tract abnormalities detected by antenatal ultrasound. Med J Aust 1994;160:633–637.
10. Gunn T R, Mora J D, Pease P. Antenatal diagnosis of urinary tract abnormalities by ultrasonography after 28 weeks gestation: incidence and outcome. Am J Obstet Gynecol 1995;172:479–486.
11. James C A, Watson A R, Twining P, Rance C H. Antenatally detected urinary tract abnormalities: changing incidence and management. Eur J Pediatr 1998;157:508–511.
12. Greig J D, Raine P A, Young D G, Azmy A F, MacKenzie J F, Danstan F, Whitle M J, McNay M B. Value of antenatal diagnosis of the urinary tract. BMJ 1989;298:1417–1419.
13. Brand I R, Kaminopatros P, Cave M, Irving H C,

Lilford R J. Specificity of antenatal ultrasound in the Yorkshire Region: a prospective study of 2261 ultrasound detected anomalies. Br J Obstet Gynaecol 1994;101:392–397.

14. Mandell J, Blyth B, Peters C, Retik A, Estroff J, Benacerraf B. Structural genitourinary defects, detected in utero. Radiology 1991;178:193–196.

15. Grignon A, Fillon R, Filitrault D. Urinary tract dilatation in utero – classification and clinical applications. Radiology 1986;160:645–647.

16. Thomas D F M. Fetal uropathy. Br J Urol 1990;66:225–231.

17. Elder J S, Duckett J W, Synder H M. Intervention for fetal obstructive uropathy, has it been effective? Lancet 1987;1007–1010.

18. Nicolaides K H, Cheng H H, Snijders R J M, Moniz C F. Fetal urine biochemistry in the assessment of obstructive uropathy. Am J Obstet Gynecol 1992;166:932–937.

19. Johnson M, Bukowski T P, Reitleman C, Isada N B, Pryde P G, Evans M I. In utero surgical treatment of fetal obstructive uropathy: a new comprehensive approach to identify appropriate candidates for vesico amniotic shunt therapy. Am J Obstet Gynecol 1994;170:1770–1779.

Embryology

20. Larsen W J. Human Embryology. London: Churchill Livingstone; 1993.

21. Wendell Smith C P, Williams P L, Treadgold S. Basic Human Embryology. London: Pitman Publishing; 1984.

Normal appearances

22. Bronshtein M, Yoffe N, Brandes J M, Blumenfeld Z. First and early second-trimester diagnosis of fetal urinary tract anomalies using transvaginal sonography. Prenat Diagn 1990;10:653–666.

23. Corteville J E, Crane J P, Gray D L. Congenital hydronephrosis: correlation of fetal ultrasonographic findings with infant outcome. Am J Obstet Gynecol 1991;165:384–388.

24. Ninosu E C, Welch C R, Manasse P R, Walkinshaw S A. Longitudinal assessment of amniotic fluid index. Br J Obstet Gynaecol 1993;100:816–819.

Renal agenesis

25. Hitchcock R, Burge D M. Renal agenesis: an acquired condition? J Pediatr Surg 1994;29:454–455.

26. Bronshtein M, Amil A, Achiron R, Noy I, Blumenfeld Z. The early prenatal diagnosis of renal agenesis: techniques and possible pitfalls. Prenat Diagn 1994;14:291–297.

27. Roodhooft A M, Birnholz J C, Holmes L B. Familial nature of congenital absence and severe dysplasia of both kidneys. N Engl J Med 1984;310:1341–1345.

28. Kuller J A, Coulson C C, McCoy C, et al. Prenatal diagnosis of renal agenesis in twin gestation. Prenat Diagn 1994;14:1090–1092.

29. Romero R, Cullen M, Graunum P, et al. Antenatal diagnosis of renal anomalies with ultrasound III.

Bilateral renal agenesis. Am J Obstet Gynecol 1985;151:38–43.

30. Potter E L. Bilateral absence of ureters and kidneys: report of fifty cases. Obstet Gynecol 1965;25:3–12.

31. Hoffman C I T, Filly R A, Callen P W. The lying down adrenal sign: a sonographic indicator of renal agenesis or ectopia in fetuses and neonates. J Ultrasound Med 1992;11:533–536.

32. DeVore G R. The value of colour Doppler sonography in the diagnosis of renal agenesis. J Ultrasound Med 1995;14:443–449.

33. Twining P. The value of transvaginal scanning in the assessment of second trimester oligohydramnios. Br J Radiol 1992;65:455–457.

34. Benacerraf B. Examination of the second trimester fetus with severe oligohydramnios using transvaginal scanning. Obstet Gynecol 1990;75:491–493.

35. Gembruch U, Hansmann M. Artificial installation of amniotic fluid as a new technique for the diagnostic evaluation of cases of oligohydramnios. Prenat Diagn 1988;8:33–45.

36. Nicolini U, Santolaya J, Hubinost C, Fisk N, Maxwell D, Rodeck C. Visualisation of fetal intra-abdominal organs in second trimester severe oligohydramnios by intraperinatal infusion. Prenat Diagn 1989;9:191–194.

37. Hackett G, Nicolaides K H, Campbell S. Doppler ultrasound assessment of fetal and uteroplacental circulation in severe second trimester oligohydramnios. Br J Obstet Gynaecol 1987;94:1074–1077.

38. Jeanty P, Romero R, Kepple D, Stoney D, Coggins T, Fleischer A. Prenatal diagnosis in unilateral empty renal fossa. J Ultrasound Med 1990;9:651–654.

Autosomal recessive (infantile) polycystic kidney disease (Potter type I)

39. Zerres K. Autosomal recessive polycystic kidney disease. Clinical Investigator 1992;70:794–901.

40. Tsuda H, Matsumota M, Imanaka M, Ogita S. Measurement of fetal urine production in mild infantile polycystic kidney disease – a case report. Prenat Diagn 1994;14:1083–1085.

41. Osathanondh V, Potter E L. Pathogenesis of polycystic kidneys. Type I due to hypoplasia of interstitial portions of collecting tubules. Arch Pathol 1964;77:466–473.

42. Blyth H, Ockenden B G. Polycystic disease of kidneys and liver presenting in childhood. J Med Genet 1971;8:257–284.

43. Guay-Woodford L M, Meucher G, Hopkins S D, Avner E D, Germino G G, Guillot A P. The severe form of autosomal recessive polycystic kidney disease maps to chromosome 6p21.1–p12: implications for genetic counselling. Am J Hum Genet 1995;56:1101–1107.

44. Romero R, Cullen M, Jeanty P, et al. The diagnosis of congenital renal anomalies with ultrasound II. Infantile polycystic kidney disease. Am J Obstet Gynecol 1984;150:259–262.

45. Wisser J, Hebisch G, Froster U, et al. Prenatal sonographic diagnosis of autosomal recessive polycystic kidney disease during the early second trimester. Prenat Diagn 1995;15:868–871.

46. Mahony B, Cullen P W, Filly R, Golbus M, Progression of infantile polycystic kidney disease in early pregnancy. J Ultrasound Med 1984;3:277–279.

47. Barth R, Guillot A, Capeless E, Clemmons J. Prenatal diagnosis of autosomal recessive polycystic kidney disease: variable outcome in one family. Am J Obstet Gynecol 1992;166:560–567.

48. Zerres K, Hansmann M, Mallmann R, Gembruck. Autosomal recessive polycystic kidney disease: problems of prenatal diagnosis. Prenat Diagn 1988;8:215–229.

49. Bronshtein M, Bar-Hava I, Blumenfeld Z. Clues and pitfalls in the early prenatal diagnosis of 'late onset' infantile polycystic kidney. Prenat Diagn 1992;12:293–298.

50. Kogutt M S, Robichaux W, Boineau F, Drake G, Simonton S. Asymmetric renal size in autosomal recessive polycystic kidney disease: a unique presentation. American Journal of Radiology 1993;160:835–836.

Multicystic renal dysplasia (Potter type II)

51. Garrett W J, Grunewald, G, Robinson D E. Prenatal diagnosis of fetal polycystic kidney by ultrasound. Aus N Z J Obstet Gynecol 1970;10:7–9.

52. Al-Khaldi N, Watson A R, Zuccollo J, Twining P, Rose D H. Outcome of antenatally detected cystic dysplastic kidney disease. Arch Dis Child 1994;70:520–522.

53. Gough D C S, Postlethwaite R J, Lewis M A, Bruce J. Multicystic renal dysplasia diagnosed in the antenatal period: a note of caution. Br J Urol 1995;76:244–248.

54. Rickwood A M K, Anderson P A M, Williams M P L. Multicystic renal dysplasia detected by prenatal ultrasonography. Natural history and results of conservative management. Br J Urol 1992;69:538–540.

55. Thomsen M S, Levine E, Meilstrup J W, et al. Renal cystic diseases. European Radiology 1997;7:1267–1275.

56. D'Alton M, Romero, Grannum P, Jeanty P. Antenatal diagnosis of renal anomalies with ultrasound IV: bilateral multicystic kidney disease. Am J Obstet Gynecol 1986;54:532–537.

57. Hashimoto B, Filly R, Callen P. Multicystic dysplastic kidney in utero: changing appearance on ultrasound. Radiology 1986;159:107–109.

58. Atiyeh B, Husmann D, Baum M. Contralateral renal abnormalities in multicystic–dysplastic kidney disease. J Pediatr 1992;121:65–67.

59. De Klerk D F, Marshall F F, Jeffs R D. Multicystic dysplastic kidney. J Urol 1977;118:306–308.

60. Diard F, le Dosseur P, Cadier L, Calabet A, Bondionny J M. Multicystic dysplasia in the upper component of the complete duplex kidney. Pediatr Radiol 1984;14:310–313.

61. Siegel R L, Rosenfeld D L, Leiman S. Complete regression of a multicystic dysplastic kidney in the setting of renal crossed fused ectopia. JCU 1992;20:466–469.

62. Wacksman J, Phipps L. Report of the multicystic kidney registry: preliminary findings. J Urol 1993;150:1870–1872.

63. Hartman G E, Smolik L M, Shocat S J. The dilemma of the multicystic dysplastic kidney. Am J Dis Child 1986;140:925–928.

64. Chen Y H, Stapleton F B, Roy S, Noe H N. Neonatal hypertension from a unilateral multicystic dysplastic kidney. J Urol 1985;133:664.

65. Homsy Y L, Anderson J H, Oudjhane K, Russo P. Wilms tumour and multicystic dysplastic kidney disease. J Urol 1997;158:2256–2260.

66. Goncalves De Oliveira-Filho A, Carvalho M H, Sbragia-Neto L, Miranda M L, Bustorff-Silva J M, Rissotode Oliveira E. Wilms tumour in a prenatally diagnosed multicystic kidney. J Urol 1997;158:1926–1927.

67. Strife J, Souza A S, Kirks D, Strife C F, Gelfand M J, Wacksman J. Multicystic dysplastic kidney in children: US follow up. Radiology 1993;186:785–788.

Autosomal dominant (adult) polycystic renal disease (Potter type III)

68. Parfrey P S, Bear J C, Morgan J, et al. The diagnosis and prognosis of autosomal dominant polycystic kidney disease. N Engl J Med 1990;323:1085–1090.

69. Michaud J, Russo P, Grignon A, et al. Autosomal dominant polycystic disease in the fetus. Am J Med Genet 1994;51:240–246.

70. Reeders S T, Breuning M H, Davies K E, et al. A highly polymorphic DNA marker linked to adult type polycystic kidney disease on chromosome 16. Nature 1985;317:542–544.

71. Kimberling W J, Kumar S, Gabow P. Autosomal dominant polycystic kidney disease: localisation of the second gene to chromosome 4q13–q23. Genomics 1995;18:467–472.

72. MacDermot K D, Saggar-Malik A K, Economides S J. Prenatal diagnosis of autosomal dominant polycystic kidney disease (PDK 1) presenting in utero and prognosis for very early onset disease. J Med Genet 1998;35:13–16.

73. Zerres K, Weis H, Bulla M, Roth B. Prenatal diagnosis of an early manifestation of autosomal dominant adult type polycystic kidney disease. Lancet 1982;2:988.

74. Pretorius D, Lee M, Manco-Johnson M, Weingast G, Sedman A, Gabour P. Diagnosis of autosomal dominant polycystic kidney disease in utero and in the young infant. J Ultrasound Med 1987;6:249–255.

75. McHugo J, Shafi M I, Rowlands D, Weaver J B. Prenatal diagnosis of adult polycystic kidney disease. Br J Radiol 1988;61:1072–1074.

76. Fick G M, Johnson A M, Strain J D, Kimberling W J, Kumar S, Manco-Johnson M L. Characteristics of very early onset autosomal dominant polycystic kidney disease. J Am Soc Nephrol 1993;3:1863–1870.

77. Sinibaldi D, Malena S, Mingarelli R, Rizzoni G. Prenatal ultrasonographic findings of dominant polycystic kidney disease and postnatal evolution. Am J Med Genet 1996;65:337–341.

78. Turco A E, Padovani E M, Chiaffoni G P, Peissel B, Rossetti S, Marcolongo A. Molecular genetics of autosomal dominant polycystic kidney disease in a newborn with bilateral cystic kidneys detected prenatally and multiple skeletal malformations. J Med Genet 1993;30:419–422.

79. Main D, Mennuti M T, Cornfield D, Coleman B. Prenatal diagnosis of adult polycystic kidney disease. Lancet 1983;2:337–338.

80. Hartman S S. Unilateral adult polycystic kidney. J Ultrasound Med 1982;1:371–374.

81. Middlebrook P F, Nizalik E, Schillinger J F. Unilateral renal cystic disease; a case presentation. J Urol 1992;148:1221–1223.

82. Ravine D, Gibson R N, Walker R G, Sheffield L J, Kincard-Smith P, Danks D M. Evaluation of ultrasonographic diagnostic criteria for autosomal dominant polycystic kidney disease 1. Lancet 1994;343:824–827.

83. Choong K L, Gruenwald S M, Hodson E. Echogenic fetal kidneys in cytomegalovirus infection. JCU 1993;21:138–132.

84. Moore B S, Pretorus D, Scioscia A, Reznik V. Sonographic findings in a fetus with congenital nephrotic syndrome of the Finnish type. J Ultrasound Med 1992;11:113–116.

85. Fishman J E, Joseph R C. Renal vein thrombosis in utero: duplex sonography in diagnosis and follow up. Pediatr Radiol 1994;24:135–136.

86. Lok J P, Hailer J O, Kassner E G, Aloni A, Glassberg K. Dominantly inherited polycystic kidneys in infants: associated with hypertrophic pyloric stenosis. Pediatr Radiol 1977;6:27–30.

Obstructive cystic dysplasia (Potter type IV)

87. Saunders R C, Nassbaum A R, Solez K. Renal dysplasia: sonographic findings. Radiology 1988;167:623–626.

88. Mahony B S, Filly R, Callen P W, Hricak H, Golbus M, Harrison M R. Fetal renal dysplasia: sonographic evaluation. Radiology 1984;152:143–146.

89. Benacerraf B, Peters C, Mandell J. The prenatal evolution of a non functioning kidney in the setting of obstructive hydronephrosis. JCU 1991; 19:446–450.

90. Avni E F, Thoua Y, Van Gansbeke. Development of the hypodysplastic kidney; contribution of antenatal US diagnosis. Radiology 1987;164:123–125.

91. Nussbaum A R, Dorst J P, Jeffs R D, Gearhart J P, Sanders R C. Ectopic ureter and ureterocoele: their varied sonographic manifestations. Radiology 1986;159:227–235.

Echogenic kidneys

92. Estroff J, Mandell J, Benacerraf B. Increased renal parenchryal echogenicity in the fetus: importance and clinical outcome. Radiology 1991;181:135–139.

93. Chitty L S, Griffin D R, Johnson P. The differential diagnosis of enlarged hyperechogenic kidneys with normal or increased liquor: report of five cases and review of the literature. Ultrasound Obstet Gynecol 1991;1:115–119.

94. Nyberg D, Hallesy D, Mahony B, Hirsch I, Luthy D, Hickok D. Meckel–Gruber Syndrome. Importance of prenatal diagnosis. J Ultrasound Med 1990;9:691–696.

Renal obstruction

95. Cendron M, D'Alton M E, Crombleholme T M. Prenatal diagnosis and management of the fetus with hydronephrosis. Semin Perinatol 1994;18:163–181.

96. Anderson N, Clautice-Engle T, Allan R, Abbott G, Wells J E. Detection of obstructive uropathy in the fetus: predictive value of sonographic measurements of renal pelvic diameter at various gestational ages. Am J Radiol 1995;164:719–723.

97. Adra A M, Mejides A A, Dennoui M S, Beydown S N. Fetal pyelectasis: is it always physiologic? Am J Obstet Gynecol 1995;173:1263–1266.

98. Ouzounian J G, Cantro M A, Fresquez M, Al-Sulyman O M, Kovacs B W. Diagnostic significance of antenatally detected fetal pyelectasis. Ultrasound Obstet Gynecol 1996;7:424–428.

99. Johnson C E, Elder J, Judge N E, Adeeb F N, Grisoni E R, Fattlar D C. The accuracy of antenatal ultrasonography in identifying renal abnormalities. Am J Dis Child 1992;146:1181–1184.

100. Dudley J A, Haworth J A, McGraw M E, Frank J D, Tizard E J. Clinical relevance and implications of antenatal hydronephrosis. Arch Dis Child 1997;76:F31–F34.

101. Barker A F, Cave M M, Thomas D F M, Lilford R J, Irvine H C, Arthur R J, Smith S E W. Fetal pelvi-ureteric junction obstruction: predictions of outcome. Br J Urol 1995;76:649–652.

102. Arger P H, Coleman B G, Mintz M C, et al. Routine fetal genitourinary tract screening. Radiology 1985;156:485–489.

103. Stocks A, Richards D, Frentzen B, Richard G. Correlation of prenatal renal pelvis anteroposterior diameter with outcome in infancy. J Urol 1996;155:1050–1052.

104. Zerin M J, Richey M L, Chang A C H. Incidental vesico-ureteral reflux in neonates with antenatally detected hydronephrosis and other renal anomalies. Radiology 1993;187:157–160.

105. Marra G, Barbieri G, Moioli C, Assael B M, Grumieri G, Caccamo M L. Mild fetal hydronephrosis indicating vesicoureteric reflux. Arch Dis Child 1994;70:F147–149.

106. Morin L, Cendron M, Crombleholme T M, Garmel S, Klauber G T, D'Alton M E. Minimal hydronephrosis in the fetus: clinical significance and implications for management. J Urol 1996;155:2047–2049.

107. Newell S J, Morgan M E I, McHugo J M, et al. Clinical significance of antenatal calyceal dilatation detected by ultrasound. Lancet 1990;372.

108. Nicolaides K H, Cheng H H, Abbas A, Snijders R J M, Gosden C. Fetal renal defects: associated malformations and chromosomal defects. Fetal Diagn Ther 1992;7:1–11.
109. Corteville J E, Dicke J M, Crane J P. Fetal pyelectasis and Down's Syndrome: is genetic amniocentesis warranted? Obstet Gynecol 1992;79:770–772.
110. Wickstrom E A, Thangavelu M, Parilla B V, Tamura R K, Sabbagha R. A prospective study of the association between isolated fetal pyelectasis and chromosomal abnormality. Obstet Gynecol 1996;88:379–382.
111. Chitty L, Chudleigh T, Campbell S, Pembray M. Incidence, natural history and clinical significance of fetal pyelectasis. Br J Radiol 1992;65:636.
112. Wickstrom E, Maizels M, Sabbagha R E, Tamura R K, Cohen L C, Pergament E. Isolated fetal pyelectasis: assessment of risk for postnatal uropathy and Down's Syndrome. Ultrasound Obstet Gynecol 1996;8:236–240.
113. Benacerraf B, Mandell J, Estroff J A, Harlow B L, Frigoletto F. Fetal pyelectasis: a possible association with Down's Syndrome. Obstet Gynecol 1990;76:58–60.
114. Snijders R J M, Nicolaides K H. Ultrasound marker for fetal chromosomal defects. Frontiers in Medicine Series. London: The Parthenon Publishing Group;1996.
115. Thomas D F M, Gordon A C. The management of prenatally diagnosed uropathies. Arch Dis Child 1989;64:58–63.
116. Reznick V M, Kaplan G W, Murphy J L. Follow up of infants with bilateral renal disease detected in utero. Am J Dis Child 1988;142:453–456.
117. Thomas D F M. Prenatally detected uropathy: epidemiological considerations. Br J Urol 1998;81:Supplement 2, 8–12.

Pelvi-ureteric junction obstruction
118. Kleiner B, Callen P W, Filly F A. Sonographic analysis of the fetus with uretero-pelvic junction obstruction. Am J Radiol 1987;148:359–363.
119. Bosman G, Reuss A, Nijman J M, Wladimiroff J W. Prenatal diagnosis, management and outcome of fetal uretero-pelvic junction obstruction. Ultrasound Med Biol 1991;17:117–120.
120. Jaffe R, Abramowicz J, Fejgin M, Ben-Aderet N. Giant fetal abdominal cyst. Ultrasonic diagnosis and management. J Ultrasound Med 1987;6:45–47.
121. Drake D P, Stevens P, Eckstein H B. Hydronephrosis secondary to uretero-pelvic obstruction in children: a review of 14 years' experience. J Urol 1978;119:649–651.
122. Gordon I, Dhillon H H, Peters A M. Antenatal diagnosis of renal pelvic dilatation – the natural history of conservative management. Pediatr Radiol 1991;21:272–275.
123. Madden N P, Thomas D F M, Gordon A C, Arthur R J, Irving H C, Smith S E W. Antenatally detected pelvic-ureteric junction obstruction. Is non operation safe? Br J Urol 1991;68:305–310.

124. Arnold A J, Rickwood A M K. Natural history of pelvic-ureteric obstruction detected by prenatal sonography. Br J Urol 1990;65:91–96.
125. O'Flynn, Gough D C S, Gupta S, Lewis M A, Postlethwaite R J. Prediction of recovery in antenatally diagnosed hydronephrosis. Br J Urol 1993;71:478–480.
126. Koff S, Campbell K D. The non operative management of unilateral neonatal hydronephrosis: natural history of poorly functioning kidneys. J Urol 1994;152:593–595.
127. Atwell J D. Familial pelvic-ureteric junction obstruction and its association with a duplex pelvicalyceal system and vesico-ureteric reflux. A family study. Br J Urol 1985;57:365–369.
128. Buscemi M, Shanke A, Mallet E. Dominantly inherited ureteropelvic junction obstruction. Urology 1985;24:568–571.

Vesico-ureteric junction obstruction
129. Dunn V, Glasier C M. Ultrasonographic antenatal demonstration of primary megaureters. J Ultrasound Med 1985;4:101–103.
130. Liu H Y A, Dhillon H K, Yeung C K, Diamond D A, Duffy P, Ransley P G. Clinical outcome and management of prenatally diagnosed primary megaureters. J Urol 1994;152:614–617.
131. Rickwood A M K, Jee L D, Williams M P L, Anderson P A M. Natural history of obstructed and pseudo-obstructed megaureters detected by prenatal ultrasonography. Br J Urol 1992;70:322–325.
132. Peters C A. Lower urinary tract obstruction: clinical and experimental aspects. Br J Urol 1998;81:Supplement 2,22–32.

Ureterocoele and ectopic ureter
133. Cremin B J. A review of the ultrasonic appearances of posterior urethral valve and ureterocoeles. Pediatr Radiol 1986;16:357–364.
134. Sherer D M, Hulbert W C. Prenatal sonographic diagnosis and subsequent conservative surgical management of bilateral ureterocoeles. Am J Perinatol 1995;12:174–177.
135. Nussbaum A R, Dorst J P, Jeffs R D, Gearhart J P, Sanders R C. Ectopic ureter and ureterocoele: their varied sonographic manifestations. Radiology 1986;159:227–235.
136. Sherer D M, Menashe M, Lebensort P, Matoth I, Basel D. Sonographic diagnosis of unilateral fetal renal duplication with associated ectopic ureterocoele. JCU 1989;17:371–373.
137. Winters W D, Lebowitz R L. Importance of prenatal detection of hydronephrosis of the upper pole. Am J Radiol 1990;155:125–129.
138. Fitzsimmons P J, Frost R A, Millward S, De Marcia J, Toi A. Prenatal and immediate postnatal ultrasonographic diagnosis of ureterocoele. Journal of Canadian Association of Radiologists 1986;37:189–191.
139. Cuplen D E, Duckett J W. The modern approach to ureterocoeles. J Urol 1995;153:166–169.

Posterior urethral valves

140. Hayden S A, Russ P D, Pretorius D H, Manco-Johnson M L, Chilwell W H. Posterior urethral obstruction. Prenatal sonographic findings and clinical outcome in fourteen cases. J Ultrasound Med 1988;7:371–375.

141. Glazer G M, Filly R, Callen P W. The varied sonographic appearance of the urinary tract in the fetus and newborn with urethral obstruction. Radiology 1982;144:563–568.

142. Hatjis C G. In utero diagnosis of spontaneous fetal urinary bladder rupture. JCU 1993;21:645–647.

143. Mandell J, Lebowitz R L, Peters G A, Estroff J, Retik A B, Benacerraf B C. Prenatal diagnosis of the megacystis-megaureter association. J Urol 1992;148:720–723.

144. Simma B, Gabner I, Brezinka C, Ellemunter H, Kreiczy A. Complete prenatal obstruction caused by congenital megalourethra. JCU 1992;20:197–199.

145. McNamara H M, Onwude J L, Thornton J G. Megacystis-microcolon-intestinal hypoperistalsis syndrome: a case report supporting autosomal recessive inheritance. Prenat Diagn 1994;14:153–154.

146. Hobbins J C, Romero R, Grannum P. Antenatal diagnosis of renal anomalies with ultrasound – I – obstructive uropathy. Am J Obstet Gynecol 1984; 148:868–873.

147. Manning F A, Harrison M R, Rodeck C H. Catheter shunts for fetal hydronephrosis and hydrocephalus. N Engl J Med 1986;315:336–342.

148. Smythe A R. Ultrasonic detection of fetal ascites and bladder dilatation with resulting prune belly. J Pediatr 1981;98:978–982.

149. Hulbert W C, Rosenberg H K, Cartwright P C, Duckett J W, McGum, Snyder H. The predictive value of ultrasonography in evaluation of infants with posterior urethral valves. J Urol 1992;148:122–124.

150. Hutton K A R, Thomas P F M, Arthur R J, Irving H C, Smith S E W. Prenatally detected posterior urethra valves: is gestational age at detection a predictor of outcome? J Urol 1994;152:698–701.

151. Glick P L, Harrison M R, Adzick N S, Noall R A, Villa R L. Correction of congenital hydronephrosis in utero IV: in utero decompression prevents renal dysplasia. J Pediatr Surg 1984;19:649–656.

152. Crombleholme T M, Harrison M R, Golbus M S, et al. Fetal intervention in obstructive uropathy: prognostic indicators and efficiency of intervention. Am J Obstet Gynecol 1990;162:1239–1244.

153. Lun A, Lenz F, Priem F, Brux B, Gross J, Bollman R. Biochemical diagnosis in prenatal uropathy. Clin Biochem 1994;27:283–287.

154. Quintero R A, Hume R, Smith C. Percutaneous fetal cystoscopy and endoscopic fulguration of posterior urethral valves. Am J Obstet Gynecol 1995;172:206–209.

Veisco-ureteric reflux

155. Marra G, Barbieri G, Dell'Agnola C A, Caccamo M L, Castellani M R, Assael B M. Congenital renal damage associated with primary vesico-ureteral reflux detected prenatally in male infants. J Pediatr 1994;124:726–730.

156. Elder J S. Commentary: importance of antenatal diagnosis of vesico-ureteric reflux. J Urol 1992;148:1750–1754.

157. Avni E F, Sopulman C C. The origin of vesico-ureteric reflux in male newborns: further evidence in favour of a transient fetal urethral obstruction. Br J Urol 1996;78:454–457.

158. Anderson P A M, Rickwood A M K. Features of primary vesico-ureteric reflux detected by prenatal sonography. Br J Urol 1991;67:267–271.

159. Scott J E S. Fetal ureteric reflux: a follow up study. Br J Urol 1993;71:481–483.

160. Stewart G D, Abluwalia A, Gowland M. Case report: diagnosis of fetal vesico-ureteric reflux as the cause of pelvicalyceal dilatation on antenatal ultrasound. Clin Radiol 1995;50:192–194.

161. Weiss R, Duckett J, Spitzer A. Results of a randomised clinical trial of medical versus surgical management of infants and children with Grades III and IV primary vesico-ureteral reflux. J Urol 1992;148:1667–1673.

Persistent cloaca

162. Jaramillo D, Lebowitz R L, Hendren W H. The cloacal malformation: radiologic findings and imaging recommendations. Radiology 1990;177:441–448.

163. Karlin G, Brock W, Rich M, Pena A. Persistent cloaca and phallic urethra. J Urol 1989;142:1056–1059.

164. Cilento B G, Benacerraf B R, Mandell J. Prenatal diagnosis of cloacal malformation. Urology 1994;43:386–388.

165. Davis G H, Wapner R J, Kurtz A B, Chibber G, Fitzsimmons J, Blocklinger A J. Antenatal diagnosis of hydrometrocolpos by ultrasound examination. J Ultrasound Med 1984;3:371–374.

166. Nussbaum Blask A R, Saunders R C, Gearhart J P. Obstructed utero-vaginal anomalies: demonstration with sonography. Radiology 1991;179:79–83.

167. Arulkumaran S, Nicolini V, Fisk N N, Rodeck C H. Fetal vesicorectal fistula causing oligohydramnios in the second trimester. Br J Obstet Gynaecol 1990;97:449–451.

Cloacal and bladder exstrophy

168. Chitril Y, Zorn B, Filidori M, Robert E, Chasseray J E. Cloacal exstrophy in monozygotic twins detected through antenatal ultrasound scanning. JCU 1993;21:339–342.

169. Wood B P. Cloacal malformations and exstrophy syndromes. Radiology 1990;177:326–327.

170. Richards D S, Langham M R, Mahaffey S M. The prenatal ultrasonographic diagnosis of cloacal exstrophy. J Ultrasound Med 1992;11:507–510.

171. Zaontz M R, Packer M G. Abnormalities of the external genitalia. Pediatr Clin North Am 1997;44:1277–1283.

172. Stolar C J, Randolph J G, Flanigan L P. Cloacal exstrophy: individualised management through a

staged surgical approach. J Pediatr Surg 1990;25:505–510.

173. Mirk P, Calisti A, Fileni A. Prenatal sonographic diagnosis of bladder exstrophy. J Ultrasound Med 1986;5:291–293.

174. Barth R A, Filly R A, Sandheimer. Prenatal sonographic findings in bladder exstrophy. J Ultrasound Med 1990;9:359–361.

Horseshoe kidney, pelvic kidney and crossed renal ectopia

175. Decter R M. Renal duplication and fusion anomalies. Pediatr Clin North Am 1997;44:1336–1341.

176. Sherer D M, Cullen J B H, Thompson H O, Metlay L A, Woods J R. Prenatal sonographic findings associated with a fetal horseshoe kidney. J Ultrasound Med 1990;9:477–479.

177. King K L, Kofinas A D, Simon N V, Clay D. Antental ultrasound diagnosis of fetal horseshoe kidney. J Ultrasound Med 1991;10:643–644.

178. Boatman D L. Congenital anomalies associated with horseshoe kidney. J Urol 1972;107:205–209.

179. Hill L, Peterson C S. Antenatal diagnosis of fetal pelvic kidneys. J Ultrasound Med 1987;6:393–396.

180. Greenblatt A M, Beretsky I, Lankin D H, Phelans L. In utero diagnosis of crossed renal ectopia using high resolution real time ultrasound. J Ultrasound Med 1985;4:105–107.

Renal tumours

181. Apuzzio J J, Unwin W, Adhate A, Nichols R. Prenatal diagnosis of fetal renal mesoblastic nephroma. Am J Obstet Gynecol 1986;154:636–637.

182. Geirsson R T, Ricketts N E M, Taylor D J, Coghill S. Prenatal appearance of a mesoblastic nephroma associated with polyhydramnios. JCU 1985;13:488–490.

183. Matsumura M, Nishi T, Sasaki Y, Yamada R, Yamamoto H, Olhama Y, et al. Prenatal diagnosis and treatment strategy for congenital mesoblastic nephroma. J Pediatr Surg 1993;28:1607–1609.

184. Fung T Y, Hedy Fung Y M, Ng P C, Yeung C K, Allan Chang M Z. Polyhydramnios and hypercalcaemia associated with congenital mesoblastic nephroma: case report and a new appraisal. Obstet Gynecol 1995;85:815–817.

185. Giulian B B. Prenatal ultrasonographic diagnosis of fetal renal tumours. Radiology 1984;152:69–70.

186. Yambao T J, Schwartz D, Henderson R, Rapp G, Anthony W, Denko J. Prenatal diagnosis of a congenital mesoblastic nephroma, a case report. J Reprod Med 1986;31:257–259.

Fetal gender

187. Elejalde B R, Mercedes de Elejalde M, Keitman T. Visualisation of the fetal genitalia, by ultrasonography. A review of the literature and ethical implication. J Ultrasound Med 1985;4:633–639.

188. Stephens J D, Sherman S. Determination of fetal sex by ultrasound. N Engl J Med 1983;309:984.

CHAPTER 14

Chromosomal abnormalities

Peter Twining

Introduction

The advent of ultrasound has meant that fetal disease can now be diagnosed. Although chromosomal disease as such cannot be treated, if a diagnosis is made before viability, then a termination of pregnancy can be offered to the mother. When the diagnosis is made late in pregnancy, it can be useful in deciding the mode of delivery. In particular, a caesarean section for fetal distress may be avoided as this is a frequent complication in certain chromosomal abnormalities.[1] In addition, the antenatal diagnosis gives the patient time to come to terms with the diagnosis and to prepare for the possibility of surgery to the baby in the neonatal period.

It is well established that although the incidence of chromosomal disease in the newborn period is relatively low, the number of fetuses with chromosomal disease in the first and second trimesters of pregnancy is considerably higher. This is due to the fact that a proportion of fetuses with chromosomal disease will not survive to term. It has been estimated that up to 30% of fetuses with trisomy 21, 74% of trisomy 18 fetuses and 71% of trisomy 13 fetuses will be lost between 16 weeks' gestation and term.[2–5] In view of this, the antenatal diagnosis of chromosomal disease is a major challenge to those carrying out obstetric ultrasound and where fetal abnormalities are seen, chromosomal disease should always be considered.

The antenatal diagnosis of chromosomal disease is based on the detection of certain fetal abnormalities. Nicolaides et al have shown a high correlation between multiple abnormalities and chromosomal disease[6,7] (Table 14.1). For example, if two or more abnormalities are seen, then the risk of chromosomal disease is 29%, whereas when five abnormalities are seen in a fetus, this risk rises to 70%.[7] There are, however, a number of patterns of abnormalities that are well established in indicating a specific chromosomal syndrome.[8] In effect, then, not only are we looking for multiple abnormalities, but also a series of specific abnormalities, a constellation of findings which fits together like pieces in a jigsaw puzzle to form the final picture.[9]

Although fetuses with multiple abnormalities have a high incidence of chromosomal disease, there are some abnormalities which, even if isolated, also carry an increased risk of chromosomal disease. The prevalence of chromosomal disease for various abnormalities is outlined in Table 14.2. It is seen that isolated cystic hygroma, nuchal oedema, duodenal atresia, omphalocoele and certain cardiac abnormalities have a high rate of chromosomal disease, whereas isolated facial clefting and talipes carry a low risk of chromosomal disease. There are also a number of other abnormalities that carry a low risk of chromosomal disease and these are outlined in Table 14.3.

It is important, however, at this stage to state that the concept of an isolated

Table 14.1
Frequency of chromosomal abnormalities and number of ultrasound detected defects

| No. of defects | Percentage of fetuses with a chromosomal abnormality | Type of chromosomal abnormality (%) | | | | | |
| | | Trisomy | | | Turner's | Triploidy | Other |
		21	18	13			
>2	29	21	30	11	13	15	8
>3	48	16	35	13	8	15	5
>4	62	12	42	15	12	12	6
>5	70	5	54	20	9	10	5
>6	72	—	62	20	14	16	9
>7	82	—	79	15	—	3	3
>8	92	—	77	18	—	—	3

Reproduced with permission from Nicolaides K, Snijders RJM, Gosden CM, et al. Ultrasonographically detectable markers of fetal chromosomal abnormalities. Lancet 1992; 340:704–707.

Table 14.2

Prevalence of fetal chromosomal defects in fetuses with isolated and multiple abnormalities

Abnormality	Isolated	Multiple
Ventriculomegaly	2%	17%
Holoprosencephaly	4%	39%
Choroid plexus cysts	<1%	48%
Posterior fossa cyst	0%	52%
Facial cleft	0%	51%
Micrognathia	—	62%
Cystic hygroma	52%	71%
Nuchal oedema	19%	45%
Diaphragmatic hernia	2%	49%
Heart defects	16%	66%
Duodenal atresia	38%	64%
Exomphalos	8%	46%
Talipes	0%	33%
Growth retardation	4%	38%

Reproduced with permission from Snijders RJM, Nicolaides K. Ultrasound markers for fetal chromosomal defects. London: Parthenon; 1996.

Table 14.3

Fetal abnormalities with a low prevalence of chromosomal abnormalities

Gastroschisis
Jejunal atresia
Large bowel obstruction
Unilateral multicystic kidney
Ovarian, duplication, mesenteric cysts
Hemivertebra
Fetal tumours
Cystic adenomatoid malformation of lung
Sequestrated segment of lung
Porencephaly
Schizencephaly

abnormality is dependent upon the skill and experience of the person carrying out the scan, the quality of the ultrasound equipment used and the stage and conditions of the pregnancy. Many early studies reported high rates of missed associated abnormalities which may, in part, have been related to the ultrasound equipment available at that time. For example, in the antenatal diagnosis of ventriculomegaly, early series indicated false-negative diagnosis of associated abnormalities in the range of 21 to 60%.[10–12] Later reports have shown considerable improvement with a 98% accuracy in the diagnosis of isolated ventriculomegaly.[13] The exclusion of associated abnormalities is a challenging task and requires a meticulous assessment of the fetus by highly trained personnel. In addition, oligohydramnios and maternal obesity can significantly hinder visualization of the fetus and can make demonstration of associated abnormalities extremely difficult. The gestational age of the fetus is also important as many anomalies, particularly cardiac abnormalities, can be missed if scanning is carried out prior to 18 weeks' gestation.

Another important point is that for a given malformation, the risk of a chromosomal abnormality may be inversely related to the severity of the defect.[7] For example, fetuses with a small omphalocoele (containing bowel only) have a much higher risk of a chromosomal defect than those with large omphalocoeles which may contain bowel and liver.[14] Similarly, fetuses with mild ventriculomegaly or mild dilatation of the renal pelvises have a higher risk of chromosomal disease than fetuses with established hydrocephalus or hydronephrosis.[15–17]

In addition to specific abnormalities, there are a number of non-specific findings that can suggest the presence of chromosomal disease. Intra-uterine growth retardation is a common finding in chromosomal disease occurring in up to 51% of fetuses with trisomy 18[18] and can occur early in the second trimester in triploidy.[19] The type of growth retardation is not specific for chromosomal disease. However, up to 30 weeks' gestation, it is more likely to be symmetrical in nature and after 30 weeks may be asymmetrical. Umbilical artery Doppler waveforms are also more likely to be normal in growth-retarded fetuses secondary to chromosomal disease.[20]

One other non-specific finding is the presence of polyhydramnios which in isolation has a low incidence of chromosomal disease; however, if growth retardation is present, then this finding not only carries a high suspicion of a chromosomal defect but should always prompt the search for fetal abnormalities associated with chromosomal disease.[47]

There has recently been considerable interest in developing markers of chromosomal disease in the first trimester of pregnancy. Nicolaides et al have reported that by measuring the subcutaneous fluid overlying the fetal cervical spine at 10 to 14 weeks, it is possible to detect over 80% of fetuses with trisomy 21, with a false-positive rate of 5%.[21] This is an extremely exciting new development and will be discussed in more detail in the section on trisomy 21 (p. 326).

In a proportion of fetuses with chromosomal disease, the signs of the condition may be so subtle that it may not be possible to make a diagnosis using ultrasound. This is most evident in trisomy 21 where at best only 33% of fetuses will demonstrate abnormalities at 18 to 20 weeks' gestation.[9,77] In trisomy 18 and trisomy 13 up to 17% and 8% of fetuses respectively may appear normal on ultrasound scanning.[35,47]

In the UK, most women are offered a routine ultrasound scan at 18 to 20 weeks' gestation[22] and this has proven to be effective in detecting fetal abnormalities.[23,24] This involves a full anatomical scan of the fetus, including assessment of the head, thorax and abdomen. Detailed ultrasound scans are reserved for high-risk pregnancies and are usually carried out at tertiary referral centres. These involve closer scrutiny of the fetus with special attention placed on visualizing the fetal face, hands, feet and heart. It is often the face, heart and extremities that may give the clue to the presence of a chromosomal defect.

When a chromosomal defect is suspected, it must always be confirmed by cytogenic analysis. Although amniocentesis has long been the mainstay for karyotyping fetuses, the main disadvantage is a 2 to 3-week delay in obtaining the result. This situation has been revolutionized with the development of chorion villus sampling or placental biopsy. The advantage of this technique is that a result can be obtained in under 2 days[25] which is extremely important when an ultrasound diagnosis is made at 18 to 20 weeks' gestation.

Cordocentesis is another technique that can be used to obtain a fetal karyotype[26] with a result available within 2 to 4 days. The overall loss rate for cordocentesis is approximately 1 to 2%;[27] however, this can rise to as much as 14 to 25% in the presence of severe growth retardation and hydrops.[28] There are, however, new cytogenic techniques such as fluorescent in situ hybridization[29] which hold the promise of a rapid karyotype, i.e. within 2 days from an amniocentesis sample.[30] Furthermore, the application of this technique to fetal cells harvested from the maternal circulation[31] holds the promise of a non-invasive means of obtaining a fetal karyotype in the future.

Trisomy 13

This condition was first described by Pattau in 1960.[32] The incidence is 1 in 5000 and the prognosis for a baby with this condition is extremely poor. 50% of babies with trisomy 13 will die within the first month, 75% die within 6 months and less than 5% survive to 3 years of age.[33] As stated earlier, the important ultrasound findings are seen in the head, face, hands and heart (Table 14.4).

Table 14.4
Frequency of abnormalities in fetuses with trisomy 13

Abnormality	Incidence (%)
Head	
Holoprosencephaly	75
Agenesis of corpus callosum	22
Dandy–Walker syndrome	20
Hydrocephalus	13
Face	
Cleft lip and palate	75
Low-set ears	
Hands/feet	
Polydactyly	65
Heart	
Ventricular septal defect	
Atrioventricular septal defect	80
Hypoplastic left heart	
Kidney	
Renal cyst dysplasia	
Hydronephrosis	30
Abdomen	
Omphalocoele	30
General	
Growth retardation	> 90

Reproduced with permission from Reid GB, Claireux AE, Cockburn F, eds. Disease of the fetus and newborn. London: Chapman and Hall Medical; 1995.

Cranial anomalies

The fetal head may show microcephaly, and intracranial abnormalities are common in fetuses with trisomy 13, in particular holoprosencephaly (Fig. 14.1). In one series of antenatally diagnosed holoprosencephaly, trisomy 13 occurred in 40% of cases.[34] The other common intracranial abnormalities are the Dandy–Walker syndrome and ventriculomegaly. Enlargement of the cisterna magna which may reflect subtle cerebellar abnormalities can be seen in fetuses with trisomy 13 and has also been described in fetuses with trisomy 18.[66] Occasionally neural tube defects may be seen in trisomy 13.

Facial anomalies

Facial clefting is a frequent observation in trisomy 13, occurring in up to 47% of cases,[35] and is often associated with holoprosencephaly.[36] The facial appearances in this condition range from cyclopia with proboscis to hypotelorism with median facial clefting and it is often stated that 'the face predicts the brain' as the changes are so characteristic. These facial abnormalities will be discussed in more detail in Chapter 15. Facial clefting may also occur in trisomy 13 without the presence of holoprosencephaly, usually in the form of bilateral cleft lip and palate.[37]

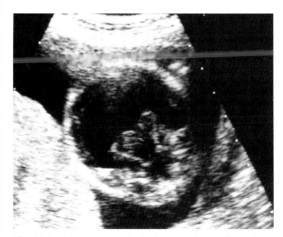

Fig. 14.1 Holoprosencephaly. A coronal scan through the fetal head of an 18-week fetus, showing a large, single, ventricular cavity typical of holoprosencephaly.

Hands and feet

Postaxial polydactyly is another common finding in trisomy 13, occurring in up to 60% of fetuses and this may affect both the hands and feet[35] (Fig. 14.2). Less frequently, one may see flexion of the fingers with or without overlapping. In addition, talipes and rocker-bottom feet may be present in up to 10% of affected fetuses.

Cardiac anomalies

The most important cardiac abnormalities are ventricular septal defects, atrioventricular septal defects and the hypoplastic left heart.[38,39] Echogenic foci within the hypoplastic left ventricle have also been described[35] (Fig. 14.3).

Abdominal anomalies

In the abdomen, an omphalocoele is the commonest abnormality and more likely to contain bowel only.[14] Cystic renal disease and hydronephrosis are also seen in approximately 30% of fetuses. In this context, it is important to differentiate Meckel's syndrome which may present with cystic renal disease, polydactyly and occipital encephalocoele with posterior fossa abnormalities.[40] The outlook for both conditions is equally poor; however, Meckel's syndrome, which has a normal karyotype, has an autosomal recessive inheritance and so an accurate diagnosis is essential in terms of counselling for future pregnancies. This point highlights the importance of obtaining a karyotype in fetuses with multiple abnormalities and its bearing on future pregnancies and genetic counselling.

As mentioned earlier, the vast majority of fetuses with trisomy 13 will also show growth retardation when seen in the late second and early third trimesters. Up to 30 weeks' gestation, symmetrical growth retardation is common but after 30 weeks, the picture is more often that of asymmetrical growth retardation. The Doppler waveforms are also likely to be normal in this situation.[20]

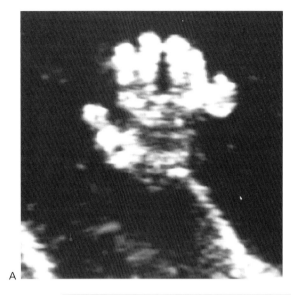

A

Fig. 14.2 Polydactyly. (A) Coronal scan through the hand of an 18-week fetus, showing postaxial polydactyly. (B) Post-mortem appearance of same fetus. (Reproduced with permission from Twining P, Zuccollo J. Ultrasound markers of chromosomal disease. Br J Radiol 1993; 66:408–414.)

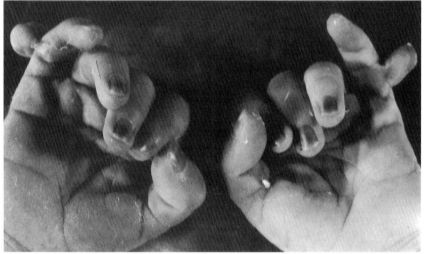

B

Polyhydramnios may also be seen and together with growth retardation are common findings in fetuses with chromosomal disease.[6]

Generalized hydrops with or without the presence of cystic hygroma can be seen in up to 24% of fetuses with trisomy 13[35] and should always prompt a karyotype examination.

A number of rare associations has also been described and these include umbilical cord cysts[41] and cholecystomegaly.[42] The author has also seen a case of multiple echogenic foci within the liver in association with persistence of the right umbilical vein

(Fig. 14.4). Achiron et al reported a similar case not associated with chromosomal disease in which pathological examination revealed that the echogenic foci represented focal areas of hepatic necrosis with calcification.[43]

Trisomy 18

Trisomy 18 was first described by Edwards in 1960[44] and has an incidence of 1 in 3000. The prognosis is extremely poor and most babies die within the first few days of life

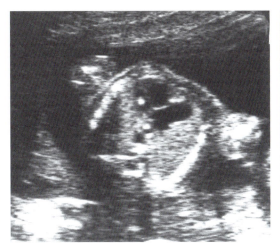

Fig. 14.3 Hypoplastic left heart syndrome with echogenic focus. Transverse scan of an 18-week fetus, showing an echogenic focus within a hypoplastic left ventricle. This is a characteristic appearance in trisomy 13.

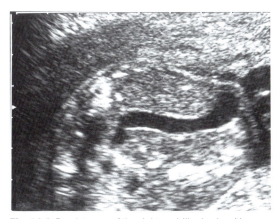

Fig. 14.4 Persistence of the right umbilical vein with echogenic hepatic foci. In this condition, the umbilical vein joins directly into the inferior vena cava. The echogenic hepatic foci represent focal areas of hepatic necrosis.

Table 14.5
Frequency of abnormalities in fetuses with trisomy 18

Abnormality	Incidence (%)
Head	
Strawberry skull	45
Choroid plexus cysts	30
Enlarged cisterna magna	19
Neural tube defects	<10
Agenesis of corpus callosum	
Hydrocephalus	
Face/neck	
Micrognathia	70
Low set 'pixie' ears	40
Cleft lip and palate	15
Hands/feet	
Flexed/overlapping fingers	80
Rockerbottom/club-foot	20
Radial aplasia	10
Heart	
Ventricular septal defect	
Atrioventricular septal defect	80
Double outlet right ventricle	
Kidney	
Cystic dysplasia	
Horseshoe kidney	15
Hydronephrosis	
Abdomen	
Omphalocoele	20
Thorax	
Diaphragmatic hernia	20
General	
Single umbilical artery	13
Growth retardation	59
Polyhydramnios	21

Reproduced with permission from Reid GB, Claireux AE, Cockburn F, eds. Diseases of the fetus and newborn. London: Chapman and Hall Medical; 1995.

from severe cardiac abnormalities.[45] The syndrome is characterized by multiple anomalies[47] (Table 14.5).

Hands and feet

One of the most striking abnormalities and a hallmark of the syndrome is fixed flexion and overlapping of the fingers (Fig. 14.5). The classical configuration is the index finger over the third finger and fifth finger over the fourth. Radial aplasia may also be seen in the hands (Fig. 14.6).[46] The feet often show talipes or rockerbottom feet (Fig. 14.7). Less common findings in the hands include hypoplasia or absence of the thumb and syndactyly. Polydactyly, although much more common in trisomy 13, is occasionally seen in trisomy 18.[8]

Facial defects

The commonest abnormality in the face is micrognathia (Fig. 14.8) and this may be seen in up to 70% of cases.[9] Facial clefting is also seen but is not so frequent as in trisomy 13. Low-set, 'pixie-type' ears are also a feature but may be more obvious in the neonatal period.

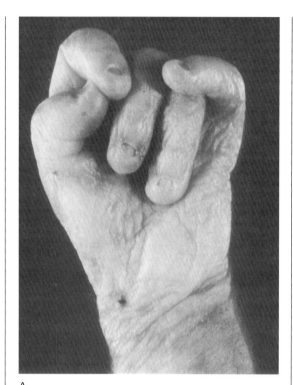

A

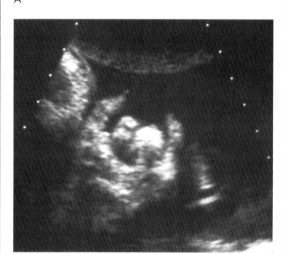

B

Fig. 14.5 Overlapping fingers of trisomy 18. (A) Postnatal photograph of the characteristic appearances of the hands in trisomy 18. The fifth finger overlaps the fourth and the second overlaps the third. Note the thumb is small. (B) Ultrasound scan through the hands of a trisomy 18 fetus, once again showing the typical overlapping appearance of the fingers.

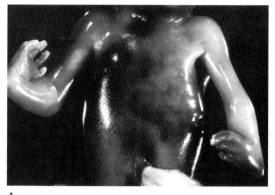

A

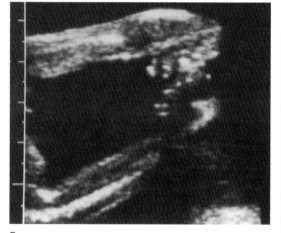

B

Fig. 14.6 Radial aplasia. (A) Post-mortem photograph of an 18-week fetus, showing bilateral radial aplasia. (B) Ultrasound scan of same fetus, showing bilateral radial aplasia. (Reproduced with permission from Twining P, Zuccollo J. Ultrasound markers of chromosomal disease. Br J Radiol 1993; 66:408–414.

Cardiac anomalies

As in all chromosomal abnormalities, cardiac disease is a frequent finding and a ventricular septal defect is the most common defect (Fig. 14.9) seen in trisomy 18.[48] Unfortunately, this abnormality is the most likely to be missed. Routine, 4-chamber scanning will detect only 38 to 40% of major cardiac anomalies.[24,49] The additional visualization of the outflow tracts increases this figure to 78%.[50]

Even in expert hands, ventricular septal defects are seen in only 65% of cases.[51] This underlines the point that although the fetal heart is a common setting for abnormality in

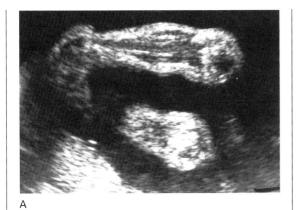

A

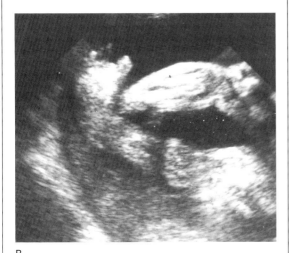

B

Fig. 14.7 Talipes. (A) and (B) show coronal scans through the lower limbs of an 18-week fetus, showing bilateral talipes.

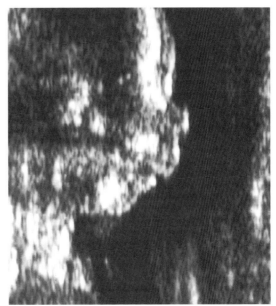

A

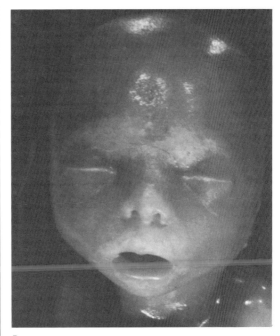

B

Fig. 14.8 Micrognathia. (A) Sagittal scan through an 18-week fetus, showing micrognathia. (B) Post-mortem photograph of same fetus, showing micrognathia and typical facial appearances of trisomy 18. (Reproduced with permission from Turner G, Twining P. The facial profile in the diagnosis of fetal abnormalities. Clin Radiol 1993; 47:389–395.)

chromosomal disease, it is often one of the most difficult organs to assess in the fetus and so extra care is needed in assessing the fetal heart when a chromosomal defect is suspected. In this respect, colour flow imaging may prove useful in assessing the patency of the fetal ventricular septum in the future.[52]

The other main cardiac abnormalities seen in trisomy 18 are atrioventricular septal defects[53] and double outlet right ventricle.[38]

Cranial anomalies

Scanning the fetal head often reveals a number of anomalies suggestive of trisomy 18. The shape of the head is important as a

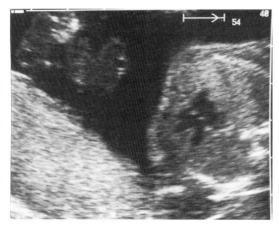

Fig. 14.9 Ventricular septal defect. Transverse scan through a 20-week fetus, showing the typical appearances of a ventricular septal defect.

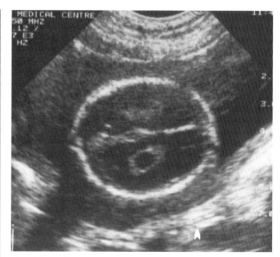

Fig. 14.11 Choroid plexus cysts. Transverse scan through an 18-week fetus, showing very typical, choroid plexus cyst.

characteristic appearance known as the 'strawberry skull' (Fig. 14.10) may be seen in up to 45% of trisomy 18 fetuses.[54] This appearance is produced by a flattened occiput and narrow frontal bones and is common in neonates with trisomy 18.[8,44] This finding, however, is not pathognomic for trisomy 18 and has been described in skeletal dysplasias[55] and may also be a normal variant.

Choroid plexus cysts

Choroid plexus cysts are another common finding in trisomy 18[57] (Fig. 14.11). First described in 1984,[56] they occur in 25 to 30% of fetuses with trisomy 18[47,58] but also occur in 1% of normal fetuses. The cysts vary in size between 3 and 16 mm, appear at about 14 to 16 weeks' gestation and resolve by 22 weeks.[46,58] The vast majority of fetuses with choroid plexus cysts and trisomy 18 have other fetal abnormalities present.[59,60] However, 17% of fetuses with trisomy 18 will have no abnormalities detectable on ultrasonography.[47] It is possible, therefore, and a few cases have been documented, to find choroid plexus cysts are the only abnormality present in a fetus with trisomy 18.[62–64] Because of this, certain groups have advocated karyotyping all fetuses with choroid plexus cysts whether abnormalities are present or not.[63,64]

At present, one would certainly offer a karyotype if choroid plexus cysts are seen in the presence of other abnormalities[46,61] as this carries a high risk of chromosomal disease. The risk of a fetus with isolated choroid plexus cysts having trisomy 18 has been calculated and maternal age-related risk estimates are available[61] (Table 14.6). The data at present, therefore, suggest that

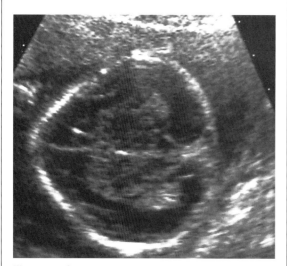

Fig. 14.10 Strawberry-shaped skull. Transverse scan through 20-week fetus, showing a strawberry skull appearance. There is flattening of the occiput with a pointed appearance to the frontal bones.

Table 14.6

Estimates of maternal age-specific risk for trisomy 18 at mid-trimester in fetuses with and without choroid plexus (CP) cysts and additional anomalies

Maternal age (years)	Overall (prior risk)	CP cysts absent	CP cysts present	
			Apparently isolated	Additional abnormalities
20	1/4576	1/8474	1/506	1/3
21	1/4514	1/8359	1/499	1/3
22	1/4435	1/8213	1/491	1/3
23	1/4333	1/8024	1/479	1/2
24	1/4204	1/7785	1/465	1/2
25	1/4045	1/7491	1/447	1/2
26	1/3850	1/7130	1/426	1/2
27	1/3619	1/6702	1/400	1/2
28	1/3351	1/6206	1/371	1/2
29	1/3050	1/5648	1/337	1/2
30	1/2724	1/5044	1/301	1/2
31	1/2385	1/4417	1/264	>1/2
32	1/2046	1/3789	1/226	>1/2
33	1/1721	1/3187	1/190	>1/2
34	1/1420	1/2630	1/157	>1/2
35	1/1152	1/2133	1/127	>1/2
36	1/921	1/1706	1/102	>1/2
37	1/727	1/1346	1/80	>1/2
38	1/567	1/1050	1/63	>1/2
39	1/439	1/813	1/49	>1/2
40	1/338	1/626	1/37	>1/2
41	1/258	1/478	1/29	>1/2
42	1/197	1/365	1/22	>1/2
43	1/149	1/276	1/16	>1/2
44	1/113	1/209	1/13	>1/2
45	1/85	1/157	1/9	>1/2

Reproduced with permission from Gupta JK, et al. Management of fetal choroid plexus cysts. Br J Obstet Gynaecol 1997; 104:881–886.

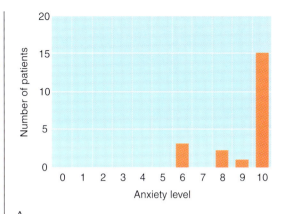

A

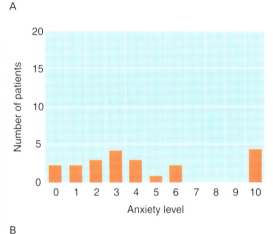

B

Fig. 14.12 Anxiety levels before and after the resolution of choroid plexus cysts. (A) Anxiety levels at initial diagnosis of choroid plexus cysts. (B) Anxiety levels after the 22-week scan at which point the choroid plexus cysts have resolved. It is clear that the anxiety levels are much reduced following the repeat scan.

isolated choroid plexus cysts are an indication for detailed scanning in order to look for ultrasound markers of trisomy 18.[60,61]

In the situation where the detailed scan is absolutely normal, the patient can be reassured that the fetus has a low risk of trisomy 18. The author also recommends a repeat scan at 22 weeks' gestation to demonstrate resolution of the cysts but also to reassess the fetus and, in particular, the heart, looking for ventricular septal defects. Another important reason for repeating the scan is that although demonstration of resolution of the choroid plexus cysts does not decrease the inherent, albeit low, risk of trisomy 18, it does produce a significant reduction in maternal anxiety levels.[65] Figure 14.12 outlines anxiety levels in patients whose fetuses have been diagnosed as

having choroid plexus cysts. There is a significant reduction in anxiety levels following resolution of the cysts.

Other cranial abnormalities associated with trisomy 18 include enlargement of the cisterna magna,[66] agenesis of the corpus callosum and hydrocephalus.[67,68] The Dandy–Walker syndrome may also be seen and the degree of associated ventriculomegaly is important as minimal or no ventricular dilatation carries a much higher risk of chromosomal disease, 77% compared to 9% when ventriculomegaly is present.[66] Neural tube defects occur in less than 10% of fetuses with trisomy 18.[47]

Chest and abdominal anomalies

In the chest and abdomen, diaphragmatic hernia[69] and omphalocoele[70,71] are often seen and it is the smaller omphalocoeles, i.e. containing bowel only, that are more likely to be associated with chromosomal disease.[72] A diaphragmatic hernia produces displacement of the heart and this can make assessment of the heart difficult and so extra vigilance is required in this situation.

Also seen in the abdomen are renal abnormalities that can occur in up to 15% of cases and range from cystic dysplasia to hydronephrosis and horseshoe kidney.[47,73]

As mentioned earlier in the text, growth retardation is seen in over 50% of fetuses with trisomy 18[74] and although it can be seen in the second trimester, it is more obvious in the third trimester. The presence of associated polyhydramnios is an ominous sign and can be seen in up to 21% of fetuses with trisomy 18.[47]

In a small number of fetuses, a cystic hygroma may be identified and occasionally generalized hydrops is seen.[6] As mentioned in the section on trisomy 13, umbilical cord cysts have also been described in fetuses with trisomy 18.[41]

Trisomy 21

Down's syndrome was first described in 1866.[75] However, it was not until 1934 that the chromosomal abnormality was recognized.[76] Trisomy 21 is the most common chromosomal abnormality with an average incidence of 1.3:1000 but it is also the most difficult to detect using antenatal ultrasound. In the best hands, scanning at 18 to 20 weeks will reveal abnormalities in only 33% of affected fetuses.[9,77] Many of these abnormalities will be subtle changes, requiring detailed ultrasound evaluation. In the UK amniocentesis is routinely offered to all women over 35 years of age. However, using this basis for screening, only 15% of affected pregnancies are likely to be detected. The introduction of serum screening has meant that up to 60% of Down's syndrome

fetuses may be detected.[78] Serum screening has also been investigated in the first trimester.[79] However, the development of nuchal translucency scanning suggests that up to 80% of Down's syndrome fetuses may be detected.[80]

Although the ultrasound diagnosis of Down's syndrome has limitations, there are a number of reliable ultrasound findings, which, if seen, should raise the possibility of Down's syndrome. In addition, over the last few years there has been a number of 'soft markers' reported which may be associated with an increased risk of Down's syndrome.[81] These will also be discussed.

The most important ultrasound findings in trisomy 21 are duodenal atresia, atrioventricular septal defects and an increased nuchal fold measurement (Table 14.7).

Table 14.7
Frequency of abnormalities in fetuses with trisomy 21

Abnormality	Incidence (%)
Head	
Mild ventriculomegaly	
Small frontal lobes	3
Face/neck	
Macroglossia	
Snub nose, prominent lips, flat profile	
Cystic hygroma	4
Nuchal oedema	16
Hands/feet	
Clinodactyly – fifth finger	28
Sandal gap	
Heart	
Atrioventricular septal defect	
Ventricular septal defect	40
Echogenic foci	
Kidney	
Mild dilatation of renal pelves	
Abdomen	
Duodenal atresia	5
Omphalocoele	2
Echogenic bowel	5
Thorax	
Pleural effusion	1
General	
Growth retardation	6
Polyhydramnios	3
Hydrops	2

Reproduced with permission from Reed GB, Claireux AE, Cockburn F, eds. Diseases of the fetus and newborn. London: Chapman and Hall Medical; 1995.

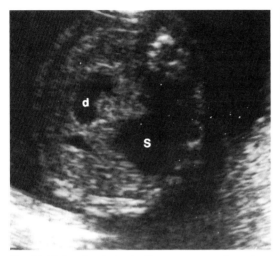

Fig. 14.13 Duodenal atresia. Transverse scan through the abdomen of a 24-week fetus, showing the typical double bubble appearance of duodenal atresia. S, stomach; d, duodenum.

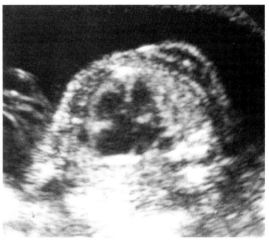

Fig. 14.14 Atrioventricular septal defect. Transverse scan through the heart of an 18-week fetus, showing a large ventricular septal defect associated with a large atrial septal defect: This combination produces the appearance of a single atrioventricular valve.

Duodenal atresia

Although duodenal atresia (Fig. 14.13) only occurs in 5% of fetuses with Down's syndrome,[77] its detection in a fetus carries a 30% risk of the syndrome.[82] Unfortunately, duodenal atresia is not usually detected with confidence before 24 weeks' gestation[82] and so its use as an early sign of Down's syndrome is limited.

Atrioventricular septal defect

Congenital heart disease occurs in about 40% of neonates with Down's syndrome[8] and the commonest abnormality detected antenatally is atrioventricular septal defect[39] (Fig. 14.14). A recent series reported Down's syndrome in 62% of fetuses demonstrating on atrioventricular septal defect.[48] This is therefore an exceptionally good sign of Down's syndrome.

Other cardiac anomalies occurring in Down's syndrome include ventricular septal defects and atrial septal defects. In addition, the presence of an isolated pericardial effusion should also raise the possibility of Down's syndrome. Sharland et al detected Down's syndrome in 26% of fetuses with isolated pericardial effusion[83] (Fig. 14.15).

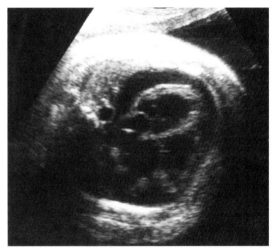

Fig. 14.15 Pericardial effusion. Transverse scan through the heart of a 32-week fetus. This fetus had an isolated pericardial effusion and was subsequently found to have trisomy 21.

Nuchal fold

Thickening of the nuchal tissues at the back of the fetal neck is a useful sign in Down's syndrome[84,85] and occurs in approximately 16% of Down's syndrome fetuses.[77] The nuchal fold measurement is carried out using a modified biparietal diameter view. The transducer is rotated into the posterior fossa to visualize the cerebellum in transverse section, ensuring that the cavum septum pellucidum is also visible (Fig. 14.16). The measurement is made from the outer edge of the occipital bone to the outer skin edge. A measurement of 6 mm or more is considered abnormal at 16 to 20 weeks' gestation.[85] Analyzing the reported series reveals that Down's syndrome will be present in 20 to 40% of fetuses with an increased nuchal fold.[84–90] This ultrasound finding therefore is of value and patients should be offered a karyotype even if it is seen in isolation in a low-risk patient.[85]

An increased nuchal fold measurement is not specific to Down's syndrome but may also be seen in cases of skeletal dysplasias, early hydrops and approximately 2 to 8.5% of the normal population.[86,87] It is important

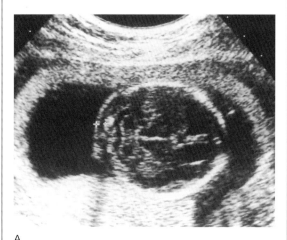

A

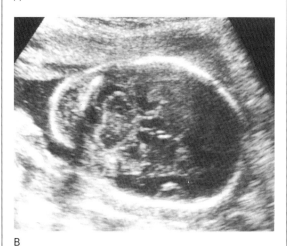

B

Fig. 14.16 Nuchal fold. (A) Normal nuchal fold measurement. (B) Increased nuchal fold measurement.

therefore to carry out a full structural survey of the fetus looking for other markers of Down's syndrome and also to exclude other causes of an increased nuchal fold.

It has recently been shown that fetuses with isolated nuchal thickening and anormal karyotype have a good outcome. However, fetuses with an increased nuchal fold, associated abnormalities and a normal karyotype have a poorer outcome.[91]

Soft markers for Down's syndrome

As a result of the frustration and difficulties encountered in making an antenatal diagnosis of Down's syndrome using ultrasound, a number of minor ultrasound findings has been proposed as potential signs of Down's syndrome. The main problem with many of these reports is that they are based predominantly on a high-risk group of patients and so it is difficult to apply the results to a low-risk population.

Furthermore, since each marker is present in 1 to 5% of all normal pregnancies, more and more fetuses will have at least one such marker.[92] The situation becomes more problematic when more than one soft marker is seen. At present, however, there seems to be insufficient evidence to indicate karyotyping fetuses in a low-risk population when an isolated soft marker is detected.

In the situation where more than one soft marker is detected, it is likely that the risk of Down's syndrome is increased; however, it is difficult to quantify this risk. Certain authors have proposed using 'scoring systems' and likelihood ratios (see sonographic approach, p. 333) in order to assess this risk. An alternative approach is to carry out biochemical testing in order to produce further information about the risk of Down's syndrome.

Short femur

It is well documented that persons with Down's syndrome have shortened long bones and there has been considerable debate in the literature as to the usefulness of the detection of a shortened femur in the second trimester diagnosis of Down's syndrome. Early papers demonstrated a clear link between Down's syndrome and a shortened femur.[93,94] However, later papers have not confirmed these findings[95–97] as there is considerable overlap with the normal population. At present, one would not routinely offer a karyotype on the basis of a shortened femur alone.

Short humerus

Benaceraff et al have proposed that a shortened humerus may be useful in the antenatal diagnosis of Down's syndrome.[18,81] Nyberg et al found significant humeral shortening in 24% of Down's fetuses and suggested that fetuses with both a short femur and humerus carried an 11-fold greater risk of Down's syndrome.[98] Johnson et al, using the ratio of humeral plus femur length divided by the foot length, correctly identified 53% of fetuses with Down's syndrome.[99] Larger studies are required, however, to confirm these findings.

Echogenic bowel

Echogenic bowel was first described by Lince et al in 1985,[100] and has an incidence of 0.2 to 0.6%. There are various definitions of echogenic bowel but the most reliable appears to be bowel that has the same echogenicity as surrounding bone[101,102] (Fig. 14.17). Early papers suggested that echogenic bowel was a normal variant with no perinatal morbidity.[100,103] However, later series have shown associations with chromosomal disease, particularly Down's syndrome, cystic fibrosis, intra-uterine growth retardation and congenital infection.[104,105] The cause of echogenic bowel is unclear, but may be related to hypoperistalsis or decreased fluid content of the meconium,[106] swallowing of amniotic fluid following intra-amniotic bleeding[107] or possibly gut ischaemia.[108]

A review by Carrol & Maxwell analyzed 599 cases of echogenic bowel and found chromosomal abnormalities in 64 cases (11%).[109] Over half of these anomalies were

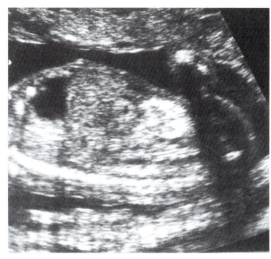

Fig. 14.17 Echogenic bowel. Sagittal scan through the thorax and abdomen of an 18-week fetus, showing a dense area of echogenic bowel in the lower abdomen. Note that the density of the bowel is similar to that of bone.

Down's syndrome; however, 75% of these fetuses also exhibited other abnormalities on ultrasound. In addition, in five out of the eleven studies reviewed, the incidence of advanced maternal age or abnormal serum biochemistry ranged from 23 to 63%. This data therefore cannot be applied to the low-risk population. The review also revealed the presence of intra-uterine growth retardation in 11% of cases, intra-uterine fetal death in 8% and neonatal death in 0.8%. Maternal serum alphafetoprotein was raised in 50% of the cases with adverse outcome. These data tend to suggest a hypothesis whereby intra-amniotic bleeding, possibly producing some placental damage and causing an elevation of the maternal serum alphafetoprotein, is swallowed by the fetus, hence producing echogenic bowel. The fetus may well be at risk of developing intra-uterine growth retardation later on in pregnancy secondary to the early placental damage.

The other main association appears to be cystic fibrosis. However, there is considerable discrepancy in the results of reported series because of the small numbers of patients studied and the variation among populations with different risks for cystic fibrosis.

At present, it would seem that isolated echogenic bowel in a low-risk population probably does warrant a karyotype procedure. If any other abnormality is present or the patient is at high risk of carrying a Down's syndrome fetus as a result of biochemical screening or advanced maternal age, then echogenic bowel should be considered an additional marker for Down's syndrome. Follow-up scans should be carried out in the third trimester to assess fetal growth and exclude intra-uterine growth retardation. The other causes of echogenic bowel such as congenital infection and cystic fibrosis should also be considered and excluded.

Mild renal pelvic dilatation

Mild renal pelvic dilatation is defined as an increase in the anteroposterior diameter of the renal pelvis without evidence of a clear-cut hydronephrosis. The measurements are best carried out on a transverse scan with the spine uppermost (Fig. 14.18). The incidence ranges between 1.6 and 2.8%.[17,110,111] The normal range has been described as greater than 4 mm up to 20 weeks' gestation, greater than 5 mm from 20 to 30 weeks and greater than 7 mm from 30 to 40 weeks' gestation.[17] In an early paper, Benaceraff et al reported 210 fetuses with mild, renal pelvic dilatation – of which 7 were found to have Down's syndrome.[17]

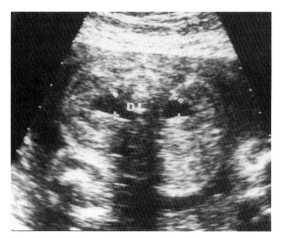

Fig. 14.18 Mild renal pelvic dilatation. Transverse scan through an 18-week fetus with the spine uppermost, showing mild dilatation of both renal pelvises.

In contrast, Nyberg et al in their review of 94 fetuses with Down's syndrome found no cases of renal pelvic dilatation.[77] Nicolaides et al reported 173 fetuses with isolated, mild hydronephrosis but only one of these fetuses was found to have Down's syndrome.[73] In a prospective study, Wickstom et al identified 121 cases of isolated, mild, renal pelvic dilatation and found one case of Down's syndrome. The authors calculated that mild, renal pelvic dilatation indicated a 3.9-fold increase in Down's syndrome risk.[112] Corteville et al reported 127 fetuses, and found mild renal pelvic dilatation in 17.4% of Down's syndrome fetuses compared to 2% in the normal population. The predictive value of renal pelvic dilatation for Down's syndrome was calculated to be 1 in 90. However, when fetuses with associated abnormalities were excluded, the predictive value fell to 1 in 340.[111] A UK multicentre study found an incidence of 1 in 150 for Down's syndrome in fetuses with mild renal pelvic dilatation.[113]

There appear to be major discrepancies within the literature as to the significance of renal pelvic dilatation with predictive values ranging from 1 in 33[17] to 1 in 340.[111] In addition, the majority of these series are from high-risk populations. At present, there seems little clear evidence to offer a karyotype in a low-risk pregnancy. If there are associated abnormalities, then a karyotype needs to be considered. In addition, fetuses with mild, renal pelvic dilatation require repeat scans in the third trimester to ensure that the dilatation has not progressed, as progression significantly increases the risk for postnatal structural renal abnormalities.[112]

Echogenic foci in the fetal heart

Echogenic foci in the fetal heart are a common finding occurring in 2 to 5% of fetuses.[114–116] The focus is usually seen in the left ventricle (Fig. 14.19) but may also be seen on the right or even both ventricles. Although the majority are single, occasionally they may be multiple; however, 95% of echogenic foci will resolve by the third trimester.[117]

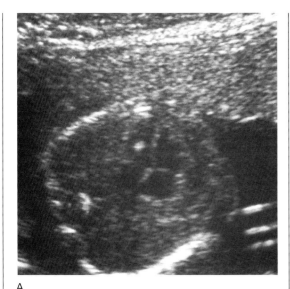

A

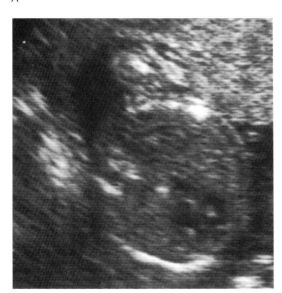

B

Fig. 14.19 Echogenic foci in the fetal heart. (A) Transverse scan through the heart of an 18-week fetus, showing the typical appearance of an echogenic focus in the left ventricle. (B) Transverse scan through the heart of a 20-week fetus, showing echogenic foci in both the left and right ventricles.

There is considerable debate within the literature as to the significance of echogenic foci. A number of papers has shown no association with Down's syndrome.[115,117–119] However, other authors have suggested echogenic foci to be a marker for Down's syndrome.[116,120,121]

A pathological study has revealed echogenic foci to be present in 16% of Down's syndrome fetuses compared to 2% in the normal population.[114] Similarly, Bromley et al reported 66 fetuses with echogenic foci and found foci present in 18% of Down's fetuses compared to 5% of normal fetuses.[116] However, this study population was from a high-risk group and extrapolation to a lower risk population did not significantly increase the risk of Down's syndrome. Sepulveda et al described seven fetuses with echogenic foci: three were found to have Down's syndrome, three trisomy 13 and one trisomy 18. All seven fetuses had other abnormalities present on antenatal ultrasound.[120] Simpson et al have reported a prospective study of 288 cases of echogenic foci in a low-risk population and found one case of Down's syndrome.[121]

Overall, the studies suggest that, although there may be an association with Down's syndrome and a higher prevalence of echogenic foci in Down's syndrome fetuses, there is insufficient evidence to offer a karyotype in the case of isolated echogenic foci in a low-risk fetus.

Hypoplasia of the middle phalanx of the fifth finger

It has been estimated that hypoplasia of the middle phalanx of the fifth finger producing clinodactyly occurs in 60% of neonates with Down's syndrome.[122] However, a study of the hand radiographs of 324 patients with Down's syndrome revealed clinodactyly of the fifth finger in only 28% and the finding was also seen in up to 3% of normal caucasian patients.[123]

Benaceraff et al described hypoplasia of the middle phalanx of the fifth finger in four out of five fetuses with Down's syndrome[124] (Fig. 14.20). In a subsequent study, Benaceraff et al devised a ratio of the size of the middle finger of the fifth finger compared to that of the fourth and using a cut-off of 0.7 detected 75% of Down's syndrome fetuses.[125] However, 18% of normal fetuses also exhibited the same finding, producing an unacceptably high, false-positive rate. In

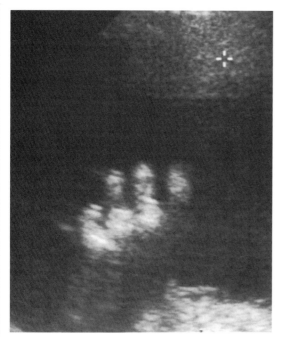

Fig. 14.20 Hypoplasia of the fifth finger. Coronal scan through the hand of a 20-week fetus, showing clinodactyly of the fifth finger. Note associated polyhydramnios. This fetus also had duodenal atresia.

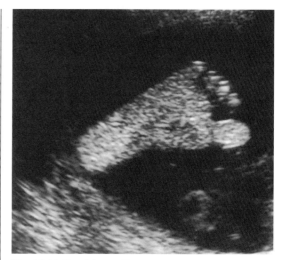

Fig. 14.21 Sandal gap. Transverse scan through the foot of a 20-week fetus, showing a wide separation between the first and second toes, typical of the sandal gap.

addition, the authors were unable to obtain the phalanx measurements in 31% of patients because of difficulty with fetal position, maternal body habitus or time constraints.[125] Although these findings may be of some value in the high-risk group, it should not be used as a marker for Down's syndrome in the low-risk population. Goldstein et al have reported measurements of the entire fifth finger in normal fetuses throughout gestation as an additional screening parameter for Down's syndrome.[126] Future studies will confirm whether measuring the entire fifth finger will refine the diagnosis any further. A simian crease has also been described in fetuses with Down's syndrome.[127]

Separation of the great toe (sandal gap)

Separation of the great toe occurs in up to 45% of children with Down's syndrome[8] (Fig. 14.21). Although there is very little data in the literature, this sign has been mentioned in a number of articles.[7,81] Wilkins et al described two fetuses with separation of the great toe who were subsequently found to have Down's syndrome following a karyotype procedure.[128] Both fetuses demonstrated other abnormalities and both women were at a high risk of carrying a Down's syndrome fetus because of raised maternal age or abnormal biochemical screening. Once again, this finding needs to be restricted to the high-risk group.

Facial findings

The facial appearances of Down's syndrome patients are well documented.[8] However, these dysmorphic appearances are often difficult to demonstrate sonographically. A number of features has been described including a flat profile[129] (Fig. 14.22), macroglossia[130] and a shortened ear length.[131]

Cranial findings

Mild ventriculomegaly may be seen in up to 3% of Down's syndrome fetuses[77] and this is likely to be caused by a degree of cerebral atrophy. Similarly, a further study has demonstrated reduced frontal lobe dimensions in fetuses with Down's syndrome.[132]

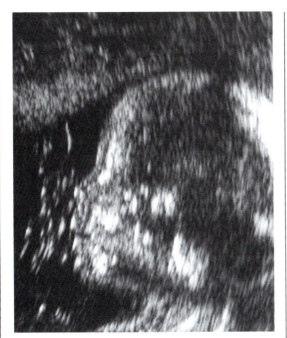

Fig. 14.22 The flat profile. Sagittal scan through the face of a 20-week fetus, showing a flattened profile typical of trisomy 21.

Table 14.8
Sonographic scoring system for the detection of trisomy 21 – fetuses with a score of 2 or more are considered at high risk for Down's syndrome

Sonographic finding	Score
Major defect	2
Nuchal fold ≥ 6 mm	2
Short femur	1
Short humerus	1
Mild renal pelvic dilatation	1
Echogenic bowel	1

Reproduced with permission from Benacerraf B. The second trimester fetus with Down's syndrome: Detection using sonographic features. Ultrasound Obstet Gynecol 1996; 7:147–155.

Sonographic scoring system

In order to quantify the risk of Down's syndrome, Benaceraf has proposed a scoring system[94,81] (Table 14.8), using both major and minor ultrasound markers for Down's syndrome. A score of 2 or more has been reported to detect 81% of fetuses with Down's syndrome. This approach, however, has not gained universal acceptance.

Adjusted risk based on an abnormal scan

Snijders & Nicolaides have suggested an alternative approach and have calculated likelihood ratios for each major and minor marker for Down's syndrome (Table 14.9). For example, in the case of echogenic bowel, this marker is reported to occur in 2.7% of Down's fetuses compared to 0.49% of normal fetuses.

Cystic hygroma and hydrops

Cystic hygroma and hydrops can be a sign of Down's syndrome and it is estimated that 5% of fetuses with a cystic hygromata and up to 12% of fetuses with hydrops may have Down's syndrome.[6]

Other findings

Occasionally, Down's syndrome fetuses demonstrate other abdominal abnormalities such as omphalocoele and anal atresia. In addition, there have been reports of increased iliac bone lengths[133] and reduced breast size in Down's fetuses.[134] In the chest, pleural effusions have been reported.

Sonographic approach to Down's syndrome

It can be seen that there are a small number of important signs of Down's syndrome and many minor markers which are present in Down's syndrome fetuses but are also seen in normal fetuses.

Table 14.9
Likelihood ratios for isolated soft markers for Down's syndrome – the likelihood ratio should be multiplied by the maternal age-specific risk (Table 14.6) to produce the modified Down's syndrome risk

Sonographic finding	Likelihood ratio
Nuchal fold ≥ 6 mm	19
Echogenic bowel	5.5
Short femur	2.3
Mild renal pelvic dilatation	1.5

Reproduced with permission from Snijders RJM, Nicolaides KH. Ultrasound markers for fetal chromosomal defects, London: Parthenon; 1996.

The likelihood ratio is therefore 2.7% ÷ 0.49 which equals 5.5.[135] This figure is then multiplied by the patient's age and gestational-age-related background risk of trisomy 21 (Table 14.10) to produce an adjusted risk based on the finding of echogenic bowel. For a 20-year-old patient at 20 weeks' gestation using this formula, the Down's syndrome risk would change from 1:1176 to 1:215 if echogenic bowel is seen. The main drawback for this system is that accurate prevalence rates for various soft markers in Down's syndrome fetuses are not available and most of this data is based on relatively small numbers of cases.

Adjusted risk based on a normal scan

The significance of a normal scan has also been investigated and the absence of ultrasound markers for Down's syndrome has been used to readjust the age-related risk and also the risk calculated using biochemical screening. Snijders & Nicolaides have suggested that a normal ultrasound scan reduces the background risk by about 40%.[135] Vintzileos & Egan have also investigated the importance of a normal ultrasound scan and suggested a reduction in risk of 28%,[136] whilst Nyberg et al found a reduction in background risk of 45%.[137] Nadel et al, however, found that, although the background risk for Down's syndrome can be reduced in the presence of a normal scan, up to 15% of Down's syndrome fetuses would be missed.[138]

The data from several studies suggest that the background risk for Down's syndrome can be reduced by about 40%. However, this may result in some babies with Down's syndrome being missed who would otherwise have been identified through karyotyping.

Table 14.10
Trisomy 21 – risk by maternal age and gestation. Estimated risk (1/number given in the table)

Age (yrs)	Gestation (wks)									
	10	12	14	16	18	20	25	30	35	Birth
20	804	898	981	1053	1117	1175	1294	1388	1464	1527
21	793	887	968	1040	1103	1159	1277	1370	1445	1507
22	780	872	952	1022	1084	1140	1256	1347	1421	1482
23	762	852	930	999	1060	1114	1227	1317	1389	1448
24	740	827	903	969	1029	1081	1191	1278	1348	1406
25	712	795	868	933	989	1040	1146	1229	1297	1352
26	677	756	826	887	941	989	1090	1169	1233	1286
27	635	710	775	832	883	928	1022	1097	1157	1206
28	586	655	705	768	805	856	943	1012	1068	1113
29	531	593	648	695	738	776	855	917	967	1008
30	471	526	575	617	655	688	758	813	858	895
31	409	457	499	536	568	597	658	706	745	776
32	347	388	423	455	482	507	559	599	632	659
33	288	322	352	378	401	421	464	498	525	547
34	235	262	286	307	326	343	378	405	427	446
35	187	210	229	246	261	274	302	324	342	356
36	148	165	180	193	205	216	238	255	269	280
37	115	128	140	150	159	168	185	198	209	218
38	88	98	107	115	122	129	142	152	160	167
39	67	75	82	88	93	98	108	116	122	128
40	51	57	62	67	71	74	82	88	93	97
41	38	43	47	50	53	56	62	66	70	73
42	29	32	35	38	40	42	46	50	52	55
43	21	24	26	28	30	31	35	37	39	41
44	16	18	20	21	22	23	26	28	29	30

Reproduced with permission from Snijders RJM, Nicolaides KH. Ultrasound markers for fetal chromosomal defects. London: Parthenon; 1996.

Nuchal translucency

It is well established that cystic hygromata and hydrops can be present in fetuses with Down's syndrome.[6,139] However, Szabo & Gellen were the first to describe an abnormal nuchal translucency thickness in the first trimester as a marker for Down's syndrome.[140] Although the physiological basis for increased nuchal translucency is unclear,[141] it is known that Down's syndrome fetuses with increased nuchal translucency have a high incidence of associated cardiac abnormalities.[142,143]

This finding suggests that fetuses with increased nuchal translucency may be suffering from a degree of heart failure which manifests as nuchal fluid.[142] In addition, pathological studies have shown an increase in hyaluronan in the extracellular matrix in the nuchal skin of Down's syndrome fetuses. This hyaluronan binds free interstitial water because of its negative charge, which leads to disorganization of the collagen scaffolding and gives the nuchal skin a spongy consistency.[144] These two factors may act together to predispose Down's syndrome fetuses to having increased nuchal fluid.

Although the main association is with Down's syndrome, an increased nuchal translucency has also been described in association with some rare genetic conditions such as Noonan syndrome, Stickler syndrome, Smith–Lemli–Opitz syndrome and arthrogryphosis.[145]

The nuchal translucency measurement is usually carried out using transabdominal scanning between 10 and 14 weeks' gestation. A sagittal section of the fetus is obtained for measurement of the crown–rump length and the maximum thickness of the subcutaneous tissue overlying the cervical spine is measured (Fig. 14.23).

A measurement greater than 3 mm is considered abnormal. However, care is taken to distinguish between the fetal skin and amnion as both structures appear as thin membranes. This is achieved by waiting for spontaneous fetal movement, by asking the mother to cough or by tapping the maternal abdomen.[145] Transvaginal scanning has also been used in some studies to measure nuchal translucency.

Studies into the reproducibility of nuchal translucency measurements have provided varying results. Roberts et al found that using different operators the nuchal translucency measurements changed classification as normal or abnormal in up to 18% of cases.[146] Pandya et al, however, showed good reproducibility with accurate measurements in 95% of patients but did stress the importance of well-trained operators carrying out the measurements.[147]

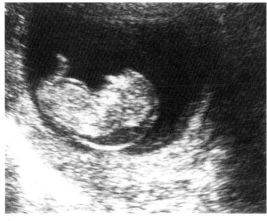

A

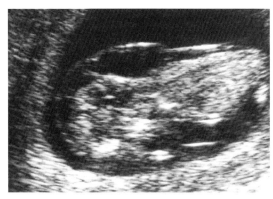

B

Fig. 14.23 Nuchal translucency. (A) Sagittal scan through a 12-week fetus, showing an increased nuchal translucency. (B) Sagittal scan through a 13-week fetus, showing an increased nuchal translucency but also generalized subcutaneous fluid. This fetus had a normal karyotype and the fluid subsequently resolved. Detailed scanning at 20 weeks, however, revealed a major cardiac abnormality, namely a truncus arteriosus.

A large number of studies has been carried out to investigate the significance of an increased nuchal translucency measurement[145,148–155] and Table 14.11 outlines these studies. It can be seen that sensitivities for the detection of chromosomal disease, of which Down's syndrome is the most frequent, range from 24% to 100%. Some of this variation will be due to differing cut-offs for the nuchal translucency measurements, differences in the gestational age at measurement, differences in the maternal ages of patients in the studies and differing uses of transabdominal and transvaginal scanning.

It is interesting to note that in two out of the three studies with sensitivity rates below 50%,[153,155] measurement rates were in the region of 60%, highlighting the importance of adequate training. In addition, transvaginal scanning does not appear to have any advantage over transabdominal scanning except in difficult cases.[150] Most studies report a detection rate for Down's syndrome of at least 50% with a false-positive rate of approximately 5%.

The largest study, however, comprising 22 076 low-risk patients in a district general hospital setting and using an algorithm based on maternal age, gestational age at time of scan and a cut-off risk of 1:300, detected 84% of Down's syndrome fetuses with a false-positive rate of 6%.[145] These results are extremely encouraging but do depend on a high level of training and careful attention to measurement technique. With this background, it would be anticipated that these results should be reproduced in further large studies.

One aspect of the early diagnosis of chromosomal disease that deserves attention is the fact that a certain proportion of aneuploid fetuses will die prior to delivery. It has been estimated that up to 40% of Down's syndrome fetuses die between 12 weeks and term.[156]

It is possible, therefore, that the early detection of Down's syndrome fetuses may be detecting a number of fetuses that would die anyway. Hyett et al reported an 11.4% loss rate for trisomy 21 fetuses with an increased nuchal translucency between 12 and 14 weeks' gestation, which was higher than the 6.9% estimated rate. Loss rates for fetuses with measurements greater than 7 mm were 23.5% compared to 8.8% for measurements of 4–6 mm.[157] In contrast,

Table 14.11
Data from nuchal translucency (NT) studies

Authors	No. in study	High risk (HR) or low risk (LR)	No. with increased NT	Gestational age (wks)	NT thickness (mm)	Sensitivity for trisomy 21	False-positive rate	% measured	Type of scan; TA, transabdominal; TV, transvaginal
Schulte-Vallentin, et al. 1992	632	HR	8	10–14	≥ 4 mm	100%	0.1%	100	—
Salvodelli, et al. 1993	1400	HR	24	9–12 mm	≥ 4 mm	54%	0.35%	100	TA
Brambati, et al. 1995	1819	HR	70	8–15	≥ 3 mm	30%	4%	100	TA/TV
Comas, et al. 1995	481	HR	51	9–13	≥ 3 mm	57%	0.7%	100	TV
Szabo, et al. 1995	3380	HR/LR	96	9–12	≥ 3 mm	90%	1.2–5.4%	100	TV
Bewley, et al. 1995	1127	LR	70	8–13	≥ 3 mm	33%	6%	62	TA
Hafner, et al. 1995	1972	LR	26	10–13	≥ 2.5 mm	50%	7.7%	100	TA
Nicolaides, et al. 1996	20 543	HR	3302	10–14	—	86%	11%	100	TA
Nicolaides, et al. 1996	22 076	LR	1316	10–14	—	84%	6%	100	TA
Kornman, et al. 1996	923	HR	36	< 13	≥ 3 mm	24%	5%	58	TA

Pandya et al followed up six Down's syndrome fetuses with an increased nuchal translucency and all six were liveborn.[156] The previous data indicate, however, that Down's fetuses with increased nuchal translucency have a much higher loss rate than those with a normal measurement. Similar findings were seen in chromosomally normal fetuses with an increased nuchal translucency[158] where 97% survived to term with a nuchal translucency measurement of 3 mm compared to only 63% with a measurement of 5 mm. In addition, 64% of fetuses developed hydrops when the nuchal translucency measurement was 7 mm or more. Traufler et al reported three cases of hydrops in 22 fetuses with an increased nuchal translucency and normal chromosomes.[159] This high loss rate may well be related to the high incidence of cardiac abnormalities present in both chromosomally normal and Down's syndrome fetuses with an increased nuchal translucency.

Sonographic approach

Screening for Down's syndrome using the nuchal translucency may well prove to be an important advance in antenatal diagnosis of Down's syndrome. However, it is not totally specific for chromosomal abnormalities. In the situation where the karyotype is normal, further follow-up is indicated with detailed scanning at 18 to 20 weeks with particular reference to cardiac abnormalities (see chapter 4).

Nuchal translucency and fetal heart rate

The importance of the fetal heart rate in the diagnosis of Down's syndrome is unclear at present. Hyett et al found the mean heart rate significantly higher in 85 fetuses with Down's syndrome and used this to improve the detection rate following nuchal translucency screening from 76% to 83%.[160]

In contrast, Martinez et al found a raised heart rate in only one of 11 fetuses with Down's syndrome and seven of the 11 had a heart rate below the 5th centile of the normal range.[161] Martinez et al have, however, suggested combining umbilical artery Doppler velocimetry with nuchal translucency measurements to improve the detection of Down's syndrome in the first trimester.[162] In this study, the combination of a nuchal translucency measurement greater than 3 mm and an abnormally high, umbilical artery pulsatility index produced a sensitivity of 88.8% for the detection of Down's syndrome.[162]

Turner's syndrome

First described by Turner in 1938, the incidence is approximately 1 in 5000 live births but it accounts for up to 10% of first trimester miscarriages.

Neonates with Turner's syndrome are often indistinguishable from normal fetuses and the diagnosis is often not made until short stature or delayed puberty becomes apparent.[8]

The hallmark of the antenatal diagnosis of Turner's syndrome is the presence of a cystic hygroma[6] (Fig. 14.24).

This abnormality is caused by an obstruction in the cervical lymphatic vessels so that lymphatic fluid collects at the back of the fetal neck; the classical appearance is of a multiseptate fluid collection in the posterior nuchal space.[163] These cystic hygromata can be very large and may be associated with generalized hydrops.

In this setting, the outlook is extremely poor.[164] It is important to differentiate cystic hygroma from an occipital encephalocoele; however, the head shape, appearances of the intracranial contents and the presence of an occipital bony defect are all important signs of an encephalocoele.[165]

The presence of a cystic hygroma, however, is not totally specific for Turner's syndrome as only 70% of fetuses with a cystic hygroma will have Turner's syndrome.[166] As mentioned previously, 5% will have trisomy 18, 5% trisomy 21 and approximately 20% will have a normal karyotype.[166] Cystic

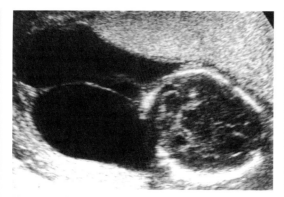

Fig. 14.24 Cystic hygroma. Transverse scan through the head of an 18-week fetus, showing a large, multi-septated cystic hygroma.

hygromata which present at other sites on the body, for example the anterior abdominal wall, have a low incidence of chromosomal disease and do not usually require karyotyping.

The other malformations which can occur in Turner's syndrome are usually cardiac which can occur in 15% of fetuses and the most common anomaly is coarctation.[48] The only other abnormality of note is renal and occasionally hydronephrosis, renal agenesis and renal hypoplasia may be seen.

It has been estimated that up to 35% of liveborn individuals may have a mosaic chromosomal defect and this may account for the relatively mild clinical signs seen in liveborn infants. In view of this and in view of the fact that not all fetuses with a cystic hygroma have Turner's syndrome, it is mandatory that a chromosomal analysis is carried out if a cystic hygroma is identified on antenatal ultrasound.

Triploidy

This condition occurs when there are three sets of chromosomes present instead of the normal two sets of diploidy. The extra set can be paternal in origin (69XXY) which is the commonest, accounting for 60% of cases or maternal (69XXX) seen in 37%. A third karyotype 69XYY is seen in about 3%.[167]

The vast majority of triploid fetuses, however, will abort in the first trimester and triploid fetuses account for approximately 10% of all first trimester abortuses. Of those that survive, the commonest finding is early growth retardation associated with oligohydramnios.[19,20,168] The condition often presents as 'small for dates' in the second trimester and abnormalities in the placenta may also be demonstrated. Hydatidiform change, although not always present in triploidy, should always prompt a karyotype if seen with growth retardation and oligohydramnios.[9] Occasionally, the placenta may be enlarged and the hydropic changes may vary from solitary large cysts to multiple small cysts.[169,170]

The presence of growth retardation and oligohydramnios makes scanning the fetus difficult and the absence of any specific patterns of abnormalities compounds the problem. Cranial abnormalities are common and in particular holoprosencephaly, hydrocephalus and agenesis of the corpus callosum may be seen. Facial clefting can occur but is often difficult to demonstrate because of the oligohydramnios as are the abnormalities of the hands and feet. In the hands, syndactyly of the third and fourth fingers (Fig. 14.25) can be seen in up to 50% of fetuses. Club-foot may also be present and

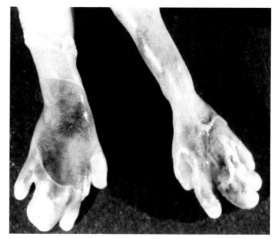

Fig. 14.25 Syndactyly of third and fourth fingers. Post-mortem photograph of the hand of a triploidy fetus, showing the typical syndactyly of the third and fourth fingers.

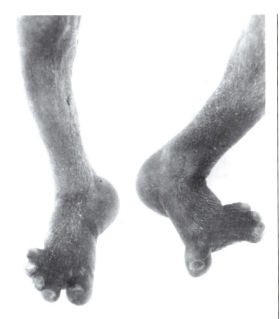

Fig. 14.26 Triploidy, separation of the first and second toes. Post-mortem photograph of a triploidy fetus, showing the typical widening and separation of the first and second toes. (Courtesy of Dr H. Andrews, Bristol Royal Infirmary.)

also a wide separation between the first and second toes (Fig. 14.26). Cardiac abnormalities are less common as are abdominal anomalies such as an omphalocoele and renal cystic dysplasia.

References

1. Schneider AS, Mennut MT, Zackai EM. High caesarean section rate in trisomy 18 births: A potential indication for late prenatal diagnosis. Am J Obstet Gynecol 1981; 140:367–370.
2. Snijders RJM, Sebire NJ, Nicolaides KH. Maternal age and gestational age specific risk for chromosomal defects. Fetal Diagn Ther 1995; 10:356–367.
3. Hook EB, Cross PK, Regal RR. The frequency of 47,+21, 47+18,47,+13 at the uppermost extremes of maternal ages: Results on 56 094 fetuses studied prenatally and comparisons with data on livebirths. Hum Genet 1984; 68:211–220.
4. Hook EB. Chromosome abnormalities and spontaneous fetal death following amniocentesis: Further data and associations with maternal age. Am J Hum Genet 1983; 35:100–116.
5. Ferguson-Smith MA, Yates JRW. Maternal age specific rates for chromosomal aberrations and factors influencing them: Report of a collaborative European study on 52 965 amniocenteses. Prenat Diagn 1984; 4:5–44.
6. Nicolaides KH, Shawa L, Brizot M, Snijders R. Ultrasonographically detectable markers of fetal chromosomal defects. Ultrasound Obstet Gynecol 1993; 3:56–69.
7. Nicolaides KH, Snijders RJM, Gosdon CM, Berry C, et al. Ultrasonographically detectable markers of fetal chromosomal abnormalities. Lancet 1992; 340:703–707.
8. Jones KL. Smith's recognisable patterns of human malformation. 4th ed. Eastbourne: WB Saunders; 1988.
9. Twining P, Zuccollo J. The ultrasound markers of chromosomal disease: A retrospective study. Br J Radiol 1993; 66:408–414.
10. Nyberg DA, Mack LA, Hirsch J. Fetal hydrocephalus: Sonographic detection and clinical significance of associated anomalies. Radiology 1987; 163:187–191.
11. Vintzileos AM, Campbell WA, Weinbaum PJ, Nochimson DJ. Perinatal management and outcome of fetal ventriculomegaly. Obstet Gynecol 1987; 69:5–11.
12. Drugan A, Kranse B, Cavaly A. The natural history of prenatally diagnosed cerebral ventriculomegaly. JAMA 1989; 261:1785–1788.
13. Filly R, Goldstein RB, Callen PW. Fetal ventricle: Importance in routine obstetric sonography. Radiology 1991; 181:1–7.
14. Getachew MM, Goldstein RB, Edge V, et al. Correlation between omphalocoele contents and karyotypic abnormalities: Sonographic study in 37 cases. Am J Radiol 1991; 158:133–136.
15. Nicolaides KH, Berry S, Snijders RJM, et al. Fetal lateral cerebral ventriculomegaly: Associated malformations and chromosomal defects. Fetal Diagn Ther 1990; 5:5–14.
16. Nicolaides KH, Cheng H, Abbas A, et al. Fetal renal defects: Associated malformations and chromosomal defects. Fetal Diagn Ther 1992; 7:1–11.
17. Benacerraf BR, Mandell J, Estroff JA, et al. Fetal pyelectasis: A possible association with Down's syndrome. Obstet Gynecol 1990; 76:58–60.
18. Benacerraf BR. Prenatal sonography of autosomal trisomies. Ultrasound Obstet Gynecol 1991; 1:66–75.
19. Edwards MT, Smith WL, Hanson J, Abu Yousef. Sonographic diagnosis of triploidy. J Ultrasound Med 1986; 5:279–281.
20. Snijders RJM, Sherod C, Gosden CM, Nicolaides KH. Fetal growth retardation: Associated malformations and chromosomal abnormalities. Am J Obstet Gynecol 1993; 168:547–555.
21. Snijders RJM, Johnson S, Sebire NJ, et al. First trimester ultrasound screening for chromosomal defects. Ultrasound Obstet Gynecol 1996; 7:216–226.
22. Royal College Of Obstetricians And Gynaecologists. Working party report on routine ultrasound examination in pregnancy; 1984.
23. Chitty LS, Hunt GH, Moore J, Lobb MO. Effectiveness of routine ultrasonography in detecting fetal structural abnormalities in a low risk population. BMJ 1991; 303:1165–1169.

24. Luck CA. Value of routine ultrasound scanning at 19 weeks: A four year study of 8849 deliveries. BMJ 1992; 304:1474–1478.

25. Ledbetter DH, Martin AO, Verlinsky Y, et al. Cytogenetic results of chorionic villus sampling. High success rate and diagnostic accuracy in the United States collaborative study. Am J Obstet Gynecol 1990; 162:495–501.

26. Nicolaides KH, Rodeck CH, Gosden CM. Rapid karyotyping in non lethal fetal abnormalities. Lancet 1986; i:283–286.

27. Daffos F, Capella P, Bovsky M, Forester F. Fetal blood sampling during pregnancy with use of a needle guided by ultrasound: A study of 606 consecutive cases. Am J Obstet Gynecol 1985; 153:655–660.

28. Maxwell DJ, Johnson P, Hurley P, et al. Fetal blood sampling and pregnancy loss in relation to indication. Br J Obstet Gynaecol 1991; 98:892–897.

29. Evans MJ, Klinger KW, Nelson B. Rapid prenatal diagnosis by fluorescent in situ hybridisation of chorionic villi. An adjunct to long term culture and karyotype. Am J Obstet Gynecol 1992; 167:1522–1525.

30. Ried T, Landes, Dackowski W. Multicolour fluorescence in situ hybridisation for the simultaneous detection of probe sets for chromosome 12, 18, 21, X and Y in uncultured amniotic fluid cells. Hum Mol Genet 1992; 1:307–313.

31. Roberts L. Fishing cuts the angst in amniocentesis. Science 1991; 254:378–379.

32. Patau K, Smith DW, Therman E. Multiple congenital anomaly caused by an extra chromosome. Lancet 1960; i:790–793.

33. Nyberg DA, Crane JP. Chromosome abnormalities. In: Nyberg DA, Mahoney BS, Pretorius DM, eds. In: Diagnostic ultrasound of fetal anomalies. Text and atlas. St Louis: Mosby Year Book; 1990:676–724.

34. Greene MF, Benacerraf BR, Frigoletto FD. Reliable criteria for the prenatal sonographic diagnosis of alobar holoprosencephaly. Am J Obstet Gynecol 1987; 156:687–689.

35. Lehman CD, Nyberg DA, Winter TC, et al. Trisomy 13 syndrome: Prenatal ultrasound findings in a review of 33 cases. Radiology 1995; 194:217–222.

36. Turner G, Twining P. The facial profile in the diagnosis of fetal abnormalities. Clin Radiol 1993; 47:389–395.

37. Benacerraf BR, Frigoletto FD, Greene MF. Abnormal facial features and extremities in human trisomy syndromes: Prenatal ultrasound appearances. Radiology 1986; 159:243–246.

38. Brown DL, Emerson DS, Shulman LP, et al. Predicting aneuploidy in fetuses with cardiac anomalies. J Ultrasound Med 1993; 3:153–161.

39. Paladini D, Calabro R, Palmieri S, D'andrea T. Prenatal diagnosis of congenital heart disease and fetal karyotyping. Obstet Gynecol 1993; 81:679–682.

40. Meckel S, Passarge E. Encephalocoele, polycystic kidneys and polydactyly as an autosomal recessive trait simulating certain other disorders: the Meckel syndrome. Ann Genet 1971; 14:97–103.

41. Sepulveda W, Pryde PG, Greb AE, et al. Prenatal diagnosis of umbilical cord pseudocyst. Ultrasound Obstet Gynecol 1994; 4:147–150.

42. Sepulveda W, Nicolaidis P, Hollingsworth J, Fisk N. Fetal cholecystomegaly: A prenatal marker of aneuploidy. Prenat Diagn 1995; 15:193–197.

43. Achiron R, Seidman DS, Afek A, et al. Prenatal ultrasonographic diagnosis of fetal hepatic hyperechogenicities: Clinical significance and implications for management. Ultrasound Obstet Gynecol 1996; 7:251–255.

44. Edwards JH. A new trisomic syndrome. Lancet 1960; i:787.

45. Carter PE, Pearn JH, Bell J, et al. Survival in trisomy 18: Life tables for use in genetic counselling and clinical paediatrics. Clin Genet 1985; 27:59–61.

46. Twining P, Zuccollo J, Clewes J, Swallow J. Fetal choroid plexus cysts: A prospective study and review of the literature. Br J Radiol 1991; 64:98–102.

47. Nyberg DA, Kramer D, Resta RG, Kapur R. Prenatal sonographic findings of trisomy 18. J Ultrasound Med 1993; 2:103–113.

48. Allan LD, Sharland GK, Chita SK. Chromosomal abnormalities in fetal congenital heart disease. Ultrasound Obstet Gynecol 1991; 1:8–11.

49. Shirley IM, Bottomley F, Robinson VP. Routine radiographer screening for fetal abnormalities by ultrasound in an unselected low risk population. Br J Radiol 1992; 65:564–569.

50. Achiron R, Glaser J, Gelernter I. Extended fetal echocardiographic examination for detecting cardiac malformations in low risk pregnancies. BMJ 1992; 304:671–674.

51. Crawford DC, Chita SK, Allan LD. Prenatal detection of congenital heart disease factors affecting obstetric management and survival. Am J Obstet Gynecol 1988; 159:352–356.

52. Devore GR, Alfi O. The use of colour Doppler ultrasound to identify fetuses at increased risk for trisomy 21: An alternative for high risk patients who decline genetic amniocentesis. Obstet Gynecol 1995; 85:378–386.

53. Copel J, Cullen M, Green JS, et al. The frequency of aneuploidy in prenatally diagnosed congenital heart disease: An indication for fetal karyotype. Am J Obstet Gynecol 1988; 158:409–413.

54. Nicolaides KH, Salveston DR, Snijders RJM, Gosden CM. Strawberry shaped skull in fetal trisomy 18. Fetal Diagn Ther 1992; 7:132–137.

55. Seymour R, Jones A. Strawberry shaped skull in fetal thanatophoric dysplasia. Ultrasound Obstet Gynecol 1994; 4:434–436.

56. Chudleigh P, Pearce JM, Campbell S. The prenatal diagnosis of transient cysts of the fetal choroid plexus. Prenat Diagn 1984; 4:135–137.

57. Ostlere SJ, Irving HC, Lilford RJ. Fetal choroid plexus cysts: A report of 100 cases. Radiology 1990; 175:753–755.

58. Nadel AS, Bromley BS, Frigoletto FD, et al. Isolated choroid plexus cysts in the second trimester fetus: Is

amniocentesis really indicated? Radiology 1992; 185:545–548.

59. Nava S, Godmilow L, Rieser S, et al. Significance of sonographically detected second trimester choroid plexus cysts: A series of 211 cases and a review of the literature. Ultrasound Obstet Gynecol 1994; 4:448–451.

60. Gross SJ, Shulman LP, Tolley EA, et al. Isolated fetal choroid plexus cysts and trisomy 18: A review and meta analysis. Am J Obstet Gynecol 1995; 172:83–87.

61. Gupta JK, Thornton JG, Lilford RJ. Management of fetal choroid plexus cysts. Br J Obstet Gynaecol 1997; 104:881–886.

62. Furness ME. Choroid plexus cysts and trisomy 18. Lancet 1987; ii:693.

63. Shields LE, Ulrick SB, Easterling TR, et al. Isolated fetal choroid plexus cysts and karyotype analysis: Is it necessary? J Ultrasound Med 1996; 15:389–394.

64. Walkinshaw S, Pilling D, Sprigg A. Isolated choroid plexus cysts: The need for routine offer of karyotyping. Prenat Diagn 1994; 14:663–667.

65. Twining P, Clewes JS. The emotional impact of the antenatal detection of choroid plexus cysts at 18–20 weeks. Fourth World Congress of Ultrasound in Obstetrics and Gynecology, Budapest. Ultrasound Obstet Gynecol 1994; (Supplement 1):200.

66. Nyberg DA, Mahoney BS, Heggs FN, et al. Enlarged cisterna vena magna and the Dandy–Walker malformation: Factors associated with chromosome abnormalities. Obstet Gynecol 1991; 77:436–442.

67. Twining P, Zuccollo J, Jaspan T. The outcome of fetal ventriculomegaly. Br J Radiol 1994; 67:26–31.

68. Nicolaides KH, Berry S, Snijders RJM, et al. Fetal lateral cerebral ventriculomegaly: Associated malformations and chromosomal defects. Fetal Diagn Ther 1990; 5:5–14.

69. Thorpe-Beeston JG, Gosden CM, Nicolaides KH. Congenital diaphragmatic hernia, associated malformations and chromosomal defects. Fetal Ther 1989; 4:21–28.

70. Nyberg DA, Fitsimmons J, Mack LA. Chromosomal abnormalities in fetuses with omphalocoele, significance of omphalocoele contents. J Ultrasound Med 1989; 8:299–308.

71. Nicolaides KH, Snijders RJM, Cheng H, et al. Fetal abdominal wall and gastrointestinal tract defects: Associated malformations and chromosomal defects. Fetal Diagn Ther 1992; 7:102–115.

72. Benacerraf BR, Saltzman DH, Estroff JA, Frigoletto FD. Abnormal karyotype of fetuses with omphalocoele: Prediction based on omphalocoele contents. Obstet Gynecol 1990; 75:317–319.

73. Nicolaides KH, Cheng H, Snijders RJM, Gosden CM. Fetal renal defects: Associated malformations and chromosomal defects. Fetal Diagn Ther 1992; 7:1–11.

74. Dicke JM, Crane JP. Sonographic recognition of major malformations and aberent growth in trisomic fetuses. J Ultrasound Med 1991; 10:433–438.

75. Down JLM. Observations on an ethnic classification

of idiots. Clinical Lecture Reports, London Hospital 1866; 3:259.

76. Bleyer A. Indication that mongoloid inbecility is a gametogenic mutation of degenerating type. Am J Dis Childhood 1934; 47:342.

77. Nyberg DA, Resta RG, Luthy DA, et al. Prenatal sonographic findings of Down's syndrome: Review of 94 cases. Obstet Gynecol 1990; 76:370–377.

78. Wald NJ, Kennard A, Densem JW, et al. Antenatal maternal serum screening for Down's syndrome: Results of a demonstration project. BMJ 1992; 305:391–394.

79. Wald NJ, George L, Smith D, et al. Serum screening for Down's syndrome between 8 and 14 weeks of pregnancy. Br J Obstet Gynaecol 1996; 103:407–412.

80. Nicolaides KH, Sebire NJ, Snijders RJM, Johnson S. Down's screening in the United Kingdom. Lancet 1996; 347:906–907.

81. Benacerraf BR. The second-trimester fetus with Down's syndrome: Detection using sonographic features. Ultrasound Obstet Gynecol 1996; 7:147–155.

82. Nelson LH, Clark CE, Fishburne JI, et al. Value of serial sonography in the in utero detection of duodenal atresia. Obstet Gynecol 1982; 59:657–660.

83. Sharland G, Lockhart S. Isolated pericardial effusion: An indication for fetal karyotyping? Ultrasound Obstet Gynecol 1995; 6:29–32.

84. Nicolaides KH, Azar G, Snijders RJM, Gosden CM. Fetal nuchal oedema, associated malformations and chromosomal defects. Fetal Diagn Ther 1992; 7:123–131.

85. Benacerraf BR, Laboda LA, Frigoletto FD. Thickened nuchal fold in fetuses not at risk for aneuploidy. Radiology 1992; 84:239–242.

86. Grandjean H, Sarramon MF. Sonographic measurement of nuchal skinfold thickness for detection of Down's syndrome in second trimester fetus: A multicenter prospective study. Obstet Gynecol 1995; 86:103–106.

87. Watson WJ, Miller RC, Menard K, et al. Ultrasonographic measurement of fetal nuchal skin to screen for chromosomal abnormalities. Am J Obstet Gynecol 1994; 170:583–586.

88. Devore GR, Alfi O. The association between an abnormal nuchal skin fold, trisomy 21 and ultrasound abnormalities identified during the second trimester of pregnancy. Ultrasound Obstet Gynecol 1993; 3:387–394.

89. Toi A, Simpson GF, Filly RA. Ultrasonically evident fetal nuchal skin thickening: Is it specific for Down's syndrome? Am J Obstet Gynecol 1987; 156:150–153.

90. Borrell A, Costa MB, Martinez J, et al. Early mid trimester fetal nuchal thickness: Effectiveness as a marker of Down's syndrome. Obstet Gynecol 1996; 175:45–49.

91. Boyd PA, Anthony MY, Manning N, et al. Antenatal diagnosis of cystic hygroma or nuchal pad – Report of 92 cases with follow up of survivors. Arch Dis Child 1996; 74:38–42.

92. Nicolaides KH. Screening for fetal chromosomal

abnormalities: Need to change the rules. Ultrasound Obstet Gynecol 1994; 4:353–354.

93. Lockwood C, Benacerraf BR, Krinsky A, et al. A sonographic screening for Down's syndrome. Am J Obstet Gynecol 1987; 157:803–808.

94. Benacerraf BR, Galman R, Frigoletto FD. Sonographic identification of second trimester fetuses with Down's syndrome. N Engl J Med 1987; 317:1371–1376.

95. Lynch L, Berkowitz GS, Chitkara U, Wickinsi A, et al. Ultrasound detection of Down's syndrome: Is it really possible? Obstet Gynecol 1989; 73:267–270.

96. Nyberg DA, Resta RG, Hickok D. Femur length shortening in the detection of Down's syndrome: Is prenatal screening feasible? Am J Obstet Gynecol 1990; 162:1247–1252.

97. Twining P, Whalley D, Lewin E, Foulkes K. Is a short femur length a useful marker for Down's syndrome? Br J Radiol 1991; 64:990–992.

98. Nyberg DA, Resta RG, Luthy DA, et al. Humerus and femur length shortening in the detection of Down's syndrome. Am J Obstet Gynecol 1993; 168:534–538.

99. Johnson MP, Michaelson JE, Barr M, et al. Combining humerus and femur length for improved ultrasonographic identification of pregnancies at increased risk for trisomy 21. Am J Obstet Gynecol 1995; 172:1229–1235.

100. Lince DM, Pretorius DH, Manco-Johnson ML, et al. The clinical significance of increased echogenicity in the fetal abdomen. AJR 1985; 145:683–686.

101. Dicke JM, Crane JP. Sonographically detected hyperechogenic fetal bowel: Significance and implications for pregnancy management. Obstet Gynecol 1992; 80:778–782.

102. Bromley B, Doubilet P, Frigoletto F, et al. Is fetal hyperechoic bowel on second trimester sonogram an indication for amniocentesis? Obstet Gynecol 1994; 83:647–651.

103. Fakhry J, Reisner M, Shapiro LR, et al. Increased echogenicity in the lower fetal abdomen: A common normal variant in the second trimester. J Ultrasound Med 1986; 5:489–492.

104. Nyberg DA, Dubinsky T, Resta RG, et al. Echogenic bowel during the second trimester: Clinical importance. Radiology 1993; 188:527–531.

105. Muller F, Dommergues M, Aubry MC, et al. Hyperechogenic fetal bowel: An ultrasonographic marker for adverse fetal and neonatal outcome. Am J Obstet Gynecol 1995; 173:508–513.

106. Stringer MD, Thornton JG, Moran GC. Hyperechogenic fetal bowel. Arch Dis Child 1996; 74:F1–F2.

107. Sepulveda W, Reid R, Nicolaidis P, et al. Second trimester echogenic bowel and intramniotic bleeding: Association between fetal bowel echogenicity and amniotic fluid spectrophotometry at 410 mm. Am J Obstet Gynecol 1996; 174:834–842.

108. Ewer AK, McHugo JM, Chapman S, Neuvell SJ. Fetal echogenic gut: A marker of intrauterine gut ischaemia? Arch Dis Child 1993; 69:510–513.

109. Carroll SG, Maxwell DJ. The significance of echogenic areas in the fetal abdomen. Ultrasound Obstet Gynecol 1996; 7:293–298.

110. Wickstrom EA, Thangavelu M, Parilla BV, et al. A prospective study of the association between isolated fetal pyelectasis and chromosomal abnormality. Obstet Gynecol 1996; 88:379–382.

111. Corteville JE, Dicke JM, Crane J. Fetal pyelectasis and Down's syndrome: Is genetic amniocentesis warranted. Obstet Gynecol 1992; 79:770–772.

112. Wickstrom E, Maizels M, Sabbagha R, et al. Isolated fetal pyelectasis assessment of risk for postnatal uropathy and Down's syndrome. Ultrasound Obstet Gynecol 1996; 8:236–240.

113. Chitly L, Chudleigh T, Campbell S, Pembray M. Incidence, natural history and clinical significance of mild fetal pyelectasis. Br J Radiol 1992; 65:636.

114. Roberts DJ, Genest D. Cardiac histologic pathology characteristic of trisomies 13 and 21. Hum Pathol 1992; 23:1130–1140.

115. Merati R, Lovotti M, Norchi S, et al. Prevalence of fetal left ventricular hyperchogenic foci in a low risk population. Br J Obstet Gynaecol 1996; 103:1102–1104.

116. Bromley B, Lieberman E, Laboda L, Benaceraff B. Echogenic intracardiac focus: A sonographic sign for fetal Down's syndrome. Obstet Gynecol 1995; 96:998–1001.

117. Petrikovski BM, Challenger M, Wyse LJ. Natural history of echogenic foci within ventricles of the fetal heart. Ultrasound Obstet Gynecol 1995; 5:92–94.

118. Levy DW, Mintz MC. The left ventricular echogenic focus: A normal variant. Am J Radiol 1987; 150:85–86.

119. How HY, Villafane J, Parihus RR, Spinnato JA. Small hyperechoic foci of the fetal cardiac ventricle: A benign sonographic finding? Ultrasound Obstet Gynecol 1994; 4:205–207.

120. Sepulveda W, Cullen S, Nicolaidis P, et al. Echogenic foci in the fetal heart: A marker of chromosomal abnormality. Br J Obstet Gynecol 1995; 102:490–492.

121. Simpson JM, Cook AC, Sharland GK. The significance of echogenic foci in the fetal heart: A prospective study of 228 cases. Ultrasound Obstet Gynecol 1996; 8:225–228.

122. Hall B. Mongolism in newborn infants. Clin Paediatr 1966; 5:4.

123. Greulich WW. A comparison of the dysplastic middle phalanx of the fifth finger in mentally normal Caucasians, mongoloids, and Negroes, with that of individuals of the same racial groups who have Down's syndrome. AJR 1973; 118:259–281.

124. Benacerraf BR, Osathanond R, Frigoletto FD. Sonographic demonstration of hypoplasia of the middle phalanx of the fifth finger: A finding associated with Down's syndrome. Am J Obstet Gynecol 1988; 159:181–183.

125. Benacerraf BR, Harlow BL, Frigoletto FD. Hypoplasia of the middle phalanx of the fifth finger.

A feature of the second trimester fetus with Down's syndrome. J Ultrasound Med 1990; 9:389–394.

126. Goldstein I, Gomiz K, Copel JA. Fifth digit measurement in normal pregnancies: A potential sonographic sign of Down's syndrome. Ultrasound Obstet Gynecol 1995; 5:34–37.

127. Jeanty P. Prenatal detection of simian crease. J Ultrasound Med 1990; 9:131–136.

128. Wilkins I. Separation of the great toe in fetuses with Down's syndrome. J Ultrasound Med 1994; 13:229–231.

129. Snijders RJM, Nicolaides KM. Ultrasound markers for fetal chromosomal defects. London: Parthenon; 1996.

130. Nicolaides KH, Salvesen DR, Snijders RJM, Gosden CM. Fetal facial defects: Associated malformations and chromosomal abnormalities. Fetal Diagn Ther 1993; 8:1–9.

131. Lettieri L, Rodis JF, Vintzileos AM, et al. Ear length in second trimester aneuploid fetuses. Obstet Gynecol 1993; 81:57–60.

132. Bahado-Singh RO, Wyse L, Dorr MA, et al. Fetuses with Down's syndrome have disproportionately shortened frontal lobe dimensions on ultrasonographic examination. Am J Obstet Gynecol 1992; 167:1009–1014.

133. Abuhamad AZ, Kolm P, Mari G, et al. Ultrasonographic fetal iliac length measurement in the screening for Down's syndrome. Am J Obstet Gynecol 1994; 171:1063–1067.

134. Petrikovsky BM, Schneider EP, Klin VR, et al. Fetal breasts in normal and Down's syndrome fetuses. J Clin Ultrasound 1996; 24:507–511.

135. Snijders RJM, Nicolaides KH. Ultrasound markers for fetal chromosomal defects. Frontiers In Medicine Series. London: Parthenon; 1996.

136. Vintzileos AM, Egan JF. Adjusting the risk for trisomy 21 on the basis of second trimester ultrasonography. Am J Obstet Gynecol 1995; 172:837–844.

137. Nyberg DA, Luthy DA, Cheng EY, et al. Role of prenatal ultrasonography in women with positive screen for Down's syndrome on the basis of maternal serum markers. Am J Obstet Gynecol 1995; 173:1030–1035.

138. Nadel AS, Bromley D, Frigoletto F, Denacerraf DR. Can the presumed risk of autosmal trisomy be decreased in fetuses of older women following a normal sonogram? J Ultrasound Med 1995; 14:297–302.

139. Elejalde BR, Elejalde MM, Leno J. Nuchal cysts syndromes: Etiology, pathogenesis and prenatal diagnosis. Am J Med Genet 1985; 21:417–432.

140. Szabo J, Gellen J. Nuchal fluid accumulation in trisomy 21 detected by vaginosonography in first trimester. Lancet 1990; 3:1133.

141. Moscoso G. Fetal nuchal translucency: Need to understand the physiological basis. Ultrasound Obstet Gynecol 1995; 5:6–8.

142. Hyett J, Moscoso G, Papapanagiotou G, et al. Abnormalities of the heart and great arteries in chromosomally normal fetuses with increased nuchal translucency thickness at 11–13 weeks of gestation. Ultrasound Obstet Gynecol 1996; 7:245–250.

143. Hyett J, Moscoso G, Nicolaides KH. First trimester nuchal translucency and cardiac septal defects in fetuses with trisomy 21. Am J Obstet Gynecol 1995; 172:1411–1413.

144. Brand-Saberi B, Epperlein HH, Romanaos E, Christ B. Distribution of extracellular matrix components in nuchal skin fetuses carrying trisomy 18 and trisomy 21. Cell Tissue Res 1994; 277:465–475.

145. Snijders RJM, Johnson S, Sabire NJ, et al. First trimester ultrasound screening for chromosomal defects. Ultrasound Obstet Gynecol 1996; 7:216–276.

146. Roberts LJ, Bewley S, Mackinson AM, Rodeck CH. First trimester fetal nuchal translucency: Problems with screening the general population 1. Br J Obstet Gynecol 1995; 102:381–385.

147. Pandya PP, Altman DG, Brizot ML, et al. Repeatability of measurement of fetal nuchal translucency thickness. Ultrasound Obstet Gynecol 1995; 5:334–337.

148. Schulte Vallentin M, Schindler H. Non-echogenic nuchal oedema as a marker in trisomy 21 screening. Lancet 1992; 339:1053.

149. Salvodelli G, Binkert F, Achermann J, Schmid W. Ultrasound screening for chromosomal anomalies in the first trimester of pregnancy. Prenat Diagn 1993; 13:513–518.

150. Brambati B, Cislaghi C, Tului L, et al. First trimester Down's syndrome screening using nuchal translucency: A prospective study in patients undergoing CVS. Ultrasound Obstet Gynecol 1995; 5:9–14.

151. Comas C, Martinez JM, Ojuel J, et al. First-trimester nuchal edema as a marker of aneuploidy. Ultrasound Obstet Gynecol 1995; 5:26–29.

152. Szabo J, Gellen J, Szemere G. First-trimester ultrasound screening for fetal aneuploides in women over 35 and under 35 years of age. Ultrasound Obstet Gynecol 1995; 5:161–163.

153. Bewley S, Roberts LJ, Mackinson AM, Rodeck CH. First trimester fetal nuchal translucency: Problems with screening the general population 2. Br J Obstet Gynecol 1995; 102:386–388.

154. Hafner E, Schuchter K, Philipp K. Screening for chromosomal abnormalities in an unselected population by fetal nuchal translucency. Ultrasound Obstet Gynecol 1995; 6:330–333.

155. Kornman LH, Morssink LP, Beekhuis JR, et al. Nuchal translucency cannot be used as a screening test for chromosome abnormalities in the first trimester of pregnancy in a routine ultrasound practice. Prenat Diagn 1996; 16:747–806.

156. Pandya PP, Snijders RJM, Johnson S, Nicolaides KH. Natural history of trisomy 21 fetuses with increased nuchal translucency thickness. Ultrasound Obstet Gynecol 1995; 5:381–383.

157. Hyett JA, Sebire NJ, Snijders RJM, Nicolaides KH. Intrauterine lethality of trisomy 21 fetuses with increased nuchal translucency thickness. Ultrasound Obstet Gynecol 1996; 7:101–103.

158. Pandya PP, Kondylios A, Hubert L, et al. Chromosomal defects: an outcome in 1015 fetuses with increased nuchal translucency. Ultrasound Obstet Gynacol 1995; 5:15–19.

159. Trauffer PML, Anderson CE, Johnson A, et al. The natural history of euploid pregnancies with first trimester cystic hygromas. Am J Obstet Gynecol 1994; 170:1279–1284.

160. Hyett JA, Noble PL, Snijders RJM, et al. Fetal heart rate in trisomy 21 and other chromosomal abnormalities at 10–14 weeks of gestation. Ultrasound Obstet Gynecol 1996; 7:239–244.

161. Martinez JM, Comas C, Ojuel J, et al. Fetal heart rate patterns in pregnancies with chromosomal disorders and subsequent fetal loss. Obstet Gynecol 1996; 87:118–121.

162. Martinez JM, Borrell A, Antohn E, et al. Combining nuchal translucency with umbilical artery Doppler velocimetry for detecting fetal trisomies in the first trimester of pregnancy. Br J Obstet Gynaecol 1997; 104:11–14.

163. Obrien WF, Cefalo RC, Bair DG. Ultrasonographic diagnosis of fetal cystic hygroma. Am J Obstet Gynecol 1980; 138:464–466.

164. Nyberg DA, Crane JP. Chromosome abnormalities. In: Nyberg DA, Mahoney BS, Pretorius DM, eds. Diagnostic ultrasound in fetal anomalies. St Louis: Mosby Year Book; 1990:676–724.

165. Goldstein R, Lapidus AS, Filly RA. Fetal cephalocoeles: Diagnosis with ultrasound. Radiology 1991; 180:803–808.

166. Azar GB, Snijders RJM, Gooden C, Nicolaides KH. Fetal nuchal cystic hygromata: Associated malformations and chromosomal defects. Fetal Diagn Ther 1991; 6:46–57.

167. Uchida IA, Freeman VCP. Triploidy and chromosomes. Am J Obstet Gynecol 1985; 151:65–69.

168. Lockwood C, Sciosa A, Stiller R. Sonographic features of the triploid fetus. Am J Obstet Gynecol 1987; 157:285–287.

169. Szulman AE, Philipp E, Bone JG, Bone A. Human triploidy: Association with partial hydatidiform moles and non molar conceptuses. Hum Pathol 1982; 12:1016.

170. Rubenstein JB, Swayne LC, Dise CA, et al. Placental changes in fetal triploidy syndrome. J Ultrasound Med 1986; 5:545–550.

CHAPTER 15

Abnormalities of the face and neck

Peter Twining

THE FETAL FACE

Introduction

The antenatal diagnosis of facial abnormalities is important for a number of reasons. Facial abnormalities are often associated with other anomalies and may be a clue to the detection of chromosomal disease[1] or a more complex syndrome.[2] This has practical implications in terms of karyotype procedures and genetic counselling. The detection of isolated facial anomalies is also important as the parents may have time to prepare themselves for the abnormality and be counselled by paediatric and plastic surgeons as to the treatment options and long-term outlook for the baby. Facial abnormalities also have a major impact in psychological and emotional terms as it is the face that is the focus of social interaction. Pruzansky has observed that:

> The face of man is his window to the world, containing the organs of sight, hearing and speech, it is the facade by which others perceive and judge the individual. Abnormalities that affect the face of man strikes at the most visible parts of his body and his most human functions such as speech.[3]

It is important therefore to make as precise a diagnosis as possible in order to give the parents a clear picture of the abnormality. In this respect the introduction of three-dimensional imaging[4] may well have an impact not only for improving the parents' understanding of the defect but also to give paediatric surgeons a clearer assessment of the problem.

Detection rates

In the UK, routine ultrasound screening is offered to the majority of women at 18 to 20 weeks' gestation[5] and it has been estimated that the fetal face is assessed in approximately 50% of examinations. Detection rates for fetal facial abnormalities vary; however, reported series range from 25% to 43% in the low-risk population.[6–8] Although detection rates in a high-risk population are difficult to assess, Pilu et al detected 12 out of 14 cases of facial malformation in 223 patients at high risk for carrying fetuses with craniofacial malformations.[9]

Embryology

The embryology of the face is a complex process but knowledge of embryology is useful in understanding some of the facial abnormalities and, in particular, facial clefting.

The human face is formed between the 4th and 10th week of pregnancy by the fusion of five facial swellings: an unpaired frontonasal process, a pair of maxillary swellings and a pair of mandibular swellings (Fig. 15.1A). The maxillary and mandibular swellings constitute dorsal and ventral regions respectively of the first pharyngeal arch and give rise to the upper and lower jaws.[10]

During the 5th week, two swellings appear on the frontonasal process which form the medial and lateral nasal processes (Fig. 15.1B). In the 6th week, the two medial nasal swellings migrate medially and by the 7th week, they fuse to form the central portion of the nose; the lateral nasal processes form the nostrils. The maxillary swellings also migrate medially so that by the 10th week they have fused in the midline to form the philtrum of the upper lip and the primary (anterior) palate (Figs 15.1C, D). The posterior or secondary palate forms from two, thin, soft tissue bands that arise from the medial walls of the maxillary swellings termed the palatine shelves. These two palatine shelves appear during the 8th and 9th week and grow medially to fuse in the midline at approximately 10 weeks. Fusion commences anteriorly and progresses posteriorly (Figs 15.2A, B) to form the secondary palate.[11] During the same period, growth of the nasal septum separates the left and right nasal passages (Fig. 15.2B).

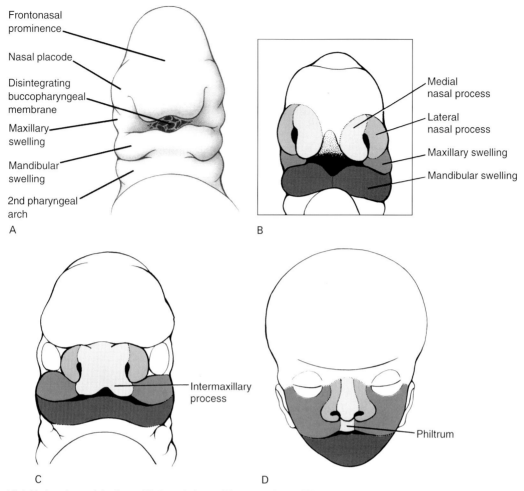

Fig. 15.1 Embryology of the face. (A) 5-week fetus. (B) 6-week fetus. (C) Late 7th week. (D) 10th week. (Reproduced with permission from Larsen WJ. Human embryology. London: Churchill Livingstone; 1993.)

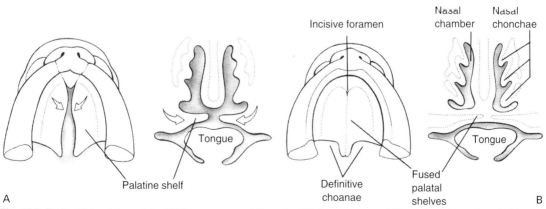

Fig. 15.2 Embryology of the palate. (A) Appearances at 8 weeks. (B) Appearances at 10 weeks. (Reproduced with permission from Larsen WJ. Human embryology. London: Churchill Livingstone; 1993.)

The eyes first appear in the 4th week in the form of a pair of lateral grooves, the optic sulci, which grow out from the primitive forebrain to reach the surface ectoderm to form the optic vesicle (Fig. 15.3). The optic vesicle differentiates into the optic cup and lens so that by the 8th week, the basic structure of the eye is established. The developing lens is supplied by the hyaloid artery which is the terminal branch of the ophthalmic artery (Fig. 15.4). The portion of the artery that crosses the vitreous degenerates at the end of the second trimester[12] and the remainder of the artery forms the central artery of the retina. The eyelids form at about 8 weeks and remain fused until approximately 20 weeks. The orbits form around the developing eye from the hypophyseal cartilages and the greater and lesser wings of the sphenoid.[10]

The ear has a complex embryology with the external and middle ears arising from the first and second pharyngeal arches whereas the inner ear develops from an epidermal tissue mass, the otic placode, which appears during the 3rd week. Development of the inner and middle ear is complete by the 8th week. The pinna of the ear is formed from six auricular swellings which appear at 6 weeks and fuse by approximately 10 weeks.

Thus, by 10 weeks, the basic structure of the face is complete.

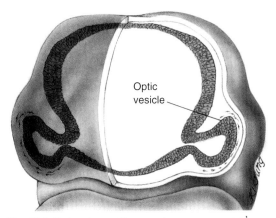

Fig. 15.3 Embryology of the eye. Appearances at $4\frac{1}{2}$ weeks. (Reproduced with permission from Larsen WJ. Human embryology. London: Churchill Livingstone; 1993.)

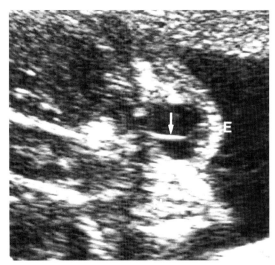

Fig. 15.4 Transverse scan through the fetal eye, showing the fetal hyaloid artery (arrow). E, eye; N, nasopharynx.

Sonographic technique

Scanning of the fetal face is essentially carried out in three planes: the transverse axial, coronal and sagittal. All three scanning planes have importance and each plane contributes different information about the face.[13]

The coronal plane is best achieved by first obtaining a standard biparietal diameter view and rotating the transducer through 90° so that one then has a coronal section through the head. By then advancing the transducer anteriorly through the fetal head, one will first scan through the anterior cranial fossa and subsequently the bony orbits and forehead. Careful scanning of the orbits should reveal the lens of the eye (Fig. 15.5).

In order to demonstrate the lips and nose, the transducer will have to be rotated around the curve of the face. Assuming the fetus is lying in a cephalic position, if the fetus is facing the person scanning, then the transducer should be moved towards the fetal chin and rotated a quarter turn clockwise. This should provide visualization of the chins, lips and nostrils (Fig. 15.6). This section is the best for demonstration of facial clefting.[16,17]

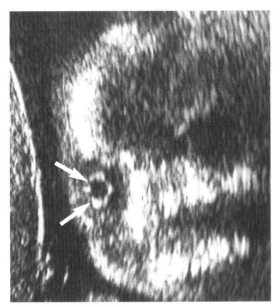

Fig. 15.5 Coronal scan through the orbit, showing the lens (arrows).

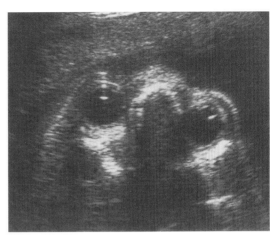

Fig. 15.7 Transverse scan through the orbits.

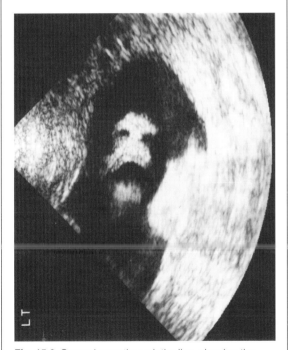

Fig. 15.6 Coronal scan through the lips, showing the upper lips and nostrils.

The transverse axial plane is achieved by first obtaining a standard biparietal diameter view. The transducer is then moved slowly towards the skull base. The bony orbits should be clearly visualized and the lenses of

the eyes will also be evident. Scanning of the orbits can be carried out with the head facing to the left or right or as in Figure 15.7 with the head facing the transducer. Accurate measurements of the orbits can be carried out and compared to standard graphs for orbital diameters and interorbital measurements (Fig. 15.8).[14]

Scanning further downwards will reveal the upper lip and maxilla. From about 16 weeks' gestation, tooth buds will be visualized, mainly those of the four incisor and the two canine teeth (Fig. 15.9). The junction between the incisor and canine teeth marks the line of fusion between the primary and secondary palate (Fig. 15.10).[15] Scanning into the mouth will reveal the tongue (Fig. 15.11) and then continuing further downwards in the transverse plane demonstrates the mandible (Fig. 15.12).

The sagittal on profile view is best obtained with the fetus facing the transducer as in Figure 15.7. In this position, simply by rotating the transducer through 90° will produce a sagittal section through the face.[13] Care must be taken to obtain a true sagittal view and in order to do this the plane of section should avoid the orbits but demonstrate the nasal bone,[18] indicating a mid-sagittal scanning plane (Fig. 15.13). The sagittal plane is the most useful in order to obtain a global view of the face and is particularly useful in detecting conditions such as micrognathia and frontal bossing. It

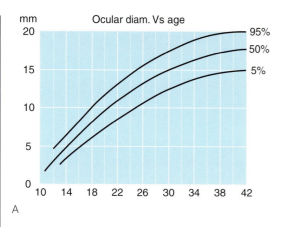

A

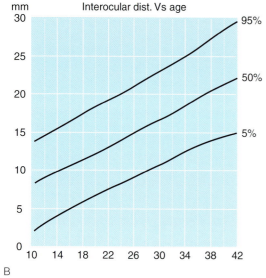

B

Fig. 15.8 Graphs of orbital measurements. (A) Ocular diameter vs gestational age. (B) Interocular distance vs gestational age. (Reproduced with permission from Jeanty P, et al. Fetal ocular biometry by ultrasound. Radiology 1982; 143:513–516.)

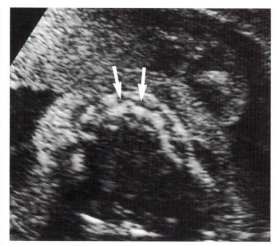

Fig. 15.9 Transverse scan through the maxilla, showing teeth buds (arrows).

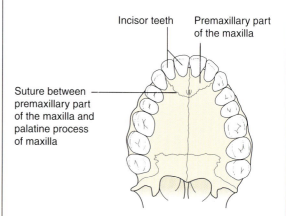

Fig. 15.10 Drawing of the human palate in the axial plane, showing the suture between the primary and secondary palate. (Reproduced with permission from Babcook CJ, et al. Evaluation of fetal mid-face anatomy related to facial clefts. Use of ultrasound. Radiology 1996; 201:113–118.)

can also provide additional information in cases of facial clefting.

The sagittal view is also of value in demonstrating the fetal ear.[19,20] By scanning laterally off the face in the sagittal plane, the ears can easily be demonstrated (Fig. 15.14). In the late second trimester, ear lobe morphology can also be assessed. Low-set ears are best demonstrated in the coronal plane where the relationship of the ear to the temporal bone and shoulder is easier to evaluate (Fig. 15.15).

Sonographic approach

The visualization of the fetal face consists of scanning the face in the three scanning planes already outlined. Demonstration of the orbits should reveal that both orbits are of equal size and that there is no evidence of hypertelorism (orbits too far apart) or hypotelorism (orbits too close together). As mentioned in the previous section, there are charts available for orbital measurements[14] but, as a rule of thumb, the interorbital

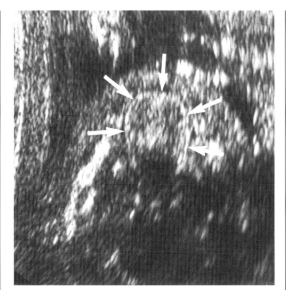

Fig. 15.11 Transverse scan through the mouth, showing the fetal tongue (arrows).

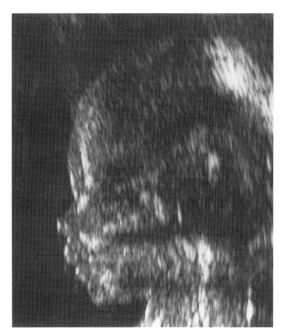

Fig. 15.13 Mid-sagittal section of the face.

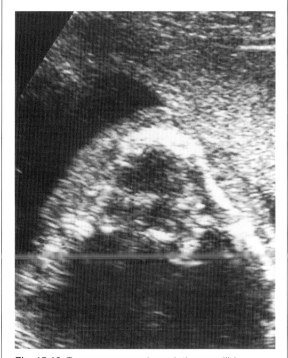

Fig. 15.12 Transverse scan through the mandible.

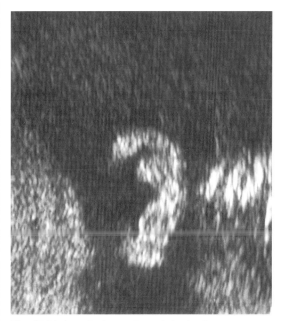

Fig. 15.14 A sagittal scan through the fetal ear.

distance is approximately equal to the orbital diameter.

Both lenses should always be demonstrated and should appear anechoic, thus excluding congenital cataracts.

Both lips should be visualized using both coronal and transverse scans to exclude facial clefting and the mandible is best assessed using the profile view to exclude micrognathia. The profile view should form a smooth curve running from forehead, nose,

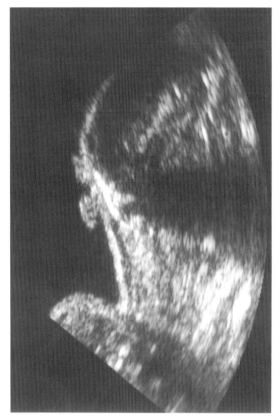
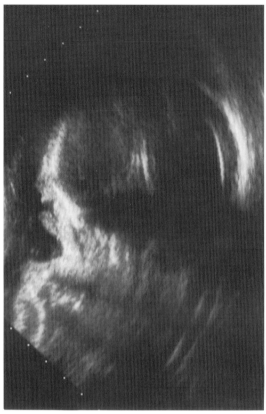

A   B

Fig. 15.15 Coronal scan through the ear and shoulder, showing relationship of ear to head and shoulder. (A) Normal appearances. (B) Low-set ears.

maxilla to mandible; any break in this smooth curve is suspicious and warrants careful assessment. In addition, an unduly flat profile is also worrying and raises the possibility of chromosomal disease.

The presence of both ears should also be established and their relationship to the temporal bone should also be assessed to exclude low-set ears.

Finally, a full assessment of the fetus should always be carried out as many facial abnormalities are often part of a more complex syndrome.

Pitfalls and artefacts

Visualization of the fetal face can be time-consuming as if the fetal head is positioned low in the pelvis or facing posteriorly, it may not be possible to obtain coronal or sagittal sections.

Turner & Twining assessed the ability to visualize the fetal face in coronal and sagittal sections and found that at 16 to 20 weeks, coronal and sagittal sections were obtained in 97% and 95% of cases respectively. However, this fell to 89% and 78% of cases at 35 to 40 weeks' gestation.[13] In addition, if the face is pressed close to the side wall of the uterus, then once again there will be difficulties in demonstrating the facial features. Occasionally, the umbilical cord can cause problems in interpretation as if the cord is draped over the upper lip in a vertical direction, then this can produce the false impression of a facial cleft. Scanning the fetus whilst opening its mouth or during fetal movement should show the cord moving away from the lip. The other alternative is to use colour flow Doppler in order to demonstrate blood flow within the cord.

Facial abnormalities

There are many different facial abnormalities and Gorlin et al have described over 150 syndromes involving the head and neck.[21] A large number of facial malformations can be classified based on pathogenesis, location of the anatomic defect and the structures involved. Stewart has proposed a classification into four major groups:[2]

1. Otocraniofacial syndromes, i.e. syndromes predominantly involving the mandible and ear, such as Treacher Collins syndrome and Goldenhar syndrome
2. Facial clefting
3. Mid-face syndromes such as holoprosencephalic malformation syndromes and frontonasal dysplasia
4. Craniosynostosis syndromes.

Although this classification will be incorporated into the discussion on facial abnormalities, the ultrasound findings will be described on an anatomic basis. The discussion starts with abnormalities of the mandible, then lips and mouth, nose and orbits, the ears and finally facial anomalies associated with abnormalities of the skull. In this way the discussion will follow a step-by-step approach, evaluating the facial structures from mandible to skull in a logical fashion.

The mandible

Micrognathia

A mild form of micrognathia may be a normal variant and is probably overlooked during routine scanning. More marked micrognathia is seen in a large number of chromosomal and genetic syndromes.

The cause of micrognathia is unclear but as the mandible is formed from the first pharyngeal arch, it is known that damage to the developing pharyngeal arch complex can cause abnormalities of the mandible, maxilla and ear. It has been postulated that ischaemic necrosis caused by an expanding haematoma arising from the stapedial artery system which provides the initial blood supply to first pharyngeal arch can produce underdevelopment of the first arch resulting in craniofacial microsomia.[10] This is thought to be the aetiology of syndromes such as Goldenhar and hemifacial microsomia[23] (see p. 355).

Jones lists 54 syndromes in which micrognathia is a common feature.[22] Turner & Twining reported nine cases of micrognathia in a series of 24 antenatal diagnoses of facial abnormalities and the majority were associated with either chromosomal disease or skeletal dysplasias.[13]

Nicolaides et al reported 146 cases of facial abnormality detected antenatally and of those there were 56 cases of micrognathia. All cases demonstrated other malformations, and chromosomal abnormalities were seen in 66%.

Bromley & Benacerraf also found a wide range of syndromes among their series of 20 fetuses with micrognathia.[24] In particular, the authors emphasized the poor outlook for fetuses with micrognathia with only 4 out of the 20 surviving the neonatal period. Nicolaides et al also reported a poor outcome in their series with only one survivor in the group of fetuses with a normal karyotype.

The main cause of death in many cases was problems related to respiratory difficulties secondary to micrognathia, and also complications secondary to associated malformations. In view of this it is important to ensure that paediatric support is present at delivery to carry out endotracheal intubation, if required. Table 15.1 outlines some of the syndromes associated with micrognathia.

Chromosomal disease

Micrognathia is a well-documented feature of certain chromosomal abnormalities. It is most commonly seen in trisomy 18 where it occurs in up to 53% of cases[1] (Fig. 15.16).

Table 15.1
Causes of micrognathia

Idiopathic	Mild form
Chromosomal disease	Trisomy 18, triploidy
Skeletal dysplasias	Camptomelic dysplasia
	Diastrophic dysplasia
	Short rib polydactyly syndrome
	Achondrogenesis
Genetic syndromes	Treacher Collins syndrome
	Goldenhar syndrome
	Hemifacial microsomia
	Pierre Robin syndrome
	Seckel syndrome
	Pena–Shokeir syndrome
	DiGeorge syndrome
	Hydrolethalus syndrome
	Roberts syndrome*
	Miller syndrome*
	Mohr syndrome*

Associated with facial clefting (see next section).

The other major chromosomal anomaly where micrognathia is a feature is triploidy where it may be seen in over 40% of cases. Micrognathia is also occasionally seen in trisomy 13. However, facial clefting is a much more common finding.[22] Bromley & Benacerraf found chromosomal disease in 25% of their series of 20 fetuses with micrognathia.[24]

Skeletal dysplasias

Bromley & Benaceraff reported two skeletal abnormalities in their series of 20 cases of micrognathia, including osteochondro-dysplasia and arthrogryposis multiplex congenita.[24] Turner & Twining described three skeletal dysplasias in their series, comprising camptomelic dysplasia, diastrophic dysplasia and short rib polydactyly syndrome.[13]

Genetic syndromes

Treacher Collins syndrome (mandibular facial dysostosis) This rare syndrome is inherited as an autosomal dominant and its gene has been mapped to the long arm of chromosome 5.[25] An antenatal diagnosis has been made on several occasions.[26–28]

The main features of the syndrome which affects structures derived from the mesenchyme of the first and second pharyngeal arches are symmetrical

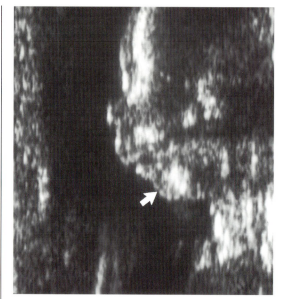

A

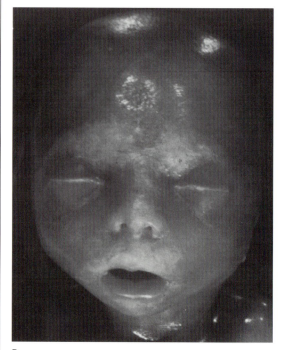

B

Fig. 15.16 Micrognathia. (A) Sagittal scan through a fetus with trisomy 18, showing micrognathia (arrow points to hypoplastic mandible). (B) Post-mortem photograph of the same fetus. (Reproduced with permission from Turner G, Twining P. The facial profile in the diagnosis of fetal abnormalities. Clin Radiol 1993; 47:389–395.)

hypoplasia of the malar bones, antimongoloid slant of the palpebral fissures, micrognathia and abnormalities of the ears. Cleft palate is seen in up to 30% of cases. Intelligence is normal in most cases.

Antenatal diagnosis in a family at risk is based on the demonstration of micrognathia associated with small malformed ears (Fig. 15.17).[27] Meizner et al reported a case where severe micrognathia was associated with an absent ear on one side and a low-set ear on the other. The fetus also had a facial cleft. Polyhydramnios may also be an accompanying feature.[28] The phenotypic expression is extremely variable and so subtle cases could be missed. Therefore normal sonographic findings do not completely exclude the syndrome.[27]

There is also a similar syndrome which has an autosomal recessive form of inheritance termed the Nager acrofacial dysostosis syndrome. This syndrome has also been detected antenatally.[29] The main differentiating feature from the Treacher Collins syndrome is the presence of hypoplasia or aplasia of the thumb. The radius may also be hypoplastic or absent.[2]

Goldenhar syndrome and hemifacial microsomia (facio–auriculo–vertebral syndrome) Whereas the Treacher Collins

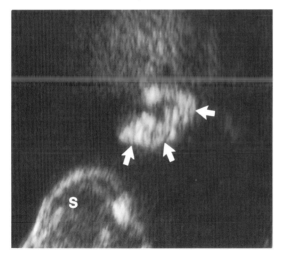

Fig. 15.17 Malformed and rotated ear. Sagittal scan through abnormal ear; the ear is rotated to lie in a horizontal position and is dysplastic. S, shoulder; arrows outline ear.

syndrome produces symmetrical deformity of the face, Goldenhar syndrome and hemifacial microsomia present with quite asymmetrical involvement of the face (Fig. 15.18A). Although most cases are sporadic, there is a 2% recurrence risk and a few autosomal dominant cases have been reported.[30] It has been estimated to have an incidence of 1:3500 deliveries.[2]

As mentioned earlier, these syndromes are secondary to underdevelopment of the first and second pharyngeal arches and produce asymmetrical and, in 70% of cases, unilateral defects. The main findings are micrognathia which may be severe (Fig. 15.18B), small deformed ears, pre-auricular tags and middle ear defects which often lead on to deafness. There may be hemivertebrae affecting the cervical spine and a fairly high incidence of cardiac abnormalities, mainly ventriculoseptal defects and Fallot tetralogy.[22] Severe central nervous system involvement is rare but hydrocephalus, encephalocoele and mental retardation have been described.

The main finding on ultrasound is micrognathia associated with asymmetrical ear abnormalities. The presence of cardiac abnormalities and the asymmetrical and often unilateral nature of the defect should help to differentiate this syndrome from the Treacher Collins syndrome. In addition, there will also be a family history of the defect in the Treacher Collins syndrome whereas Goldenhar syndrome and hemifacial microsomia are usually sporadic. The prenatal diagnosis has already been reported by Tamas et al.[31]

Pierre Robin syndrome (Robin anomalad) This syndrome is associated with micrognathia, a posteriorly positioned tongue which can produce airways obstruction in the neonate (glossoptosis) and a cleft palate or high arched palate.[32] The palatal defect is very characteristic as it has an inverted U-shape as opposed to the normal inverted V-shape and it has been postulated that the defect is produced by the posteriorly positioned tongue which prevents the normal closure of the palatine shelves which fuse to produce the normal palate (see

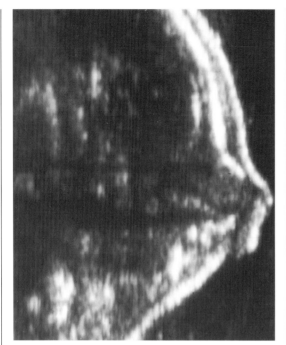

A

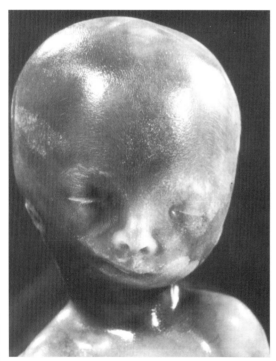

B

Fig. 15.18 Hemifacial microsomia. (A) Sagittal scan through the face, showing severe micrognathia. (B) Post-mortem photograph of the same fetus. (Courtesy of Dr J. Zuccollo, Department of Paediatric Pathology, Nottingham.)

Embryology, p. 346). The condition is usually sporadic.

The antenatal diagnosis has already been described by Pilu et al who detected micrognathia and polyhydramnios at 35 weeks' gestation in a patient who had had a previously affected child.[33] The authors stressed the importance of the antenatal diagnosis in order that paediatric support be present at the delivery to prevent airways obstruction in the neonatal period.

It is of interest that there is the potential for the mandible to catch up in growth to produce a normal appearance in later childhood.[22]

Seckel syndrome (bird-headed dwarfism)
This autosomal recessive condition is characterized by micrognathia, microcephaly, intra-uterine growth retardation, a receding forehead and a large beaked nose.[34] The ears are often malformed and low-set. The profile view is very characteristic (Fig. 15.19) and this condition is often associated with polyhydramnios. There is moderate shortening of the long bones and there may be clinodactyly of the fifth finger. There is usually moderate-to-severe mental retardation.[39]

Majoor-Krakauer et al reported a recurrence of Seckel syndrome in a patient at 20 weeks' gestation.[35] Ultrasound scanning revealed growth retardation with severe microcephaly, micrognathia and moderate shortening of the long bones. Polyhydramnios was also present. More recently, Featherstone et al confirmed a prenatal diagnosis at 30 weeks in a family without a previous history of Seckel syndrome.[36]

Pena–Shokeir syndrome This lethal condition is characterized by micrognathia, camptodactyly, multiple ankyloses, pulmonary hypoplasia and polyhydramnios. The hands show typical flexion of the fingers with overlapping and there is bilateral talipes.[37] Differentiation from chromosomal abnormalities such as trisomy 18 can be difficult but the heart is usually normal in Pena–Shokeir syndrome whereas cardiac anomalies are common in trisomy 18.

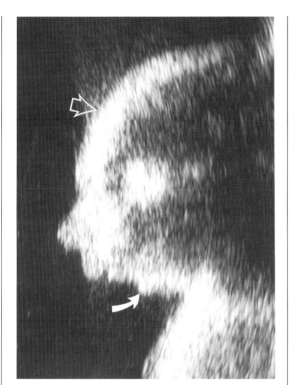

Fig. 15.19 Seckel syndrome. Profile view, showing severe micrognathia (curved arrow) and small forehead secondary to microcephaly (open arrow).

Antenatal diagnosis is based on the demonstration of micrognathia, fixed flexion of the fingers with overlapping, fixed flexion or extension deformities of the arms and legs and often bilateral talipes or rockerbottom feet. Karyotyping is required to exclude chromosomal disease. The outlook is poor and most babies die in the neonatal period from pulmonary hypoplasia.

Recurrence risks are high in the order of 10 to 15% and some cases are autosomal recessive.[38]

DiGeorge syndrome This rare condition is thought to be caused by abnormal development of the third and fourth pharyngeal arches. The syndrome comprises facial abnormalities, including micrognathia, low-set abnormal ears, hypertelorism and cleft palate. There are also cardiac anomalies, mainly persistent truncus arteriosus and interrupted aortic arch, and thirdly thymic aplasia or hypoplasia, and hypoparathyroidism.[39] About one-third of patients have partial monosomy of the proximal long arm of chromosome 22.[40]

There does appear to be significant overlap of this syndrome with Shprintzen syndrome (velo–cardio–facial syndrome) which also shows abnormalities of chromosome 22 and has similar clinical features. Micrognathia is seen but there may also be microphthalmia and microcephaly. In addition, the cardiac abnormalities are usually ventriculoseptal defects, pulmonary stenosis and double outlet right ventricle.[39] These two diagnoses should be considered when micrognathia is seen in association with cardiac abnormalities. Cytogenetic examination may be able to confirm the diagnosis.

Hydrolethalus syndrome This name was coined as although micrognathia is a prominent feature of the syndrome the other features are hydrocephalus and polyhydramnios with most cases being lethal.[41] Hypertelorism is also seen and the tongue may be small or absent. In the hands, there is postaxial polydactyly whereas, in the feet, pre-axial polydactyly is seen with a markedly angulated extra first toe a characteristic feature. Ventriculoseptal defects may be seen in up to 50% of cases and as well as hydrocephalus, an occipital encephalocoele may also be present. The syndrome can be differentiated from the Meckel–Gruber syndrome as the kidneys are normal. Inheritance is autosomal recessive.[39]

Pryde et al reported a case diagnosed at 19 weeks' gestation in a patient whose previous pregnancy had been terminated for multiple fetal abnormalities, including polyhydramnios, cleft lip and palate, micrognathia, polydactyly, severe hydrocephalus and a Dandy–Walker malformation. Scanning the current pregnancy revealed the same findings and a diagnosis of hydrolethalus syndrome was made and confirmed at post-mortem.[42]

The lips and mouth

Facial clefting

Facial clefting is the most common congenital facial abnormality with an incidence of approximately 1 per 1000 in white populations. There is however quite a wide racial variation with an incidence of 1.5–2 per 1000 in Asians and 0.5 per 1000 in blacks.[43] Cleft lip with or without cleft palate occurs twice as commonly in males as females except in the black population where boys have a very low incidence of cleft lip.[44] Unilateral cleft lip occurs twice as frequently on the left side than on the right and is more common than bilateral cleft lip and palate.

Cleft lip with or without cleft palate is a distinct entity from cleft palate alone and both have a different embryological basis. Siblings of patients with cleft lip with or without cleft palate have an increased frequency of cleft lip with or without cleft palate but not of cleft palate alone. Similarly siblings of patients with cleft palate alone only have an increased frequency of cleft palate alone and not cleft lip.[43] Recurrence risks for cleft lip and palate and cleft palate alone are outlined in Table 15.2.

There are four common combinations of facial clefting (Fig. 15.20):

1. Unilateral cleft lip
2. Unilateral cleft lip and palate
3. Bilateral cleft lip and palate
4. Isolated cleft palate.

Aetiology

Cleft lip and/or palate occurs secondary to a failure of fusion of the medial nasal swellings

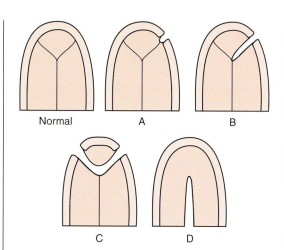

Fig. 15.20 Facial clefting. The four common types of facial clefting. (A) Unilateral cleft lip. (B) Unilateral cleft lip and palate. (C) Bilateral cleft lip and palate. (D) Isolated cleft palate.

with the maxillary swellings (see Embryology, p. 346). Although the vast majority of cases of cleft lip and/or palate are idiopathic, a number of drugs has been implicated, including phenytoin, carbamazepine, steroids and diazepam.[45] In addition, chromosomal disease and malformation syndromes are also associated with facial clefting and some of these are outlined in Table 15.3. In trisomy 13, the facial clefting is usually median (midline cleft) or bilateral cleft lip and palate and occurs in up to 65% of cases. Facial clefting is seen in 30% of triploidy, up to 15% of trisomy 18 and 0.5% of trisomy 21.[22]

Table 15.2
Recurrence risks for idiopathic cleft lip with or without cleft palate and cleft palate alone

Cleft lip with or without cleft palate	
Affected person	**Risk**
One parent	2%
One child	4–7%
One parent plus one child	11–14%
Two children	10%
Cleft palate only	
Affected person	**Risk**
One parent	7%
One child	2–5%
One parent plus one child	14–17%

Reproduced with permission from Warkany J. Congenital malformations. Chicago: Year Book; 1981.

Table 15.3
Conditions associated with cleft lip with or without cleft palate

Chromosomal defects
Trisomy 13
Trisomy 18
Trisomy 21
Triploidy

Syndromes and malformations
Amniotic band syndrome
Holoprosencephaly
Ectodermal dysplasia syndrome
Roberts syndrome*
Miller syndrome*
Mohr syndrome*
Frontonasal dysplasia

Associated with micrognathia.

Sonographic appearance

Christ & Meininger were the first to use ultrasound to diagnose cleft lip and palate in 1981,[46] and since then the technique has become well established.[17,47,48] Although antenatal diagnosis can be carried out in the early second trimester using transvaginal scanning,[49] most centres offer scanning at 18 to 20 weeks' gestation. The hallmark of unilateral cleft lip is the demonstration of a vertical transonic area within the upper lip, usually just to the left of the midline on coronal scanning.

If the palate is involved, the transonic area will extend into the nose (Fig. 15.21A). Scanning in the sagittal plane will often reveal the defect as an absent section of the upper lip (Fig. 15.21B). 3D ultrasound also is of value in the demonstration of facial clefting (Fig. 15.21C).

Bilateral cleft lip and palate is recognized by the presence of a central echodense mass in the region of the upper lip (Fig. 15.22). The presence of this mass is known as premaxillary protrusion. Nyberg et al described 10 fetuses with premaxillary protrusion[50] and 9 of the 10 proved to have bilateral cleft lip and palate.

The mass in the centre of the upper lip represents abnormal alveolar and gingival tissue resulting from uninhibited growth of the premaxilla caused by lack of continuity of the bony, gingival and lip structures. The mass itself can be large and often obscures the clefts which are present on either side. The paranasal mass appears to be most prominent at 18 to 20 weeks' gestation and becomes less obvious later in pregnancy.[50] Premaxillary protrusion is best demonstrated in the sagittal and transverse planes (Figs 15.22A, B).

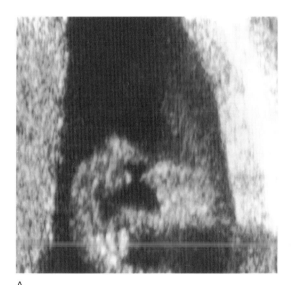

A

Fig. 15.21 Unilateral cleft lip and palate. (A) Coronal scan, showing unilateral cleft lip and palate. (B) Sagittal scan, showing absence of the upper lip (arrow). The scan plane is directed through the cleft.

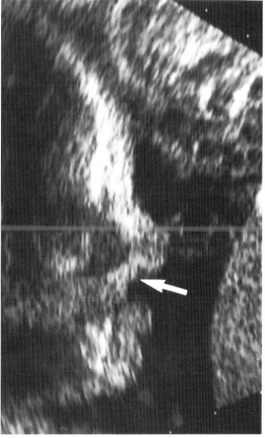

B

ABNORMALITIES OF THE FACE AND NECK

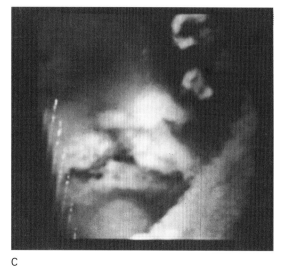

C

Fig. 15.21 Unilateral cleft lip and palate. (C) 3D ultrasound picture of right-sided cleft lip and palate. (Courtesy of Dr Benoit, Nice, France.) (D) Postnatal photograph of same fetus as Figure 15.21A. (Figs 15.21A and B reproduced with permission from Turner G, Twining P. The facial profile in the diagnosis of fetal abnormalities. Clin Radiol 1993; 47:389–395.)

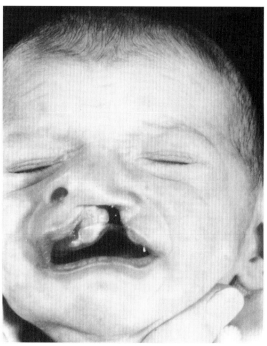

D

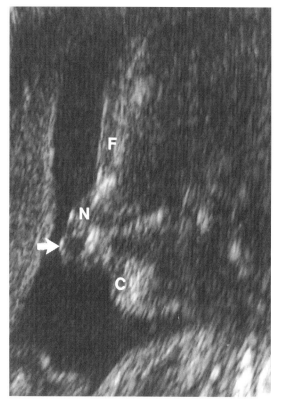

A

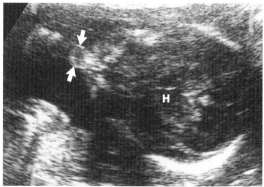

B

Fig. 15.22 Bilateral cleft lip and palate. (A) Sagittal scan, showing premaxillary protrusion (straight arrow). F, forehead; N, nose; C, chin. (B) Transverse scan, showing the premaxillary protrusion (arrows). H, head.

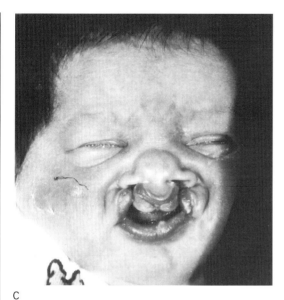

C

Fig. 15.22 Bilateral cleft lip and palate. (C) Postnatal photograph of affected fetus.

Midline or median facial clefting is often associated with chromosomal disease and holoprosencephaly and is demonstrated as a wide central gap in the upper lip involving the palate (Figs 15.23A, B). Nyberg et al have proposed a classification of facial clefts into five types (Fig. 15.24) based on the ultrasound findings. All the clefts demonstrated have been discussed apart from Type 5 which are bizarre vertical and lateral clefts, usually associated with the amniotic band syndrome (Fig. 15.27). These fetuses usually demonstrate multiple abnormalities, including encephalocoeles, anencephaly, limb and body wall defects and scoliosis.

The demonstration of an isolated cleft palate is very difficult as it is the posterior part of the palate that is usually involved (Fig. 15.20). The posterior palate can occasionally be demonstrated on the sagittal

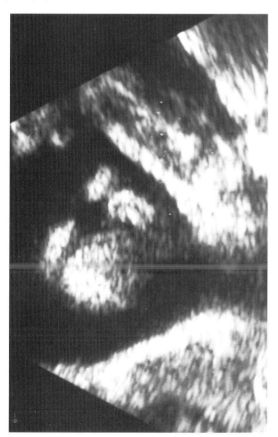

A

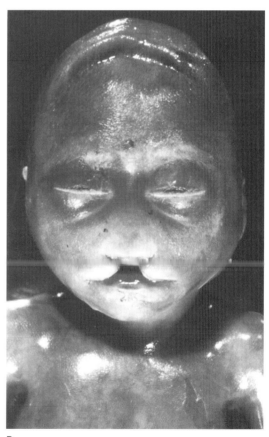

B

Fig. 15.23 Median facial clefting. (A) Coronal scan through the upper lip, showing a median cleft lip. (B) Post-mortem photograph of affected fetus, showing median clefting. (Courtesy of Dr J. Zuccollo, Department of Paediatric Pathology, Nottingham.)

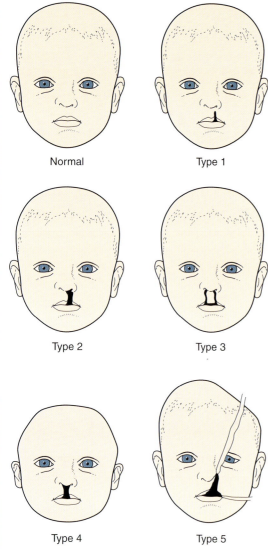

Fig. 15.24 Ultrasound classification of facial clefts. (Reproduced with permission from Nyberg et al. Fetal cleft lip and palate: Ultrasound classification and correlation with outcome. Radiology 1995; 195:677–684.)

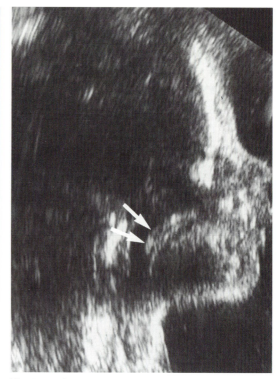

Fig. 15.25 Sagittal scan through the fetal face, showing amniotic fluid within the oropharynx. Arrows point to the posterior part of the soft palate.

scan when the pharynx contains amniotic fluid and this can outline the soft palate (Fig. 15.25).

Brundy et al have suggested that polyhydramnios and a small stomach bubble may indicate the presence of a cleft palate[51] but more recent reports stress the importance of colour flow Doppler in demonstrating palatal clefts.[52,53] Colour flow Doppler carried out during fetal breathing reveals flow in both the mouth and nasopharynx (Fig. 15.26).

The demonstration of flow across the palate would indicate the presence of a palatal defect.

Sonographic approach

Once a diagnosis of facial clefting has been made, then a thorough search should be carried out for other anomalies, particularly features of trisomies 13 and 18 and triploidy. The presence of multiple abnormalities carries a high risk of chromosomal disease; however, isolated cleft lip and palate has a low incidence of chromosomal defects.[1]

In the situation where there is facial clefting and other abnormalities and the karyotype is normal, then the more uncommon syndromes should be considered.[53] Some of these are outlined in Table 15.3 and will be discussed in the following section.

In addition, special attention should always be paid to the heart as patients with cleft lip and palate have a high incidence of also lateral or vertical facial clefts[57] (Fig. 15.27). These clefts correspond to Type 5 in Figure 15.24.

The defects typically are severe and often bizarre in nature. Encephalocoeles are situated in a lateral position as opposed to the normal midline location and may even resemble anencephaly if the defect is extensive. Amputation defects involve the limbs and there may be large abdominal wall defects which can also affect the chest wall (gastropleuroschisis).[58] There may also be severe spinal involvement with kyphosis, scoliosis and marked angulation deformities. The combination of a severe spinal deformity and an abdominal wall defect is diagnostic of amniotic band syndrome.[57] Cases are sporadic with a low incidence of recurrence. The outlook is extremely poor.

Holoprosencephaly

Midline or median facial clefting is common as is bilateral cleft lip and palate. This condition will be discussed in more detail on page 368.

Ectrodactyly-ectodermal dysplasia-clefting (EEC) syndrome

This autosomal dominant syndrome combines cleft lip and palate with limb defects usually involving the hands and feet.[59] The characteristic findings are cleft hand or foot with wide separation of the fingers sometimes described as the lobster claw deformity (Fig. 15.28). One may also see syndactyly and reduced numbers of fingers. Diagnosis has been described in the early second trimester utilizing transvaginal scanning.[60] Urinary anomalies may also be seen including hydronephrosis and vesicoureteric reflux.[39] The features may be very variable so confident exclusions of the syndrome using ultrasound may be difficult.

Roberts syndrome

This syndrome comprises cleft lip with or without cleft palate, micrognathia, prominent premaxilla, prominent eyes and malformed ears. In addition, there are also major limb reduction defects which range from phocomelia to moderately severe limb

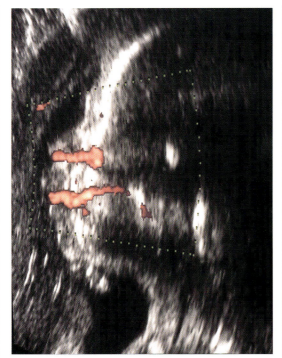

Fig. 15.26 Sagittal scan through the fetal face, showing flow through the nose and mouth demonstrated by colour flow Doppler.

cardiac abnormalities, estimated to be in the region of 7%.[53]

Amniotic band syndrome and limb–body wall complex

The amniotic band syndrome and limb–body wall complex are two conditions with similar features which appear to be related to early amnion rupture. A vascular disruption theory has also been proposed as in some cases amniotic bands have not been identified as a cause for the abnormalities.[54] The incidence has been estimated between 1 in 1200 to 1 in 15 000 liveborn pregnancies[55] but probably accounts for up to 1 in 50 spontaneous abortions.[56]

The main abnormalities are thought to occur following amnion rupture, allowing the embryo to enter the chorionic cavity and fetal parts may then become entrapped by the fibrous septa that traverse the chorionic space. These septa or bands entangle the fetus and produce amputation defects, atypical encephalocoele, omphalocoele and

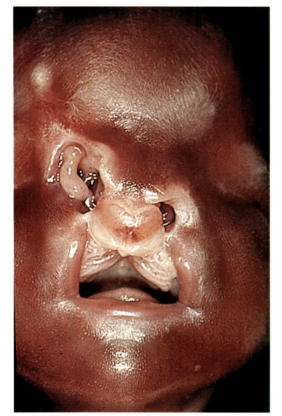

A

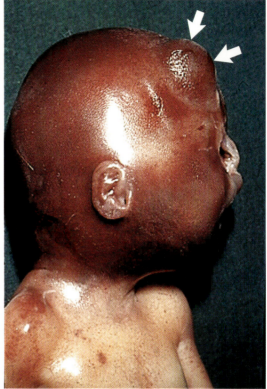

B

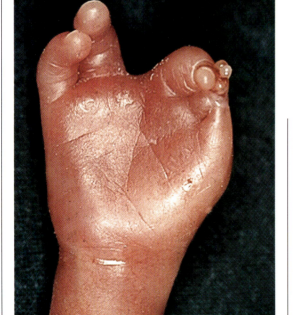

C

Fig. 15.27 Amniotic band syndrome. (A) Post-mortem photograph of the face, showing vertical fetal facial clefting. (B) Side view of head, showing lateral encephalocoele (arrows). (C) Post-mortem photograph of the hand, showing the amputation of digits with fusion secondary to amniotic band.

shortening with radial or humeral aplasia. Typically the limb defects are more severe in the upper limbs.[22]

The profile view of the face is often bizarre, produced by the combination of micrognathia and severe facial clefting (Fig. 15.29). Other defects include congenital heart disease and cystic dysplasia of the kidneys.[39] Prenatal diagnosis has been reported in both the second and first trimesters.[61,62] The outlook overall is very poor with most babies dying in the neonatal period. A proportion of survivors will show mental retardation. Inheritance is autosomal recessive. Centromeric straining of

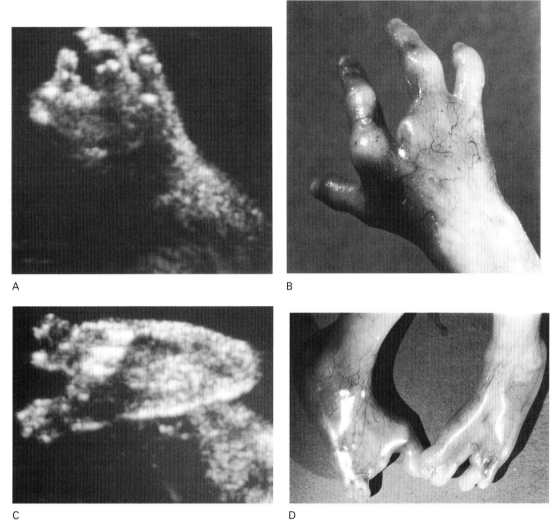

A

B

C

D

Fig. 15.28 Ectrodactyly-ectodermal dysplasia-clefting syndrome. (A) Scan through the hand, showing separation of the third and fourth fingers with abnormal positioning of the fingers. (B) Post-mortem photograph of the hand. (C) Scan showing cleft foot. (D) Post-mortem photograph showing cleft feet.

chromosomes shows premature centromere separation (chromosome puffs) and this can be used for prenatal diagnosis.[63]

Miller syndrome (acrofacial dysostosis with postaxial defects)

This autosomal recessive syndrome comprises micrognathia, cleft lip, prominent eyes and absence of the fifth digits on all four limbs. The forearms are often incurving with ulnar and radial hypoplasia. Intelligence is normal.[39]

Mohr syndrome (orofacial digital syndrome)

The main features of this autosomal recessive condition are a midline cleft of the upper lip, micrognathia, a high or cleft palate, postaxial polydactyly in the hands and both pre- and postaxial polydactyly in the feet. The tibiae are severely hypoplastic. The chest is relatively normal allowing survival.[39]

Suresh et al reported a prenatal diagnosis at 20 weeks in a patient who had had a previous baby with the syndrome. The ultrasound findings included micrognathia,

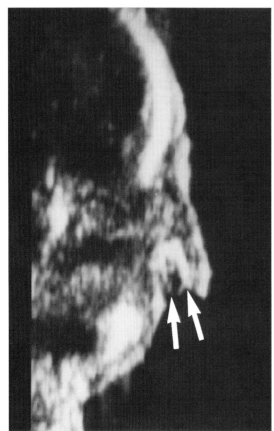

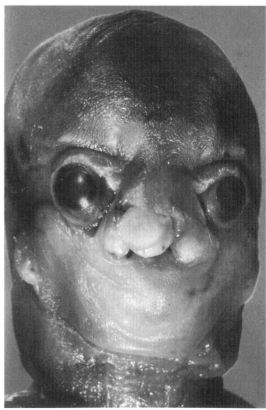

A   B

Fig. 15.29 Roberts syndrome. (A) Sagittal scan through the face, showing micrognathia and bizarre appearance secondary to facial clefting (arrows). (B) Post-mortem photograph of same fetus. (Courtesy of Dr J. Zuccollo, Department of Paediatric Pathology, Nottingham.)

postaxial polydactyly in both hands, polydactyly, talipes and double hallux in the feet. Post-mortem examination revealed clefting of the upper lip, a bifid nasal tip and low-set ears.[64]

Abnormalities of the tongue

Macroglossia

The two most important associations of macroglossia are with trisomy 21 and Beckwith–Wiedemann syndrome. Nicolaides et al reported a group of 13 fetuses with macroglossia and of the 13, 9 were found to have trisomy 21 and 2 Beckwith–Wiedemann syndrome.[1]

Beckwith–Wiedemann syndrome is characterized by macroglossia, omphalocoele and enlargement of the liver, spleen, kidneys and adrenals. Prenatal diagnosis is based on the demonstration of macrosomia, visceromegaly, omphalocoele and macroglossia.[65,66] Nicolaides et al also reported the presence of adrenal cysts and Chambers noted a hepatic cyst during prenatal diagnosis.[67]

This syndrome carries an increased risk of malignancy in childhood, particularly Wilms' tumour. Intelligence is usually normal.

Nicolaides et al have also reported a case of Coffin–Lowry syndrome characterized by macroglossia, hypertelorism, a constantly open mouth, thoracolumbar scoliosis and cavum excavatum. This syndrome is associated with severe mental retardation.

Tumours and masses involving the mouth

Epignathus (nasopharyngeal teratoma)

Fetal teratomas occur with an incidence of approximately 1 in 20 000 to 1 in 40 000 live births. Teratomas of the head account for 40% and the neck approximately 5%. Teratomas of the nasopharynx are even rarer.[67]

Nasopharyngeal teratoma arises from the palate and usually extends through the mouth to protrude into the amniotic fluid (Fig. 15.30). The tumours tend to have solid and cystic components and are usually benign histologically. The tumours can become very large and are often associated with polyhydramnios because of difficulty with fetal swallowing.[68] Occasionally, intracranial teratomas can extend through the skull base into the oropharynx and mouth. Shipp et al reported three such cases and none of these fetuses survived.[69]

Overall survival rates are poor with most babies dying in the neonatal period from respiratory complications as a result of compression of the airway.[67]

In view of this, Chervenak has advocated an aggressive management approach.[68] In cases of polyhydramnios, serial amniocentesis can be carried out to delay delivery until pulmonary maturity has been achieved. Delivery should be by caesarean section to avoid dystocia or avulsion of the tumour. Paediatric and surgical support should be available at delivery in order to perform a tracheostomy if endotracheal intubation is not possible.[68]

Epulis (congenital gingival granular cell tumour)

This rare, but benign, soft tissue tumour arises from the maxillary alveolar ridge anteriorly. Unlike teratomas, the tumours are usually of homogeneous echodensity and appear sonographically as a rounded mass arising from the mouth and displacing the lips and tongue. Hulett et al noted bright internal echoes within such a tumour diagnosed at 39 weeks' gestation, suggesting the presence of calcification.[70] The tumour

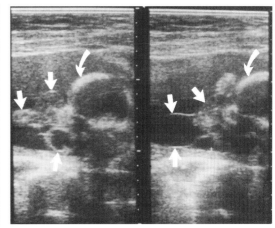

A

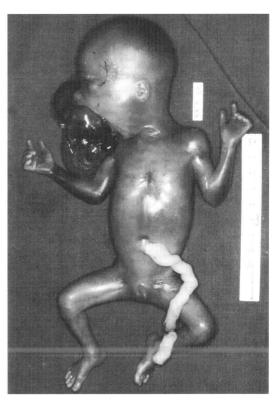

B

Fig. 15.30 Nasopharyngeal teratoma. (A) Scans through the head, showing mixed cystic and solid tumour arising through the mouth (curved arrow points to skull, straight arrows point to tumour). (B) Post-mortem photograph of the fetus with nasopharyngeal teratoma.

can be pedunculated or broad based and is covered by smooth, non-ulcerated mucosa. Surgical excision in the neonatal period is successful with no reports of post-surgical recurrence. Most authors suggest delivery at a centre with paediatric and surgical support in case of airways obstruction post-delivery.[69,70]

Cephalocoele

The majority of encephalocoeles involve the occipital bone with protrusion of meninges and/or brain tissue posteriorly. In approximately 10% of cases, encephalocoeles can involve the frontal bones[71] and rarely the skull base to protrude into the oropharynx and mouth.[72] Carlon et al reported a case of cephalocoele which had herniated through the clivus into the oropharynx and sonographically appeared as a cystic mass surrounded by an echogenic rim protruding through the mouth. There was associated ventriculomegaly and polyhydramnios. At delivery, intubation was not possible and the baby did not survive.

The differential diagnosis of a cystic mass within the mouth should include a salivary gland cyst. Shipp et al diagnosed a salivary gland cyst in a fetus at 22 weeks' gestation.[69] Sonographically, salivary gland cysts appear as simple cysts within the mouth. The case reported by Shipp et al remained unchanged in size during pregnancy and was aspirated in the neonatal period. The cyst did not recur. An important factor in the diagnosis would be the presence of normal intracranial anatomy, whereas in the case of a cephalocoele involving the mouth the intracranial anatomy would be abnormal.[72]

The nose and orbits

The most important group of malformations to affect the orbits, nose and, to a certain extent, the upper lip, is the mid-face syndromes which include holoprosencephaly and frontonasal dysplasia syndrome.

Holoprosencephaly

Holoprosencephaly is a complex intracranial abnormality produced by incomplete separation of the prosencephalon to form the two cerebral hemispheres. The result is a monoventricular cavity, fused thalami, and absence of midline structures such as the corpus callosum and falx cerebri.[73] There is usually microcephaly and the striking and often dramatic facial abnormalities seen in holoprosencephaly are due to defects of the facial structures arising from the frontonasal prominence (see Embryology, p. 346). Failure of the medial nasal processes to form results in agenesis of the intermaxillary process and the reduction or absence of other mid-facial structures such as the nasal bones, nasal septum and ethmoid. The consequence may be cebocephaly (single nostril), hypotelorism, ethmocephaly, cyclopia and facial clefting (Fig. 15.31).[10] The findings in the face are so characteristic that it prompted De Meyer et al to state that in holoprosencephaly the face predicts the brain.[74] The converse, however, is not true as the face can be entirely normal in holoprosencephaly.

Cyclopia

Cyclopia is seen in 10 to 20% of fetuses with holoprosencephaly and represents varying degrees of ocular fusion.[73,75] In most cases, the fusion is not complete and two fused eyes can be seen within a single orbit (Fig. 15.32). The nose is situated above the eye in the form of a proboscis. The mouth may be small or absent and the ears are often low-set.

Ethmocephaly

Ethmocephaly is probably the least common facial abnormality seen in holoprosencephaly and comprises severe hypotelorism associated with a proboscis at the level of the orbits. This is likely to represent a less severe form of cyclopia.

Cebocephaly

Cebocephaly is characterized by a single nostril and marked hypotelorism (Fig. 15.33). The profile view is very variable but tends to be flattened. The single nostril produces a rudimentary nose which is supposed to resemble the platyrrhinic monkey face.[73]

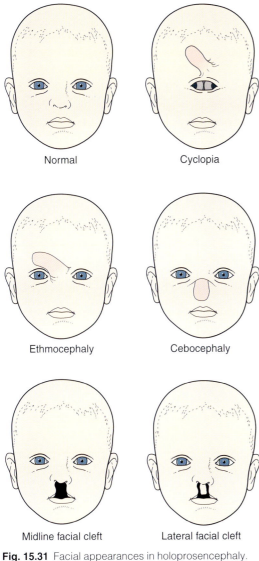

Normal

Cyclopia

Ethmocephaly

Cebocephaly

Midline facial cleft

Lateral facial cleft

Fig. 15.31 Facial appearances in holoprosencephaly. (Reproduced with permission from Nyberg BA, ed. Diagnostic ultrasound of fetal anomalies: Text and atlas. St Louis: Mosby Year Book; 1990.)

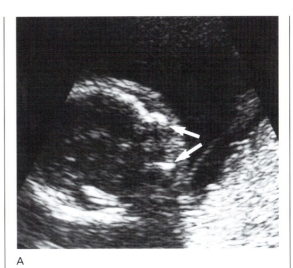

A

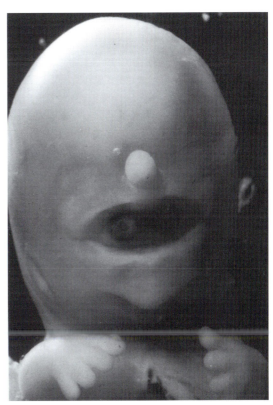

B

Fig. 15.32 Cyclopia. (A) Transverse scan through a single orbit (arrows). (B) Post-mortem photograph of a fetus, showing cyclopia and a proboscis. (Courtesy of Dr J. Zuccollo, Department of Paediatric Pathology, Nottingham.)

Hypotelorism

Hypotelorism may be the only finding associated with holoprosencephaly and may be very mild. There are very few other syndromes in which hypotelorism is a frequent finding. It is an occasional feature of the Meckel–Gruber syndrome but is the characteristic finding in holoprosencephaly.

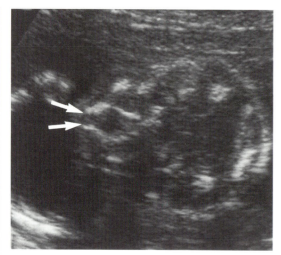

A

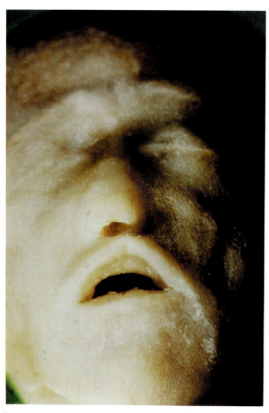

B

Fig. 15.33 Cebocephaly. (A) Transverse scan through the fetal face, showing a single nostril (arrows). (B) Post-mortem of same fetus, showing hypotelorism and a single nostril. (Reproduced with permission from Turner G, Twining P. The facial profile in the diagnosis of fetal abnormalities. Clin Radiol 1993; 47:389–395.)

Median clefting

Median clefting is common in holoprosencephaly and is often associated with hypoplasia of the nose and hypotelorism (Fig. 15.34). This is often difficult to demonstrate in the coronal plane as the profile of the face is so flat. Bilateral cleft lip and palate is also seen in holoprosencephaly but is less common than median clefting. McGahan et al have also reported two cases of unilateral cleft lip associated with holoprosencephaly.[73]

Holoprosencephaly can be an isolated finding but is often associated with other fetal abnormalities and chromosomal disease, in particular trisomy 13, trisomy 18 and triploidy.[76]

Frontonasal dysplasia (median cleft syndrome)

Frontonasal dysplasia is the other important mid-face syndrome but whereas hypotelorism is the major feature of holoprosencephaly, it is hypertelorism which is the hallmark of frontonasal dysplasia.[77] Other syndromes are associated with hypertelorism and these are outlined in Table 15.4. The main feature of frontonasal dysplasia is marked hypertelorism with a broad nasal tip which is frequently cleft. There may also be a median cleft lip[78] (Fig. 15.35). Most cases are sporadic but a few autosomal dominant cases have been reported. Frattarelli et al reported a case diagnosed in a dizygotic twin pregnancy at 21 weeks' gestation. The affected fetus

Table 15.4
Syndromes associated with hypertelorism

Frontonasal dysplasia
Frontal encephalocoeles
Craniosynostosis syndromes
   Apert syndrome
   Saetre–Chotzen syndrome
   Pfeiffer syndrome
   Crouzon syndrome
DiGeorge syndrome
Hydrolethalus syndrome
Coffin–Lowry syndrome
Noonan syndrome
Larsen syndrome

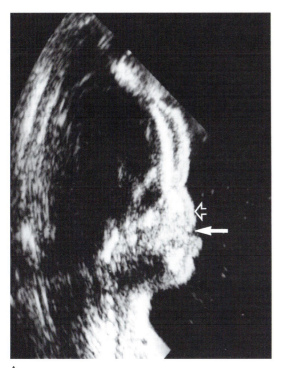
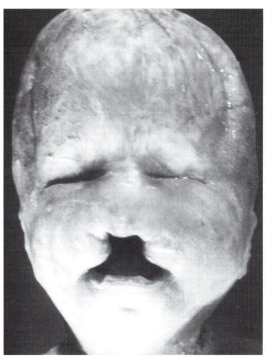

A   B

Fig. 15.34 Median clefting. (A) Sagittal scan through a fetus with holoprosencephaly, showing a flat profile, nasal hypoplasia and absence of the upper lip, indicating median clefting (straight arrow points to absence of the upper lip; open arrow, hypoplastic nose). (B) Post-mortem photograph, showing median clefting. (Reproduced with permission from Turner G, Twining P. The facial profile in the diagnosis of fetal abnormalities. Clin Radiol 1993; 47:389–395).

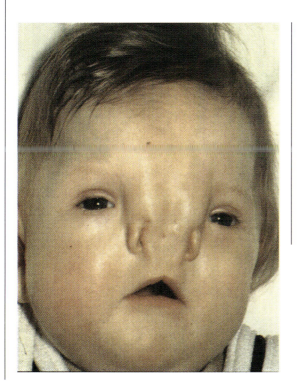

demonstrated marked hypertelorism, an abnormal wide nose with separation of the nostrils and an occipital encephalocoele.[79] Intelligence is normal where the abnormality is isolated and craniofacial reconstructive surgery can produce good cosmetic results.

Frontal encephalocoele

Encephalocoeles have an incidence of approximately 1 in 5000 to 1 in 10 000 live births. Frontal encephalocoele, however, accounts for only 10% of the total.[80] Although rare in the western world, frontal

Fig. 15.35 Frontonasal dysplasia. Photograph of a child with frontonasal dysplasia. Note the severe hypertelorism and cleft nose. (Reproduced with permission from Baraitser M, ed. Colour atlas of congenital malformation syndromes. London: Mosby Wolfe; 1996.)

encephalocoeles are far more common in the East and are associated with a better outcome than that for posterior encephalocoele.[81] The main disabilities in children with frontal encephalocoeles are facial disfigurement, anosmia and visual problems, which can be present in up to 50% of cases.[81]

Sonographically, frontal encephalocoele presents as quite marked hypertelorism associated with an anterior midline calvarial defect (Fig. 15.36). Brain tissue may herniate into the defect and there may be associated intracranial anomalies such as hydrocephalus, agenesis of the corpus callosum and microcephaly. Orbital abnormalities such as anophthalmia may be associated as might facial clefting.

Craniosynostosis syndromes

These syndromes are discussed on page 375.

Microphthalmia

Microphthalmia is a rare condition which is associated with chromosomal disease, genetic syndromes and also intracranial abnormalities.

It is estimated to occur in 1 in 5000 live births.[86] Clinically, it may be difficult to differentiate severe microphthalmia from cases of true anophthalmia. However, this distinction should be possible sono-graphically in the fetus. In microphthalmia, the orbit is small but the lens should be present. If the lens is absent, then anophthalmia is the more likely diagnosis.[82]

Bronshtein et al reported eight cases of orbital abnormalities which included two cases of microphthalmia. The two cases were associated with both intracranial abnormalities (hydrocephalus) and other extracranial anomalies. Both cases were diagnosed between 15 and 17 weeks' gestation.[82]

Microphthalmia is demonstrated as an asymmetry of the orbital diameters in unilateral or bilaterally small orbits if both orbits are affected (Fig. 15.37). Reference should always be made to nomograms of orbital measurements in order to confirm the diagnosis (Fig. 15.8). In mild cases, it may not be possible to make a prenatal diagnosis.

Schauer et al reported a case of bilateral microphthalmia and hypertelorism at 18 weeks' gestation in a fetus with Fraser syndrome.[83] The fetus also demonstrated oligohydramnios secondary to bilateral renal agenesis and enlarged echodense lungs secondary to laryngeal atresia. Syndactyly of the fingers is a further, frequent finding.

Clearly, if microphthalmia is seen in utero, then a careful assessment of the orbit should be made to establish the presence of the lens. In addition, the remainder of the fetus should be assessed for further abnormalities and a karyotype considered if found. In the situation of a normal karyotype, genetic syndromes should be considered such as the Lenz Microphthalmia syndrome and Oculo–Dento–Digital

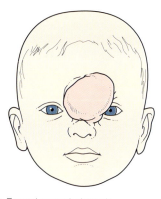

Fig. 15.36 Frontal encephalocoele.

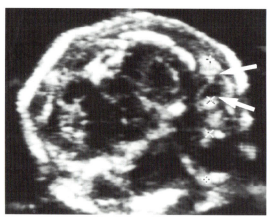

Fig. 15.37 Microphthalmia. Transverse scan through the fetal head, showing microphthalmia (arrows).

syndrome. The outlook for the fetus to a large extent depends on the associated abnormalities or syndrome. Reconstructive surgery can be carried out to improve the cosmetic appearance.

Anophthalmia

Anophthalmia is a rare condition which is estimated to have an incidence of 1 in 20 000 live births.[84] Most cases are sporadic but an autosomal recessive form has been described.[85] Anophthalmia, like microphthalmia, may also form part of a number of rare genetic syndromes.[22]

Primary anophthalmia is caused by failure of formation of the optic pit and optic outgrowths from the forebrain. This produces absence of the lens, optic nerves and chiasma.

Sonographically, anophthalmia is diagnosed when there is a small orbit with absence of the lens. Bronshtein et al in their series[82] reported two cases of isolated anophthalmia, both occurring in patients with a family history of anophthalmia syndromes. It is of interest to note that in both cases the fetal orbits and lenses were normal in the first trimester. This prompted the authors to suggest that in some cases, anophthalmia may occur later in pregnancy and may be related to premature occlusion of the hyaloid artery producing secondary degeneration of the fetal eye.[82] In view of this, it would certainly be prudent to carry out scans later in pregnancy if the initial scans are normal in any patient with a family history of microphthalmia or anophthalmia. In addition, if a positive diagnosis of anophthalmia is made, then a careful search should be carried out for other abnormalities.

Congenital cataracts

Congenital cataracts account for 30% of congenital eye malformations in liveborn babies and have an estimated incidence of 1 in 5000 to 1 in 10 000 births.[86] Causes of cataracts include congenital infections such as rubella, cytomegalovirus and toxoplasmosis (36%), enzymatic disorders such as G6PD deficiency, galactokinase deficiency, homocystinuria and galactosaemia (23%), genetic syndromes such as Lowe syndrome, Hallerman–Streiff, Alport and Smith–Lemli–Opitz syndromes in 9% and 32% for which there is no known cause.[87]

Monteagudo describes three sonographic appearances of fetal cataracts: the first is when the normal lens is completely hyperechoic; the second is a double ring appearance where the outer ring represents the border of the lens and the inner ring the cataract; and the third is where there is a central hyperechoic area within the lens[86] (Fig. 15.38). More recently, Drysdale et al reported a case of congenital cataract also in a patient with a strong family history of congenital cataracts.[88]

Dacrocystocoele

Dacrocystocoeles are cysts of the lacrimal duct and most of the cysts that present at birth resolve spontaneously in the first few months of life.[89] Approximately 30% of all newborns have a nonpatent nasolacrimal duct but because of mild or absent symptoms and the tendency for spontaneous resolution, dacrocystocoeles are under-reported.

The cysts are typically located inferomedially to the orbit and are completely transonic. In contrast to a frontal encephalocoele, the orbital anatomy and interorbital distance is normal. Battaglia et al reported two cases that resolved spontaneously during pregnancy.[89] Most dacrocystocoeles measure no more than 1 cm in diameter. Shipp et al reported a case of bilateral dacrocystocoeles in which one dacrocystocoele resolved spontaneously

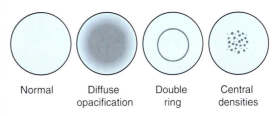

Normal   Diffuse opacification   Double ring   Central densities

Fig. 15.38 The three different ultrasound appearances of fetal cataracts.

during pregnancy, the second persisted and the diagnosis was confirmed in the neonatal period. Most dacrocystocoeles are diagnosed after 30 weeks' gestation.[69]

The ear

The ear has received little attention in the ultrasound literature and this is probably because visualization of the ears is not part of the routine assessment of the fetus. Even in detailed scanning, the ears can be overlooked if other major anomalies are present.

Birnholz described the normal appearance of the fetal ear and noted abnormally shaped ears in four cases of lethal dwarfism.[90] Jones lists 88 causes of malformed ears and 20 causes of low-set ears; most of these, however, are rare genetic syndromes with well-documented recurrence risks. Birnholz & Farrell also documented ear length[20] and found a correlation between small ears and chromosomal disease. More recently this was confirmed by Lettieri et al.[91]

Sonographically, the detail of the ear is best demonstrated in the sagittal plane (Fig. 15.14). However, low-set ears are more easily appreciated on the coronal plane where the relationship to the temporal bone and shoulder can be assessed (Fig. 15.15).

Visualization of the ears should be attempted wherever a fetal anomaly is demonstrated, particularly a facial abnormality, as useful information may be detected which could narrow the differential diagnosis (Fig. 15.17).

The forehead

Frontal bossing

Frontal bossing is seen when the forehead is very prominent with depression of the nasal bridge and has been described in a number of syndromes. Some of these are outlined in Table 15.5. Frontal bossing is best demonstrated on the sagittal plane where the relationship of the forehead to the mid-face

Table 15.5 **Syndromes associated with frontal bossing**
Skeletal dysplasias Achondroplasia Thanatophoric dysplasia Achondrogenesis
Craniosynostosis syndromes Crouzon syndrome Pfeiffer syndrome Craniofrontonasal dysplasia
Other syndromes Russell Silver syndrome Robinson syndrome Hurler syndrome

can be readily appreciated (Fig. 15.39). Turner & Twining reported three cases of frontal bossing: two associated with thanatophoric dysplasia and the third with heterozygous achondroplasia.[13] The authors noted that in the case of heterozygous achondroplasia the frontal bossing was not evident until the third trimester. The other main associations are with the

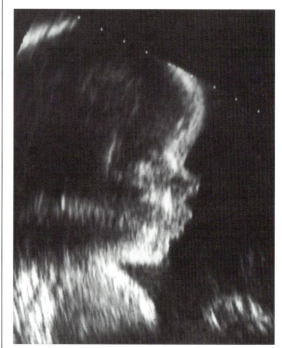

Fig. 15.39 Frontal bossing. Sagittal scan through a fetus with achondroplasia. Scan was taken at 28 weeks' gestation. Please note that the appearances were normal at 20 weeks. (Reproduced with permission from Turner G, Twining P. The facial profile in the diagnosis of fetal abnormalities. Clin Radiol 1993; 47:389–395.)

craniosynostosis syndromes and some rare genetic syndromes.

The flat profile

In contrast to frontal bossing, a flat profile shows a flat facial contour. This appearance has been described in a number of conditions[22] but an important association is Down's syndrome (see Ch. 14).

Facial abnormalities associated with abnormalities of the skull

Craniosynostosis syndromes

Craniosynostosis or premature fusion of the sutures is a non-specific abnormality which can be isolated or associated with various syndromes. This occurs when there is premature fusion of the cranial bones with subsequent limitation of expansive growth normally accommodated by that suture.[2] This premature fusion can lead on to secondary changes in the brain through the effects of raised intracranial pressure and subsequent deformation. Patel et al have described the normal appearance of the cranial sutures in utero.[92] Sonographically, the sutures appear as linear translucencies within the skull and have a characteristic location and distribution (Fig. 15.40). Prenatal diagnosis of asymmetrical craniosynostosis[93] and also of craniofacial syndromes has already been documented.[94–97]

All the sutures remain open until the fourth decade except the metopic suture which fuses between 18 months and 2 years. Premature fusion of a cranial suture produces a characteristic appearance with increased growth of the skull parallel to the fused suture. In the case of premature fusion of the sagittal suture, an elongated or dolicocephalic skull shape is produced (Fig. 15.41A).

In contrast, premature fusion of the coronal sutures produces a rounded

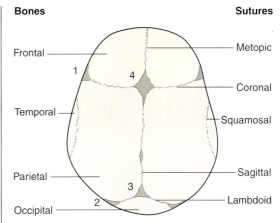

Fig. 15.40 Diagram of the skull, showing the position of the sutures. (Published with permission from Romero R, ed. Prenatal diagnosis of congenital anomalies. New York: Appleton and Lang; 1988.)

(brachycephalic) skull shape with a pointed appearance to the vertex (acrocephaly or turricephaly): in the case of the clover-leaf skull, this is produced by premature closure of all the sutures in association with hydrocephalus (Fig. 15.42).

There are a number of syndromes associated with craniosynostosis and these include Carpenter syndrome, Apert syndrome, Crouzon syndrome, craniofronto-nasal dysplasia, Pfeiffer syndrome and Saethre–Chotzen syndrome. The main features of these syndromes are outlined in Table 15.6. The prenatal diagnosis is based predominantly on the demonstration of an abnormal head shape in association with facial abnormalities which include hypertelorism, exophthalmos, mid-face hypoplasia, frontal bossing and digital abnormalities such as polydactyly and syndactyly.[98–101]

Ashby et al[94] reported an antenatal diagnosis of Carpenter syndrome at 20 weeks' gestation in a twin pregnancy where only one twin was affected. The sonographic features included a 'diamond-shaped' head, pre-axial polydactyly of the feet and syndactyly in the hands. Scanning at 29 weeks also demonstrated proptosis and apical peaking (acrocephaly) of the skull. The diagnosis was confirmed postnatally.[94] Gollin et al [95]diagnosed a case of Crouzon syndrome at 23 weeks' gestation based on the findings

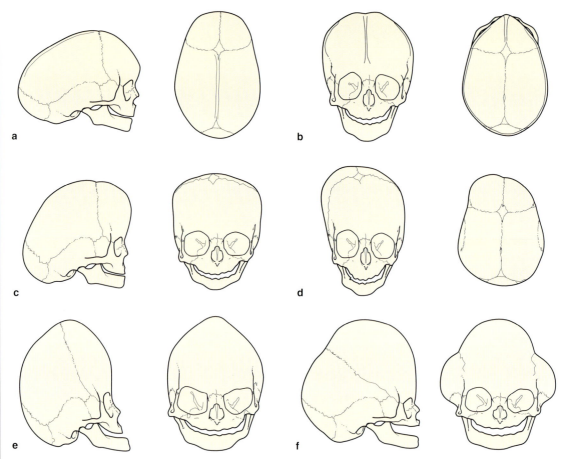

Fig. 15.41 The common appearances of craniosynostosis. (A) Premature fusion of the sagittal suture. (B) Premature fusion of the metopic suture. (C) Premature fusion of the coronal sutures. (D) Unilateral fusion of the coronal suture. (E) Premature fusion of the coronal and sagittal sutures. (F) Clover-leaf skull. Premature fusion of all sutures with hydrocephalus. (Reproduced with permission from Romero R, ed. Prenatal diagnosis of congenital anomalies. New York: Appleton and Lang; 1988.)

of hypertelorism, proptosis, ventriculo-megaly and the clover-leaf skull deformity. Although the clover-leaf skull deformity is commoner in Pfeiffer syndrome (Fig. 15.42), the absence of digital abnormalities such as syndactyly made Crouzon syndrome more likely.[95] Menashe et al reported a case of Crouzon syndrome at 35 weeks' gestation where exophthalmos was the only sonographic finding of note.[96] The clover-leaf skull deformity was also reported by Bernstein et al[97] in their case of Pfeiffer syndrome diagnosed at 27 weeks' gestation. The fetus also demonstrated hypertelorism, a flattened nasal bridge and in the feet there was a wide gap between the first and second

toes. Natarajan et al reported an antenatal diagnosis of craniofrontonasal dysplasia in a patient with a previously affected child. The antenatal sonogram demonstrated hypertelorism, cranial asymmetry, nasal hypoplasia with a broad nasal tip and contractures at the elbows, knees and ankles. There were also broad thumbs and big toes with a wide space between the first and second toes.[102]

It would seem that there is a lot of clinical overlap between these syndromes and specific antenatal diagnosis may well be very difficult. In addition, subtle or mild forms of these conditions may not be amenable to prenatal diagnosis by ultrasound.

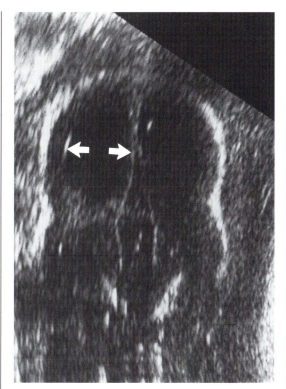

A

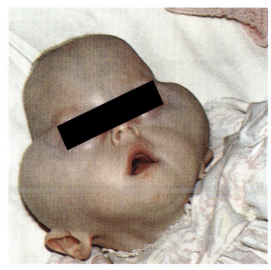

B

Fig. 15.42 Clover-leaf skull. (A) Coronal scan, showing clover-leaf skull (arrows point to dilated ventricles). (B) Postnatal photograph of an infant with clover-leaf skull. (Reproduced with permission from Baraitser M, ed. Colour atlas of congenital malformation syndromes. London: Mosby Wolfe; 1996.)

Diprosopus

Diprosopus (two faces) is a rare form of symmetric conjoined twins consisting of a single neck and body and a spectrum of duplication of craniofacial structures. In its mildest form, isolated duplication of the nose occurs; in the most severe forms, the fetus has two complete faces. The term tetrophthalmos is applied to a fetus with four eyes. The two median eyes may be partially fused and separate but share a central orbit or may occupy completely separate orbits.[103]

Okajaki et al reported a case at 28 weeks' gestation demonstrating four eyes with the two median globes sharing the same orbit. The intracranial structure was partially duplicated with two pairs of lateral ventricles, one set of which was dilated, and a single large cystic structure involving the posterior fossa. Dextrocardia was noted but no other abnormality was present. Three weeks later the fetus died in utero and a stillborn female diprosopus infant was delivered by caesarean section. Fontanorosa et al[104] diagnosed a case in the first trimester associated with craniorachischisis and case reports of diprosopus have shown a common association with both neural tube defects and anterior duplication.[105]

When the diagnosis is made prior to viability, then a termination of pregnancy can be offered to the parents. Later diagnosis can allow for counselling of the patient in terms of the prognosis and of the possibility that caesarean section may be necessary as a result of cephalopelvic disproportion. If significant hydrocephalus is the major cause of macrocephaly, cephalocentesis under sonographic guidance may be offered to avoid caesarean section.[103]

Anencephaly

Anencephaly is the commonest form of neural tube defect and results from failure of closure of the anterior portion of the neural groove.[22] This produces absence of the cerebral hemispheres and related skull bones. The midbrain and brain stem are present as is the skull base. The facial

Table 15.6
Craniosynostosis syndromes

Syndrome	Inheritance	Features	Intelligence

Apert syndrome	Autosomal dominant	Hypertelorism turricephaly
		Prominent eyes
		Syndactyly of digits 2–5 and occasionally
		  the thumb
		Syndactyly of toes
			50% mental
			  retardation

Carpenter syndrome	Autosomal recessive	High forehead Mid-facial hypoplasia Flat facial profile Postaxial polydactyly in hands Pre-axial polydactyly in feet	Variable Can be normal IQs range from 54–104
Crouzon syndrome	Autosomal dominant	Proptosis, hypertelorism Frontal bossing, premature closure of coronal sutures Beaked nose Occasionally clover-leaf skull	Usually normal

Pfeiffer syndrome	Autosomal dominant	Craniosynostosis or coronal suture but
		  clover-leaf skull is common
		Broad or duplicated big toes
		Broad thumbs
		Variable soft tissue syndactyly
			Neurological
			  compromise is
			  common
			Clover-leaf skull has a
			  poor prognosis

Saethre–Chotzen
  syndrome
	Autosomal dominant	Hypertelorism
		Mid-face hypoplasia
		High flat forehead
		Craniosynostosis of coronal, lambdoid
		  sutures
		Small ears
			Most normal

Craniofrontonasal dysplasia	X-linked dominant	Females more severely affected than males Hypertelorism, frontal bossing Syndactyly of fingers and toes	Usually normal

appearances are characteristic with absence of the cranial vault above the level of the orbits (Fig. 15.43A). The profile view shows nasal hypoplasia and a receding forehead (Fig. 15.43B). Residual brain tissue is often seen in the skull base. Cleft lip and palate is seen in up to 10% of cases.

Otocephaly

Otocephaly (synotia) is a rare, complex malformation which, in its simplest form, represents marked under-development of the mandible. There are many forms of otocephaly and some forms resemble cyclopia. In isolated otocephaly, the brain is not involved. Other forms represent true combinations of otocephaly and cyclopia.[107]

Cayea et al reported a case at 26 weeks' gestation with a large anterior encephalocoele associated with absent orbits and nose. Both ears were situated anteriorly in the midline.[106] Sonographically, this condition would be most likely to resemble anencephaly, but the absence of orbits and opposition of the ears anteriorly in the midline should suggest the diagnosis.

Facial tumours

Teratoma

Teratomas are rare, but they probably represent the commonest type of facial tumour. Nasopharyngeal teratoma has already been discussed. Shipp et al reported a nasal teratoma in their series of ten facial masses, which arose from the nasal septum and sonographically appeared as a solid mass arising from the tip of the nose. The mass enlarged from 2.5 cm in diameter at 20

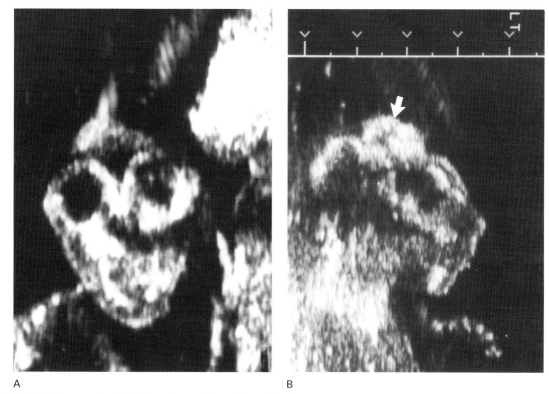

Fig. 15.43 Anencephaly. (A) Coronal scan through the orbit, showing the typical appearances. (B) Sagittal scans through the face, showing the shortened forehead and residual brain tissue (arrow).

weeks' gestation to 7 cm at 36 weeks. The mass was removed surgically without complication in the neonatal period.[69]

Haemangioma

Craniofacial haemangiomata are benign tumours that arise from the skin and usually have a good prognosis. Haemangiomata can occur on the cheek[108] the soft tissues overlying the skull,[69,109–111] or the neck.

Sonographically, the masses are of mixed or homogeneous echodensity and often show either flow in the periphery of the lesion[110] or, as in the case of a giant cavernous haemangioma, a high-flow waveform secondary to arteriovenous shunting.[110] The masses may remain unchanged in size or can gradually increase in size during pregnancy.[111,112]

Masses overlying the skull bones should always be differentiated from encephalocoeles by the demonstration of intact skull bones beneath the lesion. Confusion with cranial sutures should be avoided by the characteristic location of sutures and their distribution (Fig. 15.40).

Most haemangiomata can be excised in the neonatal period. However, if these tumours are large and show considerable arteriovenous shunting, then they can lead to cardiac decompensation and death.[111]

In view of this, these tumours should be carefully assessed using colour flow and Doppler velocimetry looking for low-resistance waveforms and high-flow states. This would suggest significant arteriovenous shunting and the risk of cardiac decompensation. The fetus may then be regularly monitored for signs of cardiac decompensation or fetal distress.

Harlequin ichthyosis

This autosomal recessive condition is characterized by thickened skin which is fissured and separated into polygonal plaques. It is these plaques which may resemble the diamond pattern on the costume of the archetypal harlequin that are responsible for the name of this disorder. Ectropion (eyelid eversion) and eclabium (eversion of the lips) are typically present.[113]

The diagnosis can be established by fetal skin biopsy,[114] but the ultrasound features are characteristic. Sonographically, the fetal skin may be thickened and Milalko et al reported a thickened membrane of skin floating freely in the amniotic fluid but attached to the anterior abdominal wall. This represented sloughed, abnormally thickened skin.[113] The mouth is held fixed and open and is 'O'-shaped with the lips everted. Cystic masses are seen anterior to the orbits[115] because of the pronounced ectropion. In addition, the markedly thickened skin can also produce flexion deformities of the limbs.

The outlook is very poor and most affected neonates die within hours or days after birth. Causes of death include sepsis, mechanical restriction of breathing and electrolyte imbalance.[113]

THE FETAL NECK

Introduction

Abnormalities of the fetal neck are uncommon. However, the most important anomalies are cystic hygroma, occipital encephalocoele, cervical meningomyelocoele and cervical teratoma. Rarely, a haemangioma or a fetal goitre may be detected.

Ultrasound examination of the neck may include assessment of the occipital region of the head, the cervical spine, the oropharynx (Fig. 15.25) and vessels of the neck.

Sonographic approach

Most neck abnormalities are masses that are predominantly either cystic or solid. Careful

attention to the position and extent of a neck mass should provide sufficient information to narrow the differential diagnosis.

Posterior neck masses are usually either a cystic hygroma or occipital encephalocoele. Rarely, a cervical meningomyelocoele may be seen. Most anterior masses are teratomas; haemangiomas can occur anywhere but may have characteristic Doppler signals. Most teratomas and haemangiomas are solid and cystic hygromata are always cystic and multiseptate. Occipital encephalocoeles may be cystic, solid or of mixed echotexture; however, there will always be either associated intracranial abnormalities or a skull defect. Rarely, an anterior neck mass may be due to a fetal goitre.

Neck abnormalities

Cystic hygroma

This is the commonest neck abnormality occurring in 0.5% of spontaneous abortions[116] and up to 1 in 700 low-risk pregnancies[117] but is seen rarely in the neonate.

Cystic hygroma is a lymphatic malformation which produces a multiseptated cystic mass in the posterior cervical area. It is thought to represent overdistension of the jugular lymphatic sacs as a consequence of failure of communication with the internal jugular vein. Secondary dilatation of the lymphatic channels draining the chest and limbs results in peripheral lymphoedema and development of non-immune hydrops.[116]

Sonographically, the appearances are of a multiseptate cystic mass affecting the back of the fetal neck. There is always a midline septum which extends into the cystic hygroma (Fig. 15.44). Bronshtein et al have described two types of cystic hygromata, septated and non-septated.[118]

The septated cystic hygromas are similar to those previously described. However, the non-septated hygromas appear as small unilocular sonolucent sacs, located bilaterally in the anterolateral cervical region. Bronshtein et al found that non-septated

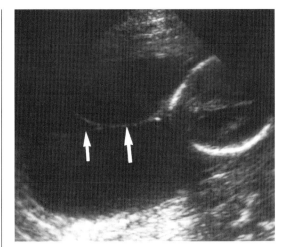

Fig. 15.44 Cystic hygroma. Transverse scan, showing large cystic hygroma (arrows outline midline septum).

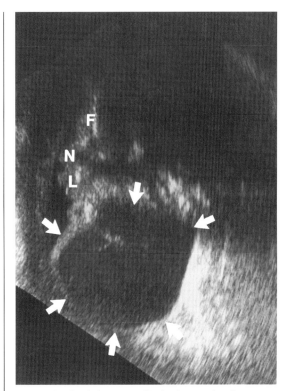

Fig. 15.45 Cystic hygroma. Sagittal scan, showing anterior cystic hygroma (arrows outline the cystic hygroma; F, forehead; N, nose; L, lips.)

cystic hygromata had a better prognosis and much lower incidence of chromosomal disease than septated cystic hygromata.[118]

Cystic hygroma has a high incidence of chromosomal disease, cardiac abnormalities and hydrops. The commonest chromosomal abnormality is Turner's syndrome which occurs in 75%, trisomy 18 occurs in 5% and trisomy 21 in 5%. The remaining fetuses may have a normal karyotype.

The main cardiac abnormality seen in fetuses with cystic hygromata is coarctation of the aorta, and this can be seen in up to 48% of fetuses with Turner's syndrome.[116]

Hydrops is a common association with cystic hygromata and is seen in up to 68% of fetuses with Turner's syndrome and 82% of chromosomally normal fetuses.[116]

The outlook for fetuses with cystic hygroma and hydrops is poor with an estimated mortality in the region of 80 to 90%.[119] Isolated cystic hygromata with a normal karyotype may have a good prognosis with surgical removal in the neonatal period; a similar good prognosis is seen in cystic hygromata presenting in the third trimester.[116]

Occasionally, cystic hygromata may occur anteriorly (Fig. 14.45), laterally or elsewhere on the body. Anteriorly positioned cystic hygromata increase the risk of respiratory problems in the neonatal period and it is recommended that paediatric support is present at delivery.

Although chromosomal disease is the commonest association, cystic hygromata have also been reported in association with Noonan syndrome, fetal alcohol syndrome and familial pterygium colli.[120]

Occipital encephalocoele

Encephalocoeles have an incidence of between 1:5000 and 1:10 000 pregnancies and 80% occur in the occipital region.[121] The abnormality is produced by incomplete closure of the anterior neuropore producing a midline skull defect which is associated with herniation of meninges (meningocoele) or brain tissue (encephalocoele) through the defect.[80]

Sonographically, there is always a cranial defect usually in the midline in the occipital region. Occasionally, it may be difficult to demonstrate the defect if small (Fig. 15.46A)

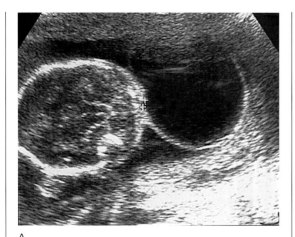

A

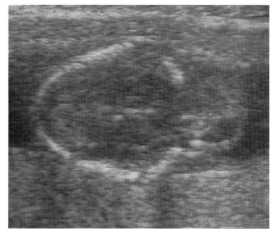

Fig. 15.47 Encephalocoele. Transverse scan through the fetal head, showing a herniation of brain tissue into a large encephalocoele sac.

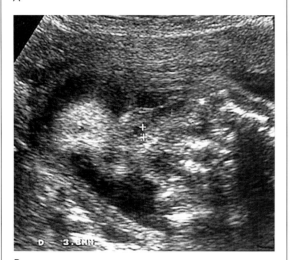

B

Fig. 15.46 Encephalocoele. Cranial meningocoele. (A) Transverse scans through the head, showing a cystic structure arising from the occipital region. (B) Coronal scan shows the small bony defect-calipers.

but careful scanning in the transverse plane with the occiput at 90° to the ultrasound beam or scanning in the coronal plane should reveal the defect (Fig. 15.46B).

When only meninges have herniated through the defect, the appearances will be of a cystic mass (Fig. 15.46). An encephalocoele, however, will demonstrate solid brain tissue extending through the skull defect (Fig. 15.47).

There is often associated microcephaly, hydrocephalus and an abnormally shaped skull. Other associated intracranial abnormalities include the Arnold–Chiari

malformation, Dandy–Walker syndrome, cerebellar hypoplasia, agenesis of the corpus callosum, migrational abnormalities and cervical rachischisis.[80] A lateral encephalocoele should always suggest the presence of the amniotic band syndrome and a search should be made for the associated features.[57, 58]

The presence of polydactyly and cystic dysplastic kidneys would indicate the Meckel–Gruber syndrome which has an autosomal recessive inheritance. In this respect, it is always important to consider a karyotype procedure if other extracranial abnormalities are present as an encephalocoele can also be part of the features of trisomy 13, trisomy 18 and triploidy.

The outlook for fetuses with an encephalocoele is generally poor, with an overall survival of 55%[81] and of these 74% of babies are likely to be mentally retarded. The main reason for this is the high association of other intracranial abnormalities, many of which may not be amenable to prenatal ultrasound diagnosis.[80]

The outcome for cranial meningocoele is better than that for occipital encephalocoele with an overall survival rate of 75 to 90%[81] and up to 48% of fetuses may have normal outcome.

Cervical meningocoele

Neural tube defects are rare in the neck and there are few reports in the literature.[122, 123] The typical appearances resemble meningomyelocoele elsewhere in the spine with splaying of the posterior elements of the spine associated with a meningomyelocoele sac. The Arnold–Chiari malformation is frequently associated, producing the 'lemon' head and 'banana' cerebellum.[124]

The presence of associated abnormalities always raises the possibility of chromosomal disease and would prompt a karyotype procedure. As with neural tube defects elsewhere in the spine, talipes may be present.

The outlook for cervical myelomeningocoele is thought to be better than that for an encephalocoele but worse than that of an occipital meningocoele.[119]

Cervical teratoma

Cervical teratomas are rare tumours and account for 5% of all teratomas. The majority of cervical teratomas detected in the neonatal period are benign and are often large, producing airways obstruction. The converse is true in adults where the tumours are often small with a high incidence of malignancy.[125]

The tumours are situated in the anterior or anterolateral aspect of the neck and are thought to arise from embryonic thyroid tissue. The tumours often become large, producing hyperextension of the neck, and are associated with polyhydramnios in 20 to 40% of cases[126] because of oesophageal compression.

Sonographically, the tumours are usually solid with cystic components (Fig. 15.48) and typically, if large, produce hyperextension of the neck.[127–129] The differential diagnosis includes an anterior cystic hygroma (Fig. 15.45), a haemangioma and a goitre. A cystic hygroma, however, does not usually contain solid areas and does not typically produce hyperextension of the neck. A haemangioma may show characteristic Doppler signals and a goitre is relatively small with a bi-lobed appearance.[132]

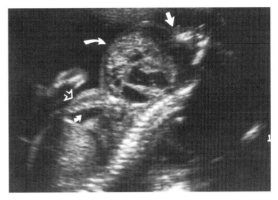

A

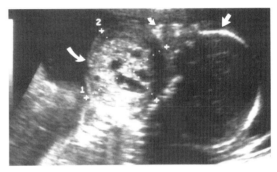

B

Fig. 15.48 Cervical teratoma. (A) Profile scans, demonstrating a complex neck mass (curved arrow), chin (solid arrow) and anterior chest wall (open arrow). Small pleural effusion is also noted (small curved arrow). (B) Profile view, demonstrating forehead (solid arrow). Mandible (small curved arrow) and mass (large curved arrow). (Reproduced with permission from Langer J, et al. Management of prenatally diagnosed tracheal obstruction: Access to the airway in utero prior to delivery. Fetal Diagn Ther 1992; 7:12–16.)

Postnatally, up to 50% of cervical teratomas contain calcification, but this has not been seen prenatally.[126] A number of associated abnormalities has been described which include one case each of cystic fibrosis, imperforate anus, chondrodystrophia fetalis, hypoplastic left ventricle and pulmonary hypoplasia.[125]

The outcome for fetuses with cervical teratoma is poor unless urgent treatment is instituted in the immediate neonatal period to establish an airway. Jordan et al documented a mortality of 43% for neonates demonstrating respiratory distress at birth.[125] In view of this, most fetuses with cervical teratoma will need to be delivered by caesarean section in order to improve the chances of survival. Longer et al proposed endotracheal intubation of the fetus during caesarean section and prior to cord ligation[129] as a means of obtaining access to the airway. In view of this, full paediatric and surgical support needs to be present at delivery in order to achieve early airways access and improve the outcome for the infant.

Haemangioma

Haemangioma of the neck is a rare tumour with few antenatal reports.[130,131] Most tumours show a mixed cystic and solid appearance and these tumours may lead on to hydrops if the lesions are large. Evaluation of the tumour with colour flow Doppler and spectral Doppler may reveal arterial and venous pulsations within the mass which may help in the antenatal diagnosis.[131] A haemangioma can occur anywhere in the neck.

Goitre

Congenital hypothyroidism occurs in approximately 1:5000 live births[132] and is usually caused by treatment with antithyroid drugs for maternal thyrotoxicosis.[133] Antithyroid agents can easily cross the placenta and if this occurs during the period of fetal thyroid development at 10 to 16 weeks' gestation, it can produce fetal hypothyroidism and goitre. Occasionally, the cause of the fetal hypothyroidism is unknown.[132]

Fetal goitre can cause polyhydramnios and occasionally fetal neck extension. More importantly, it can cause intra-uterine growth retardation, fetal bradycardia and delayed appearances of ossification centres.

Sonographically, the appearance is of a bi-lobed, predominantly solid mass affecting the anterior neck. Abuhamad et al described a homogeneous mass in the neck whereas Noia et al reported an echogenic bi-lobed anterior neck mass.[132, 133] Earlier reports of goitre indicated cystic masses or cystic solid neck masses.[134, 135]

Although treatment can be initiated in the neonatal period in cases of congenital hypothyroidism, some authors have advocated intra-uterine therapy with thyroxine in the form of intra-amniotic injection of thyroxine.[132]

Malignant tumours

Metastatic deposits have been reported involving the neck; one case report documented neuroblastoma deposits appearing as a solid anterior neck mass in a hydropic fetus,[136] while the second described a case of malignant melanoma involving the back and neck in a 30-week fetus. Sonographically, the appearance was of a mixed cystic and solid mass.[137] The outcome for these cases was extremely poor with one neonatal death and one stillbirth.

References

1. Nicolaides KH, Salvesen DR, Snijders RJ, Gosden CM. Fetal facial defects: Associated malformations and chromosomal abnormalities. Fetal Diagn Ther 1993; 8:1–9.
2. Stewart RE. Craniofacial malformations: Clinical and genetic considerations. Pediat Clin North Am 1978; 25(3):485–515.
3. Pruzansky S. Clinical investigation of the experiments in nature. ASHA Reports 1973; 8: Orofacial anomalies: Clinical and research implications.
4. Lee A, Deutinger J, Bernaschek G. Three dimensional ultrasound: Abnormalities of the fetal face in surface and volume rendering mode. Br J Obstet Gynaecol 1995; 102:302–306.
5. Report of the Royal College of Obstetricians and Gynaecologists Working Party on routine ultrasound examination in pregnancy. Royal College of Obstetrics and Gynaecology; 1991.
6. Anderson N, Boswell O, Duff G. Prenatal sonography for the detection of fetal anomalies. Results of a prospective study and comparison with prior series. Am J Radiol 1995; 165:943–950.
7. Chitty LS, Hunt GH, Moore J, Lobb M. Effectiveness of routine ultrasonography in detecting fetal structural abnormalities in a low risk population. BMJ 1991; 303:1165–1169.
8. Shirley IM, Bottomley F, Robinson V. Routine radiographer screening for fetal abnormalities by ultrasound in an unselected low risk population. Br J Radiol 1992; 65:564–569.
9. Pilu G, Reece A, Romero R, et al. Prenatal diagnosis of craniofacial malformations with ultrasonography. Am J Obstet Gynecol 1986; 155:45–50.

10. Larsen WJ. Human embryology. London: Churchill Livingstone; 1993.

11. McLachlan J. Medical embryology. Wokingham: Addison-Wesley; 1994.

12. Birnholz JC, Farrell EE. Fetal hyaloid artery: Timing of regression with ultrasound. Radiology 1988; 166:781–783.

13. Turner G, Twining P. The facial profile in the diagnosis of fetal abnormalities. Clin Radiol 1993; 47:389–395.

14. Jeanty P, Dramaix-Wilmet M, Van Gansbeke D, Van Regemorter N, Rodesch F. Fetal ocular biometry by ultrasound. Radiology 1982; 143:513–516.

15. Babcook CJ, McGahan JP, Chong BW, et al. Evaluation of fetal midface anatomy related to facial clefts: use of ultrasound. Radiology 1996; 201:113–118.

16. Meizner I, Katz M, Bar-Ziu J, Insler V. Prenatal sonographic detection of fetal facial malformations. Isr J Med Sci 1987; 23:881–885.

17. Benacerraf BR, Frigoletto FD, Bieber FR. The fetal face; ultrasound examination. Radiology 1984; 153:495–497.

18. Guis F, Ville Y, Vincent S, et al. Ultrasound evaluation of the length of the fetal nasal bones throughout gestation. Ultrasound Obstet Gynecol 1995; 5:304–307.

19. Birnholz JC. The fetal external ear. Radiology 1983; 147:819–821.

20. Birnholz JC, Farrell EE. Fetal ear length. Paediatrics 1988; 81:555–558.

21. Gorlin R, Pindborg JJ, Cohen MM. Syndromes of the head and neck. 3rd ed. New York: McGraw-Hill; 1990.

22. Jones KL. Smith's recognisable patterns of human malformation. London: WB Saunders; 1997.

23. Poswillo D. The aetiology and pathogenesis of craniofacial deformity. Development 1988; 103 (Supplement):207–212.

24. Bromley B, Benacerraf BR. Fetal micrognathia: associated anomalies and outcome. J Ultrasound Med 1994; 13:529–533.

25. Dixon MJ, Read AP, Donnai D. The gene for Treacher Collins syndrome maps to the long arm of chromosome 5. Am J Hum Genet 1991; 49:17–22.

26. Nicolaides KH, Johansson D, Donnai D, Rodeck CH. Prenatal diagnosis of mandibulofacial dysostosis. Prenat Diagn 1984; 4:201–205.

27. Crane J, Beaver H. Mid trimester diagnosis of mandibulofacial dysostosis. Am J Med Genet 1986; 25:251–255.

28. Meizner I, Carmi R, Katz M. Prenatal ultrasonic diagnosis of mandibulofacial dysostosis. J Clin Ultrasound 1991; 19:124–127.

29. Benson CB, Pober BR, Hirsch MP, Doubilet PM. Sonography of Nager acrofacial dysostosis syndrome in utero. J Ultrasound Med 1988; 7:163–167.

30. Robinow M, Reynolds JF, Fitzgerald J, Bryant JA. Hemifacial microsomia, ipsilateral facial palsy and malformed auricle in two families: an autosomal dominant malformation. Am J Med Genet 1986; Supplement 2:129–133.

31. Tamas DE, Mahoney BS, Bowie JD. Prenatal sonographic diagnosis of hemifacial microsomia (Goldenhar Syndrome). J Ultrasound Med 1986; 7:163–167.

32. Dennison WM. The Pierre Robin syndrome. Paediatrics 1965; 36:336–342.

33. Pilu G, Romero R, Reece A, et al. The prenatal diagnosis of Robin Anomalad. Am J Obstet Gynecol 1986; 154:630–632.

34. Majewski F, Goecke T. Studies of microcephalic dwarfism: approach to delineation of the Seckel syndrome. Am J Med Genet 1982; 12:7–21.

35. Majoor-Krakauer DF, Wladimiroff JW, Stewart PA. Microcephaly, micrognathia and bird headed dwarfism: Prenatal diagnosis of a Seckel like syndrome. Am J Med Genet 1987; 27:183–188.

36. Featherstone LS, Sherman SJ, Quigg MM. Prenatal diagnosis of Seckel syndrome. J Ultrasound Med 1996; 15:85–88.

37. Shenker L, Reed K, Anderson C, Hauck L, Spark R. Syndrome of camptodactyly, anklyoses, facial anomalies and pulmonary hypoplasia (Pena Shokeir syndrome). Obstetric and ultrasound aspects. Am J Obstet Gynecol 1985; 152:302–307.

38. Hall JG. Analysis of Pena Shokeir phenotype. Am J Med Genet 1986; 25:99–117.

39. Baraitser M, Winter RM. Colour atlas of congenital malformation syndromes. London: Mosby Wolfe; 1996.

40. Wilson DI, Cross I, Goodship J. A prospective cytogenetic study of 36 cases of Di George syndrome. Am J Hum Genet 1992; 51:957–963.

41. Salonen R, Herva R. Syndrome of the month – hydrolethalus syndrome. J Med Genet 1990; 27:756–759.

42. Pryde PG, Qureshi F, Hallak M, Kupsky W. Two consecutive hydrolethalus syndrome affected pregnancies in a nonconsanguinous black couple: discussion of problems in prenatal differential diagnosis. Am J Med Genet 1993; 46:537–541.

43. Nyberg DA, Sickler GK, Hegg F, et al. Fetal cleft lip with and without cleft palate: ultrasound classification and correlation with outcome. Radiology 1995; 195:677–684.

44. Das SK, Runnels RS, Smith JC, Cohly HH. Epidemiology of cleft lip and cleft palate in Mississippi. South Med J 1995; 8:437–442.

45. Koren G, Edwards MB, Miskin M. Antenatal sonography of fetal malformations associated with drugs and chemicals: a guide. Am J Obstet Gynecol 1987; 176:79–84.

46. Christ JE, Meininger MG. Ultrasound diagnosis of cleft lip and cleft palate before birth. Plast Reconstr Surg 1981; 68:854–859.

47. Seeds JW, Cefalo RC. Technique of early sonographic diagnosis of bilateral cleft lip and palate. Obstet Gynecol 1983; 62:25–75.

48. Saltzman DH, Benacerraf BR, Frigoletto FD.

Diagnosis and management of fetal facial clefts. Am J Obstet Gynecol 1986; 155:377–379.

49. Bronshtein M, Blumenfeld I, Kohn J, Blumenfeld Z. Detection of cleft lip by early second trimester transvaginal sonography. Obstet Gynecol 1994; 84:73–76.

50. Nyberg DA, Hegge FN, Kramer D, et al. Premaxillary protrusion: A sonographic clue to bilateral cleft lip and palate. J Ultrasound Med 1993; 12:331–335.

51. Bundy AL, Saltzman DH, Emerson D, Fine C. Sonographic features associated with cleft palate. J Clin Ultrasound 1986; 14:486–489.

52. Monni G, Ibba RM, Olla G, Cao A. Colour Doppler ultrasound and prenatal diagnosis of cleft palate. J Clin Ultrasound 1995; 23:189–191.

53. Pashayan HM. What else to look for in a child born with a cleft of the lip and/or palate. Cleft Palate J 1983; 20:54–82.

54. Moerman P, Fryns JP, Vandenberghe K, Lauweryns J. Constrictive amniotic bands, amniotic adhesions and limb body wall complex: discrete disruption sequences with pathogenetic overlap. Am J Med Genet 1992; 42:470–479.

55. Fiedler JM, Phelan JP. The amniotic band syndrome in monozygotic twins. Am J Obstet Gynecol 1983; 146:864–865.

56. Kalouseck DK, Bamforth S. Amnion rupture in previable fetuses. Am J Med Genet 1988; 31:63–73.

57. Burton DJ, Filly RA. Sonographic diagnosis of the amniotic band syndrome. Am J Radiol 1991; 156:555–558.

58. Mahony BS, Filly RA, Callen PW, Golbus MS. The amniotic band syndrome: antenatal sonographic diagnosis and potential pitfalls. Am J Obstet Gynecol 1985; 152:63–68.

59. Rodini E, Richieri-Costa A. Ectrodactyly-ectodermal dysplasia clefting syndrome: report on 20 new patients, clinical and genetic considerations. Am J Med Genet 1990; 37:42–53.

60. Bronshtein M, Gershoni-Baruch R. Prenatal transvaginal diagnosis of the ectrodactyly ectodermal dysplasia, cleft palate (EEC) syndrome. Prenat Diagn 1993; 13:519–552.

61. Robins DB, Ladda RL, Thieme GA. Prenatal detection of Roberts SC phocomelia syndrome, report of two siblings with characteristic manifestations. Am J Med Genet 1989; 32:390–394.

62. Stioui S, Privitera O, Brambati B. First trimester prenatal diagnosis of Roberts syndrome. Prenat Diagn 1992; 12:145–149.

63. Paladini D, Palmieri S, Lecora M, et al. Prenatal ultrasound diagnosis of Roberts syndrome in a family with negative history. Ultrasound Obstet Gynecol 1996; 7:208–210.

64. Suresh S, Rajesh K, Suresh I, Raja V. Prenatal diagnosis of orofaciodigital syndrome: Mohr type. J Ultrasound Med 1995; 14:863–866.

65. Shah YG, Metlay L. Prenatal ultrasound diagnosis of Beckwith–Wiedeman syndrome. J Clin Ultrasound 1990; 18:597–600.

66. Chambers J. Prenatal diagnosis of Beckwith–Wiedemann syndrome. Br Med Ultrasound Bull 1994; 2(2):44.

67. Teal LN, Angtuaco TL, Jimenez JF, Quirk JG. Fetal teratomas: Antenatal diagnosis and clinical management. J Clin Ultrasound 1988; 16:329–336.

68. Chervenak FA, Isaacson G, Touloukian R, et al. Diagnosis and management of fetal teratomas. Obstet Gynecol 1985; 66:666–671.

69. Shipp TD, Bromley B, Benacerraf B. The ultrasonographic appearance and outcome for fetuses with masses distorting the fetal face. J Ultrasound Med 1995; 14:673–678.

70. Hullett RL, Bowerman RA, Marks T, Silverstein A. Prenatal ultrasound detection of congenital gingival granular cell tumour. J Ultrasound Med 1991; 10:185–187.

71. Jeanty P, Shah D, Zaliski W, et al. Prenatal diagnosis of fetal cephalocoele: A sonographic spectrum. Am J Perinatol 1991; 8:144–149.

72. Carlan SJ, Angel JL, Leo J, Feeney J. Cephalocoele involving the oral cavity. Obstet Gynecol 1990; 75:494–495.

73. McGahan JP, Nyberg DA, Mack LA. Sonography of facial features of alobar and semilobar holoprosencephaly. Am J Radiol 1990; 154:143–148.

74. De Meyer W, Zeman W, Palmer CA. The face predicts the brain: Diagnostic significance of median facial anomalies for holoprosencephaly (arrhinencephaly). Paediatrics 1964; 34:256–264.

75. Hsieh FJ, Lee CN, Wu CC, et al. Antenatal ultrasound findings of craniofacial malformations. J Formos Med Assoc 1991; 90:551–554.

76. Benacerraf BR, Frigoletto FD, Greeve MF. Abnormal facial features and extremities in human Trisomy syndromes: Prenatal ultrasound appearance. Radiology 1986; 159:243–246.

77. Fryberg JS, Persing JA, Lin KY. Frontonasal dysplasia in two successive generations. Am J Med Genet 1993; 46:712–714.

78. Chervenak FA, Tortora M, Mayden K, Mesologites T. Antenatal diagnosis of median cleft face syndrome: sonographic demonstration of cleft lip and hypertelorism. Am J Obstet Gynecol 1984; 149:94–97.

79. Frattarelli JL, Boley TJ, Miller RAC. Prenatal diagnosis of frontonasal dysplasia. Median cleft syndrome. J Ultrasound Med 1996; 15:81–83.

80. Goldstein RB, Lapidus AS, Filly RA. Fetal cephalocoeles: diagnosis with ultrasound. Radiology 1991; 180:803–808.

81. Brown M, Sheridan-Pereira M. Outlook for the child with a cephalocoele. Paediatrics 1992; 90:914–919.

82. Bronshtein M, Zimmer E, Gershoni-Baruch R, et al. First and second trimester diagnosis of fetal ocular defects and associated anomalies: report of eight cases. Obstet Gynecol 1991; 77:443–449.

83. Schauer GM, Dunn LK, Godmilow L, et al. Prenatal diagnosis of Fraser syndrome at 18.5 weeks gestation, with autopsy findings at 19 weeks. Am J Med Genet 1990; 37:583–591.

84. Gilbert R. Clusters of anophthalmia in Britain. BMJ 1993; 307:340–341.

85. Pearce WG, Nigam S, Rootman J. Primary anophthalmos: histological and genetic features. Can J Ophthalmol 1974; 9:141–145.

86. Monteagudo A, Timor-Tritch IE, Friedman AH, Santos R. Autosomal dominant cataracts of the fetus: early detection by transvaginal ultrasound. Ultrasound Obstet Gynecol 1996; 8:104–108.

87. Gaary EA, Rawnsley E, Marin-Padilla JM, et al. In utero detection of fetal cataracts. J Ultrasound 1993; 4:234–236.

88. Drysdale K, Kyle PM, Sepulveda W. Prenatal detection of congenital inherited cataracts. Ultrasound Obstet Gynecol 1997; 9:62–63.

89. Battaglia C, Artini PG, D'Ambrogio G, Genazzani AR. Prenatal ultrasonographic evidence of transient dactrocystocoeles. J Ultrasound Med 1994; 13:897–900.

90. Birnholz JC. The fetal external ear. Radiology 1983; 147:819–821.

91. Lettieri L, Rodis JF, Vintzileos A, et al. Ear length in second trimester aneuploid fetuses. Obstet Gynecol 1993; 81:57–60.

92. Patel MD, Swinford AE, Filly RA. Anatomic and sonographic features of the fetal skull. J Ultrasound Med 1994; 13:251–257.

93. Meilstrup JW, Botti JJ, Mackay DR, Johnson DL. Prenatal sonographic appearance of asymmetric cranio-synostosis. J Ultrasound Med 1995; 14:307–310.

94. Ashby T, Rouse GA, De Longe M. Prenatal sonographic diagnosis of Carpenter syndrome. J Ultrasound Med 1994; 13:905–909.

95. Gollin YG, Abuhamad AZ, Inati MN, et al. Sonographic apperance of craniofacial dyostosis (Crouzon syndrome) in the second trimester. J Ultrasound Med 1993; 12:625–628.

96. Menashe T, Baruch B, Rabinovitch O, et al. Exophthalmos – Prenatal ultrasonic features for diagnosis of Crouzon syndrome. Prenat Diagn 1989; 9:805–808.

97. Bernstein PS, Gross SJ, Cohen DJ, et al. Prenatal diagnosis of type 2 Pfeiffer syndrome. Ultrasound Obstet Gynecol 1996; 8:425–428.

98. Robinson LK, James HE, Mubarak SJ, Allen EJ. Carpenter syndrome: Natural history and clinical spectrum. Am J Med Genet 1985; 20:461–469.

99. Cohen MM. Pfeiffer syndrome update, clinical subtypes, and guidelines for differential diagnosis. Am J Med Genet 1993; 45:300–307.

100. Cohen MM. Genetic and family study of the Apert syndrome. J Cranial and General Dev Biol 1991; 11:7–17.

101. Reardon W, Winter RM. Saethre–Chotzen syndrome. J Med Genet 1994; 31:393–396.

102. Natarajan U, Baraitser M, Nicolaides KH, Gosden C. Craniofrontonasal dysplasia in two male siblings. Clin Dysmorphol 1993; 2:360–364.

103. Okajaki JR, Wilson JL, Holmes SM, Vandermark LL. Diposopus: diagnosis in utero. Am J Radiol 1987; 149:147–148.

104. Fontanarosa M, Bagnoli G, Golini P, et al. First trimester sonographic diagnosis of diposopus twins with craniorachischisis. J Clin Ultrasound 1992; 20:69–71.

105. Amr SS, Hammouri MF. Craniofacial duplication (diposopus): Report of a case with a review of the literature. Eur J Obstet Gynecol Reprod Biol 1995; 58:77–80.

106. Cayea PD, Bieber FR, Ross MJ. Sonographic findings in otocephaly (synotia). J Ultrasound Med 1985; 4:377–379.

107. Warkany J. Congenital malformations. Chicago: Year Book Medical; 1981.

108. Meizner I, Bas-Ziv J, Holberg G, Katz M. In utero prenatal diagnosis of fetal facial tumour – haemangioma. J Clin Ultrasound 1985; 13:345–347.

109. Sherer DM, Perillo AM, Abramowicz JS. Fetal haemangioma overlying the Temporal Occipital Suture. Initially diagnosed by ultrasonography as an encephalocoele. J Ultrasound Med 1993; 12:691–693.

110. Bulas DI, Johnson D, Fonda-Allen J, Kapur S. Fetal haemangioma. Sonographic and colour flow Doppler findings. J Ultrasound Med 1992; 11:499–501.

111. Lasser D, Preis O, Dor N, Tancer ML. Antenatal diagnosis of giant cystic cavernous haemangioma by Doppler velocimetry. Obstet Gynecol 1988; 72:476–477.

112. Pennell RG, Baltarowick OH. Prenatal diagnosis of fetal facial haemangioma. J Ultrasound Med 1986; 5:525–528.

113. Milalko M, Lindfors KK, Grix AW, et al. Prenatal sonographic diagnosis of harlequin ichthyosis. Am J Radiol 1989; 153:827–828.

114. Suzumori K, Kanzaki T. Prenatal diagnosis of harlequin ichthyosis by fetal skin biopsy. Report of two cases. Prenat Diagn 1991; 11:451–457.

115. Meizner I. Prenatal ultrasonic features in a rare case of congenital ichthyosis (harlequin fetus). J Clin Ultrasound 1992; 20:132–134.

116. Azar GB, Snijders RJM, Gosden C, Nicolaides KH. Fetal nuchal cystic hygromata: Associated malformations and chromosomal defects. Fetal Diagn Ther 1991; 6:46–57.

117. Marchese C, Savin E, Dragone E, et al. Cystic hygroma: Prenatal diagnosis and genetic counselling. Prenat Diagn 1985; 5:221–227.

118. Bronshtein M, Barlana I, Blumenfeld I, et al. The difference between septated and nonseptated nuchal cystic hygroma in the early second trimester. Obstet Gynecol 1993; 81:683–687.

119. Nyberg DA, Mahony BS, Pretamus DH. Diagnostic ultrasound of fetal anomalies: Text and atlas. St Louis: Mosby Year Book; 1990.

120. Chervenak FA, Isaacson G, Blakemore K, et al. Fetal cystic hygroma. Cause and natural history. N Engl J Med 1983; 309:822–825.

121. Lorber J, Schofield JK. The prognosis of occipital meningocoele. Z Kinderchir 1979; 28:347–351.

122. Sabbagha RE, Depp R, Grasse D. Ultrasound diagnosis of occipitothoracic meningocoele at 22

weeks gestation. Am J Obstet Gynecol 1978; 131:113–114.

123. Sabbagha RE, Tamura RK, Dal Compos S. Fetal cranial and craniocervical masses: Ultrasound characteristics and differential diagnosis. Am J Obstet Gynecol 1980; 138:511–517.

124. Campbell J, Gillbert WM, Nicolaides KH. Ultrasound screening for spina bifida: Cranial and cerebellar signs in a high risk population: Obstet Gynecol 1987; 70:247–250.

125. Jordan RB, Ganderer MW. Cervical teratomas: An analysis, literature review and proposed classification. J Paediatr Surg 1988; 23:583, 591.

126. Patel RB, Gibson JY, D'Cruz CA, Burklafter JL. Sonographic diagnosis of cervical teratoma in utero. Am J Radiol 1982; 139:1220–1222.

127. Trecet JC, Clarmunt V, Larraz J. Prenatal ultrasound diagnosis of fetal teratoma of the neck. J Clin Ultrasound 1984; 12:509–511.

128. Thurkow AL, Visser GMA, Oosterhuis JW. Ultrasound observations of a malignant cervical teratoma of the fetus in a case of polyhydramnios – Case history and review. Eur J Gynaecol Reprod Biol 1983; 13:375–384.

129. Langer JC, Tabb T, Thompson P, et al. Management of prenatally diagnosed tracheal obstruction: access to the airway in utero, prior to delivery. Fetal Diagn Ther 1992; 7:12–16.

130. Lewis BD, Doubilet PM, Meller VL, et al. Cutaneous and visceral haemangiomata in the Klippel–Tenamnary–Weber syndrome: Antenatal sonographic detection. Am J Radiol 1986; 147:598–600.

131. McGahan JP, Schneider JM. Fetal neck haemangioendothehoma with secondary hydrops fetalis: Sonographic diagnosis. J Clin Ultrasound 1986; 14:384–388.

132. Abuhamad AZ, Fisher DA, Warsof SL, et al. Antenatal diagnosis and treatment of fetal goitrous hypothyroidism: Case report and review of the literature. Ultrasound Obstet Gynecol 1995; 6:368–371.

133. Noia G, De Santis M, Tucci A, et al. Early prenatal diagnosis and therapy of fetal hypothyroid goitre. Fetal Diagn Ther 1992; 7:138–143.

134. Waner S, Scharf JI, Bolognese RJ. Antenatal diagnosis and treatment of a fetal goitre. J Reprod Med 1980; 24:39–42.

135. Pekonen F, Teratoma K, Makisen T. Prenatal diagnosis and treatment of fetal thyrotoxicosis. Am J Obstet Gynecol 1984; 150:893–894.

136. Gadwood KA, Reynes CJ. Prenatal sonography of metastatic neuroblastoma. J Clin Ultrasound 1983; 11:512–515.

137. Campbell WA, Storlazzi E, Vintzileos AM. Fetal malignant melanoma: Ultrasound presentation and review of the literature. Obstet Gynecol 1987; 70:434–439.

CHAPTER 16

Abnormalities of twin pregnancies

A. Pat M. Smith

Introduction

Twins and twin pregnancy have been a world-wide source of fascination throughout history. Rome was said to have been founded in 753 BC by the twins Romulus and Remus who were suckled by a she-wolf. Many rituals surround twins.[1] The North American Indian tribes considered twins to be supernatural and developed great rituals surrounding them. In Nigeria in one area, both mother and twins might be killed whilst in another, they would be revered. As recently as 1910, in Rhodesia, parents were put on trial for the ritual murder of their twins and in 1920, in Basutoland, parents were put on trial for a similar crime.[2] In mediaeval Europe, it was believed that the mother was unfaithful to her husband because twins implied two fathers.[3] In Wales, twins were associated with good luck and increased fertility whilst, in England and Scotland, it was thought that infertility followed a twin pregnancy and that the twins would be infertile.[3] Until the introduction of routine ultrasound into a pregnant population, twins were often not diagnosed until delivery. Grennert et al demonstrated that by routinely scanning a pregnant population the mean gestational age for diagnosis fell from 33 to 19 weeks.[4]

Embryology

Zygosity

Monozygotic twin rates appear to be fairly constant at around 3 to 5/1000 maternities throughout the world whereas the dizygotic rates vary from 1.3 to 49/1000 (Table 16.1). This can be partly explained by the embryogenesis.

Monozygotic twins result from the fertilization of one ovum. Thus, they are the same sex and are genetically identical. It has been postulated that they occur because of an oxygen lack as a result of delayed implantation.[5] It is generally believed that their occurrence is not associated with

Table 16.1
Twinning rates per 1000 maternities by zygosity in different countries

	Monozygotic	Dizygotic	Total
Nigeria	5.0	49.0	54.0
USA			
black	4.7	11.1	15.8
white	4.2	7.1	11.3
England and			
Wales	3.5	8.8	12.3
India	3.3	8.1	11.4
Japan	3.0	1.3	4.3

Adapted from MacGillivray I. Epidemiology of twin pregnancy. Semin Perinatol 1986; 10(1).

hereditary factors but there have been reports of an increased incidence of monozygotic twinning in some families.[6,7]

Dizygotic twins result from the fertilization of two ova by two different sperms and have different genetic 'make up'. They result from multiple ovulation owing to over-stimulation by the hormone follicle stimulating hormone (FSH). It has been found that women who have given birth to dizygotic twins tend to have higher levels of FSH and luteinizing hormone than those who have given birth to singletons.[8,9] It is interesting to note that the Yoruba tribe in Nigeria has a high incidence of dizygotic twins (Table 16.1) and this is thought to be due to their diet. They eat a variety of yam which contains substances with oestrogen-like properties and these may induce ovulation through the secretion of high levels of FSH.[10] Certain fertility drugs, such as clomiphene, cause a rise in the serum FSH and induce multiple ovulation and this results in an increased incidence of multiple births.[11] In 1994, the overall national twin pregnancy rate was 28% for in vitro fertilization.[12]

Chorionicity

80% of twins are **dizygotic** and 20% **monozygotic**. There are two types of placentation in twin pregnancies: **monochorionic** and **dichorionic**. In monochorionic placentas there may be vascular anastomosis between the twins but with dichorionic placentas there are two

Table 16.2
Different monozygotic twin types

Time of division	Type of twinning
< 4 days	Dichorionic diamniotic
4–8 days	Monochorionic diamniotic
8–13 days	Monochorionic monoamniotic
> 13 days	Conjoined twins

placentas and the circulation between the twins is usually separate. Dizygotic twins always have dichorionic placentas whereas monozygotic twins may have dichorionic placentas (80%) or monochorionic placentas (20%) depending when the division occurred[13] (Table 16.2).

Three different types of fetal membrane pattern can be seen with monozygotic placentas (Fig. 16.1) depending on the time of division of the embryonic cell mass. The different types of monozygotic twinning are as follows:

a. a zygote which divides 4 days after fertilization results in a **dichorionic diamniotic** gestation
b. a zygote which divides between 4 and 8 days after fertilization will result in a **monochorionic, diamniotic** gestation.
c. a zygote which divides after 8 days results in a **monochorionic monoamniotic** gestation.
d. division of the embryonic disc 13 days or more after conception results in **conjoined twins**.

It is now possible and important to assess chorionicity antenatally using ultrasound. In an early study transabdominal ultrasound was used to assess chorionicity.[14] Although the workers were good at predicting dichorionic diamniotic twin pregnancies, they were less good at predicting monochorionic monoamniotic gestations. Transvaginal assessment appears to be better than transabdominal in determining chorionicity in the first trimester.[15] If no membrane is visualized between the twins in

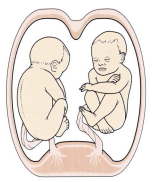

Monoamniotic
Monochorionic

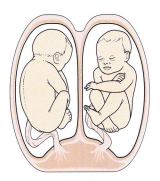

Monochorionic
Diamniotic

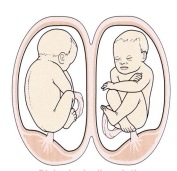

Dichorionic diamniotic
[fused placenta]

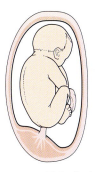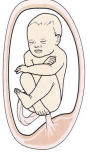

Dichorionic diamniotic
[separate placenta]

Fig. 16.1 Different types of fetal membrane pattern in twinning.

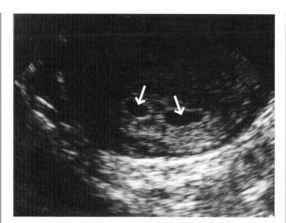

Fig. 16.2 Twin gestation sacs (arrows) at $4\frac{1}{2}$ weeks.

the first trimester on transabdominal assessment, then transvaginal evaluation of chorionicity is recommended.

Twin gestation sacs can be seen from approximately 4½ weeks (Fig. 16.2). The amnion cannot be seen clearly until 8 weeks (Fig. 16.3). Therefore, chorionicity should only be determined after 8 weeks' gestation by the transvaginal approach. The optimal time for determination of chorionicity is between 9 and 10 weeks.[15]

a. **Dichorionic diamniotic** twins (Fig. 16.4) are relatively easy to diagnose. The gestational sacs are separated by a thick membrane which is made up of two chorionic and two amniotic layers. Dichorionic diamniotic pregnancies will always have two placentas.

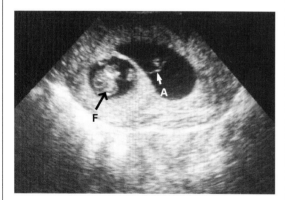

Fig. 16.3 Twin gestation sacs at 8 weeks. The amniotic membrane is clearly marked by arrow. A, amnion; F, fetus.

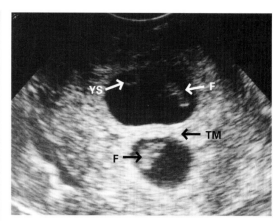

Fig. 16.4 Dichorionic diamniotic twin pregnancy. 'Twin peak' or lambda sign can be clearly seen. F, fetus; TM, thick membrane; YS, yolk sac.

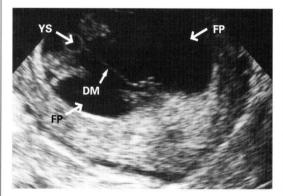

Fig. 16.5 Monochorionic diamniotic twin pregnancy. The diamniotic membrane (DM) between the twins is shown. FP, fetal pole; YS, yolk sac.

b. **Monochorionic diamniotic** twins have a thick chorion surrounding the two gestation sacs (Fig. 16.5). There is a very thin membrane between the twins which is composed of two amniotic layers and there is only one placenta (chorion).

c. **Monochorionic monoamniotic** twins are rare and the twins are surrounded by a single chorion and amnion. It is not possible to see a membrane between the twins (Fig. 16.6).

The transvaginal approach can be used to assess chorionicity up to 14 weeks' gestation. In later pregnancy, determination of chorionicity using ultrasound has been described by several workers.[16–20] If there are two separate placentas, then the pregnancy is dichorionic. If only one placenta is visualized

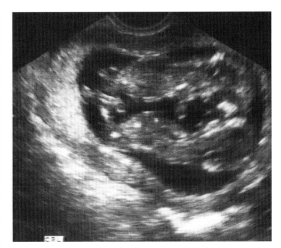

Fig. 16.6 Monochorionic monoamniotic twins. Membrane between twins not visualized.

monochorionic is around 10 to 14 weeks' gestation.[24] As gestation progresses, it becomes increasingly difficult to visualize the lambda sign and it disappears by 20 weeks[25] in 7% of dichorionic twin pregnancies with fused placentas. Therefore, if the lambda sign is not present after 20 weeks, it cannot be diagnostic of monochorionicity and other ultrasound features of chorionicity should be used. Chorionicity should be determined antenatally because if twins are different sizes, then the reason for this difference should be established. If the twins are dichorionic, then the reason for the size difference is growth retardation of the smaller twin but if they are monochorionic, then the most likely explanation is twin–twin transfusion syndrome.

Clinical significance

Only 1% of monozygotic twin pregnancies are monoamniotic,[13] i.e. sharing the one amniotic and chorionic cavity. There has been an increased incidence of monochorionic twins resulting from assisted reproductive techniques. There was an eight-fold increase in monochorionicity above the background rate in these women and this is thought to be due to a delay in early development processes or abnormal hatching.[26]

It is important to assess chorionicity antenatally because monochorionic twin pregnancies are associated with an increased risk of prematurity, fetal malformations, twin–twin transfusion and consequent increased perinatal morbidity and mortality. The highest death rates have been reported in monozygotic pairs with monochorionic placentas, while unlike-sex dizygotic pairs with separate placentas have the lowest mortality.[27] In the north-east of Scotland the perinatal death rate in monozygotic twins was 50/1000 compared to 31.9/1000 for dizygotic twins.[28] Vascular connections between the two fetal circulations are present in virtually all monochorionic placentas.[16] This is important for the management of particular problems such as fetal

and the twins are of a different sex, then the placenta is dichorionic. Fetal sex, however, cannot always be accurately determined in the second trimester.[21] If only one placenta is visualized and the twins are the same sex, then careful examination of the membrane should be undertaken. If two layers (two amnions) are demonstrated, then the diagnosis of monochorionic diamniotic placentation is made. If four layers (two amnions and two chorions) are seen, then the diagnosis of dichorionic diamniotic placentation is made.[17]

Obviously, the resolution of the ultrasound machine has to be good to count the layers of membranes between the twins. The separating membrane in dichorionic twins is much thicker than in monochorionic twins. It is easier to measure membrane thickness and some workers have used this to establish chorionicity.[18,20,22] It has been found that dichorionic membranes have a mean thickness of 2.4 mm compared with monochorionic membranes which have a mean thickness of 1.4 mm and that a membrane thickness of < 2 mm can predict a monochorionic placenta with a sensitivity and specificity of 90%.[20] Another method of determining chorionicity is known as the 'twin peak' or lambda sign. It is a sign of dichorionicity[23] (Fig. 16.4). The optimal gestational age to identify this sign and classify twins into dichorionic or abnormality, intra-uterine death of one twin or discordant growth. If, for example, one of the twins has an abnormality such as spina bifida, then selective fetocide of the affected fetus may be undertaken. However, this should only be attempted if the placenta is dichorionic because the likelihood of vascular anastomoses is negligible. In monochorionic twin pregnancies selective fetocide is not recommended as there is a risk that the normal fetus may succumb. Recently, however, a case of anastomoses between dichorionic monozygotic twins has been described. Therefore caution should be exercised when considering selective fetocide.[29]

If fetal death occurs in one twin and the pregnancy is monochorionic, then there is a risk that embolization of thromboplastins could occur from the dead twin to the survivor. Some workers believe that the surviving twin should be delivered as soon as there is a reasonable chance of viability because it may develop a coagulopathy.[16]

Diagnosis of twin pregnancy

Normal

The diagnosis of twin pregnancy is straightforward. It is made when two fetal poles are visualized simultaneously. Overdiagnosis of twins can occur as a result of artefacts such as a bicornuate uterus, retromembranous haematoma or an empty second sac. The misdiagnosis of twins should be less frequent because of improved resolution of ultrasound equipment and the introduction of transvaginal ultrasound.

Abnormal

VANISHING TWIN

Incidence

Some pregnancies begin as twin pregnancies and end up as singletons. It is thought that 21% of twin pregnancies have the 'vanishing twin' phenomenon.[30] It is uncertain as to what proportion of these pregnancies are chromosomally or structurally abnormal.

Diagnosis

The patient often gives a history of vaginal bleeding and when scanned, an empty second sac may be visualized next to a healthy viable pregnancy (Fig. 16.7). The phenomenon may have been overdiagnosed in the past because of poor resolution of ultrasound equipment.

Many of the diagnoses of the so-called 'vanishing twins' may have been the result of retromembranous haematoma (Fig. 16.8), chorioamniotic separation and occasionally the yolk sac in the first trimester. The diagnosis of 'vanishing twin' can only be made with *absolute certainty* when a previous scan showed a live fetus with pulsations. The

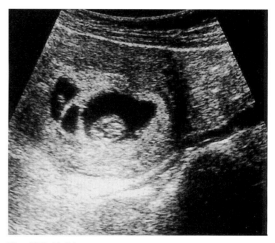

Fig. 16.7 Viable pregnancy next to two empty sacs.

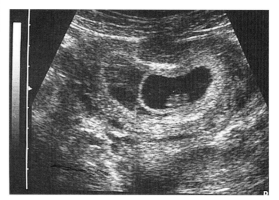

Fig. 16.8 Retromembranous haematoma adjacent to viable pregnancy.

overdiagnosis of this condition should be less since the introduction of transvaginal ultrasound and improved resolution of equipment.

Management

Conservative management is recommended as the surviving twin will continue to develop normally.

Outcome

Often the empty second sac disappears by the time that the patient is scanned again and the outlook for the surviving twin is good.[30]

FETAL DEATH OF ONE TWIN

Fetus papyraceous occurs when one fetus of a twin pregnancy dies after the 8th week of pregnancy and before the end of the second trimester. It may be noticed at delivery when the remains of the fetus (fetus papyraceous) is found in the placenta of the surviving twin (Fig. 16.9). Death of one twin in the first trimester is not uncommon and, as discussed previously, has little effect on the mother or surviving twin. However, when the death of a twin occurs in the second or third trimester, it is associated with an increased risk to the surviving twin and of maternal disseminated intravascular coagulation.[31,32]

Incidence

It is thought that the incidence is 1 in 12 000 live births[33] or 1 in 200 twin pregnancies[34]

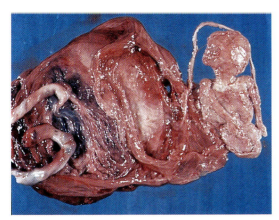

Fig. 16.9 Fetus papyraceous. (Courtesy of Dr E. Gray.)

although reports vary from 0.5 to 6.8%.[32,35] Single fetal death in a twin pregnancy has been found to be more common in monochorionic twin pregnancies.[36] In monochorionic twins death may be due to twin–twin transfusion syndrome or, in monoamniotic twins, to cord entanglement. However, some of these fetuses are dichorionic and it is thought that a velamentous insertion of the cord may increase the risk of fetal death.[37] Death of one twin in the second or third trimester is a rare complication. The incidence of antepartum death amongst monochorionic twins was 3.7%.[38]

Diagnosis

The diagnosis may be made by ultrasound when a twin pregnancy is confirmed in the first trimester and a later scan confirms fetal death of one of the fetuses.

Management

If death occurs in one twin and conservative management is adopted, then regular ultrasonic follow-up is recommended for the surviving twin.[39] The purpose of this is to recognize any changes in the surviving twin as a result of thromboplastins from the dead twin. Brain lesions which can be recognized on ultrasonic examination include ventriculomegaly, porencephalic cyst formation, microcephaly and cerebral atrophy. It is difficult to be exactly sure if and when brain damage occurs in the surviving monozygotic twin, and so the timing and mode of delivery of the surviving twin are still debatable. Delivery by caesarean section has not demonstrated an improved perinatal mortality or morbidity[40,41] and so vaginal delivery should be anticipated. The decision on timing of delivery will be based on the gestational age of the twins. A recent study has advocated expectant management in twin pregnancies complicated by single fetal death.[36]

Outcome

If one fetus dies in early pregnancy in monochorionic twins, emboli may be transferred from the dead to the surviving twin. This may cause disruption or ischaemia to the developing organs of the surviving twin. A variety of anomalies has been reported as being secondary to the intra-uterine death of a co-twin with a monochorionic placenta. The type of anomaly seen in the surviving twin depends on the gestation at which the co-twin dies.[38] Death of the co-twin in early pregnancy results in atresia and tissue loss; death in later pregnancy results in tissue infarction. The most common complication appears to affect the central nervous system followed by the gastrointestinal system, kidneys and lungs.[42,43] It has been shown that there was a striking difference in outcome in monochorionic compared to dichorionic twins in terms of morbidity and survival.[44] The majority of survivors in dichorionic twin pregnancies were normal, whereas 26% of the surviving fetuses in monochorionic twin pregnancies had neurological damage. Many authors have described a variety of abnormalities following the death of a co-twin but this appears to be confined to monochorionic twin pregnancies.[44]

Brain damage to the surviving twin is a possibility which parents should be aware of and they should be adequately counselled.

Growth in twin pregnancies

Normal

The detection of growth retardation in twins antenatally is inherently more difficult than in singletons. Even in singletons, detection of intra-uterine growth by conventional clinical methods (e.g. abdominal palpation, girth measurements, fundal height) has been less than satisfactory.[45,46] Owing to the increased liquor and numerous fetal parts in twin pregnancies, the diagnosis of the growth-retarded twin is made even more difficult. Ultrasound has proved useful in the assessment of fetal growth in twin pregnancies[47–49] and singleton growth charts may be used up to 28 weeks' gestation.[50]

After that time controversy exists as to what is the normal growth pattern for twins. From our own work in Aberdeen,[51] based on serial measurements on 162 sets of twins, it was found in the third trimester that there was slowing of growth in both the biparietal diameter and abdominal circumference measurements compared to singletons. It was also found that abdominal circumference was the most useful parameter for assessing fetal growth in twins as it was consistently obtainable. It is the incremental growth in abdominal circumference that is important in the detection of growth problems.[52]

Abnormal

Discordant growth is defined as the birthweight difference between co-twins expressed as a proportion (or percentage) of the larger twin's birthweight. This is important because a birthweight difference of 25% or greater between the twins has been shown to be associated with an increased perinatal morbidity and mortality in the smaller twin.[53,54] Several workers have used various ultrasonic parameters to detect discordant growth between the twins and it has been found that an abdominal circumference difference (Fig. 16.10) between the twins of 20 mm or more is a useful 'cut-off' level for detecting discordancy[55] and this is our own experience. From a total group of 162 sets of twins, 26 showed discordant growth at delivery. The range of

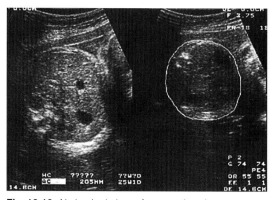

Fig. 16.10 Abdominal circumferences in twins, demonstrating discordant growth.

discordant growth was 20 to 48%. Out of this group, 2 had unknown zygosity, 11 were monozygotic (45.8%) and 13 were dizygotic (54.1%). The neonatal outcome for the 26 sets of discordant twins was studied (Fig. 16.11); comparing the smaller with the larger of each set, 15 were induced because of discordancy, 5 being preterm before 37 weeks. A further 7 delivered preterm after the spontaneous onset of labour. 23 of the smaller twins were light for dates. Of the 26 smaller twins, 2 were intra-uterine deaths and the remaining 24 were admitted to the neonatal unit, 1 having a lethal abnormality (anencephaly) and dying after 1 hour. Of the 26 larger twins, 14 were admitted to the neonatal unit. Not surprisingly, the smaller had a higher incidence of hypothermia, hypoglycaemia and acidosis.[51]

Once the diagnosis of discordant growth has been made, then intensive monitoring of the smaller twin using Doppler ultrasound should be undertaken.

Fetal abnormalities in twin pregnancies

Incidence

With the increased use of routine ultrasound in pregnancy, not only is it possible to diagnose twins at an earlier stage but it is useful in the prenatal diagnosis of fetal anomalies which are commoner in multiple pregnancy. Lethal congenital anomalies contribute to the perinatal mortality of twins. From the Scottish Stillbirth and Neonatal Death Report (1994) congenital anomalies contributed 1.4/1000 to the perinatal death rate in singletons compared to 3.7/1000 in multiples.[56] Between 1989 and 1994 the perinatal mortality rate attributable to congenital anomalies was greater in multiples than singletons (Fig. 16.12). In twin gestations, Wenstrom & Gall[57] found a 2% incidence of major malformation and 4% incidence of minor malformation. From a study at our own hospital from 1984–91, there were 306 twin pregnancies and of these 1.3% had major abnormalities and 2.5% had minor abnormalities (Table 16.3). The overall incidence of anomalies is higher in twin pregnancies, tends to be confined to those of like sex,[58] and is higher in monozygotic twins.[59–62] Concordance rates differ for various anomalies and, even in monozygotic

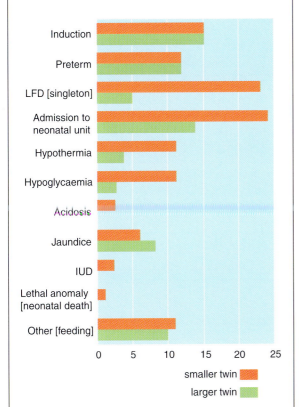

Fig. 16.11 Outcome for discordant twins. IUD, intra-uterine death; LFD, light for dates.

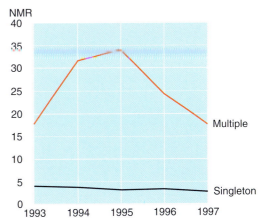

Fig. 16.12 Perinatal mortality rate (PNMR) attributable to congenital anomalies in singletons and multiples. (Statistics from Scottish Stillbirth and Neonatal Death Report 1994.[56])

Table 16.3
Abnormalities in twin pregnancies (Grampian twin study 1984–91)

Major abnormalities – 8/612
- Cardiovascular system
  — Ivemark syndrome (1)
  — Transposition of the great vessels (1)
  — Acardiac monster (2)
  — Hypoplastic left heart (2)
- Central nervous system
  — Anencephaly (1)
  — Cystic hygroma (1)

Minor abnormalities – 15/612
- Hydrocele (4)
- Clicking hip (3)
- Ovarian cyst (1)
- Single umbilical artery (2)
- Undescended testes (3)
- Hypospadias (1)
- Single palmar crease (1)

twins, it is possible for one twin to have an abnormality and the other twin to be perfectly normal.[63]

Congenital heart abnormalities

Congenital heart defects are commoner in monozygotic twin pregnancies.[64] From a study which combined data from two large series of twins, it was found that the incidence of cardiac defects was 18.9/1000 in monozygotic twins, 7.4/1000 in dizygotic twins and 7.4/1000 in like-sex twins of unknown zygosity. The incidence among singletons was 6/1000 and this excluded persistent patent ductus arteriosus.[64]

There appears to be a susceptibility to disturbance of the heart formation by the twinning process. The mechanism whereby this occurs is thought to be a disturbance of laterality. In early development the heart tube fails to make a precise bend to the right. In order for this step to take place, the left–right axis of the embryo must be clearly defined. The left side of the embryo acts as a reference point from which cells to the right derive their orientation. If, however, twinning occurs after this gradient has formed, then the right half of the pair is separated from the point of reference and the laterality gradient is disturbed.[64] A detailed cardiac scan should be undertaken in all twin pregnancies.

Gastrointestinal abnormalities

It has been found that oesophageal atresia with or without tracheo-oesophageal fistula is commoner in twin pregnancies.[65] Another study[66] found a five-fold increase in this abnormality in twins and 95% were discordant for this anomaly.

Central nervous system abnormalities

Some studies have reported an increased incidence of neural tube defects in twins[67] whereas others have not found this to be so.[68] The incidence of anencephaly has been reported to be higher in twins than singletons whereas the incidence of spina bifida is lower.[63] Neural tube defects usually only affect one twin and the other is perfectly normal. A study from pooled literature[68] showed that the concordance rate for anencephalus was 4.1% and for spina bifida 5.1%. It has been shown that there is a relationship between upper neural tube defects and twinning,[69] found in twins of the same sex or monozygotic twins. The reason for this is unknown but, as the upper neural tube forms earlier than the lower, then a factor acting on early embryonic life in the form of a development delay might be the explanation.

Several studies have shown an increased incidence of hydrocephalus in twin pregnancies.[61,70] The problem with diagnosis is that many cases are not recognized until after delivery. Many of these cases will be as a result of intraventricular haemorrhage or meningitis as a consequence of prematurity which is common in twins.

Management

A woman faced with the prospect of one abnormal twin and a normal fetus has a particularly difficult choice to make. She may continue with the pregnancy as it is delivering both a normal and an affected fetus. Termination of the pregnancy is another option but this will result in the loss of the normal as well as the affected fetus. Lastly, it is possible to undertake 'selective termination' of the abnormal twin. Chorionicity of the pregnancy should be ascertained before undergoing this procedure, otherwise it may lead to the loss of both the normal and affected fetus. The woman who has to make this unenviable decision should be fully counselled about all the possible outcomes. She should understand that there is a risk that the normal twin may well be lost as a result of the technique. Parents having to make this choice will require much support before and after the procedure. The prevalence of anencephaly is much higher in monochorionic than dichorionic twin pregnancies.[71] Anencephaly is associated with a high rate of intra-uterine death which in monochorionic twins is accompanied by the death of the normal co-twin.[71] There is a high risk of preterm delivery because of polyhydramnios in twin pregnancies complicated by anencephaly. If the pregnancy is dichorionic, then selective fetocide is a management option but this is also associated with mortality of the normal twin.[71]

Abnormalities unique to monochorionic twinning

Twin–twin transfusion syndrome

Incidence

The twin–twin transfusion syndrome occurs in approximately 15% of monozygotic twin pregnancies.[72,73] In a review of 306 twin pregnancies delivered in Grampian from 1989–91, the incidence of twin–twin transfusion syndrome was 1.6% (6/306) of all twin pregnancies. There is an increased perinatal mortality associated with the twin–twin transfusion syndrome and this anomaly is unique to monochorionic twin pregnancies. It is a result of fetofetal transfusion and although cross-circulation may be demonstrated in dichorionic placentas, it is very rare.[74] The vascular anastomoses between the twins may be superficial, deep or a combination of both and twin–twin transfusion syndrome results when these anastomoses become

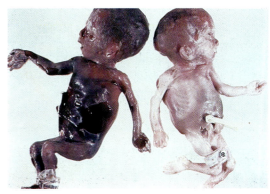

Fig. 16.13 Twin–twin transfusion syndrome, demonstrating the anaemic donor and the plethoric recipient. (Courtesy of Dr E. Gray.)

'unbalanced', and so not all monochorionic twin pregnancies develop twin–twin transfusion syndrome.[74,75] The twin–twin transfusion syndrome results in shunting of blood from the donor twin to the recipient twin (Fig. 16.13, Table 16.4). The donor becomes anaemic and hypovolaemic and the recipient hypervolaemic. Thus the recipient may develop 'high output' cardiac failure and an increased urine output resulting in polyhydramnios and likely preterm labour. The donor twin becomes hypovolaemic and hypotensive and the reduced renal blood flow may result in oligohydramnios. Since all the nutrients are shunted from it, the donor twin resembles a growth-retarded fetus by comparison. The recipient twin has a larger heart, liver, pancreas and adrenal cortex compared to the donor twin.[75]

Diagnosis

The diagnosis may be made antenatally when there is a significant difference in abdominal circumference measurements between the twins (Fig. 16.10). It has been

Table 16.4
Features of twin–twin transfusion syndrome

Donor twin	Recipient twin
Anaemia	Hypervolaemia
Hypovolaemia	Cardiac failure
Oligohydramnios	Polyhydramnios
Growth retardation	Enlargement of heart, liver and pancreas; occasionally hydrops

suggested that a twin abdominal circumference difference of more than 20 mm may alert the clinician to the possibility of the syndrome.[55] The twin–twin transfusion may present acutely in the second trimester with polyhydramnios (Fig. 16.14). This is associated with a high perinatal mortality rate, either because of spontaneous abortion or very preterm delivery of growth-retarded babies or babies with hydrops.[75] Ultrasound will detect polyhydramnios or oligohydramnios in the different sacs. An important sign associated with these findings is that of the 'stuck twin', which is a growth-retarded fetus surrounded by oligohydramnios. This sign was found in 6 out of 10 cases of twin–twin transfusion syndrome.[76] In this same series, the commonest finding in twin–twin transfusion syndrome was discrepancy in the amniotic fluid volume but fetal hydrops was an infrequent finding. Therefore, if there is discordant fetal size or a discrepant amniotic fluid volume, the differential diagnosis is twin–twin transfusion or growth retardation of one twin. If the twins are dichorionic, then growth retardation of one twin is the likely diagnosis.[76] Again, this emphasizes the importance of determining chorionicity before problems occur. Doppler ultrasound has been used with varying degrees of accuracy in the diagnosis,[77,78] but it appears difficult to differentiate between the donor and recipient twin using this method. Some workers have found that an increased nuchal translucency at 10 to 14 weeks is associated with four-fold increased risk of developing the twin–twin transfusion syndrome.[79]

Management

Twin–twin transfusion syndrome has a very high perinatal mortality and because of this various treatments have been attempted ranging from amniocentesis to selective fetocide.

Serial amniocenteses. This treatment has been recommended by several workers in cases of acute polyhydramnios as a result of the twin–twin transfusion syndrome. It has been reported to be effective in increasing survival rates.[80–84] In many cases, the twins were subjected to repeated amniocenteses as the polyhydramnios reaccumulated. In some cases, serial amniocenteses has resulted in normal fluid levels in both sacs.[82] There are risks associated with serial amniocenteses and these are: amnionitis; rupture of membranes; abruptio placentae; onset of labour; amniotic fluid embolism and inadvertent puncture of the fetus or the cord. The last complication should not occur if the procedure is undertaken using ultrasonic guidance.

Selective fetocide. Selective fetocide stops the shunting of blood from one twin to the other but requires the death of a twin. This raises difficult moral and ethical issues for the mother. The procedure has been accomplished successfully by injecting normal saline to disrupt the fetal heart of the smaller donor twin.[85] This was carried out at 25 weeks with a successful outcome. The technique raises concern about embolization of substances from the deceased twin to the living one. It is also recognized that prolonged retention of a dead fetus can cause depletion of coagulation factors in the mother.[85] Generally, the technique is recognized as potentially dangerous and should not be recommended.[86] More

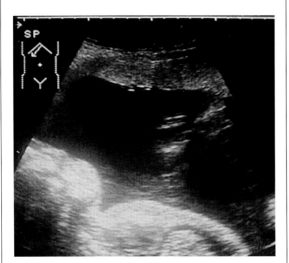

Fig. 16.14 Polyhydramnios with hydrops in the recipient twin.

recently, different techniques have been developed to achieve fetocide in one of the twins which blocks the placental communication with the surviving twin,[87] avoiding the passage of toxic material from one twin to the other. The technique involved blocking both the umbilical vein and heart and/or ascending aorta and thus occluding both sides of the vascular system of the terminated fetus. This was undertaken in four sets of twins with severe forms of the twin–twin transfusion syndrome and there were three live births as a result.

Laser surgery. Laser coagulation has been used to obliterate the communicating placental vessels[88,89] between the twins. This was undertaken in 45 women carrying twins at 15 to 28 weeks' gestation. In each case, there was severe hydramnios in one fetus caused by the twin–twin transfusion syndrome. 48 fetuses (53%) survived to delivery and 32 of the 45 pregnancies (71%) had at least one survivor. Although this is a very invasive procedure, the preliminary results appear encouraging.

Outcome

When acute twin–twin transfusion syndrome occurs in the second trimester, the perinatal mortality can be as high as 95% in the absence of treatment.[84,90] Severe disparity in the amniotic fluid between the twins is associated with a poor outcome for both twins with a survival rate of less than 20%.[90] Premature labour develops in almost all cases as a result of secondary uterine distension because of polyhydramnios. Death of one of the twins, usually the donor, causes severe haemodynamic changes in the surviving twin, resulting in death or brain damage.[91] Serial therapeutic amniocenteses in cases of polyhydramnios have improved the survival rate to 69% compared with 16% in those not treated with amniocenteses.[90] The survival rate depends on the gestation at which the polyhydramnios occurs,[84,90] being poorest before 20 weeks. The technique of selective fetocide carries a considerable risk of losing both twins. Endoscopic laser surgery appears, from the preliminary reports, to be the most promising in terms of treatment for this condition. However, not every centre has the endoscopic laser facilities. Therapeutic amniocentesis offers an alternative option for severe cases in centres where laser facilities are not available.

Conjoined twins

Incidence

This is a very rare condition occurring in 1 in 50 000 to 1 in 100 000 deliveries[92] (Fig. 16.15). The frequency of this condition is independent of maternal age and parity and occurs sporadically. Conjoined twins are frequently female[93] which is interesting as the majority of monozygotic twins are male. Polyhydramnios is commonly present.

Embryology

Conjoined twins only occur in monozygotic twin pregnancies. If division of the embryonic disk occurs 13 days after

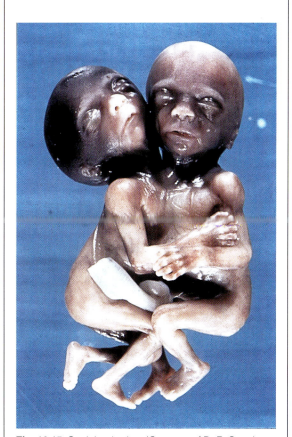

Fig. 16.15 Conjoined twins. (Courtesy of Dr E. Gray.)

Table 16.5
Different types of conjoined twins

Type of union	Features	Prognosis
Craniopagus	Classified according to area joined. Parietal craniopagus most common	Depends on degree of connection between the brains
Thoracopagus	Most common type; congenital heart defects found in 75% of cases	Depends on degree of fusion
Omphalopagus–xiphopagus	Liver conjoined in 81%; associated with malformations of the abdominal wall (usually omphalocoele) and congenital heart defect	Better than thoracopagus as less likely to have cardiac defect
Pyopagus	Accounts for 20% of conjoined twins; joined at buttocks and lower spine; may share rectum bladder and urethra	Good as no major organ systems shared
Ischiopagus	5% of all conjoined twins joined at sacrum and coccyx; common large pelvic ring; may have three or four legs; single colon, bladder and urethra not uncommon as are vaginal and rectovaginal anomalies	Unknown

fertilization and is incomplete, conjoined twins will result. There is only one chorion and one amnion in conjoined twins. There are five main types of conjoined twins (Table 16.5, Fig. 16.16).

Diagnosis

The first report of the diagnosis of conjoined twins using ultrasound was made in 1976[94] and before this time, the diagnosis was suspected only by failure to progress during labour. Although magnetic resonance imaging and computer tomography have also been used in prenatal diagnosis, ultrasound is still considered to be the most accurate diagnostic technique[95,96] (Fig. 16.17). The possible diagnosis of conjoined twins should be considered if an interamniotic membrane cannot be visualized as they are all monoamniotic. Therefore, if a membrane is seen or there are two placentas, the diagnosis is excluded. Other ultrasound signs include difficulties in completely separating the twins, fetal spines in unusual extension or proximity, more than three vessels in the cord and a single cardiac motion. There is a high frequency of associated anomalies and echocardiography is indicated as congenital heart disease is a major prognostic factor for survival.[97] Neural tube defects, orofacial clefts, imperforate anus and diaphragmatic hernia are commonly found in conjoined twins. Serial scans are recommended to monitor fetal growth, detect hydrops and diagnose fetal demise.[97] It is important to avoid misdiagnosis and the ultrasound examination should be repeated at least once, looking carefully for a membrane between the twins. This can sometimes be difficult to see and in the first trimester, transvaginal ultrasound should be undertaken to confirm the diagnosis. Diagnosis of conjoined twins in the third trimester can be missed, especially if the joining bridge between the fetuses is small. A careful search should be made for duplication of organs and limbs.[98]

Management

If the diagnosis is made before viability, then the parents should be offered termination of pregnancy. If the diagnosis is made after 24 weeks' gestation, then careful ultrasonic assessment of the twins should be made to determine where they are conjoined so that appropriate counselling with regard to prognosis can be given to the parents. The recommended mode of delivery should be caesarean section to prevent dystocia. Vaginal delivery should be reserved for stillbirths and those conjoined twins who will not survive.[99] Most obstetricians may never see a case of conjoined twins in their lifetime but it is important to be aware of the condition and if they are delivered after viability, then it should be at a centre

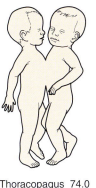
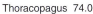

Thoracopagus 74.0

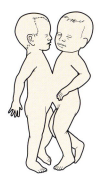

Omphalopagus and xiphopagus 0.5

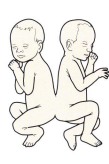

Pygopagus 18.0

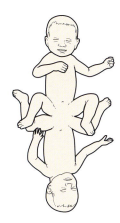

Ischiopagus 6.0

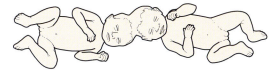

Craniopagus 1.0

Fig. 16.16 Types of conjoined twins.

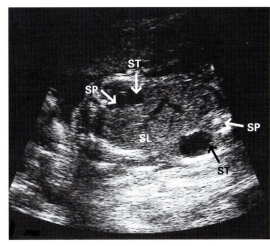

Fig. 16.17 Ultrasound image of conjoined twins. SL, shared liver; SP, spine; ST, stomach. (Courtesy of Dr S. Russell.)

with appropriate paediatric and surgical facilities.

Outcome

The majority deliver preterm, 40% are stillborn and 35% die within 24 hours.[99] Survival depends on where the twins are joined and the presence of other abnormalities. It is also important to identify the degree of conjoining as this will help rational decision-making and minimize the shock for the parents. Early diagnosis and assessment allow the determination of

postnatal viability.[99] Postnatal viability depends on the organs shared and whether surgical correction is possible. Table 16.5 shows the different types of conjoined twins. In omphalopagus, the twins have a reasonable chance of survival but the prognosis is worse if an omphalocoele is present.[100] In thoracopagus, the degree of fusion of the heart determines the outcome. If there is a common heart between the twins, then the outlook is very poor[101] and even separation in these cases with the loss of one twin did not improve the prognosis. Xiphopagus has a better prognosis than thoracopagus because the former has a lower incidence of cardiac lesions. The outcome for craniopagus is unpredictable and depends on the degree of fusion of the intracranial structures and the extent of the venous connections at the junction sites.[97] A cerebral connection is present in 43% of cases but unfortunately cannot be reliably diagnosed pre-operatively. The peri-operative mortality rate for craniopagus is 36%. The worst outcome was for those who had unions between the temporoparietal and occipital junctions compared with the frontal and parietal regions. However, if the separation is successful, the outlook is good.[102] Pyopagus has a good outlook because the twins do not share organs critical for life.[98] However, they may need further surgery to correct problems of a shared genitourinary and intestinal systems.

All conjoined twins will require surgery if they survive the neonatal period. Often, it is difficult to be absolutely certain of the prognosis and quality of life for the survivors and parents will require much support during this period.[99]

Twin reversed arterial perfusion (TRAP) syndrome

The condition is also known as acardius, acardiac monster, acephalus, pseudocardiac anomaly, acephalus acardia and holocardius.

Incidence

The incidence of this condition is 1 in 35 000 deliveries and 1 in 100 monozygotic twins (Fig. 16.18). TRAP is a lethal abnormality for both twins in early pregnancy and it is only found in twin pregnancies with fused placentas. 75% occur in monozygotic triplet pregnancies and the rest in monozygotic twins.[103] The condition is characterized by vascular anastomoses between twins in combination with partial, or complete, lack of development of the heart of one of them.[104–107]

Embryology

This syndrome is a unique complication of monozygotic twinning. The normal twin is known as the 'pump' twin. This twin provides circulation for both itself and the

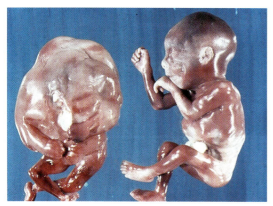

Fig. 16.18 Twin reversed arterial perfusion (TRAP) syndrome, demonstrating the 'pump' or normal twin and the acardiac twin. (Courtesy of Dr E. Gray).

acardiac twin. The acardiac twin is the perfused twin. The vascular communications between the twins are highly complicated but there must be at least arterial-to-arterial and venous-to-venous communications present to complete the circuit. The aetiology of the condition is unknown but the 'vascular reversal perfusion theory' is the most widely accepted hypothesis. During early embryogenesis, large vascular anastomoses develop leading to competition between the two circulations. When arterial pressure in one twin exceeds that of the other, reversed circulation in one twin develops with secondary disruption and reduction of the morphogenesis, resulting in the acardiac anomaly.[108] The perfused twin has no direct vascular connection with the placenta and the blood enters directly through a single umbilical artery and exits through the umbilical vein. This is known as the twin reversed arterial perfusion sequence. The lower part of the body receives better oxygenated venous blood through the hypogastric artery and consequently the most severe abnormalities are in the upper part of the body. There are four different types of acardiac twins:

- **acardiac acephalus** – this is the commonest type and is characterized by an absent cranium; the upper limbs may be absent and often the intrathoracic and abdominal organs are rudimentary
- **acardiac anceps** – in this case, there may be a partially developed head and brain; the body and limbs may be present
- **acardius amorphous** – here the twin is an amorphous mass or 'blob'-like
- **acardius acormus** – in this case, the head is present and the umbilical cord is directly attached to the head or the head is directly attached to the placenta.

Diagnosis

The diagnosis can be made antenatally using ultrasound (Fig. 16.19). The following may be features: absence of cardiac activity; amorphous shape of the cephalic pole; poor definition of trunk and extremities; diffuse subcutaneous oedema; abnormal cystic areas

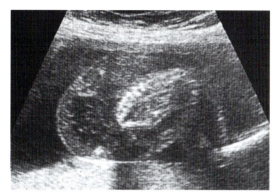

Fig. 16.19 Acardiac twin (acardiac acephalus).

in the upper part of the body. Often the diagnosis can be difficult and the acardiac fetus may be mistaken for a 'missed abortion' in a twin pregnancy. Occasionally, a heart beat may be seen which may be a rudimentary heart.[109] There is often associated polyhydramnios.

Management

The incidence of fetal malformation in the 'pump' twin is 10%[110] and a detailed anomaly scan should be undertaken. Serial ultrasonic assessment of the pregnancy is recommended. This should be undertaken to assess the growth and cardiovascular status of the pump twin. Signs of cardiac failure such as cardiac enlargement, ascites, hydrothorax, pericardial effusion, hepatomegaly and polyhydramnios should be looked for at each ultrasound examination. Congestive cardiac failure in the normal 'pump' twin is a poor prognostic sign. Maternal digoxin has been shown to be effective in the treatment of fetal cardiac failure in these cases.[111] Therapeutic amniocentesis has been recommended if polyhydramnios[112] develops as has administration of maternal indomethacin[113] which will reduce the amniotic fluid volume. Vascular occlusion of the vessels between the twins has been reported.[114] In this case, the insertion of a helical metal coil was used to induce thrombosis in the umbilical artery of the acardiac twin. The co-twin survived and was delivered at 39 weeks. A conservative approach in selected cases has been recommended. The most important

prognostic factor is the twin weight ratio. If the ratio is above 70%, then the incidence of preterm delivery, polyhydramnios and congestive cardiac failure in the pump twin is significantly higher than in cases with a ratio below 70%.[115] It is recommended that M-mode echocardiography and Doppler should be undertaken to assess cardiac function in the pump twin.

Outcome

The mortality of the acardiac twin is 100% and that of the pump twin is 50%. The main causes of death are preterm delivery as a consequence of polyhydramnios and congestive cardiac failure in the pump twin. The condition is sporadic and familial tendencies have not been reported.[107]

Monoamniotic non-conjoined twins

It is important to identify these twins antenatally because monochorionic monoamniotic twin pregnancies have the highest mortality of otherwise uncomplicated twin pregnancies.[116] This is due to the increased incidence of congenital anomalies, cord entanglement, prematurity and twin–twin transfusion syndrome.

Incidence

This happens in less than 2% of monozygotic twin pregnancies.[116]

Embryology

The division of the blastocyst occurs more than 8 days after fertilization. The twins have a single placenta, and a common chorionic and amniotic sac (Fig. 16.1).

Diagnosis

The diagnosis can be made where it is not possible to visualize a membrane between the twins. Since the advent of transvaginal ultrasound, it is possible to visualize the dividing membrane in the first trimester[15] when the diagnosis should be made.

Management

The pregnancy should be monitored closely using ultrasound. The purpose of this is to identify the development of twin–twin transfusion syndrome. There is controversy as to the mode of delivery with some believing that the twins should be delivered by caesarean section to avoid cord entanglement and delivery trauma.[117]

Outcome

Monochorionic monoamniotic twins have a fetal death rate of 10 to 40%[118,119] and in many cases fetal demise will have occurred by 24 weeks' gestation.[16] This is mainly attributable to cord entanglement and delivery-related trauma.

Conclusion

There has been an increase in the number of twin pregnancies with the advent of assisted reproductive techniques. The diagnosis of twin pregnancy is made by ultrasound. The importance of determining chorionicity antenatally has been emphasized and this is probably easiest to determine in the first trimester using transvaginal ultrasound. The majority of twins are dizygotic but it is monozygotic and, in particular, monochorionic twins which have the highest perinatal morbidity and mortality. The main cause is preterm labour although growth retardation and congenital anomalies may contribute. Abnormalities unique to the twinning process such as fetal acardia and conjoined twins have a poor outlook. It is important that parents are fully informed about the possible outcomes. Parents have a particularly difficult decision to make when an abnormality is detected in one of the twins and selectively terminating one may result in the loss of both twins. As twins are recognized as belonging to a 'high-risk' group, we have made the following recommendations for scanning twins:

- All twins should have a detailed anomaly scan at 20 weeks to exclude fetal anomaly and, if not already established, determine chorionicity.
- Monochorionic twins should have fortnightly growth scans from 24 weeks to look for signs of twin–twin transfusion
- Dichorionic twins should have 3-weekly growth scans from 28 weeks to detect growth discordancy.

It has still to be shown that routine scanning will decrease the perinatal morbidity or mortality of twins but complications such as twin–twin transfusion syndrome or growth retardation will be detected and therefore increased surveillance and appropriate intervention may be undertaken.

References

1. Corney G. Mythology and customs associated with twins. In: MacGillivray I, Nylander PPS, Corney G, eds. Human multiple reproduction. London: WB Saunders; 1975:4–15.
2. Harris JR. A recent twin murder in South Africa. Folklore 1922; 33:214–223.
3. Giles P. Abandonment and exposure. In: Hastings J, ed. Encyclopaedia of religion and ethics, vol 1. Edinburgh: Clark; 1908.
4. Grennert L, Persson PH, Gennser G. Benefits of ultrasonic screening of a pregnant population. Acta Obstet Gynecol Scand Suppl 1978; 78:5–14.
5. Stockard CR. Developmental rate and structural expression. I. An experimental study of twins, double monsters and single deformities and the interaction among embryonic organs during their origin and development. Am J Anat 1921; 28:115–277.
6. Shapiro LR, Zemek L, Shulman MJ. Familial monozygotic twinning: an autosomal dominant form of monozygotic twinning with variable penetrance. In: Nance WE, Allen G, Parisi P, eds. Twin research: Biology and epidemiology. New York: Alan R. Liss; 1978:61–63.
7. Parisi P, Gatti M, Prinzi G, Caperna G. Familial incidence of twinning. Nature 1983; 304:626–628.
8. Nylander PPS. Serum levels of gonadotrophin in relation to multiple pregnancy in Nigeria. J Obstet Gynaecol Brit Cwlth 1973; 80:651–653.
9. Martin NG, El Beaini JL, Olsen MC, Bhatnagar AS, Macourt D. Gonadotrophin levels in mothers who had two sets of DZ twins. Acta Genet Med Gemellol 1984; 33:131–139.
10. Hardman R. Pharmaceutical products from plant steroids. Trop Sci 1969; 11:196.
11. Gemzell C, Roos P. Pregnancies following treatment with human gonadotrophins with special reference to the problem of multiple births. Am J Obstet Gynecol 1966; 94:490–496.
12. Human Fertilisation and Embryology Authority. Fifth Annual Report, London; 1996.

13. Benirschke K, Chung KK. Multiple pregnancy. Part II. N Engl J Med 1973; 288:1329–1336.

14. Kurtz A, Wapner RJ, Mata J, Johnson A, Morgan P. Twin pregnancies: Accuracy of first trimester abdominal ultrasound in predicting chorionicity and amnionicity. Radiology 1992; 185:759–762.

15. Monteagudo A, Timor-Tritsch IE. Early and simple determination of chorionic and amniotic type in multifetal gestations in the first fourteen weeks by high frequency transvaginal sonography. Am J Obstet Gynecol 1994; 170:824–829.

16. Barss VA, Benacerraf BR, Frigoletto FD. Ultrasonographic determination of chorion type twin gestation. Obstet Gynecol 1985; 66:779–782.

17. D'Alton ME, Dudley DK. The ultrasonographic prediction of chorionicity in twin gestation. Am J Obstet Gynecol 1989; 160:557–561.

18. Hertzberg BS, Kurtz AB, Choi HY, et al. Significance of membrane thickness in the sonographic evaluation of twin gestations. AJR 1987; 148:151–153.

19. Mahony BS, Filly RA, Callen PW. Amnionicity and chorionicity in twin pregnancies: prediction using ultrasound. Radiology 1985; 155:205–209.

20. Winn HN, Gabrielli S, Reece EA. Ultrasonographic criteria for the prenatal diagnosis of placental chorionicity in twin gestations. Am J Obstet Gynecol 1989; 161:1540–1542.

21. Harrington K, Armstrong V, Freeman J, Aquilina J, Campbell S. Fetal sexing by ultrasound in the second trimester: maternal preference and professional ability. Ultrasound Obstet Gynecol 1996; 8:318–321.

22. Townsend RR, Simpson GF, Filly RA. Membrane thickness in ultrasound prediction of chorionicity of twin gestations. J Ultrasound Med 1988; 7:327–332.

23. Finberg HJ. The twin peak sign: reliable evidence of dichorionic twinning. J Ultrasound Med 1992; 11:571–577.

24. Sepulveda W, Sebire NJ, Hughes K, Odibo A, Nicolaides KH. The lambda sign at 10–14 weeks of gestation as a predictor of chorionicity in twin pregnancies. Ultrasound Obstet Gynecol 1996; 7:421–423.

25. Sepulveda W, Sebire NJ, Hughes K, Kalogeropolous A, Nicolaides KH. Evolution of the lambda or twin chorionic peak sign in dichorionic twin pregnancies. Obstet Gynecol 1997; 89:439–441.

26. Wenstrom KD, Syrop CH, Hammit DG, Van Voorhis BJ. Increased risk of monochorionic twinning associated with assisted reproduction. Fertil Steril 1993; 60:510–514.

27. Wharton B, Edwards JH, Cameron AH. Monoamniotic twins. Br J Obstet Gynaecol 1968; 75:158–163.

28. Thompson B, Pritchard C, Corney G. Perinatal mortality in twins by zygosity and placentation. Paper given at Fourth Congress of International Society for Twin Studies, London; 1983 (unpublished).

29. King AD, Soothill PW, Montemagno R, Young MP, Sams V, Rodeck CH. Twin to twin blood transfusion in a dichorionic pregnancy without the oligohydramnios-polyhydramnios sequence. Br J Obstet Gynaecol 1995; 102:334–335.

30. Landy HJ, Weiner S, Corson SL, et al. The 'vanishing twin': Ultrasonographic assessment of fetal disappearance in the first trimester. Am J Obstet Gynecol 1986; 155:14–19.

31. Hanna JH, Hill JM. Single intrauterine fetal demise in multiple gestation. Obstet Gynecol 1984; 63:126–130.

32. Enbom JA. Twin pregnancy with intrauterine death of one twin. Am J Obstet Gynecol 1985; 152:424–429.

33. Saier F, Burden D, Cavanagh D. Fetus papyraceous. An unusual case with congenital anomaly of the surviving fetus. Obstet Gynecol 1975; 45:217–220.

34. Baker VV, Doring MC. Fetus papyraceous; an unreported congenital anomaly of the surviving infant. Am J Obstet Gynecol 1982; 143(2):234.

35. Burke MS. Single fetal demise in twin gestation. Clin Obstet Gynecol 1990; 33:69–78.

36. Santema JG, Swaak AM, Wallenberg HCS. Expectant management of a twin pregnancy with single fetal death. Br J Obstet Gynaecol 1995; 102:26–30.

37. Daw E. Fetus papyraceous – 11 cases. Postgrad Med J 1983; 59:598–600.

38. Melnick M. Brain damage in a survivor after in utero death of monozygous co-twin. Lancet 1977; ii:1287.

39. Filly RA, Goldstein RB, Callen PW. Monochorionic twinning: sonographic assessment. AJR 1989; 154:459–469.

40. Bell D, Johansson D, McLean FH, Usher RH. Birth asphyxia, trauma and mortality in twins: has caesarian section improved the outcome? Am J Obstet Gynecol 1986; 154:253–259.

41. D'Alton ME, Newton ER, Cetrulo CL. Intrauterine fetal demise in multiple pregnancy. Acta Genet Med Gemellol 1984; 33:43–49.

42. Hoyme HE, Higgenbottom MC, Jones KL. Vascular aetiology of disruptive structural defects in monozygotic twins. Paediatrics 1981; 67:288–291.

43. Szymonowizc W, Preston H, Yu V. The surviving monozygotic twin. Arch Dis Child 1986; 61:454–458.

44. Fusi L, Gordon H. Twin pregnancy complicated by single intrauterine death. Problems and outcome with conservative management. Br J Obstet Gynaecol 1990; 97:511–516.

45. Rosenberg K, Tweedie I, Grant J, Aitchison T, Gallacher F. Measurement of fundal height as a screening gest for fetal growth retardation. Br J Obstet Gynaecol 1982; 89:447–450.

46. Belizan JM, Villaw J, Mardin JC. Diagnosis of intra-uterine growth retardation by a simple clinical method: measurement of uterine height. Am J Obstet Gynecol 1978; 131:643–646.

47. Houlton MCC, Marivate M, Philpott RH. The prediction of fetal growth retardation in twin pregnancy. Br J Obstet Gynaecol 1981; 88:264–273.

48. Neilson JP. Detection of the small for dates twin fetus by ultrasound. Br J Obstet Gynaecol 1981; 88:27–32.

49. Secher NJ, Kaern J, Hansen PK. Intrauterine growth in twin pregnancies: prediction of fetal growth retardation. Obstet Gynecol 1985; 66:63–67.

50. D'Alton ME, Dudley DKL. Ultrasound in the antenatal management of twin gestation. Semin Perinatol 1986; 10:30–37.

51. Smith APM. The role of ultrasound in the evaluation of growth, the estimation of fetal weight and cervical length in twin pregnancies. University of Aberdeen; MD thesis; 1994.

52. Harrison SD, Cyr DR, Patten RM, Mack LA. Twin growth problems: causes and sonographic analysis. Semin Ultrasound CT MR 1993; 14:1:56–67.

53. Erkkola R, Ala-Melleo S, Picroinen O, Kero P, Sillampää M. Growth discordancy in twin pregnancies: a risk factor not detected by measurement of biparietal diameter. Obstet Gynecol 1985; 66:203–206.

54. Babson SG, Phillips DS. Growth and development of twins dissimilar in size at birth. N Engl J Med 1973; 298:937–940.

55. Storlazzi E, Vintzileos AM, Campbell WA, Nochimson BJ, Weinbaum PJ. Ultrasound diagnosis of discordant fetal growth in twin gestations. Obstet Gynecol 1987; 69:363–367.

56. Scottish Stillbirth and Neonatal Death Annual Reports (1989–94) Edinburgh: Scottish Health Service Common Services Agency.

57. Wenstrom KD, Gall SA. Incidence, morbidity and mortality and diagnosis of twin gestation. Clin Perinatol 1988; 15(1):1–11.

58. Bryan E, Little J, Burn J. Congenital anomalies in twins. Baillière's Clin Obstet Gynaecol 1987; 1(3):697–715.

59. Cameron AH, Edwards JH, Derom R, Thiery M, Boelaert R. The value of twin surveys in the study of malformations. Eur J Obstet Gynecol Reprod Biol 1983; 14:347–356.

60. Corney G, MacGillivray I, Campbell DM. Congenital anomalies in twins in Aberdeen and North East Scotland. Acta Genet Gemellol 1983; 32:31–35.

61. Myrianthopoulos MC. Congenital malformation in twins: epidemiological survey. Birth Defects 1975; XI(8):1–39.

62. Myrianthopoulos MC. Congenital malformations. The continuation of twin studies. Birth Defects 1978; XIV:151–165.

63. Little J, Bryan E. Congenital anomalies in twins. Semin Perinatol 1986; 10:50–64.

64. Burn J, Corney G. Congenital heart defects and twinning. Acta Genet Med Gemellol 1984; 33:61–69.

65. Van Staey M. Familial congenital oesophageal atresia: personal case report and review of the literature. Hum Genet 1984; 66(2–3):260–266.

66. Fraeser FC, Nora JJ. Genetics of man. Philadelphia: Lea and Febiger; 1975.

67. Hay S, Wehrung DA. Congenital malformation in twins. Am J Hum Genet 1970; 22:662–678.

68. Elwood JM, Elwood JH. Epidemiology of anencephalus and spina bifida. Oxford: Oxford University Press; 1980:205–221.

69. Garabedian BH, Fraser FC. A familial association between twinning and upper neural tube defects. Am J Hum Genet 1994; 55:1050–1053.

70. Layde PM, Erickson JD, Falek A, McCarthy BJ. Congenital malformation in twins. Am J Hum Genet 1980; 32:69–78.

71. Sebire NJ, Sepulveda W, Hughes KS, Noble P, Nicolaides KH. Management of twin pregnancies discordant for anencephaly. Br J Obstet Gynecol 1997; 104:216–219.

72. Patten RM, Mack LA, Harvey D, Cyr DR, Pretorious DH. Disparity of amniotic fluid volume and fetal size: problem of the stuck twin – US studies. Radiology 1989; 172:153–157.

73. Weir PE, Ratten GJ, Beischer NA. Acute polyhydramnios: A complication of monozygous twin pregnancy. Br J Obstet Gynaecol 1979; 86:849–853.

74. Robertson EG, Neer KJ. Placental injection studies in twin gestation. Am J Obstet Gynecol 1983; 147:170–173.

75. Blickstein I. The twin–twin transfusion syndrome. Obstet Gynecol 1990; 76:714–722.

76. Brown DL, Benson CB, Driscoll SG, Doubilet PM. Twin–twin transfusion syndrome: sonographic findings. Radiology 1989; 170:61–63.

77. Saldana LR, Eads MC, Schaefer TR. Umbilical blood waveforms in fetal surveillance of twins. Am J Obstet Gynecol 1987; 157(3):712–715.

78. Yamada A, Kasugal M, Ohno Y. Antenatal diagnosis of twin–twin transfusion by Doppler ultrasound. Obstet Gynecol 1991; 78:1058–1061.

79. Sebire NJ, D'Ercole C, Hughes K, Carvalho M, Nicolaides K. Increased nuchal translucency thickness at 10–14 weeks of gestation as a predictor of severe twin to twin transfusion syndrome. Ultrasound Obstet Gynecol 1997; 10:86–89.

80. Saunders NJ, Snijders RJM, Nicolaides KH. Therapeutic amniocentesis in twin–twin transfusion syndrome appearing in the second trimester of pregnancy. Am J Obstet Gynecol 1992; 166:820–824.

81. Reisner DP, Mahony BS, Petty CN. Stuck twin syndrome: outcome in thirty seven consecutive cases. Am J Obstet Gynecol 1993; 169:991–995.

82. Elliot JP, Urig MA, Clewell WH. Aggressive therapeutic amniocentesis for treatment of twin–twin transfusion syndrome. Obstet Gynecol 1991; 77:537–540.

83. Pinette MG, Pinette PY, Stubblefield PG. Treatment of twin–twin transfusion syndrome. Obstet Gynecol 1993; 82:841–846.

84. Saunders NJ, Snijders RJM, Nicolaides KH. Therapeutic amniocentesis in twin–twin transfusion syndrome appearing in the second trimester of pregnancy. Am J Obstet Gynecol 1992; 166:820–824.

85. Wittmann BK, Farquharson DF, Thomas WD, Baldwin VJ, Wadsworth LD. The role of feticide in the management of severe twin transfusion syndrome. Am J Obstet Gynecol 1986; 155:1023–1026.

86. Mahone PR, Sherer DM, Abramowicz JS, Woods JR. Twin–twin transfusion syndrome: Rapid development of severe hydrops of the donor following selective feticide of the hydropic recipient. Am J Obstet Gynecol 1993; 169:166–168.

87. Dommergues M, Mandelbrot L, Delezoide AL et al. Twin to twin transfusion syndrome: selective feticide by embolisation of the hydropic fetus. Fetal Diagn Ther 1995; 10:26–31.

88. De Lia JE, Cruikshank DP, Keye WR. Fetoscopic neodymium: YAG laser occlusion of placental vessels in severe twin-twin transfusion syndrome. Obstet Gynecol 1990; 75:1046–1053.

89. Ville Y, Hyett J, Hecher K, Nicolaides K. Preliminary experience with endoscopic laser surgery for severe twin–twin transfusion syndrome. N Engl J Med 1995; 332:224–227.

90. Mahony BS, Petty CN, Nyberg DA, Luthy DA, et al. The 'stuck twin' phenomenon: ultrasonographic findings, pregnancy outcome, and management with serial amniocentesis. Am J Obstet Gynecol 1990; 163:1513–1522.

91. Bejar R, Viggliocco G, Gramajo H, et al. Antenatal origin of neurological damage in newborn infants. II: Multiple gestations. Am J Obstet Gynecol 1990; 162:1230–1236.

92. Hanson JW. Incidence of conjoined twins. Lancet 1975; ii:1257.

93. Apuzzio JJ, Ganesh V, Landau I: Prenatal diagnosis of conjoined twins. Am J Obstet Gynecol 1984; 148(3):343–344.

94. Wilson RL, Cetrulo CL, Shaub MS. The prepartum diagnosis of conjoined twins by the use of diagnostic ultrasound. Am J Obstet Gynecol 1976; 126(6):737.

95. Benson CB, Doubilet PM. Sonography of multiple gestations. Radiol Clin North Am 1990; 28(1):149–161.

96. Turner RJ, Hankins GVD, Weinreb JC, et al. Magnetic resonance imaging and ultrasonography in the antenatal evaluation of conjoined twins. Am J Obstet Gynecol 1986; 155(3):645–649.

97. Romero R, Pilu G, Jeanty P, Ghidini JC, Hobbins JC. Prenatal diagnosis of congenital anomalies. Norwalk: Appleton and Lange; 1988:405–408.

98. van den Brand SF, Nijhuis JG, van Dongen WJ. Prenatal ultrasound diagnosis of conjoined twins. Obstet Gynecol Survey 1994; 49:656–662.

99. Sakala EP. Obstetric management of conjoined twins. Obstet Gynecol 1986; 67:21–25.

100. Vottler TP. Conjoined twins. In: Welch KJ, Randolph JG, Ravitch MM, eds. Pediatric surgery. Chicago: Year Book; 1986:771–779.

101. Razavi-Encha F, Mulliez N, Benhaiem-Sigaux N. Cardiovascular abnormalities in thoracopagus twins: Embryological interpretation and review. Early Hum Dev 1987; 15(1):33–34.

102. Bucholz RD, Yoon KW, Shively RE. Temperoparietal craniopagus: case report and review of the literature. J Neurosurg 1987; 66(1):72–79.

103. James WH. A note on the epidemiology of acardiac monsters. Tetralogy 1977; 16(2):211–216.

104. Berniscke K, Kim CK. Multiple pregnancy. N Engl J Med 1973; 288:1276–1329.

105. Napolitani FD, Schreiber I. The acardiac monster. A review of the world literature. Am J Obstet Gynecol 1960; 80:582.

106. Van Allen MI, Smith DW, Shepard TH. Twin reversed arterial perfusion (TRAP) sequence: a study of fourteen twin pregnancies with acardius. Semin Perinatol 1983; 7(4):285–293.

107. Wilson EA. Holocardius. Obstet Gynecol 1972; 40(5):740–748.

108. Sepulveda WH, Quiroz VH, Giuliano A. Prenatal ultrasonographic diagnosis of acardiac twin. J Perinat Med 1993; 21:241–246.

109. Romero R, Pilu G, Jeanty P, Ghidini JC, Hobbins JC. Prenatal diagnosis of congenital anomalies. Norwalk: Appleton and Lange; 1988:409–411.

110. Keith LG, Papiernik E, Keith DM, Luke B. Twin–twin transfusion syndrome. In: Multiple pregnancy. New York: Parthenon; 1995.

111. Simpson PC, Trudinger BJ, Walker A, Baird PJ. The intrauterine treatment of cardiac failure in twin pregnancy with an acardiac, acephalic monster. Am J Obstet Gynecol. 1983; 147(7):842–844.

112. Platt LD, DeVore GR, Bieniarz P, Benner PR, Rao R. Antenatal diagnosis of acephalus acardia: a proposed management scheme. Am J Obstet Gynecol 1983; 146(7):857–859.

113. Ash K, Harman CR, Gritter H. TRAP sequence successful outcome with indomethacin treatment. Obstet Gynecol 1990; 76(5):960–962.

114. Porreco RP, Barton SM, Haverkamp AD. Occlusion of umbilical artery in acardiac, acephalic twin. Lancet 1991; 337:326–327.

115. Moore TR, Gale S, Benirschke K. Perinatal outcome of forty nine pregnancies complicated by acardiac twinning. Am J Obstet Gynecol 1990; 163(3):907–912.

116. Bernischke K. The placenta in twin gestation. Clin Obstet Gynecol 1990; 33:18–30.

117. Dorum A, Nesheim B. Monochorionic monoamniotic twins – the most precarious of twin pregnancies. Acta Obstet Gynecol Scand 1991; 70:381–383.

118. Carr SR, Aronson MP, Coustan DR. Survival rates of monoamniotic twins do not decrease after 30 weeks gestation. Am J Obstet Gynecol 1990; 163:719–722.

119. Wensinger JA, Daly RF. Monoamniotic twins. Am J Obstet Gynecol 1962; 83:1254–1256.

CHAPTER 17

Non-immune fetal hydrops

Stephen A. Walkinshaw

Introduction

Fetal hydrops is the result of a number of pathophysiological mechanisms. Hydrops secondary to iso-immunization with red cell antibodies (immune hydrops) was the commonest cause of fetal hydrops prior to the use of prophylactic anti-D immunoglobulin, but now accounts for less than 20% of cases. All other causes are described as non-immune in aetiology.

The incidence of non-immune fetal hydrops is essentially unknown as there are no published, population-based data across all gestations. Published figures suggest incidences between 1 in 1500 and 1 in 4000. With recognition of early hydrops through increased use of both first trimester dating ultrasound and routine ultrasound screening at 18 to 22 weeks, the incidence is likely to be at least 1 in 1500, and is probably more. This would be our local experience.

Hydrops is strictly defined as the presence of excess fluid in more than one body cavity – a combination of at least two from subcutaneous oedema, hydrothorax, pericardial effusion and ascites being required (Figs 17.1, 17.2). Some authors[1] include polyhydramnios and placental oedema within the definition. In other publications, isolated fluid collections, particularly fetal ascites, are included as 'hydrops'. In some texts, cystic hygroma is included in the definition.[2] The aetiologies of

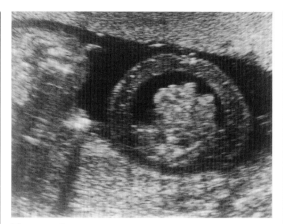

Fig. 17.2 Cross-sectional view through fetal abdomen, showing ascites and skin oedema.

fetal ascites[3] and pericardial effusions[4] are closely related to that of non-immune hydrops but not exclusively so. Wherever possible, data are confined to hydrops as defined above. The special circumstances of hydrops in monochorionic twin–twin transfusion syndrome will not be included in this chapter.

Causes

There are many causes of non-immune hydrops. No standardization exists over aetiological classification and various groups have classified the condition in differing ways.[1,2,5,6] Comparison of the causes of this condition across time and geography are hampered as a consequence.

The situation is further complicated by referral patterns and special interests, by how groups prioritize coexistent pathology in the fetus, by the intensity and expertise utilized before and after birth to reach a diagnosis, and above all by the gestation at diagnosis. Even where an anatomical diagnosis is reached, attribution of non-immune hydrops cannot be assumed. Many structural defects found in non-immune hydrops cases are commonly found in non-hydropic fetuses and neonates, and attribution of hydrops to that abnormality may not be appropriate.[7,8] Table 17.1, drawn

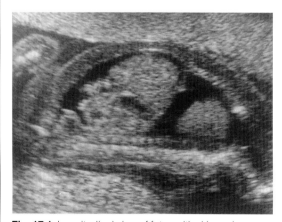

Fig. 17.1 Longitudinal view of fetus with skin oedema, hydrothorax and ascites.

Table 17.1
Causes of non-immune fetal hydrops

No. cases	Ref. 5 740	Ref. 2 386	Ref. 9 600	Ref. 10 77	Ref. 11 246	Ref. 12 53	Ref. 13 64	Ref. 7 64
Years	80–89	79–88	82–89	83–93		76–88	83–88	85–90
Chromosomal	10.8	14.0	15.7	16.0	29.2	33.9	34.3	21.9
Cardiovascular	27.1	18.4	17.0	23.0		3.7	12.5	15.6
Pulmonary	7.6	10.1	3.5	13.0				3.1
GI tract	2.9	2.3						
GU tract	3.4	2.5						
Hygroma	2.3	12.1						15.6
Skeletal	2.4		4.0			5.6		
Multiple		4.7				3.7		10.9
Akinesia	2.1		3.3					
Genetic	1.0					5.6		
Anaemia	6.2	10.1	10.3					
Infection	4.2	2.8	4.5		2.4	5.7	17.1	1.6
Misc.	4.4	5.9						4.7
No diagnosis	23.5	16.7	15.5	22.0	23.1	35.8	9.4	26.5

GI, gastrointestinal; GU, genitourinary.

from large series published since 1989, demonstrates the variety of causes and proportions seen.

The major causes are chromosomal abnormality, structural cardiovascular disease, cardiac rhythm disorders, chest anomalies, haematological disease and infection. These account for more than half of all cases.[2,5,7,9–13] No explanation could be found in 13.4 to 35.8% of cases,[2,5,7,9–13] though generally 15 to 20% remain unexplained. Groups, particularly in specialist centres, reporting smaller series have described smaller proportions of unexplained cases.[8,14,15]

Tables 17.2 and 17.3 show the effect of gestational age at diagnosis on the proportions of the various causes. The most

Table 17.3
Causes of non-immune fetal hydrops at less than 20 weeks' gestation

Abnormality group	% cases
Chromosomal cause	65.6
Infection	7.3
Cardiovascular cause	2.1
Fetal akinesia	8.3
Multiple malformation	2.1
Other anatomical defect	3.1
Haematological cause	1.1
Unknown cause	10.4

Derived from references 13, 15, 16, 17.

striking effect is the increasing incidence of chromosomal abnormalities with decreasing gestational age.[2,10,12,16] As a result, it is unusual not to find a cause in early hydrops[16,17] (Fig. 17.3).

Advances in clinical and laboratory genetics and in fetal medicine have also contributed to changes in diagnostic complexity over time.[9] Increasing numbers of chromosomal abnormalities appear in recent reports. Lesser proportions of cardiovascular disease and higher numbers of metabolic disease[12] and fetal akinesia[9] are recognized. Specific causes now run to several pages of any review or text (see reference 1 for recent detailed listing) but in many cases the diagnosis is paediatric, clinical genetic or pathological in origin.

Table 17.2
Proportion of causes by gestation

	Less than 24–28 weeks %	More than 24–28 weeks %
Chromosomal cause	29.6	5.0
Cardiovascular cause	10.2	25.1
Genetic or syndromal cause	3.7	7.9
Infective cause	1.6	4.0
Pulmonary cause	6.4	14.5
Unknown cause	17.1	20.1

Derived from references 2, 10, 12.

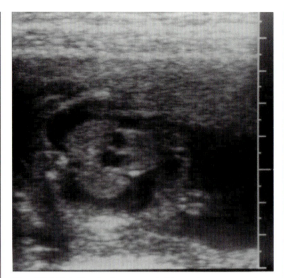

Fig. 17.3 Fetal hydrothorax and skin oedema secondary to trisomy 21 at 19 weeks' gestation.

Utilizing advances in the understanding of the pathophysiology of hydrops, and more widespread availability of both fetal medicine and specialist perinatal pathology, the classification system in Table 17.4 is suggested. This tries to prioritize pathology

where possible, and acknowledge the difficulties in attribution. In one series[8] the authors found that 1 in 8 cases had a structural anomaly which did not account for the presence of hydrops.

Pathophysiology

Hydrops is an end state for many pathologies and requires an imbalance between intra- and extravascular fluid. The driving force out of the vascular space is the difference between the capillary hydrostatic pressure and the colloid oncotic pressure of interstitial fluid. The driving force into the vascular space is the difference between the interstitial hydrostatic pressure and the plasma oncotic pressure. Colloid oncotic pressure in turn depends on both the concentration of osmotically-active molecules and the efficacy with which differences in oncotic pressure can cause water shifts.

There are a number of features in the fetus which make extrapolation of infant and adult

Table 17.4
Classification of causes of non-immune fetal hydrops

Chromosomal abnormality	Classify as this irrespective of other pathology
Cardiovascular abnormality	Classify where lesion physiologically likely to be associated with hydrops or where antenatal evidence of cardiac dysfunction known to occur in hydrops
Pulmonary abnormality	Where isolated, thoracic, space-occupying lesion or where either documented progression from isolated hydrothorax or resolution of hydrops after thoracocentesis/shunting
Gastrointestinal abnormality	Where isolated anomaly. Ascites must be present
Genitourinary abnormality	Where isolated anomaly likely to result in ascites or where evidence of bladder or renal pelvic rupture
Cystic hygroma	Where non-chromosomal or syndromal cause. Presence of oedema alone sufficient
Skeletal malformation	Where recognized skeletal dysplasia
Multiple malformation syndrome	Multiple anomalies where no specific diagnosis reached
Miscellaneous anatomical abnormality	Where anatomical abnormality detected, but, in the opinion of the investigators, no good evidence that anomalies seen could cause hydrops
Fetal akinesia syndrome	Specific syndromes or where documented evidence of akinesia in utero or contractures
Specific anatomical syndromes	Where known genetic anatomical syndrome or recognized non-genetic malformation sequence
Genetic metabolic disease	Specify conditions
Haematological causes	Non-infective causes of fetal anaemia. Include genetic causes of anaemia
Infection	Where infection demonstrably causes pathology known to be associated with hydrops
Tumours	Include both fetal and placental tumours
Idiopathic recurrent	Where no other cause determined
Unknown cause	Where no cause identified. Specify extent of investigations normally performed

physiology unreliable. Capillaries are more permeable, thus colloid oncotic pressure is a less effective driver, and the distribution of body water is less sensitive to changes in oncotic pressure. Capillary filtration coefficients are raised, resulting in a higher water flux for a given driving force. The fetal interstitial space is more compliant, and therefore there is less rise in hydrostatic pressure with a given volume change (see reference 18 for detailed account). This could result in the loss of large volumes to the interstitium before a rise in interstitial colloid oncotic pressure checked the flux. All of these mechanisms allow more rapid correction of changes in intravascular volume than in the adult. This is confirmed in utero by the finding of a four- to five-fold increase in lymph flow in the fetus.[19]

Clearance of lymph fluid is dependent on the outflow pressure in the great veins of the neck, largely the same as central venous pressure (CVP). So long as negative pressure is maintained then lymph flow occurs. Once the pressure is positive, there is a linear decrease in lymph flow with increasing venous pressure, with no flow at pressures above 11.5 mmHg.[19] There is approximately a 12% reduction in flow for every 1 mm increase in venous pressure. It can be predicted that a 4 mm rise in venous pressure could result in the accumulation of 360 ml in 24 hours. As a result of these sorts of experiments, it is felt that the final common pathway for most causes of hydrops is raised CVP.

This has been confirmed by both experimental findings and human in vivo work. Rapid onset of anaemia results in a rise in CVP and the development of hydrops.[20] Fetal lamb models for supraventricular tachycardia also show rapid and large CVP rises.[21] Models for the development of hydrops secondary to cystic adenomatoid lung lesions have similarly found rises in CVP coincident with the development of hydrops.[22]

That CVP is elevated in the human fetus with hydrops has been confirmed by Weiner & Moise[23,24] by measuring umbilical venous pressure in a wide range of differing pathologies. Venous pressure was elevated in fetuses hydropic secondary to thoracic disease, anaemia, cardiac disease and infection. It was not elevated in cases of supraventricular tachycardia without hydrops. Human fetuses with cardiac anomalies which result in a raised right atrial pressure are more likely to develop hydrops.

Venous pressure can be elevated by various means. Pump failure (hypoxia, infection, arrhythmia), high output failure (anaemia, tumours), or obstruction (thoracic lesions, organomegaly or lysosome storage disease) could all bring about a raised CVP. A raised CVP raises capillary hydrostatic pressure, driving fluid out of the vascular space. Hypoxia secondary to anaemia, or endothelial damage secondary to infection, may cause capillary endothelial damage resulting in increased capillary permeability at lesser values of CVP. Alterations in colloid oncotic pressure may occur through hepatic damage or infiltration, through accumulation of osmotically active lactic acid secondary to hypoxia or anaemia,[25] or through modification of osmotically important proteins by linkage with disease by-products.[24] Atrial natriuretic factor may play some role in vascular permeability here[26] with resultant increase in extracellular volume, although the effects on lymph ducts are complex.

Because of the interplay of factors, and the multiplicity of possible causes, it is important to try to link a pathological mechanism which makes sense to the proposed cause of hydrops in each case.

Specific causes

Chromosomal abnormality

In current practice this is the commonest cause of non-immune hydrops. The incidence changes dramatically with gestation as shown in Tables 17.2 and 17.3. Population data from Australia[27] emphasizes this with 52% of cases prior to 20 weeks having a karyotypic anomaly compared with 28% of those diagnosed after 20 weeks. A wide range of abnormalities has been described.[5,9,12,13,28] Commonest are trisomy 21 and monosomy X, but trisomies 13, 16 and 18 and triploidy are not infrequent.[5,16] Various structural rearrangements have been described in case reports.

The proportion of monosomy X and trisomies 21 and 18 may alter with gestation, with the autosomal trisomies being more common earlier in gestation. Iskaros[16] et al found 24 cases of trisomy 18 or 21 in 45 cases of hydrops under 20 weeks, but only 6 cases of monosomy X. This preponderance of trisomies has been noted in some earlier studies[17] but not in others.[13] A diagnosis is clearly important as there are implications for follow-up and recurrence risks.

The exact mechanism of hydrops varies. Many fetuses with monosomy X have severe disruption of lymphatic drainage and/or marked outlet obstruction of the left heart. The mechanism in trisomy 21 is less clear in many cases. Some are associated with cardiac malformation[2] but others have no obvious structural defect to account for the development of hydrops. It is assumed that the mechanism involves alterations in lymphatic drainage.

Cardiovascular disease

The combination of structural cardiac disease, tachyarrhythmias and bradyarrhythmias makes cardiovascular disease the second commonest group of causes (Table 17.5). Many are associated with chromosomal abnormality.[2,5,29,30] They present throughout pregnancy.[2,10,16] In some cases, the structural malformation is clearly responsible for hydrops, but in many cases, the anomaly may more usually present as mild heart failure in the neonatal period. Attribution to structural cardiovascular cause may be inappropriate in these circumstances unless antenatal or neonatal echocardiography can demonstrate a mechanism by which hydrops may have developed.

Lesions which raise right atrial pressure are the most likely to lead to fetal hydrops.[30] Hydrops appears more likely in a given

Table 17.5
Cardiovascular causes of non-immune fetal hydrops
Obstruction or restriction of left ventricular outflow
Hypoplastic left heart syndrome
Coarctation of the aorta
Aortic stenosis/atresia
Mitral stenosis
Tumour
Restrictive cardiomyopathy
Primary increase in right atrial pressure
Restriction/closure foramen ovale
Pulmonary atresia/severe stenosis
Tricuspid atresia/severe stenosis
Hypoplastic right ventricle
Severe atrioventricular regurgitation
Ebstein's anomaly
Atrioventricular canal defect
Pulmonary insufficiency
Dilated cardiomyopathy
Arrhythmias
Atrioventricular re-entrant tachycardia
Atrial flutter
Congenital heart block
Atrial fibrillation
Sinus bradycardia
Other causes
Tumours
Myocardial infarction
Idiopathic arterial calcification

defect if there is increased preload,[31] or where there are reduced peak descending aortic velocities.[32]

Lesions with significant left-sided obstruction are commonest as they result in increased right ventricular flow.[5] Restriction of both ductus arteriosus or the foramen ovale may further contribute.[30] Right-sided obstruction or hypoplasia may be determined by the relative restriction of the foramen ovale (Fig. 17.4). Other defects where a mechanism is likely include premature closure or restriction of the foramen ovale or ductus arteriosus, Ebstein's anomaly where there is significant tricuspid regurgitation or arrhythmia, atrioventricular canal defects where there is marked mitral regurgitation directed towards the right atrium and severe pulmonary insufficiency.[5,30] Hydrops has been described with septal defects, transposition of the great vessels, tetralogy of Fallot and truncus arteriosus but these may be associations rather than causal, and care should be taken to demonstrate functional problems which could lead to hydrops.

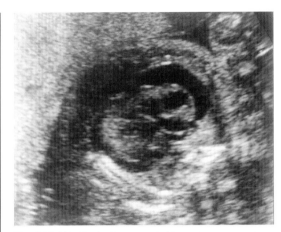

Fig. 17.4 Fetal hydrothorax and skin oedema secondary to hypoplastic right heart syndrome.

Tachyarrhythmias are the next commonest group.[5] There is good experimental evidence that hydrops develops as a consequence of raised venous pressure[21] and the degree of mitral and tricuspid regurgitation. Supraventricular tachycardias are commonest, accounting for around 50% of hydrops owing to this cause[30] but hydrops can arise from paroxysmal tachycardia in cases with isolated extrasystoles. This group is atrioventricular re-entrant tachycardias, usually either Wolff–Parkinson–White syndrome or concealed atrioventricular connections. Atrial flutter is less common, and is usually a 2:1 block. It can be secondary to atrial dilatation. Atrial fibrillation and ventricular tachycardias are rare. In many cases, even detailed fetal echocardiography will not differentiate with complete certainty unless there is clear atrioventricular dissociation.

Fetal bradyarrhythmias are the least common. They are associated either with structural disease or with connective tissue disease.[33,34] Most fetuses with congenital heart block do not develop hydrops.

Other cardiac causes include tumours,[35] usually rhabdomyomata, but harmartomas, haemangiomas and teratomas have been reported. These produce hydrops by either restriction of function or by obstruction. Cardiomyopathies of restricted and dilated types have been reported in fetal life as causes of hydrops. Very rare causes are idiopathic arterial calcification and myocardial infarction.[36]

The outlook for structural heart disease with hydrops is extremely poor[37] with few survivors. Theoretically treatment with inotropes and diuretics could improve function and this might be worth considering where the defect is in the group where a causal relationship is less clear.

Fetuses with hydrops secondary to arrhythmias have the best outlook of all causes of non-immune hydrops. Spontaneous resolution of both tachyarrhythmia and hydrops has been described.[38] First choice therapy in the presence of hydrops should be flecainide[39] as cardioversion appears more likely than with digoxin. Alternatives include direct fetal therapy with digoxin or in resistant cases, successful chemical cardioversion with adenosine has been reported.[40]

The outcome of hydrops in congenital heart block of non-structural origin is poor. Therapy with maternal infusion of sympathomimetics,[41] maternal administration of high-dose steroids,[42] direct fetal drug therapy[43] and transvenous fetal pacing[44] have all been attempted with varying success.

Pulmonary abnormality

Thoracic causes of hydrops include cystic adenomatoid malformation of the lung (Fig. 17.5), congenital diaphragmatic hernia, pulmonary sequestration and isolated hydrothorax.[3,5,6] However, any space-occupying lesion in the chest can lead to hydrops, and tracheal atresia, pulmonary lymphangiectasia, bronchogenic cysts and intrapulmonary tumours have all been described in a few cases.[5]

Animal work has shown that space-occupying lesions result in significant rises in CVP[22] which impairs lymphatic return. Umbilical venous pressure has been demonstrated to be elevated in six human fetuses with a thoracic aetiology for hydrops.[23] In an interesting small series, one group has shown torsion of extralobar

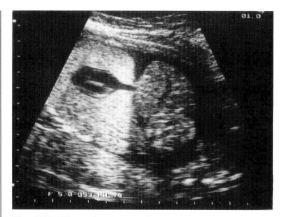

Fig. 17.5 Bilateral, microcystic, congenital cystic adenomatoid malformation with skin oedema and ascites.

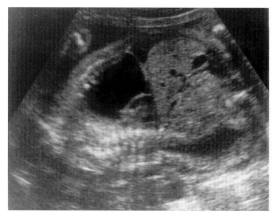

Fig. 17.6 Severe hydrothorax and ascites. This case started as moderate, isolated, right-sided hydrothorax and progressed over 2 weeks. Hydrops resolved after pleuro-amniotic shunting at 26 weeks' gestation.

pulmonary sequestration resulting in hydrothorax, presumably as a result of occlusion of lymphatics.[45]

The prognosis of pulmonary lesions with hydrops is poor. All cases associated with sequestration reported up till 1992 died[46] although, subsequently, survivors have been reported.[47] The development of fetal hydrops is one of the major determinants of survival for cystic adenomatoid malformation. Of 20 survivors reported by Thorpe-Beeston[48] diagnosed before 22 weeks, only two had hydrops. Survival in those diagnosed after 24 weeks was 17% compared with 93% for those without hydrops.[48] Similar results have been reported by others.[49,50]

Such poor results have led to attempts at fetal therapy, including open resection of lesions in fetal life[51] with limited success. Drainage of large cysts in macrocystic cases may also result in reversal of hydrops.[52] Where there is good evidence of progression from isolated hydrothorax to hydrops then pleuro-amniotic shunt placement can result in resolution of hydrops[10,53] (Fig. 17.6).

Gastrointestinal abnormalities

These are uncommonly associated with hydrops but they may arise following meconium perforation and peritonitis, fetal volvulus and hepatic fibrosis or dysplasia. Extensive hepatic disruption, as occurs in polycystic disease of the liver, has also been reported as a cause. For most gastrointestinal causes of hydrops, care must be taken to actually establish a likely mechanism for hydrops.

Genitourinary abnormalities

These are rare, but any severe obstructive uropathy leading to urinary ascites could cause the development of hydrops. Renal vein thrombosis may result in hydrops. Other genitourinary abnormalities attributed as causes of hydrops should be viewed with suspicion.

Skeletal dysplasia

This accounts for 2 to 5% of cases. Over 20 types of dysplasia have been described in cases of hydrops.[1,12] They largely include those syndromes which have marked thoracic restriction as part of the phenotype and it is presumed that the pathophysiology is similar to that of a space-occupying chest lesion.

Fetal akinesia syndrome

These are a group of disorders which are increasingly recognized as a cause of hydrops. No cases were identified in a 1982 review[54] but subsequently between 2 and 3%

of cases are due to these disorders.[5,9] They have been described in early pregnancy.[16]

The commonest causes are lethal multiple pterygium syndrome, arthrogryposis multiplex congenita, Neu–Laxova syndrome, Pena–Shokeir syndrome and myotonic dystrophy. Other neuronal migration disorders may also present in this way.[55] A particular variant of akinesia is the Finnish type which occurs in 1 in 19 000 births.[56] Almost all cases have hydrops, and this typically develops around 14 weeks.

These are lethal disorders and important diagnoses. Myotonic dystrophy is inherited as an autosomal dominant trait, whereas all the others are inherited as autosomal recessive disorders.

Genetic disease

van Maldergem[12] cited 64 different genetic causes of fetal hydrops in 1992. Excluding chromosomal causes, genetic causes account for 10 to 15% of all non-immune hydrops. Where genetic disease results in anaemia, skeletal disease or akinesia then these should be classified under those headings. This leaves two main groups – metabolic disease and recognized multiple malformation syndromes.

Of the heterogeneous group of syndromes, Noonan syndrome is the commonest.[5] Others include Opitz–Frias syndrome, Cornelia de Lange syndrome, tuberous sclerosis, Mohr syndrome (orofaciodigital syndrome type II) and angio-osteohypertrophy. Again these are important diagnoses as recurrence risks are high. Idiopathic familial recurrent hydrops,

recurrent cystic hygroma, and Elejalde syndrome (multiple nuchal cysts extending into the abdomen) are other recessively inherited causes of hydrops.[1]

There are a large number of metabolic disorders which have been described as associated with hydrops. These largely consist of lysosomal storage disorders[1,5,28] such as the mucopolysaccharidoses, Niemann–Pick disease, Gaucher's disease and galactosialidosis. Others include GM1 gangliosidosis and carnitine deficiency which can present as a cardiomyopathy.

The precise mechanism of hydrops in these diseases is unclear. It may be hypoalbuminaemia secondary to hepatic dysfunction, obstructed venous return as a result of organomegaly or obstruction of sinusoids by swollen liver cells.

The range of possible diseases makes testing extremely problematical unless there is a good family history. Detailed information is needed as frequently different tissues are needed for diagnosis.

Fetal anaemia

Fetal anaemia is one of the commonest causes of non-immune hydrops (see Table 17.1), especially if infection by human parvovirus B19 is included. Table 17.6 lists the common haematological causes.

Alpha-thalassaemia is seen in 1 in 300 births in some parts of South-East Asia, and can account for up to one-quarter of all perinatal deaths.[57] The carrier rate is 5 to 15% in some areas. It is rare in the Afro Caribbean population and there is a small carrier rate in Mediterranean countries. It

---

Table 17.6
Haematological causes of non-immune fetal hydrops

Alpha-thalassaemia	
Red cell enzyme disorders	Glucose phosphate isomerase deficiency, pyruvate kinase deficiency, glucose-6-phosphate deficiency
Red cell membrane defects	
Myeloproliferative disease	Transient myeloproliferative disorder, congenital leukaemia
Red cell aplasia or dyserythropoiesis	Blackfan–Diamond syndrome, Fanconi anaemia, congenital dyserythropoietic anaemia
Fetal bleeding	Fetomaternal haemorrhage, spontaneous fetal haemorrhage
Infection	Human parvovirus B19, cytomegalovirus
Miscellaneous	Kasabach–Merritt syndrome, haemorrhage into tumours

classically presents in the late second and early third trimesters[58] as up till then tetramers of embryonic fetal haemoglobin may allow survival. The absence of alpha chains in the third trimester rapidly results in the formation of haemoglobin Barts (a gamma tetramer) which has an extremely high affinity for oxygen. Tissue hypoxia rapidly results. Hydrops is a consequence of both tissue hypoxia with ensuing endothelial damage, and raised venous pressure secondary to myocardial failure. Stillbirth usually follows.

Alpha-thalassaemia can now be diagnosed using molecular genetic techniques. In the absence of these, placental thickness has proved a sensitive indicator and occurs before hydrops.[59] It is lethal although there have been reports of survival by aggressive antenatal transfusion.[60] However, life-long transfusion therapy is then needed.

Glucose-6-phosphate dehydrogenase deficiency affects a substantial number of the world's population and the neonatal syndrome is frequently reported.[61] However, fetal hydrops is rare and appears to be related to maternal ingestion of a triggering factor.[62] There have been case reports of hydrops secondary to other enzyme defects.[63,64]

Transient myeloproliferative disorder (TMD) is often indistinguishable from true congenital leukaemia. It is commonly seen in neonates with trisomy 21 and cases of hydrops in trisomy 21 fetuses have been reported.[65,66] Although if the anaemia is severe it can lead to stillbirth, the natural history of this disorder is gradual resolution. There have been cases of true congenital leukaemia presenting as hydrops.[67] The mechanism of hydrops is mixed. Most are linked with severe anaemia, but infiltration of the liver and increased peripheral resistance have also been implicated. Rare aplasias have been reported usually in single families.

Fetomaternal haemorrhage is well described as a cause of hydrops[5] as a result of chronic anaemia. Prenatal fetal bleeding into the brain or into tumours is another reported cause.

The mechanism by which fetal anaemia causes hydrops is complex and requires quite severe anaemia (usually less than 5 g.dl^{-1}). Umbilical venous pressure was elevated in one case of anaemia secondary to fetomaternal haemorrhage in Weiner's series[23] and in the sheep model, rapid production of anaemia was associated with a rise in central venous pressure and the development of hydrops.[20] Atrial natriuretic protein has been reported as elevated in cases where hydrops is a result of anaemia,[68] and this may drive fluid from the intravascular to the extravascular space, especially if the anaemia is severe enough to cause tissue hypoxia and endothelial damage. Other possibilities are analogous to immune hydrops. Here, although there is also a rise in CVP,[24] there are marked changes in colloid oncotic pressure and the gradient between venous and colloid oncotic pressure, which could result in quite large fluid shifts. Similarly, severe immune anaemia results in a marked lactic acidosis. In experimental animal models, it has been suggested that this accumulation of a powerful oncotic substance which does not cross the placenta results in large fluid shifts across the placenta and to increases in fetal urine production[25] and extracellular fluid. This accounts for the hydramnios seen in many such cases. However, if there is tissue hypoxia, then the fetal kidney will cope poorly with these increases in fluid and this could ultimately result in hydrops.

Hydrops secondary to anaemia is one of the few reliably treatable causes of non-immune hydrops, although it must be borne in mind both that some of these conditions are lethal after birth and that mortality from fetal blood sampling and transfusion in the presence of hydrops is high.[69]

Fetal infection

Fetal infection figures prominently in most series (see Table 17.1) as a cause of fetal hydrops, with around 5% of cases having this as an underlying aetiology. It is now felt that many 'unexplained' hydrops are due to

Table 17.7
Infectious causes of non-immune fetal hydrops

Common	Rare
Parvovirus B19	Herpes simplex virus
Cytomegalovirus	*Listeria monocytogenes*
Adenovirus	*Chlamydia trachomatis*
Syphilis	Rubella
Coxsackie virus	Respiratory syncytial virus
Toxoplasma gondii	Influenza B

infection.[11,13] Table 17.7 describes the common agents implicated.

The mechanism by which fetal infection results in hydrops varies. Some bacterial infection results in disseminated damage to capillaries and to endothelial cells which could result in fluid shifts. Others, particularly coxsackie virus, may act by primary myocardial failure as a result of myocarditis. Hepatic damage can occur in some infections such as syphilis, whilst erythroid damage is sustained in cytomegalovirus and parvovirus infection.

Cytomegalovirus infection is present in virtually all large series. It may present in the first half of pregnancy[11,16] but is more usually diagnosed later. Overall survival appears better than with many causes of hydrops[70] and spontaneous resolution has been described.[71] However, long-term outcome in survivors is poor. There is little experience with specific treatment such as ganciclovir during pregnancy.

Toxoplasmosis causing hydrops is uncommon but appears commoner after infection in early pregnancy, which is the time of lowest maternal transmission risk. Maternal therapy with combinations of spiramycin, pyrimethamine and sulfadiazine are successful in reducing the risk of long-term sequelae from intra-uterine infection, but there are few data on use in the presence of fetal hydrops.

There are isolated reports of disseminated infection with herpes simplex virus, *Listeria*, *Chlamydia* and other bacterial infections leading to the development of hydrops.[5,70,72] Syphilis can cause hydrops[73] and, as a result of the prozone phenomenon, hydrops can be an indication of fetal syphilis in the absence of maternal serological evidence of infection.

Successful resolution of hydrops secondary to syphilis following maternal administration of high-dose parenteral penicillin has been described and it is felt that the overall outcome of therapy can be good.[74]

Other viruses may be important. Coxsackievirus has been described as a cause. Adenovirus was isolated from 6 of 14 cases of hydrops or ascites using molecular genetic techniques.[75] Both of these viruses are common causes of neonatal myocarditis.

The commonest single infectious cause of hydrops is parvovirus B19 infection (Fig. 17.7).[76] This virus binds to the P antigen system present on red cells, erythroblasts, endothelium, placenta, fetal liver and heart. Tropism for erythroid progenitor cells results in lytic destruction and severe red cell aplasia. This generally occurs 4 to 6 weeks after primary infection[77] but can be delayed. The most vulnerable time is 16 to 24 weeks which coincides with the largest increase in fetal red cell mass.[70] However, hydrops secondary to parvovirus infection has been described in the first trimester[78] and is presumed to be due to direct myocardial infection.

The overall risk of maternal parvovirus infection resulting in fetal hydrops is low.[76,77] Therapy by fetal transfusion is well described and results in better outcome than conservative management in severe disease. However, unlike anaemia secondary to immune hydrops, mild anaemia in parvovirus infection can be associated with hydrops as a result of myocardial

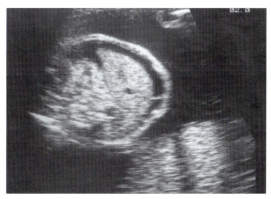

Fig. 17.7 Fetal ascites and mild skin oedema secondary to fetal parvovirus infection.

dysfunction. The effect on red cell mass is transient and spontaneous resolution is common,[76] especially if fetal haemoglobin values are more than 8 g.dl⁻¹ or where there is a marked reticulocytosis. Conservative management may be appropriate in these circumstances. Where anaemia is severe, there seems little doubt that transfusion is the treatment of choice.[76,79] Long-term outcome appears normal.[80]

Investigation

The wide range of conditions presenting as hydrops makes investigation difficult. The best approach involves both exclusion of those aetiologies which are common and core investigations which are applied to all cases (Table 17.8). However, all investigations should have a recognized purpose.

Investigation begins with maternal history. The increasing numbers of cases linked to infectious and genetic causes make this an important part of the investigation protocol. Racial background is important for some genetic disease. A detailed genetic family history should be obtained, including details of past pregnancy losses. Information on consanguinity should be actively sought. Occupational history may highlight possible infectious causes. Medical history such as systemic lupus erythematosus or maternal anaemia may guide other investigations. Pregnancy problems such as antepartum haemorrhage or rash can also aid diagnosis. If hydramnios or Ballantyne syndrome is a feature, then the timing of onset of these complications may be helpful.

The mainstay of the investigation is detailed real time ultrasound of the fetus and placenta. Fetal anatomy including structural echocardiography should be performed. The distribution of hydrops should be noted. Amniotic fluid volume should be assessed and umbilical arterial Doppler undertaken. Fetal status can be assessed either by cardiotocography or by ultrasound biophysical assessment at the time of the anatomical survey. In view of increasing

attempts to treat non-immune hydrops of uncertain aetiology in utero, non-invasive assessment of fetal cardiac function by both conventional and colour flow Doppler is useful. M-mode echocardiography should be reserved for where there is a clear arrhythmia.

In the absence of a clear anatomical cause, or where chromosomal abnormality is strongly suspected, then invasive fetal testing is required. In the first half of pregnancy where the risk of chromosome anomaly is very high, then sampling by chorion villus biopsy offers the quickest result, although modern culture techniques are resulting in amniocentesis culture results in 7 to 9 days. Amniocentesis may be preferred as, in addition, it allows sampling for viral or bacterial culture. It also allows metabolic testing such as that for Gaucher's disease. Arrangements should be available to store liquor and cultured cells for future testing if the aetiology is unclear.

Beyond 18 weeks, fetal blood sampling is the preferred investigation, yielding the maximum information, although amniocentesis may still be required if there is strong suspicion of a viral aetiology. Blood sampling in the presence of hydrops carries increased risk of loss.[69] Where there is known genetic risk, then samples may be needed for specific assays. It may be useful to have a system by which additional blood cells and serum are stored.

Where fetal fluid collections are present, these should be sampled; this is particularly important if there is pleural fluid, and allows distinction between transudate and exudate.

Maternal investigations should be carried out at this time. These may be general as in Table 17.8, or be directed. Thus haemoglobin electrophoresis, anti-RNA antibodies, red cell enzyme status or biochemistry may be needed.

Where a diagnosis is not reached before delivery, then in survivors, neonatal investigations should be as extensive as the prenatal investigations. Aid from clinical genetics services is important at this stage. Where there is perinatal loss, placental histology, full autopsy, radiology and clinical genetics input is needed. It is wise to prepare

Table 17.8
Investigation of non-immune fetal hydrops

Maternal history	Racial background, occupation, genetic family history, personal and family history of pregnancy loss, consanguinity, medical disease, illness in pregnancy, onset of symptoms
Ultrasound examination	Anatomy, liquor, biophysical assessment, echocardiography including Doppler
Maternal investigations	Blood group and antibody screen, full blood count, Kleihauer–Betke test, VDRL, virology (parvovirus, cytomegalovirus, adenovirus, toxoplasma)
Fetal blood sampling	Full blood count, blood group and direct Coombs' test, karyotype, protein, viral IgM, parvovirus and cytomegalovirus DNA
Amniocentesis	Karyotype, cytomegalovirus culture, toxoplasma DNA
Fetal effusions	Lymphocyte count, protein

and store DNA from fetal and placental tissue. Some consideration may be given to storing cultured fibroblasts or liver biopsy material.

Management

Non-immune hydrops may present at any time during pregnancy, and there is no standard management. The prognosis remains grim, especially where the diagnosis is made in the first half of pregnancy. Management initially centres on reaching a diagnosis. However, there may be other pregnancy problems to contend with. Hydramnios is common, and increases the risk of preterm delivery, malpresentation, cord prolapse and abruptio placentae. Occasionally, uterine decompression by amnioreduction may be necessary on symptomatic grounds.

Severe oedema and proteinuric hypertension, Ballantyne syndrome, may occur and it has been described in many aetiologies of hydrops.[81] Resolution of the hydrops can result in improvement.[82]

Preterm delivery should be avoided unless there is clear deterioration in the fetal condition. Termination of pregnancy is clearly an option where the diagnosis is made early. The role of late termination has not been extensively explored, but it may be an option where multiple malformations, chromosomal anomaly, known genetic syndrome or structural cardiac disease are the underlying causes. It would seem

difficult to justify late termination where there is no known cause.

Increasingly fetal treatment is an option (Table 17.9). Where there is no specific directed therapy, some general techniques have been explored on empirical grounds. In cases where the predominant fluid collection is in the thorax, there has been a number of reported cases of resolution of hydrops after pleuro-amniotic shunting[10,14,53] and this should be considered more frequently, especially where early delivery is not a realistic option (Fig. 17.8). Using similar arguments, a case could be made for peritoneo-amniotic shunting for ascites, but this is not reported. Another approach is to try to improve cardiac output by the use of inotropic agents. One group has reported success in unexplained hydrops using maternal digoxin therapy in conjunction with aggressive amnioreduction.[83] This approach warrants further investigation. It also may be

Table 17.9
Specific therapy for non-immune fetal hydrops

Fetal transfusion	Parvovirus, red cell disorders, fetomaternal haemorrhage
Anti-arrhythmic agents	Supraventricular tachycardias, atrial tachycardias
Beta-mimetics/steroids	Congenital heart block
Antibiotics	Syphilis, toxoplasmosis, *Listeria*
Antiviral agents	Cytomegalovirus
Antithyroid agents	Fetal thyrotoxicosis
Pleuro-amniotic shunting	Large cystic CAM, primary hydrothorax, congenital diaphragmatic hernia
Open fetal surgery	Microcystic CAM

CAM, cystic adenomatoid malformation.

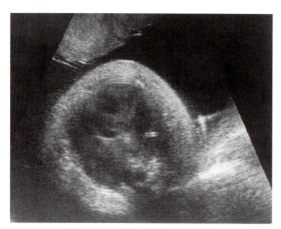

Fig. 17.8 A case of severe non-immune fetal hydrops of unknown cause at 30 weeks' gestation. Pleuro-amniotic shunting, shown here, resulted in partial resolution of hydrops with delivery and survival 3 weeks later.

worth considering this in cases secondary to structural heart disease where the link between the lesion and hydrops is less clear.

References

1. Jones DC. Nonimmune fetal hydrops: Diagnosis and management. Semin Perinatol 1995; 19:447–461.
2. Hansmann M, Gembruch U, Bald R. New therapeutic aspects in nonimmune hydrops fetalis based on four hundred and two prenatally diagnosed cases. Fetal Ther 1989; 4:29–36.
3. Shah YP, Hadlock FP. Hydrops and ascites. In: Nyberg DA, Mahony BS, Pretorius DH, eds. Diagnostic ultrasound of fetal anomalies: text and atlas. St Louis: Mosby Year Book; 1990:563–591.
4. Shenker L, Reed KL, Anderson CF, Kern W. Fetal pericardial effusions. Am J Obstet Gynecol 1989; 160:1505–1508.
5. Machin GA. Hydrops revisited: Literature review of 1414 cases published in the 1980s. Am J Med Genet 1989; 34:366–390.
6. Ryan G, Whittle MJ. Immune and non-immune hydrops. In: Diseases of the fetus and newborn. Pathology, imaging, and management. 2nd ed., vol 2. London: Chapman and Hall; 1995:1257–1266.
7. Santolaya J, Alley D, Jaffe R, Warsof SL. Antenatal classification of hydrops fetalis. Obstet Gynecol 1992; 79:256–259.
8. Ruiz-Villaespesa A, Suarez-Mier MP, Lopez-Ferrer P, Alvarez-Baleriola I, Rodriguez-Gonzalez J. Nonimmunologic hydrops fetalis: an etiopathogenetic approach through the postmortem study of 59 patients. Am J Med Genet 1996; 35:274–279.
9. Jauniaux E, van Maldergem L, De Munter C, Moscoso G, Gillerot Y. Nonimmune hydrops fetalis associated with genetic abnormalities. Obstet Gynecol 1990; 75:568–572.
10. McCoy MC, Katz VL, Gould N, Kuller JA. Nonimmune hydrops after 20 weeks gestation: Review of 10 years' experience with suggestions for management. Obstet Gynecol 1995; 85:578–582.
11. Sebire NJ, Bianco D, Snijders RJM, Zuckerman M, Nicolaides KH. Increased fetal nuchal thickness at 10–14 weeks: is screening for maternal–fetal infection necessary? Br J Obstet Gynaecol 1997; 104:212–215.
12. van Maldergem L, Jauniaux E, Forneau C, Gillerot Y. Genetic causes of hydrops fetalis. Pediatrics 1992; 89:81–86.
13. Boyd AA, Keeling JW. Fetal hydrops. J Med Genet 1992; 29:91–97.
14. Ayida GA, Soothill PW, Rodeck CH. Survival in nonimmune hydrops fetalis without malformation or chromosome abnormality after invasive treatment. Fetal Diagn Ther 1995; 10:101–105.
15. Smoliniec J, James D. Predictive value of pleural effusions in fetal hydrops. Fetal Diagn Ther 1995; 10:95–100.
16. Iskaros J, Jauniaux E, Rodeck CH. Outcome of nonimmune hydrops fetalis diagnosed during the first half of pregnancy. Obstet Gynecol 1997; 90:321–325.
17. Wilson RD, Venir N, Farquharson DF. Fetal nuchal fluid – physiological or pathological? – in pregnancies less than 17 menstrual weeks. Prenat Diagn 1992; 12:755–763.
18. Apkon M. Pathophysiology of hydrops fetalis. Semin Perinatol 1995; 19:437–446.
19. Brace RA. Effects of outflow pressure on fetal lymph flow. Am J Obstet Gynecol 1989; 160:494–497.
20. Blair DK, Vander Straten MC, Gest AL. Hydrops in fetal sheep from rapid induction of anaemia. Paed Res 1994; 35:560–564.
21. Gest AL, Martin CG, Moise AA, Hansen TN. Reversal of venous blood flow with atrial tachycardia and hydrops in fetal sheep. Paed Res 1990; 28:223–226.
22. Rice HE, Estes JM, Hendrick MH, Bealer JF, Harrison MR, Adzick NS. Congenital cystic adenomatoid malformation: a sheep model of fetal hydrops. J Paed Surg 1994; 29:692–696.
23. Weiner CP. Umbilical pressure measurement in the evaluation of nonimmune hydrops fetalis. Am J Obstet Gynecol 1993; 168:817–823.
24. Moise KJ, Carpenter RJ, Hesketh DE. Do abnormal Starling forces cause fetal hydrops in red blood cell alloimmunisation? Am J Obstet Gynecol 1992; 167:907–912.
25. Powell TL, Brace RA. Elevated fetal plasma lactate produces polyhydramnios. Am J Obstet Gynecol 1991; 165:1595–1607.
26. Silberbach M, Woods L, Hohimer AR, Shiota T, Matsuda Y, Davis LE. Role of endogenous atrial natriuretic peptide in chronic anaemia in the ovine fetus: Effect of a non-peptide antagonist for ANP receptor. Paed Res 1995; 38:772–778.

27. Halliday J, Lumley J, Bankier A. Karyotype abnormalities in fetuses diagnosed as abnormal on ultrasound before 20 weeks gestational age. Prenat Diagn 1994; 14:689–697.

28. Steiner RD. Hydrops fetalis: Role of the geneticist. Semin Perinatol 1995; 19:516–524.

29. Eronen M. Outcome of fetuses with heart disease diagnosed in utero. Arch Dis Child 1997; 77:F41–F46.

30. Knilans TK. Cardiac abnormalities associated with hydrops fetalis. Semin Perinatol 1995; 19:483–492.

31. Kanzaki T, Chiba Y. Evaluation of the preload condition of the fetus by inferior vena caval bloodflow pattern. Fetal Diagn Ther 1990; 5:168–174.

32. Chiba Y, Kobayashi H, Kanzaki T, Murakami T. Quantitative analysis of cardiac function in nonimmune hydrops fetalis. Fetal Diagn Ther 1990; 5:175–185.

33. Wladimiroff JW, Stewart PA, Tonge HM. Fetal bradyarrhythmia: Diagnosis and outcome. Prenat Diagn 1988; 8:53–57.

34. Litsey SE, Noonan JA, O'Connor WN, et al. Maternal connective tissue disease and congenital heart block: Demonstration of immunoglobulin in cardiac tissue. N Engl J Med 1985; 312:98–100.

35. Groves AMM, Fagg NLK, Cook AC, Allen LD. Cardiac tumours in intrauterine life. Arch Dis Child 1992; 67:1189–1192.

36. Jones DED, Pritchard KI, Gioannini CA, et al. Hydrops fetalis associated with idiopathic arterial calcification. Obstet Gynecol 1972; 39:435–440.

37. Forouzan I. Hydrops fetalis: Recent advances. Obstet Gynecol Survey 1997; 52:130–138.

38. Smoliniec J, Martin R, James DK. Intermittent fetal tachycardia and fetal hydrops. Arch Dis Child 1991; 66:1160–1161.

39. Frohn-Mulder IM, Stewart PA, Witsenburg M, DenHollander NS, Wladimiroff JW, Hess J. The efficacy of flecainide versus digoxin in the management of fetal supraventricular tachycardia. Prenat Diagn 1995; 15:1297–1302.

40. Blanch G, Walkinshaw SA, Walsh K. Cardioversion of fetal tachyarrhythmia with adenosine. Lancet 1994; 344:1646.

41. Groves AMM, Allen LD, Rosenthal E. Therapeutic trial of sympathomimetics in 3 cases of complete heart block in the fetus. Circulation 1995; 92:3394–3396.

42. Bierman FZ, Baxi I, Jaffe I, et al. Fetal hydrops and congenital complete heart block: response to maternal steroid therapy. J Pediatr 1988; 112:646–648.

43. Anandakumar C, Biswas A, Chen SSL, Chia D, Wong YC, Ratnam SS. Direct fetal therapy for hydrops secondary to congenital atrioventricular heart block. Obstet Gynecol 1996; 87:835–837.

44. Walkinshaw SA, Welch CR, McCormack J, Walsh K. In utero pacing for fetal congenital heart block. Fetal Diagn Ther 1994; 9:183–185.

45. Hernanz-Schulman M, Stein SM, Neblett WW, et al. Pulmonary sequestration: diagnosis with color Doppler sonography and a new theory of associated hydrothorax. Radiology 1991; 180:817–821.

46. Dolkart LA, Reimers FT, Helmuth WV, Porte MA, Eisinger G. Antenatal diagnosis of pulmonary sequestration: a review. Obstet Gynecol Survey 1992; 47:515–520.

47. da Silva O, Ramanan R, Romano W, Bocking A, Evans M. Nonimmune hydrops fetalis, pulmonary sequestration and favourable neonatal outcome. Obstet Gynecol 1996; 86:681–683.

48. Thorpe-Beeston JG, Nicolaides KH. Cystic adenomatoid malformation of the lung: prenatal diagnosis and outcome. Prenat Diagn 1994; 14:677–688.

49. Harrison M, Adzick N, Jennings R, et al. Antenatal intervention for congenital cystic adenomatoid malformation. Lancet 1990; 336:965–967.

50. Taguchi T, Suita S, Yamanouchi T, et al. Antenatal diagnosis and surgical management of congenital cystic adenomatoid malformation of the lung. Fetal Diagn Ther 1995; 10:400–407.

51. Adzick NS, Harrison MR, Hake AW, Howell LJ, Golbus MS, Filly RA. Fetal surgery for cystic adenomatoid malformation of the lung. J Paed Surg 1993; 28:806–812.

52. Clark SL, Vitale DJ, Minton SC, et al. Successful fetal therapy for cystic adenomatoid malformation associated with second trimester hydrops. Am J Obstet Gynecol 1987; 157:294–297.

53. Morrow RJ, MacPhail S, Johnson J-A, Ryan G, Farine D, Knox Ritchie JW. Midtrimester thoracoamniotic shunting for the treatment of fetal hydrops. Fetal Diagn Ther 1995; 10:92–94.

54. Turkel SB. Conditions associated with nonimmune hydrops fetalis. Clin Perinatol 1982; 9:613–625.

55. Herva R, Conradi NG, Kalimo H, Leisti J, Sourander P. A syndrome of multiple congenital contractures: neuropathological analysis on five fetal cases. Am J Med Genet 1988; 29:67–76.

56. Vuopala K, Herva R. Lethal congenital contracture syndrome: further delineation and genetic aspects. J Med Genet 1994; 31:521–529.

57. Cong KI, Shong HP. Hydrops fetalis and haemoglobinopathy. Chinese J Obstet Gynecol 1982; 17:226–228.

58. Tan SL, Tseng AMP, Thong T-W. Bart's hydrops fetalis – clinical presentation and management – an analysis of 25 cases. Aust NZ J Obstet Gynaecol 1989; 29:233–237.

59. Ghosh A, Tang MHY, Lam YH, et al. Ultrasound measurement of placental thickness to detect pregnancies affected by homozygous alpha-thalassaemia-1. Lancet 1994; 344:988–989.

60. Carr S, Rubin L, Dixon D, et al. Intrauterine therapy for homozygous alpha-thalassaemia. Obstet Gynecol 1995; 85:876–879.

61. Arcasoy MO, Gallagher PG. Haematological disorders and nonimmune hydrops fetalis. Semin Perinatol 1995; 19:502–515.

62. Mentzer WC, Collier E. Hydrops fetalis associated with erythrocyte G-6-PD deficiency and maternal ingestion of fava beans and ascorbic acid. J Pediatr 1975; 86:565–567.

63. Gilsanz F, Vega MA, Gomez-Castillo E, et al. Fetal anaemia due to pyruvate kinase deficiency. Arch Dis Child 1993; 69:523–524.

64. Ravindranath Y, Paglia DE, Warrier I, et al. Glucose phosphate isomerase deficiency as a cause of hydrops fetalis. N Engl J Med 1987; 316:258–261.

65. Donnenfeld AE, Scott SC, Henselder-Kimmel M, Dampier CD. Prenatally diagnosed nonimmune hydrops caused by congenital transient leukaemia. Prenat Diagn 1994; 14:721–724.

66. Hendricks SK, Sorensen TK, Baker ER. Trisomy 21, fetal hydrops, and anaemia: prenatal diagnosis of transient myeloproliferative disorder? Obstet Gynecol 1993; 82:703–705.

67. Nunez E, Varela S, Cervilla K, et al. Hydrops fetalis caused by congenital leukaemia. Rev Child Pediatr 1991; 62:186–188.

68. Ville Y, Proudler A, Abbas A, Nicolaides KH. Atrial natriuretic factor concentration in normal, growth retarded, anemic and hydropic fetuses. Am J Obstet Gynecol 1994; 171:777–783.

69. Maxwell DJ, Johnson P, Hurley P, et al. Fetal blood sampling and pregnancy loss in relation to indication. Br J Obstet Gynaecol 1991; 98:892–897.

70. Barron SD, Pass RF. Infectious causes of hydrops fetalis. Semin Perinatol 1995; 19:493–501.

71. Fadel HE, Ruedrich DA. Intrauterine resolution of nonimmune hydrops associated with cytomegalovirus infection. Obstet Gynecol 1988; 71:1003–1005.

72. Im SS, Rizos N, Jouts P, et al. Nonimmunological hydrops fetalis. Am J Obstet Gynecol 1984; 148:566–569.

73. Barton JR, Thorpe EM, Shaver DC, et al. Nonimmune hydrops fetalis associated with maternal infection with syphilis. Am J Obstet Gynecol 1992; 167:56–58.

74. El Tabbakh GH, Elejalde BR, Broekhuizen FF. Primary syphilis and nonimmune hydrops in a penicillin-allergic woman. J Reprod Med 1994; 39:412–414.

75. Towbin JA, Griffith LD, Martin AB, et al. Intrauterine adenoviral myocarditis presenting as nonimmune hydrops fetalis: diagnosis by polymerase chain reaction. Pediatr Infect Dis J 1994; 13:144–150.

76. Levy R, Weissman A, Blomberg G, Hagay ZJ. Infection by parvovirus B19 during pregnancy: a review. Obstet Gynecol Survey 1997; 52:254–259.

77. Rodis JF, Quinn DL, Gary W Jnr, et al. Management and outcomes of pregnancies complicated by human B19 parvovirus infection: a prospective study. Am J Obstet Gynecol 1990; 163:1168–1171.

78. Petrikovsky BM, Baker D, Schneider E. Fetal hydrops secondary to human parvovirus infection in early pregnancy. Prenat Diagn 1996; 16:342–344.

79. Fairley CK, Smoleniec JS, Caul OE, Miller E. Observational study of effect of intrauterine transfusion on outcome of fetal hydrops after parvovirus B19 infection. Lancet 1995; 346:1335–1337.

80. Sheikh AU, Ernest JM, O'Shea M. Long term outcome in fetal hydrops from fetal parvovirus B19 infection. Am J Obstet Gynecol 1992; 167:337–341.

81. Carbillon L, Oury J-F, Guerin J-M, Azancot A. Clinical biological features of Ballantyne's syndrome and the role of placental hydrops. Obstet Gynecol Survey 1997; 52:310–314.

82. Duthie J, Walkinshaw SA. Parvovirus associated fetal hydrops: reversal of pregnancy induced proteinuric hypertension by in utero transfusion. Br J Obstet Gynaecol 1995; 102:1011–1013.

83. Pinette MG, Pan Y, Pinette SG, Blackstome J, Stubblefield PG. A new approach to the treatment of nonimmune hydrops associated with polyhydramnios using therapeutic amniocentesis and maternal digoxin. J Maternal Fetal Investigation 1995; 5:254–259.

CHAPTER 18

Intra-uterine therapy

Mark D. Kilby
Martin J. Whittle

Introduction

The continuing improvements in ultrasound technology have enhanced our ability to inspect and examine the fetus which now has a similar status to that of any other patient. This has led to a revolution in fetal diagnosis. Ultrasonography enables the specialist to perform tests and other investigations which confirm or refute the provisional diagnosis and so consider methods of treatment (some intra-uterine) that might improve fetal prognosis.

As with all treatment modalities, intra-uterine therapy may be medical, transplacental or direct pharmacological or surgical therapy in which ultrasound is used to guide needles and catheters into fetal body cavities. The introduction of fetal surgical procedures also means that the natural history of some disorders can be modified. This has transformed the way that we now think about fetal disease and has raised a number of complex moral and ethical questions about the risks and benefits of such therapy.

The impetus for fetal therapy has come from a number of directions. Paediatricians and paediatric surgeons have been frustrated by caring for babies with diseases that were already uncorrectable at birth. In addition, ultrasonographers have been increasingly able to identify and diagnose the presence of fetal disease and considered the possibility that intervention in utero may improve survival by influencing the natural history of the disorder. Before fetal therapy can be considered, there are a number of important points to establish. The natural history of the disease process (either congenital or acquired) should be understood and studied by serial examinations of the untreated fetus. Understanding is often enhanced by experimental work using animal models to assess the feasibility of fetal therapy. Such work is multidisciplinary, involving the skills and talents of doctors from all branches of perinatal medicine as part of a team which includes obstetricians, radiologists, geneticists, paediatricians and paediatric surgeons. The critical importance of counselling by the provision of accurate information and psychological support cannot be over-emphasized. Because of its multidisciplinary approach, fetal therapy is often performed in specialized 'tertiary referral' centres. All work performed should be strenuously audited. The acquisition of case details in the form of a prospective database will aid both assessment and potential improvements in practice.[1]

This chapter reviews both established and novel forms of fetal therapy and discusses the use of such therapy in the light of our knowledge of pathogenesis.

General aspects

Prior to any consideration of intra-uterine therapy, a detailed assessment of both the maternal and fetal condition should be made. It is also vital that the views and wishes of the mother are taken into account. It should be possible from both history and examination to ascertain maternal risk factors (both causative, as in the case of maternal red cell alloimmunization or coexistent) whilst the assessment of the fetal prognosis may be enhanced by the use of further investigations. The clear 'visualization' of the fetus using ultrasound is obviously extremely important. Systematic examination will provide important information, including the gestational age, the number of fetuses, their viability and the presence and severity (morphologically) of any structural anomaly. Such information will of course determine both the suitability of the fetus for potential treatment and influence the parents' decision to have further investigations performed prior to undertaking specific therapy.

Factors, such as the exclusion of karyotypic anomalies, will be important and need to be discussed in some depth with the parents. It may be that the type of structural abnormality carries a specific risk of a chromosomal anomaly which adversely affects prognosis, as in congenital diaphragmatic hernia[2] or that ultrasound 'markers' or maternal age increase the chance of a coexistent anomaly.[3] Under these circumstances, a relatively rapid method of fetal karyotyping is often chosen (i.e. fetal blood sampling), the risk of which is dependent upon the 'wellbeing' of the fetus.[4] This and other techniques of fetal karyotyping are discussed elsewhere in this text.

Multiple pregnancies carry their own particular problems, mainly as a result of chorionicity and the presence of other risk factors,[5,6] such as the chance of chromosome anomaly and potential interventions such as selective reduction.[7] The prospective identification of monochorionicity is important in pathologies such as the twin–twin (feto–fetal) transfusion syndrome.

The general 'wellbeing' of the fetus is also an important factor to establish. The co-existence of fetal hydrops with a unilateral hydrothorax may indicate the need for intervention such as drainage, whereas a small 'rim' of pleural effusion in an otherwise healthy fetus may be more appropriately observed, although karyotyping would be considered.

Counselling prospective parents is a vital part of fetal medicine and is essential, prior to the initiation of any in utero therapy. It involves imparting accurate information to both the woman and her partner and, if appropriate, to the wider family and helping these individuals to understand the problems affecting their baby. This process involves often frank, detailed discussion and the provision of considerable psychological support. The benefits and risks of potential therapies need to be discussed, often using a multidisciplinary approach, along with the anticipated results and alternative strategies for management. The practical aspects of any procedures must be carefully explained both prior to and during any therapy in order that informed consent is obtained. It is the habit of the authors to obtain written informed consent. Such discussions should be performed in an unhurried, calm environment where both privacy and confidentiality are guaranteed. It is important that such information is provided in understandable language; due consideration must be given to the patient's education and ethnic background. Such discussions are often usefully reinforced by trained counselling nursing/midwifery staff. The couple should feel that they are not under pressure to make a rapid decision and should be given time to reflect. There is some evidence that a taped copy of the discussions surrounding the case given to the parents to keep and re-play at a later date may enhance understanding (Dr G. Rylance, personal communication).

Because of the multidisciplinary nature of fetal assessment and therapy, expertise will usually be concentrated in teaching hospitals although some tertiary referral centres do exist in big District General Hospitals. Regardless of the site, considerable experience in all aspects of obstetric ultrasound and high-risk pregnancy management is required if appropriate action is to be taken in any given circumstance. It is essential that obstetric units offering such a service audit their work and maintain sufficient experience to both maintain expertise and minimize risks to the fetus.

Specific examples of fetal therapy

In general terms, intra-uterine therapy can be given either indirectly (via pharmacological treatment given to the mother) or directly, either as a medical or surgical intervention to the fetus.

Fetal cardiovascular disease

Fetal dysrhythmias

The majority of disturbances of fetal cardiac rhythm are noted either incidentally during auscultation of the fetal heart or during sonographic examination. Such fetuses require careful evaluation to establish the electrophysiological mechanism of the arrhythmia. The type of arrhythmia can be established using fetal M-mode echocardiography, duplex-pulsed Doppler imaging and colour-encoded M-mode echocardiography. Ultrasound, in experienced hands, can exclude serious structural cardiac anomalies and make a prospective diagnosis with good sensitivity and specificity.[8,9] Such determination is of course different from the sensitivity and specificity described for 'screening' programmes. Correct diagnosis is obviously of importance, so that suitable therapy can be considered and instituted. The overall condition of the fetus and the ultrasound exclusion of hydrops are important both in terms of the choice of therapies and in delineating the overall prognosis.

One of the most common pathological fetal dysrhythmias is supraventricular tachycardia (SVT), most often caused by reciprocating or atrioventricular re-entrant tachycardia.[10] The ventricular rate is always rapid (240–260 beats.min^{-1}) and if incessant may cause heart failure and fetal hydrops. The need for therapy must be based upon the logical analysis of a number of factors. These include gestational age, the presence or absence of fetal hydrops and the duration of the tachycardia. The presence of fetal hydrops indicates a severe or long-standing problem which carries with it a considerable risk of perinatal mortality and as such, these fetuses are often better candidates for in utero rather than postnatal therapy.

In the absence of hydrops, the assessment of whether the arrhythmia is continuous or intermittent may be ascertained by the use of ultrasound and continuous fetal heart rate monitoring for a prolonged period. Doppler studies of the venous circulation, especially the inferior vena cava, may indicate the presence of sustained retrograde flow during atrial ectopy or increased venous flow secondary to premature, partial closure of the foramen ovale, both of which may precede the early onset of hydrops fetalis.[11]

Treatment in the prenatal period relies upon the use of pharmacological agents, many of them chosen because of their success in neonatal/infant life. Physical techniques which transiently increase vagal tone, such as cord compression, may cause short-term atrioventricular block and cessation of the arrhythmia,[12] but such techniques are

intermittent in their success and are not usually appropriate. Maternal oral digoxin therapy induces resolution of this dysrhythmia in 60% of cases and is probably still the mainstay therapy because of its longstanding use, efficacy and safety and the fact that it is a positive inotropic agent.[10] The dose required to achieve therapeutic serum levels (1.5–2 ng.ml^{-1}) is often relatively high, 0.5–1 mg.day^{-1}. The problems with 'transplacental' therapy are the unreliable pharmacodynamics and kinetics which may be affected at a number of levels and may adversely affect efficacy. Maternal pharmacokinetics of drugs are altered in pregnancy as a result of the increased volume of distribution and clearance whether renal or hepatic.[13] Placental transfer of drugs is complex and depends upon the structure and hydrophilic properties of the molecule to be transferred. In addition, the drug itself may undergo metabolism within the placenta and all of these mechanisms may be significantly altered in the presence of hydropic change in the placenta itself.[14] Because of these and fetal pharmacokinetic alterations,[15] other pharmacological agents and possibly direct, parenteral administration to the fetus are sometimes necessary. In the 40% of fetuses that do not demonstrate a sustained response to maternal oral digoxin therapy, second line drugs such as flecainide[16,17] or verapamil[18] are required. Alternatively, drugs such as digoxin may be given directly into the fetal circulation by intravascular infusion. This approach bypasses the problems of maternal–placental drug transfer[19] and has proved effective in some cases. The increasing use of 'medical cardioversion' of SVT with adenosine in the postnatal period[20] has led to the direct instillation of adenosine into the fetal venous circulation with resolution of the dysrhythmia and survival of the fetus.[21]

Other fetal tachydysrhythmias require equally careful assessment and management. These are much rarer but the clinical experience using anti-arrhythmic drugs is well described.[22] Fetal bradycardias are relatively rare and are defined as a fetal heart rate which is persistently below

100 beats.min^{-1}. The most frequently seen bradycardia is that of complete heart block. Again, careful fetal assessment, especially to exclude a structural cardiac anomaly such as left or right atrial isomerism, is vital. When complicated by fetal hydrops, there is a high perinatal mortality.[23] The association with maternal autoimmune disease and specifically the presence of circulating maternal anti-SSA/R$_0$ and anti-SSB/L$_a$ is well described, with their antibodies having a particular predilection for the fetal cardiac conduction system.[24] The detection of such maternal antibodies is important as there is the potential for therapy. The use of maternally administered dexamethasone (4 mg each day) has been described in a very small study with evidence of fetal ventricular response.[25] A large study would be required but the rareness of the condition would make placebo-controlled trials impractical. Unfortunately, other approaches such as the use of pro-arrhythmic agents[26] and direct fetal pacing have not demonstrated sustained success[27] and carry risks of maternal morbidity and mortality.

Structural fetal cardiac anomalies

Techniques to gain access to the fetal heart in utero are rare and much of the literature describes the transcutaneous placement of an intracardiac catheter in the attempted management of complete heart block. However, serial fetal echocardiography has indicated how critical outflow (aortic or pulmonary) stenosis can affect ventricular development. Percutaneous placement of catheters into the fetal ventricles, either left[28] or right,[29,30] to allow dilatation of the outflow valvular obstruction has been described, with seemingly improved ventricular development. However, such operations are experimental and carry fetal mortality.

Maternal alloimmunization syndromes

Red cell alloimmunization

Direct fetal therapy. In alloimmune red cell haemolytic disease, the fetus becomes anaemic from the transplacental passage of relevant maternal antibodies. In the 1990s, the process is mostly commonly due to anti-D but anti-C may also produce severe problems. Anti-Kell antibodies[31] can cause severe anaemia in utero through a combination of both increased red cell destruction and erythroid cell hypoplasia.

This condition carries a high perinatal loss rate and its treatment represents one of the earliest attempts at in utero therapy in the human fetus and it was Liley[32] who first described intraperitoneal transfusion via a catheter placed under fluoroscopic control into the fetal peritoneal cavity.

Initial attempts to gain access to the fetal circulation were by open hysterotomy. The more recent advances of fetoscopic blood sampling[33] and subsequently ultrasound-guided fetal blood sampling[34] meant that for the first time there was direct access to the fetal circulation. Bang et al[35] reported a successful intravascular transfusion via the intrahepatic tract of the umbilical vein (Fig. 18.1). Daffos[34] described the technique

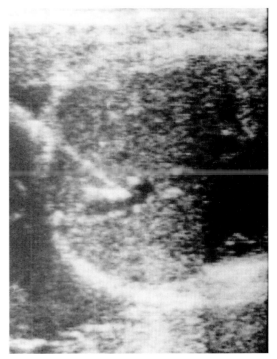

Fig. 18.1 The percutaneous insertion of a 21 gauge needle under ultrasound guidance into the fetal intrahepatic vein.

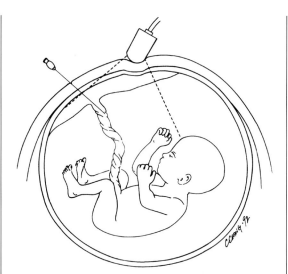

Fig. 18.2 Cordocentesis involves fetal blood sampling by the placement of an ultrasound-guided needle into the umbilical cord.

of fetal blood sampling using a 20 gauge needle inserted transplacentally or transamniotically into the umbilical cord (Fig. 18.2). Ultrasound-directed fetal cardiac puncture was also introduced in 1983 with the insertion of a 1.2 mm diameter into the fetal thorax; and a second 0.7 mm needle being advanced into the right or left ventricle of the fetal heart, thus allowing pure blood sampling and transfusion.[36] This was only advocated in extreme circumstances when other circulatory sites were not accessible.

Ultrasound-guided fetal blood transfusion is now a widely practised technique. Fetal blood sampling is always undertaken as a prelude to transfusion to assess the need for treatment.[37–39] Whatever the site of access to the fetal circulation, fetal blood sampling is generally performed as an outpatient procedure, with local anaesthesia and sedation rarely being necessary. Antibiotic prophylaxis and administration of β-mimetics, although adopted by some centres, are of unproven value. An aseptic technique, with the transducer wrapped in a sterile plastic bag, is commonly, but not universally preferred. Just prior to the procedure, the preferred site of sampling is identified. A variety of ultrasound transducers have been advocated (sector,

linear and curvilinear). It seems, however, that excellent resolution, rather than a specific field of view, is the main variable when choosing the ultrasound equipment. Either a single- or two-operator technique is used. Confirmation that uncontaminated fetal blood has been aspirated is provided immediately by comparing the sample's mean cell volume distribution in a particle size analyzer to that of the mother and estimation of the fetal haemoglobin performed. Some operators use transient fetal paralysis usually with vecuronium to reduce potential injury to either viscera or the umbilical cord.[40] The needle insertion should be visualized by the operator throughout the procedure and checks on cardiac activity should be made. Careful arrangements should be made to label specimens obtained from the fetus and their urgent transportation to the relevant laboratories. Concise but accurate information should accompany these samples, so that results may be interpreted in the light of clinical information.

When a transfusion is considered necessary, the blood products (usually fresh, antigen negative, irradiated, cytomegalovirus- and HIV-negative) are packed to reduce the volume needed for transfusion, typically to a haematocrit of between 70 and 80%. The rationale for this has been that the fetal heart is more able to cope with large changes in haematocrit rather than fetoplacental volume, although recent evidence both in anaemic fetal sheep[41] and in humans,[42] questions this. The rapid infusion of blood produces ultrasonically visible 'turbulence'. The volume of donor blood required to achieve a satisfactory final fetal haematocrit (usually between 35 and 45%) is dependent upon the donor blood haematocrit, the initial fetal haematocrit and the estimated fetoplacental volume.[43] However, when the fetus is severely anaemic and hydropic, the final haematocrit should not exceed 25% or four times the initial haematocrit, so as to minimize perinatal loss owing to cardiac overload.[44] The inter-transfusion interval can usually be increased with successive procedures, as the proportion of circulating cells caused by transfusion increases (Fig. 18.3).

Following intrahepatic vein sampling, an intra-abdominal echo-free area detected by ultrasonography suggests intraperitoneal bleeding, an event described in only 2% of fetuses.[45] In contrast with extravasation during transfusion at the placental cord insertion, it is of little consequence and is usually absorbed within a few days. The trans-hepatic approach is undoubtedly safer, extravasation in the cord producing bradycardia and often fetal death. After withdrawing the needle, bleeding into the amniotic cavity is almost always seen on ultrasound when the site of sampling is the umbilical cord with a posterior placenta. Overall, most series have reported a 12 to 41% frequency of intra-amniotic bleeding. When the sample is transplacental, bleeding into the amniotic fluid is rarely observed. However, fetomaternal haemorrhage occurs in approximately 70% of patients, and the mean volume of blood, which is lost with this mechanism, is estimated at around 3% of the total fetoplacental blood volume.[46]

Difficulties in sampling from the placental cord insertion may arise in cases of polyhydramnios, oligohydramnios, maternal obesity or when the fetus obscures a posterior cord insertion. Occasionally, it may be helpful to empty or fill the maternal bladder, or to perform external manipulation to move the fetus.

Each transfusion procedure carries a perinatal loss rate of approximately 3%. The survival of babies with fetal anaemia that undergo transfusion is dependent upon the experience of the operator, the gestation and the condition of the fetus at diagnosis. Hydropic fetuses have a survival of at least 80% compared to 90% in those without hydrops.[47] There is evidence also, that the fetuses treated in utero demonstrate normal growth velocity, so that at delivery the birthweights of the transfused babies were not significantly different from gestationally-matched controls.[48] Similarly, small prospective studies of neurodevelopmental follow-up in these babies indicate no long-term morbidity in the transfused fetuses if they survive.[49]

Other therapies. Many alternative therapies for alloimmune fetal anaemia have been described either used in isolation or to supplement intravascular transfusions. Oral administration of both promethazine[50] and rhesus-positive erythrocyte membranes[51] have been tried but have not proved advantageous. Plasmophoresis and plasma exchange therapy have been advocated in women with very high circulating antibody levels,[52] and although it has not significantly reduced the need for intravascular transfusion, it may delay the gestational age at which transfusions are started. Clearly, the later the better, the procedure having significantly lower mortality at 24 weeks compared with 20 weeks. Alternatively, intraperitoneal transfusions could be used from 16 weeks to reduce fetal anaemia until 20 to 24 weeks' gestation when intravascular transfusions could be initiated. The use of maternal administration of hyperimmune globulin has been described in two dose regimens of 1 g.kg^{-1} weekly[53,54] and 0.4 g.kg^{-1} every 2 weeks intravenously.[55] Such therapy is very expensive and, given current evidence, of doubtful efficacy. The mechanism of action is thought to be through the saturation of the F$_c$-transporter system on the placenta, thus reducing

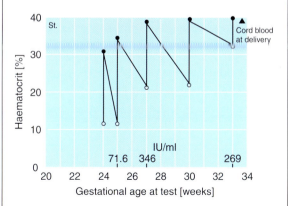

Fig. 18.3 A 'transfusogram', indicating the fetal haematocrit pre- and post-intra-uterine, intravascular transfusions (IVT). The 'inter-transfusion interval' increases (commonly) with successive IVT as a result of suppression of endogenous fetal haematopoiesis.

endogenous IgG transfer to the fetoplacental circulation.

Haemopoietic stem cell transplantation is a theoretical possibility in the fetus affected by maternal red cell alloimmunization. The fetus, in the first trimester, has immune tolerance to a foreign antigen, resulting in the induction of specific transplantation tolerance.[56] Long-standing haematopoietic chimerism in primates has been achieved without the need for immunosuppression[57] and the resulting chimeric cell line is capable of responding to anaemia-induced stress.[58]

Fetal alloimmune thrombocytopaenia

Alloimmune thrombocytopaenia is the platelet equivalent of rhesus disease caused commonly by the presence of either anti-human platelet antigen (HPA)1 or HPA2 (although other membrane-related glycoprotein antigens exist: HPA1 to 5). As with rhesus disease, in the HPA-positive father it is essential to investigate the paternal genotype, so that zygosity can be confirmed. Clinically, the fetus may be asymptomatic at birth, or may have objective minor sequelae such as purpura or echymosis. Major morbidity exists in the form of prenatal intracerebral haemorrhage in approximately 23% of cases[59] or mortality of 2%. These major complications have been described as early as 20 weeks' gestation. Thus, prolonged prenatal fetal therapy is required. As with rhesus disease, this may take the form of maternal therapy, such as hyperimmune globulin (1 g.kg^{-1} given intravenously weekly[54] or oral low-dose dexamethasone therapy.[60] A randomized prospective study indicates that dexamethasone confers no particular advantage and is not recommended. The direct therapeutic approach requires fetal blood sampling and serial platelet transfusions, if the fetal platelet count is less than 50 000 mm^3. The circulating half-life of platelets is 11 days and thus rationally this therapy will need to be repeated every 7 to 10 days. Such therapy carries significant risks of exsanguination from the site of blood sampling. It may be that combined therapy reduces the inter-transfusion interval, although little objective evidence presently exists concerning such treatment.

Fetal urinary tract obstruction

Urine sampling and the placement of vesico-amniotic shunts

Bladder obstruction arises usually as a result of posterior urethral valves in a male fetus. This typically produces the ultrasound appearances of a distended, often thick-walled, bladder and posterior urethra, associated with bilateral hydronephrosis and hydroureters.[61] A catheter or shunt may be inserted into the fetal bladder or dilated renal filling system to drain urine into the amniotic cavity, thus bypassing the obstruction and preventing fetal kidney damage.

Although it is possible to bypass the obstruction by the insertion of shunts, the efficacy of this procedure remains in doubt for two main reasons. Firstly, there are considerable difficulties in selecting appropriate cases. Secondly, the ability to evaluate renal function is generally unsatisfactory. Oligohydramnios, although associated with a generally poor prognostic sign, may relate more to the degree of obstruction than the severity of renal damage. The ultrasound appearances of fetal kidneys have a low sensitivity and specificity in the diagnosis of renal dysplasia. Renal cysts are only visualized in 44% of dysplastic kidneys, and only 40% of kidneys without ultrasound evidence of cysts are free of dysplastic change.[62] The conventional indices of poor renal function in the adult are normal in fetal blood, even in the most severe forms of renal failure, so that analytes in aspirated urine from the fetal bladder, or selectively from each renal pelvis are an objective method in the assessment of renal function.

The dilated portion of the urinary tract is usually easy to sample and the procedure can be repeated at regular intervals, in order to provide sequential data and therefore significant trends in the analytes.[63] Longer delay is necessary if serial evolution of renal function needs to be assessed in doubtful cases. The value of urinary electrolytes in the prediction of long-term renal outcome remains in doubt.[64]

Ranges of different biochemical indices in fetal urine with gestation have been produced from cross-sectional data of individually sampled fetuses with normal renal function.[65] Urinary sodium and phosphate have been found to decrease, while creatinine increases with gestational age, possibly reflecting progressive maturation of tubular function and increase in glomerular filtration rate. In fetuses with lower urinary tract obstruction, urine sodium, calcium and phosphate have been prospectively demonstrated to show a significant correlation with the degree of renal impairment, with the best sensitivity achieved by urinary calcium and the highest specificity by sodium.

Urine biochemistry of fluid aspirated from large fetal cystic renal masses, unassociated with bladder dilatation, may help to distinguish hydronephrosis from multicystic kidney in difficult cases in which mis-identification has been reported in more than 50% of cases. Whereas urinary phosphate is normal in all fetuses with hydronephrosis, irrespective of the degree of renal damage, all those with multicystic kidney have raised levels. Given the different outcome and risk of chromosomal abnormalities between the two conditions, sampling an uncertain renal mass may thus help counselling and perinatal management.

Drainage procedures, however, are restricted to very specific situations. If normal liquor is consistently present and the degree of dilatation of the urinary tract remains constant or only unilateral renal obstruction is present, there seems little need for vesico- or reno-amniotic shunting. The risks of the procedure are considerable and the benefits poorly defined. However, in one study of 40 cases who had vesico-amniotic shunting procedures, 38% (15 cases) ended in abortion/intra-uterine fetal death.[66] Such 'pigtailed' shunts (Rodeck catheter, Rocket Ltd, London: Fig. 18.4) are inserted under direct ultrasound guidance with maternal sedation and local anaesthesia, using the Rocket trochar system (Fig. 18.5).

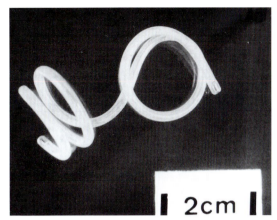

Fig. 18.4 A 'pigtail' catheter for insertion into a fetal viscous or body cavity.

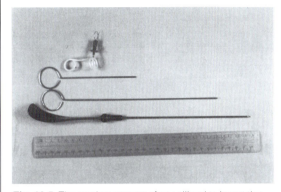

Fig. 18.5 The trochar system often utilized to insert the 'pigtail' catheter.

The uncertainty arises in bilateral hydronephrosis which is increasing in severity together with worsening oligohydramnios. There are difficulties, however, as in certain cases when the obstruction has been present from an early stage in pregnancy, permanent renal damage will have occurred in the form of renal dysplasia. As has already been discussed, the predictive ability of ultrasound to identify accurately such dysplasia is relatively poor. Renal dysplasia may be severe at an early gestation and thus objective renal function will not recover (even after a shunting procedure to relieve the obstruction). Aspiration of urine from the fetal bladder and assessing the sodium and chloride concentrations can be useful in assessing renal function. A sodium content of less than

100 mEq.l^{-1} and a chloride content of less than 90 mEq.l^{-1} carry a favourable prognosis and indicate that the kidneys are functioning, but again sensitivity and specificity have been variably described.[67] The vesico-amniotic shunting procedure therefore is limited to very specific situations where liquor is decreasing, the hydronephrosis is deteriorating and the urinary sodium and chloride are normal. It should also be stated quite clearly that little prospective information is available in the form of a postnatal register indicating long-term prognosis and morbidity.

There is an urgent need for multicentred data to be collected so that the natural history of such conditions and their long-term morbidity and mortality can be accurately defined. The paucity of such data at the present time gives little objective evidence to indicate an advantage to vesico-amniotic shunt procedures.

Fetal cystoscopy

With advances in high-resolution ultrasound and fibre optics, the use of a flexible endoscope (< 0.7 mm) down an 18 gauge needle has allowed video-fetoscopy to be performed. These techniques have been extended to fetal cystoscopy, for direct inspection of the trigone, ureteric orifices and the upper urethra (Fig. 18.6). Such visualization would technically allow laser or diathermization of a congenital bladder neck obstruction.[68] The risks of thin-gauge flexible fetoscopy are evident in terms of amniotic leakage (10%), infection (0.5%) and fetal death (2%). Again, although such techniques are potentially exciting, their use should be audited and tempered until the natural history of the underlying condition is fully elucidated.

Pleural effusions

Fetal pleural effusions (Fig. 18.7) occur in approximately 1 per 10 000 pregnancies and may be either primary, when they are usually caused by a chylothorax,[69] or secondary as a result of aneuploidy or infection. They are often associated with non-

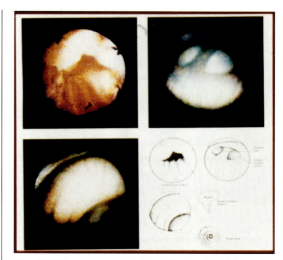

Fig. 18.6 The cystoscopic view of the fetal bladder 'trigone'. The fetoscope was inserted into the fetal bladder via an ultrasound-guided needle. (Reproduced by permission of the Editor of *The Lancet*.)

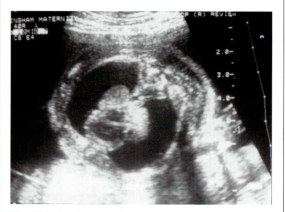

Fig. 18.7 An ultrasound image, demonstrating bilateral pleural effusions in a transverse section of the fetal chest.

immune hydrops fetalis. The outcome for fetal pleural effusions depends on four factors: the aetiology, the presence of hydrops fetalis, the timing of the delivery and prenatal therapy. A full assessment of the fetus must be carried out first to determine aetiology, including detailed ultrasonography to exclude coincidental abnormalities. Fetal echocardiography should exclude cardiac anomalies and a fetal karyotyping is recommended because of the high association with aneuploidy.[70] The overall perinatal mortality is approximately 50% and associated anomalies are seen in 40%.

The pleural fluid initially can be aspirated and analysis may give an indication as to its aetiology. The presence of high mononuclear counts is diagnostic of a chylothorax,[71] although with variable sensitivity.

Overall, spontaneous resolution occurs in about 10% of cases. When effusions are seen before 32 weeks, the management may be conservative if there is no evidence of fetal hydrops and is probably appropriate as long as the effusion is stable or decreasing.

Fetal hydrops is initially visualized or develops in 50% of cases and 61% of these fetuses eventually die. With the development of fetal ascites and hydrops or if the hydrothorax is increasing, then therapy should be considered, in the form of either serial thoracocentesis (Fig. 18.8) or the placement of a thoraco-amniotic shunt (Fig. 18.9). Some data indicate that in the non-hydropic fetus, those treated conservatively have a survival rate of 83% and in hydropic babies the survival was as low as 12%. However, serial thoracocentesis and thoraco-amniotic shunt insertion improve survival, especially in the hydropic cohort.[72] Such therapy may reverse fetal hydrops and polyhydramnios thus reducing the risk of preterm delivery. The extent to which it improves lung development and prevents pulmonary hypoplasia is unknown. Again, little long-term follow-up data in terms of neonatal/childhood survival and

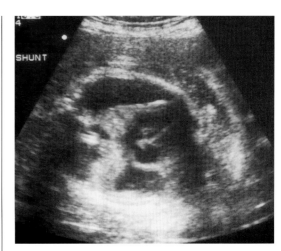

Fig. 18.9 The ultrasound image, post-insertion of a 'pigtail' catheter into the fetal thorax with a hydrothorax.

morbidity are known and prospective evaluation is required.

The management of oligohydramnios/polyhydramnios

The amniotic fluid surrounds the fetus and is in constant homeostasis with the epithelial surfaces like the skin and the lining of the respiratory and gastrointestinal systems and the amniotic membrane lining the uterine cavity and placenta.[73] Changes in amniotic fluid volume are constantly occurring and alter with gestational age. However, this delicate homeostasis may be disturbed in a heterogeneous group of aetiologies of fetal, placental and maternal origin. The alteration of this balance and the appearance of either too much amniotic fluid (polyhydramnios) or too little (oligohydramnios) have an adverse and quantifiable effect on perinatal morbidity and mortality.[74,75] The rationale for treatment is very much dependent on the underlying aetiology of the anomaly. The detailed assessment of the fetus should exclude potentially lethal structural anomalies, such as renal agenesis and associated chromosomal abnormalities. However, there is a small and well-defined cohort of fetuses in which oligohydramnios is present (i.e. early pre-labour rupture of membranes or bladder outflow obstruction with good renal function) for which

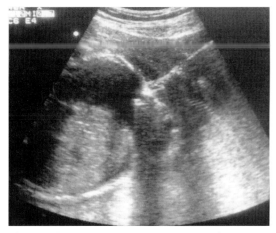

Fig. 18.8 The ultrasound-guided placement of a percutaneous needle into the fetal thorax for investigation and drainage of a pleural effusion.

treatment modalities may be of some use, mainly in an attempt to prevent pulmonary hypoplasia.

In polyhydramnios arising as a result of salvageable structural anomalies, or occasionally in idiopathic cases, both medical and surgical therapy to reduce amniotic fluid may be attempted in a bid to prevent preterm labour, and also to make the mother more comfortable. Of special note is the management of oligohydramnios/ polyhydramnios sequence in monochorionic twinning, often secondary to feto–fetal transfusion.

Oligohydramnios

Amniotic fluid instillation. This technique has been used by a number of workers both as a diagnostic and a therapeutic procedure in oligohydramnios. Whatever the cause of severe oligohydramnios, the prognosis is generally poor and, in the absence of chromosomal or structural anomalies, is mainly related to pulmonary hypoplasia. The actual risk of pulmonary hypoplasia with gestational age in pregnancies complicated by oligohydramnios has been objectively defined.[76] If there is a calculated high probability of associated pulmonary hypoplasia, then termination of pregnancy should be discussed as the prognosis is poor. In selected cases, serial transabdominal amnioinfusions may be considered in an attempt to prevent the progression of pulmonary hypoplasia. It should be stated that the ultrasound predictors of pulmonary hypoplasia, other than severe oligohydramnios, are extremely poor. Prerequisite is a correct ultrasound diagnosis, which is often difficult, because of poor ultrasound visualization of fetal anatomy. Adequate 'views' are often impeded by the lack of an acoustic window and a frequently abnormal lie.

Transabdominal instillation of artificial amniotic fluid has recently been proposed to improve the ultrasound image. Following amnioinfusion, diagnosis of the aetiology of oligohydramnios was correctly revised in 13% of cases[77] but the use for this approach diminished with the use of both colour flow and power Doppler to visualize the renal arteries.[78] In the first reported series,[79] rupture of membranes and preterm labour occurred in 10.5% of cases following a single intra-amniotic infusion and in 28.9% overall, thus suggesting that amnioinfusion may be a potentially hazardous procedure. However, when intra-amniotic pressure was monitored throughout the procedure and excessive increase in intra-uterine pressure was avoided,[80] vaginal leakage did not occur in any of 32 diagnostic or therapeutic amnioinfusions in patients with urinary tract disorders. An alternative explanation for the previously reported high frequency of amniotic fluid leakage is that pre-existing rupture of membranes may have been unmasked by amnioinfusion. Indeed, a history of vaginal leakage following rupture of membranes in early pregnancy is often unclear, possibly because of the small volume of amniotic fluid lost at this stage of gestation. Fisk[77] undertook 14 infusions on 9 women with severe oligohydramnios. Of these, 3 neonates survived, and 5 of the 6 fetuses who died in the perinatal period had normal lungs with no evidence of pulmonary hypoplasia. So amniotic fluid replacement may be useful as a form of treatment for the fetus with oligohydramnios to try to prevent the development of pulmonary hypoplasia. However, the potential maternal complications of acute infection must not be underestimated. The use of techniques such as maternal hydration remain anecdotal and of unproven benefit. This prenatal therapy should be differentiated from intrapartum amnioinfusion which meta-analysis has suggested may be of value in decreasing morbidity and mortality in cases where meconium staining of the liquor is present.[81]

Polyhydramnios

This is defined as excessive amniotic fluid volume and occurs in 3.2% of pregnancies.[75] Again, the aetiologies are diverse and careful ultrasound examination with the exclusion of fetal karyotypic abnormalities (5% of cases) and maternal disease such as glucose intolerance is essential. The association with fetal hydrops may indicate a possible karyotypic or viral aetiology to this process. This condition is associated with considerable excess perinatal mortality because of the association between fetal structural anomaly, uteroplacental perfusion abnormality and preterm labour. The intra-uterine pressure rises significantly once the maximal pool depth is greater than 120 ml.[77] Medical therapies have included the use of prostaglandin synthetase inhibitors, such as indomethacin,[82] which probably works via arginine vasopressin mechanism[83] to reduce fetal urine output. The potential side effects are both maternal, in terms of gastrointestinal irritation, fluid retention and potential coagulopathies and fetal, in terms of premature closure of the ductus arteriosus and cerebral vasoconstriction. The effects are dose-dependent and different regimens exist in the USA (200–400 mg.day^{-1}) and UK (75–100 mg.day^{-1}). It has a further disadvantage, in that it often takes 7 to 10 days before the excessive liquor starts to lessen. Other medical therapies, such as sulindac, are of interest, although they require further evaluation. Regular, intermittent amnioreduction is of benefit in the management of polyhydramnios and certainly reduces intra-amniotic pressure significantly. However, the procedure does carry risk of infection, preterm delivery and abruptio placentae.[84]

Amnioreduction is a feature of the management of feto–fetal transfusion in monochorionic twins. When the oligohydramnios/polyhydramnios sequence (OPS) presents in the mid-second trimester, it carries a high perinatal mortality.[85] The overall prognosis has been described as being dependent upon the gestation at onset, fetal growth discordance and amniotic fluid changes.[86] Several treatment options have been advocated for the management of the OPS twin syndrome. Medical treatment with indomethacin[87] or digoxin has been advocated, but widespread use has been made of serial amnioreductions[88] and more recently fetoscopic laser ablation of placental vessels.[89,90] Certainly, amnioreduction has the advantage of being relatively cheap and simple to perform, but there have been

concerns regarding the long-term neurodevelopmental outcomes of the surviving fetuses.[91] Our own series indicated an overall perinatal mortality rate of 44%, which is in concordance with other studies utilizing this method of therapy.[88,92] Much recent interest has focused on the fetoscopic laser ablation of aberrant fetoplacental vasculature.[89,90] A recent collaborative study has been reported comparing serial amniodrainage (n = 25) to laser coagulation (n = 75). This study used the same entry criteria for both treatment modalities[93] and thus a relatively homogenous sample was assumed, although the very heterogeneous aetiology of the 'stuck twin' syndrome makes this questionable.[94] However, the most important significant finding was of a reduced neurological handicap rate from 5% in the amnioreduction group as compared to 1.3% in those pregnancies undergoing laser coagulation. In the small prospective study reported here, only one surviving fetus suffered major demonstrable neurological pathology prior to its demise at 22 days post-delivery. Its co-twin also died in the early neonatal period. Of the eight remaining fetuses born alive all had no apparent ultrasound evidence of brain damage and ongoing follow-up has not to date indicated neurodevelopmental delay (range 3 to 11 months). It is conceded though, that a more formal neurological assessment at 2 and 5 years will be required.

Hydrocephalus/ventriculomegaly

In the early 1970s there was considerable interest in the antenatal treatment of hydrocephalus to improve eventual outcome. The rationale behind this treatment was based on the fact that as the cerebral ventricles increase in size, pressure is increased on the cerebral tissue leading to oedema of the white matter and eventual irreversible brain damage. If this sequence of events could be interrupted, then the amount of brain damage seen in babies with hydrocephalus could be reduced. Certain centres set up strict criteria for the in utero ventriculo-amniotic shunting of hydrocephalus. Unfortunately, not all centres adhered to these strict criteria and so shunts were placed in a number of inappropriate cases. The overall results of shunting were no better than conservative management and so for the last 10 years there has been an international moratorium on in utero treatment for fetal hydrocephalus.[95]

Fetal surgery

Open operations

The main work in this field has been carried out by Professor Michael Harrison, a paediatric surgeon at the Fetal Treatment Center in San Francisco. The main experience in this type of operation has been with congenital diaphragmatic herniae. These occur because there is a failure in closure of the pleuroperitoneal canal at 8 to 10 weeks' gestation. However, the herniae do not form a homogenous group and the diaphragmatic defects are in fact variable in aetiology. The overall prognosis is dependent upon when and to what extent viscera herniate into the chest, the coexistence of other structural and chromosomal anomalies.[2] If the hernia is large and occurs before 16 weeks, then this lesion may be associated with significant pulmonary hypoplasia. This fact contributes to the very high perinatal mortality rate in this condition with a range of 50 to 80%.

Professor Harrison pioneered the research and first created congenital diaphragmatic herniae in lambs and then repaired them at different intervals so proving that early intervention could modify the development of hypoplasia. Other possible therapeutic, prenatal surgery included the formation of an iatrogenic gastroschisis.[96] Such in utero surgery was marked with reasonable success in the animal model. Data have been collected on 'open' in utero surgery (in which a hysterotomy was performed to gain access to the fetus) in the human fetus with this condition. By 1993, 14 babies had open fetal surgery performed to correct the diaphragmatic hernia, but with only four survivors. Preterm labour remains an intractable problem. There have been five deaths from intra-operative problems, three

post-surgical in utero deaths and two neonatal deaths.[97] These data are of interest, since in the absence of fetal surgery, the prognosis of babies with diaphragmatic herniae (1989–94), once coexistent anomalies are excluded, led to an overall survival rate to the late neonatal period of 50%.[2] Such comparative data need to be examined, along with a data registry of cases of open surgery performed so that maternal morbidity may be minimized.

The same team has also carried out fetal surgery on cystic adenomatoid malformation of the lung and of the six babies who had a partial lung resection performed, five have survived. The results therefore are more promising but comparisons need to be made with conservative management in these conditions.

Minimal invasive fetal surgery

In an attempt to minimize fetal 'stress' and the theoretical risks of open operation (such as maternal anaesthetic risks), the concept of attempting minimally invasive procedures on the fetus has been developed.[98,99] The major technique described is that of **plug** (**p**lug the **l**ung **u**ntil it **g**rows). The fetal lungs associated with diaphragmatic herniae are small and immature. The rationale for this operation is to obstruct laryngeal/tracheal flow of amniotic fluid, increasing pressure within the lungs which in turn increases lung size and pushes viscera back out of the chest.[100] This produces a situation which is similar to the effects seen in laryngeal atresia.[101] Such tracheal obstruction has been achieved by ligature or by needle-guided placement of umbrellas/micro-balloons. However, although this iatrogenic obstruction can be simply removed at birth, there are concerns that this treatment produces large alveoli with reduction of type II pneumocytes and lamellar bodies, thus not enhancing pulmonary function. Again, prospective evaluation is required, with improved understanding of the pathogenesis of the condition using animal models and possibly by the use of a randomized controlled study if human procedures continue.

Fetal analgesia

There is considerable ethical and scientific debate over the issue of fetal pain.[102] Certainly there has been some evidence that the fetus undergoing intrahepatic fetal blood sampling as opposed to cordocentesis shows a greater response in its cortisol and β-endorphin levels.[103] However, such transient hormonal changes may not constitute 'pain', which is a learned response involving cerebration (in terms of higher centres' function).[104] The possibility that the fetus can feel and interpret painful stimuli is of course important as it raises the possibility of providing in utero analgesia or anaesthesia. There are no recommendations or practical guidelines to date, but the evidence for its use and anecdotal experiences are beginning to be discussed (Northern Fetal Society 1997: personal communications).

Ethics of fetal therapy

With the widespread use of many of the previously described techniques, reference to the fetus becoming a 'patient' is more accepted. Clinical ethical judgement and decision-making about invasive and transplacental fetal therapy are complex matters.[7] Despite their complexity, these matters are conceptually and clinically manageable with the application of concepts and language of medical ethics. The clarified obligations owed to the pregnant woman and to the fetal patient are mandatory. They provide the basis for the identification of when it is appropriate to recommend or offer such therapy and to whom. Finally, these 'guidelines' can be applied to other complex ethical/clinical problems such as multifetal reduction. As experience grows in the management of complex problems in utero, the concepts and language of medical ethics will be an essential dimension of the developing field of invasive/transplacental fetal therapy. In our own centre, we have convened a Fetal Ethics Committee (comprising an obstetrician, perinatologist, neonatologist and layperson). The physician may thus refer 'difficult and complex' cases for discussion to this group.

Conclusions

The advent of high-resolution ultrasound imaging has allowed perinatologists to visualize their patients and thus to make both a biomorphological and biophysical assessment of fetal wellbeing. This has allowed the development of structural anomalies in utero to be more closely defined and for a greater understanding of the pathogenesis of fetal illnesses to be delineated. Such data have allowed in utero treatment protocols to be developed. These require constant evaluation and audit, with perinatal outcomes being evaluated in the light of the pathogenesis of the underlying disease process.

References

1. Harrison MR, Filly RA, Globus MS, et al. Fetal treatment. N Engl J Med 1982; 307:1651–1652.
2. Howe DT, Kilby MD, Sirry H, et al. Structural chromosome anomalies in congenital diaphragmatic hernia. Prenatal Diagn 1996; 16(11):1003–1009.
3. Whittle MJ. Ultrasonographic 'soft markers' of fetal chromosomal defects. BMJ 1997;314(7085):918.
4. Maxwell D, Johnson P, Hurley P, Neales K, Allan LD, Knott P. Fetal blood sampling and pregnancy loss in relation to indication. Br J Obstet Gynaecol 1991; 98:892–897.
5. Fisk NM, Bryan E. Routine prenatal determination of chorionicity in multiple gestation: a plea to the obstetrician. Br J Obstet Gynaecol 1993; 100:975–977.
6. Snijder MJ, Wladimiroff JW. Fetal biometry and outcome in monochorionic vs. dichorionic twin pregnancies; a retrospective cross-sectional matched-control study. Ultrasound in Medicine & Biology 1998; 24(2):197–201.
7. Smith-Levitin M, Kowalik A, Birnholz J, et al. Selective reduction of multifetal pregnancies to twins improves outcome over nonreduced triplet gestations. American Journal of Obstetrics & Gynecology 1996; 175(4 Pt 1): 878–882.
8. Kleinman CS, Copel JA. Electrophysiologic principles and fetal anti-arrhythmic therapy. Ultrasound Obstet Gynecol 1991; 1:286–297.
9. Rustico MA, Berettoni A, D'Ohavio G, et al. Fetal heart screening in low risk pregnancies. Ultrasound Obstet Gynecol 1995; 6:313–319.

10. Kleinman CS, Copel JA, Weinstein EM, Santulli TV, Hobbins JC. Treatment of supraventricular tachycardias. J Clin Ultrasound 1985; 13:265–273.

11. Buis-Liem TN, Ottenkamp J, Meerman RH, Verway R. The concurrence of fetal supraventricular tachycardia and obstruction of the foramen ovale. Prenat Diagn 1987; 7(6):425–431.

12. Fernandez C, De Rosa GE, Guevara E, et al. Reversion by vagal reflex of a fetal paroxysmal atrial tachycardia detected by echocardiography. Am J Obstet Gynecol 1988; 159:860–861.

13. Noschel H, Pieker G, Muller B, et al. Pharmacokinetics during pregnancy and delivery. Int J Biol Res 1982; 3:66–73.

14. Rayburn WF, Holsztynska EF, Dommino E. In utero drug therapy. Pharmacol Ther 1993; 58:237–247.

15. Mirkin BL, Singh S. Placental tranfer of pharmacologically active molecules. In: Mirkin BL, ed. Perinatal pharmacologic therapy. New York: Academic Press; 1976:1–77.

16. Wren C, Hunter SC. Maternal administration of flecainide to terminate and suppress fetal tachycardia. BMJ 1988; 296:249–250.

17. Perry JC, Ayres NA, Carpenter RJ Jr. Fetal supraventricular tachycardia treated with flecainide acetate. J Pediatr 1991; 118:303–305.

18. Allan LD, Chita SK, Sharland GK, et al. Flecainide in the treatment of fetal tachyarrhythmias. Br Heart J 1991; 65:46–48.

19. Weiner CP, Thompson MI. Direct therapy of supra-ventricular tachycardia after failed transplacental therapy. Am J Obstet Gynecol 1988; 158:570–573.

20. Camm AJ, Garrett GJ. Adenosine and supraventricular tachycardia. N Engl J Med 1991; 325:1621–1629.

21. Blanch G, Walkinshaw SA, Walsh K. Cardioversion of fetal tachyarrhythmia with adenosine. Lancet 1994; 344(8937): 1646.

22. Blandon R, Leandro I. Fetal heart arrhythmia. Clinical experience with anti-arrhythmic drugs. In: Doyle EF, Engle WM, eds. Pediatric cardiology. Proceedings of 2nd World Congress. New York: Springer-Verlag; 19:483–484.

23. Wladimiroff JW, Stewart JW, Tonge HM. Fetal bradyarrhythmias, diagnosis and outcome. Prenat Diagn 1988; 8:53–57.

24. Maxwell D, Allan L, Tynan MJ. Balloon dilatation of the aortic valve in the fetus: a report of two cases. British Heart Journal 1991; 65(5): 256–258.

25. Copel JA, Buyon JP, Kleinman CS. Successful in-utero treatment of fetal heart block. Am J Obstet Gynecol 1994; 170:280.

26. Morganroth J. Risk factors for the development of pro-arrhythmic events. Am J Cardiol 1987; 150:324–326.

27. Carpenter RJ, Strasburger JF, Garson A, et al. Fetal ventricular pacing for hydrops fetalis secondary to complete atrio-ventricular block. J Am Coll Cardiol 1986; 8:1434–1436.

28. Maxwell D. In-utero balloon valvuloplasty in critical aortic stenosis. Br Heart J 1994

29. Wright J, Beattie RB, Welch R, Whittle MJ. Pulmonary valvuloplasty in utero for the management of critical pulmonary stenosis. Procedings of IFMSS 1994 (abstract).

30. Kilby MD, Whittle MJ. Fetal surgery. BMJ 1996

31. Caine ME, Mueller-Heubach E. Kell sensitisation in pregnancy. Am J Obstet Gynecol 1986; 154:85–90.

32. Liley AW. In-utero transfusion of the fetus with Rhesus disease. BMJ 1961; ii:1107–1109.

33. Rodeck CH, Kemp RJ, Holman CA, Whimore DN, Karnicki J, Austin MJ. Direct intravascular fetal blood transfusion by fetoscopy in severe rhesus isoimmunisation. Lancet 1981; i:625–627.

34. Daffos F, Capella-Pavlovsky M, Forestier F. Fetal blood sampling via the umbilical cord using a needle guided by ultrasound. Report of 66 cases. Prenat Diagn 1983; 3:271–277.

35. Bang J, Bock JE, Trolle D. Ultrasound guided fetal intravenous transfusion for severe rhesus haemolytic disease. BMJ 1982; 284:373–374.

36. Bang J. Intrauterine needle diagnosis. In: International Ultrasound. Eds. J Bang. Copenhagen, Munksgaard, Denmark. 1983, 122–128.

37. Grannum PA, Copel JA, Plaxe SC, Scioscia AL, Hobbins JC. In utero exchange transfusion by direct intravascular injection in severe erythroblastosis fetalis. N Engl J Med 1986; 314:1431–1434.

38. Berkowitz RL, Chitkara U, Goldberg JD, Wilkins I, Chervenak FA, Lynch L. Intrauterine transfusions for severe red cell alloimunisation: ultrasound guided percutaneous approach. Am J Obstet Gynecol 1986. 155:574–581.

39. Poissonier MH, Brossard Y, Demedeiros N, et al. Am J Obstet Gynecol 1989; 161:709–713.

40. de Crespigny L, Robinson HP, Quinn M, Doyle L, Ross A, Cauchi M. Ultrasound guided fetal blood transfusion for severe rhesus isoimmunisation. Obstet Gynecol 1985; 66:529–532.

41. Kilby MD, Szwarc R, Benson L, Morrow RJ. Left ventricular hemodynamics in anemic fetal lambs. J Perinat Med 1998; 26(1):5–12.

42. Welch R, Rampling MW, Anwar A, Talbert DG, Rodeck CH. Changes in hemorheology with fetal intravascular transfusion. Am J Obstet Gynecol 1994; 170:726–732.

43. Mandlebrot L, Daffos F, Forrestier F, MacAleese J, Descombey D. Assessment of fetoplacental blood volume for computer assisted management of in-utero transfusion. Fetal Ther 1988; 3:60–66.

44. Radunovic N, Lockwood CJ, Alverez M, et al. The severely anaemic and hydropic isoimmune fetus: changes in fetal hematocrit associated with in-utero death. Obstet Gynecol 1992; 79:390–393.

45. Nicolini U, Nicolaidis P, Fisk NM, Tannirandorn Y, Rodeck CH. Fetal blood sampling from the intrahepatic vein: analysis of safety and clinical experience with 214 procedures. Obstet Gynecol 1990; 6:47–53.

46. Nicolini U, Kochenour NK, Greco P, et al. Consequences of fetomaternal haemorrhage after intrauterine transfusion. BMJ 1988; 297:1379–1381.

47. Proceedings of the Fourth International Conference

on Percutaneous Fetal Umbilical Blood Sampling. Philadelphia, USA; October 1989.

48. Roberts A, Graanum P, Belanger K, et al. Fetal growth and birthweight in iso-immunised pregnancies after intravenous intrauterine transfusion. Fetal Ther Diagn. 1993; 8:407–411.

49. Doyle LW, Kelley EA, Rickards AL, Ford G, Callanan C. Sensineural outcome at two years for survivors of erythroblastosis treated by in-utero transfusion. Obstet Gynecol 1993; 81:931–935.

50. Gudson JP, Witherow C. Possible ameliorating effects of erythroblastosis by promethazine. Am J Obstet Gynecol 1973; 117:1101–1108.

51. Gold WR, Queenan JT, Woody J, Sacher R. Oral desensitisation in Rhesus disease. Am J Obstet Gynecol 1983; 146:980–981.

52. Graham-Pole J, Barr W, Willoughby ML. Continuous-flow plasmophoresis in management of severe rhesus disease. BMJ 1977; 1:1185–1188.

53. Chitkara U, Bussel J, Alverez M, et al. High-dose intravenous gamma globulin: does it have a role? Obstet Gynecol 1990; 76:703–708.

54. Bussel JB, Berkavitz RL, Lynch L, et al. Antenatal management of alloimmune thrombocytopenia with IV IgG: A randomised trial of the addition of low-dose steroid to IVIG. Am J Obstet Gynecol 1996; 174:1414–1423.

55. Maguiles M, Voto L, Mathet E, Marguiles M. High dose intravenous IgG for the treatment of Rhesus disease. Vox Sang 1991; 61:181–189.

56. Zanjani ED. Adult haematopoietic cells transplanted into sheep fetuses. Continue to produce adult globulin. Nature 1982; 295:244.

57. Flake AW, Harrison M, Adzick N, Zanjani ED. Transplantation of fetal hemopoietic stem cells in utero: the creation of hemopoietic chimeras. Science 1986; 233:776–778.

58. Duncan et al, 1992

59. Kaplan C, Dehan M, Tchernia G. Fetal and neonatal thrombocytopenia. Platelets 1992; 3:61–67.

60. Murphy MF, Pullon HWM, Metcalfe P, et al. The management of fetal alloimune thrombocytopenia by weekly in-utero platelet transfusions. Vox Sang 1990; 58;45.

61. Glazier GM, Filly RA, Callen PW. The varied ultrasound appearance of the urinary tract in the fetus and neonate with urethral obstruction. Radiology 1982; 144:563–568.

62. Mahoney BS, Filly RA, Callen PW, Hricak H, Globus MS, Harrison MR. Fetal renal dysplasia: sonographic evaluation. Radiology 1984; 152:143–146.

63. Nicolini U, Tannirandorn Y, Vaughan J, Fisk NM, Nicolaidis P, Rodeck CH. Further predictors of renal dysplasia in fetal obstructive uropathy: bladder pressure and biochemistry of 'fresh' urine. Prenat Diagn 1991; 71:159–166.

64. Wilkins IA, Chitkara U, Lynch L, et al. The non-predictive value of the fetal urinary electrolytes:preliminary report of outcomes and correlations with pathologic diagnosis. Am J Obstet Gynecol 1987; 157:694–698.

65. Nicolini U, Fisk NM, Beacham J, Rodeck CH. Fetal urine biochemistry: An index of renal maturation and dysfunction. Br J Obstet Gynaecol 1992; 99:46–50.

66. Crombleholme TM, Harrison MR, Globus MS, et al. Fetal intervention in obstructive uropathy: prognostic indicators and efficacy of intervention. Am J Obstet Gynecol 1990; 162:1239–1244.

67. Berkowitz R, Glickman MG, Smith GJW, et al. Fetal urinary tract obstruction: what is the role of surgical intervention in-utero? Am J Obstet Gynecol 1982; 144:367–375.

68. Quintero RA, Johnson MP, Romero R, et al. In utero percutaneous cystoscopy in the management of fetal lower obstructive uropathy. Lancet 1995; 346:537–540.

69. Chernick V, Reed MH. Pneumothorax and chylothorax in the neonatal period. J Pediatr 1970; 76:624–632.

70. Rodeck CH, Fisk NM, Frazer DI, Nicolini U. Long-term in utero drainage of fetal hydrothorax. N Engl J Med 1988; 319:1135–1138.

71. Benacerraf B, Frigoletto FD, Wilson M. Successful midtrimester thoracocentesis with analysis of the lymphocyte population in the pleural effusions. Am J Obstet Gynecol 1986; 155:398–399.

72. Nicolaides KH, Azar GB. Thoraco-amniotic shunting. Fetal Diagn Ther 1990; 5:153–164.

73. Parmley TH, Seeds AE. Fetal skin permeability to isotopic water in early pregnancy. Am J Obstet Gynecol 1970; 108:128–129.

74. Chamberlain P, Manning FA, Morrison I, Harman CR, Lange IR. Ultrasound evaluation of AFV: I. The relationship of marginal and decreased AFVIs and perinatal outcome. Am J Obstet Gynecol 1984; 150:245–249.

75. Chamberlain P, Manning FA, Morrison I, Harman CR, Lange IR. The ultrasound evaluation of AFV: II. The relationship of increased AFV and outcome. Am J Obstet Gynecol 1984; 150:250–254.

76. Vergani P, Ghildini A, Locatelli A, et al. Risk factors of pulmonary hypoplasia in second trimester premature ruptured membranes. Am J Obstet Gynecol 1994; 170:1359–1364.

77. Fisk NM, Ronderos-Dumit D, Soliani A, Nicolini U, Vaughan J, Rodeck CH. Diagnostic and therapeutic transabdominal amnioinfusion in oligohydramnios. Obstet Gynecol 1991; 78:270–278.

78. Sepulveda W, Stangiannis K, Flack N, Fisk N. Prenatal diagnosis of renal agenesis using colour flow imaging in severe second trimester oligohydramnios. Am J Obstet Gynecol 1995; 173:1788–1792.

79. Gembruch U, Hansmann M. Artificial instillation of amniotic fluid as a new technique for the diagnostic evaluation of cases of oligohydramnios. Prenat Diagn 1988; 8:33–36.

80. Nicolini U, Santolaya J, Hubinont C, Fisk NM, Maxwell D, Rodeck CH. Visualization of fetal intra-abdominal organs in second trimester severe oligohydramnios by intraperitoneal infusion. Prenat Diagn 1989; 9:191–194.

81. Hofmeyer GJ. Prophylactic versus therapeutic amnioinfusion for intrapartum oligohydramnios. In: Keirse M, et al. Pregnancy and childbirth module. London: BMJ.

82. Millard RW, Baig H, Vatner SF. Prostaglandin control of the renal circulation in response to hypoxaemia in the fetal lamb. Circ Res 1979; 45:172–179.

83. Walker MP, Moore TR, Brace RA. Indomethacin and arginine vasopressin interaction in the fetal kidney: mechanisms of oliguria. Am J Obstet Gynecol 1994; 171:1234–1241.

84. Feingold M, Cetrulo CL, Newton E, Weiss J, Shakar C, Shmoys S. Serial amniocentesis in the treatment of twin–twin transfusion syndrome complicated by acute polyhydramnios. Acta Genet Med Gemellol 1986; 35:107–113.

85. Benirschke K, Kim CK. Multiple pregnancy. N Engl J Med 1973; 288:1276–1284.

86. Bromley B, Frigoletto FD, Estroff JA, Benaceraff BR. The natural history of oligohydramnios/polyhydramnios sequence in monochorionic diamniotic twins. Ultrasound Obstet Gynecol 1992; 2:317–320.

87. Jones JM, Sbarra AJ, Dililko L. Indomethacin in severe twin–twin transfusion. Am J Perinatol 1993; 10:24–26.

88. Elliot JP, Urig MA, Clewell WH. Aggressive therapeutic amniocentesis for the treatment of twin–twin transfusion syndrome. Obstet Gynecol 1991; 77:537–540.

89. Ville Y, Hecher K, Ogg D, et al. Successful outcome after Nd:YAG laser separation of chorioangiopagus twins under sonoendoscopic control. Ultrasound Obstet Gynecol 1990; 2:429–431.

90. De Lia J, Kuhlmann R, Harstad T, et al. Fetoscopic laser ablation of placental vessels in severe pre-viable twin-to-twin transfusion syndrome. Am J Obstet Gynecol 1995; 172:1202–1211.

91. Mahony BS, Petty CN, Nyberg DA, et al. The stuck twin phenomenon: ultrasonic findings, pregnancy outcome and management with serial amniocentesis. Am J Obstet Gynecol 1990; 163:1513–1522.

92. Kilby MD, Howe DT, McHugo J, Whittle MJ. Bladder visualisation as a prognostic sign in oligohydramnios–polyhydramnios sequence in twin pregnancies treated using therapeutic amniocentesis. Br J Obstet Gynaecol 1997; 104:939–942.

93. Nicolaides KH, Hyett J, Ville Y, Hecher K. Management of severe twin-to-twin transfusion and reverse arterial perfusion sequence. In: Ward RH, Whittle MJ, eds. Multiple pregnancy. London: RCOG Press; 1995:251–266.

94. Weiner CP, Ludomirski A. Diagnosis, pathophysiology and treatment of chronic twin-to-twin transfusion. Fetal Diagn Ther 1994; 9:283–290.

95. Clewell WH, Manch-Jones ML, Manchester DK. Diagnosis and management of fetal hydrocephalus. Clin Obstet Gynecol 1986; 29:514–522.

96. Montgomerry LD, Belfort MA, Saade GR, et al. Iatrogenic gastroschisis decreases the incidence of pulmonary hypoplasia in an ovine model of congenital diaphragmatic hernia. Fetal Diag Ther 1995; 10:119–126.

97. Harrison M, Langer JC, Adzick NS, et al. Correction of CDH in utero: the initial experience. J Pediatr Surg 1990; 25:47–57.

98. Estes JM, Brown RA, Helms P, et al. Techniques of in-utero endoscopic surgery. A new approach to fetal intervention. Surg Endosc 1992; 6:215–218.

99. Deprest J, Luks FI, Vanderberge K, Lerut T, Brosens IA, Van Asche FA. Intrauterine video-endoscopic creation of the lower urinary tract obstruction in the fetal lamb. Am J Obstet Gynecol 1994; 170:274.

100. Wilson JM, Di Fiore J, Peters CA. Experimental fetal tracheal ligation prevents pulmonary hypoplasia asssociated with fetal nephrectomy. The possible role in CDH. J Pediatr Surg 1993; 28:1433–1440.

101. Wigglesworth JS, Desai R, Hislop AA. Fetal lung growth in congenital laryngeal atresia. Ped Pathol 1987; 7:515–525.

102. Glover V, Fisk N. Do fetuses feel pain? BMJ 1996; 313:796.

103. Giannakoulopoulos X, Selpulveda W, Ksurtis P, Glover V, Fisk N. Fetal plasma cortisol and beta-endorphin response to intrauterine needling. Lancet 1994; 344:77–81.

104. Anand KJS, Hickey PR. Pain and its effects in the human neonate and fetus. N Engl J Med 1987; 317:1321–1329.

CHAPTER 19

Abnormalities of the placenta and membranes

Anne S. Garden

Introduction

Whereas the benefits to be gained from careful, systematic ultrasound examination of the fetus are obvious, the information that may be obtained from imaging of the placenta may not be immediately so evident. Important clinical information, however, can be obtained. Ultrasound examination of the placenta should include examination of the texture of the placenta, its size, the presence of abnormalities and its position. In addition, the retroplacental area, the umbilical cord and membranes should be studied.

Development and structure

After implantation and up to 6 weeks' gestation, the embryo is completely surrounded by trophoblast and can be visualized using transvaginal ultrasound scanning (TVS). At this stage, differentiation of the gestational sac from thickened endometrium or from the decidual reaction seen with an ectopic pregnancy can be difficult, but careful scanning may reveal the 'double halo' appearance produced by the two layers of the decidua and the trophoblast in the presence of an intra-uterine pregnancy. Measurement of the gestational sac is necessary in the diagnosis of early pregnancy viability. At 5 weeks' gestation, using TVS, a gestational sac with a mean diameter of 10 mm can be seen and at 5½ weeks, the yolk sac can also be identified. Embryonic heart activity can be identified when the mean gestational sac diameter is 2 cm and embryonic body movements can be seen when the gestational sac is greater than 3 cm.[1] This has led to the recommendations by the Royal College of Radiology and Royal College of Obstetricians and Gynaecologists and others[2,3] that the appearance, on TVS, of a gestational sac of mean diameter greater than 20 mm with no evidence of an embryo or yolk sac, is highly suggestive of a blighted ovum. They recommend that, in addition to the mean sac diameter, the regularity of the sac outline and the presence of the yolk sac are noted and that doubt about the viability of a pregnancy is confirmed by two transvaginal scans at least 7 days apart.

By 6 to 7 weeks' gestation, the differentiation of the trophoblast into the echogenic chorion frondosum, which in later pregnancy forms the placenta, and the chorion laeve, which becomes the chorionic membrane, begins – a process which is complete by around 10 to 12 weeks' gestation – and which can be visualized on ultrasound examination.

The process of placental maturation can be seen on ultrasound and has been described in four stages by Grannum et al.[4] Grade 0 described a placenta where the chorionic plate was smooth and straight and the placental substance homogenous and devoid of outstanding echoic areas. A grade I placenta was described as having subtle undulations in the chorionic plate and scattered echoic areas present in the placental substance, while in a grade II placenta these changes are more marked with the placental substance incompletely divided by linear or comma-like echogenic densities contiguous with the indentations of the chorionic plate. Grade III was described as representing a mature placenta with the chorionic plate interrupted by indentations which run the thickness of the placenta to the basal layer, dividing the placenta into cotyledons (Fig. 19.1). The central area of these compartments displays an echo-free or 'fall-out' area with dense echogenic areas near the chorionic plate. The initial study by Grannum et al related these appearances to fetal lung maturity. Subsequent work refuted this but the descriptions in the changes in appearance of the placenta with gestation are valid and are of clinical significance.

Premature placental calcification is associated with maternal smoking (Fig. 19.2). The mean gestational age for the finding of a grade III placenta was 34.4 weeks in smokers compared to 38.3 weeks in non-smokers.[5] More significantly, the finding of a grade III placenta prior to 34 weeks' gestation is associated with an increased incidence of

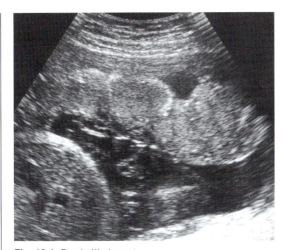

Fig. 19.1 Grade III placenta.

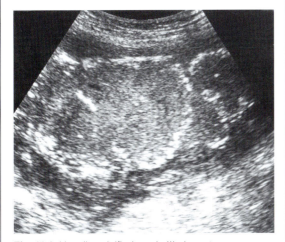

Fig. 19.2 Heavily calcified grade III placenta.

the thickness of the placenta. If such a measurement is performed, the upper limit of normal is 3 cm before 20 weeks' gestation and between 4 and 5 cm up to 40 weeks' gestation.[8] Jauniaux et al found a significant correlation between placental size (thickness, circumference and volume) and gestational age in uncomplicated, second trimester pregnancies. They also reported a significant correlation between placental circumference and the fetal abdominal circumference.[9]

An increase in the thickness of the placenta may be a normal pregnancy finding but occurs more frequently in pregnancies complicated by rhesus isoimmunization (when it may appear before the fetus becomes hydropic), non-immune hydrops, diabetes and severe maternal anaemia and in triploidy. Chronic infection has also been reported as a cause of thickening of the placenta; 11 out of 89 cases of confirmed prenatal toxoplasmosis had a placenta of increased thickness.[10]

A smaller than average placenta may be seen in pregnancies complicated by pregnancy-induced hypertension, fetal intra-uterine growth retardation, fetal trisomies and in insulin-dependent diabetes with vascular pathology. Studies of placental area in mid-pregnancy have been shown to be useful in the prediction of intra-uterine growth retardation.[11] Abnormalities of placental volume have been reported as preceding abnormal growth of the biparietal diameter and abdominal circumference but is not clinically useful owing to the length of time taken for the studies.[12]

problems in labour, low birthweight, poor condition at birth and perinatal death. Improved pregnancy outcome was found when the finding of a grade III placenta in the third trimester was reported to the clinicians, allowing closer monitoring of the pregnancy.[6] This is one of the few trials of ultrasound assessment in low-risk pregnancies to yield strong evidence of improved fetal outcome.[7]

Placental size

Ultrasound examination in most centres does not usually involve a formal measurement of

Placental position

Accurate definition of the site of the placenta or chorion frondosum is obviously of importance when performing invasive obstetric techniques such as chorionic villus sampling, amniocentesis or cordocentesis. Localization of the placenta is also of importance in making or refuting the diagnosis of placenta praevia.

Placenta praevia is traditionally defined

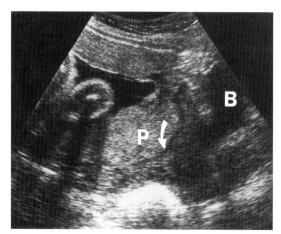

Fig. 19.3 Placenta praevia. Sagittal scan through lower uterus, showing placenta (P) completely covering the internal os (curved arrow). B, bladder.

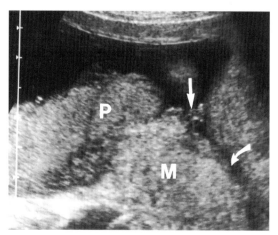

Fig. 19.4 Myometrial contraction. Sagittal scan through lower uterus, showing myometrial contraction bringing lower edge of placenta apparently close to internal os (straight arrow). Real position of internal os is shown by curved arrow. M, myometrium; P, placenta.

as a placenta which is wholly or partially situated in the lower segment of the uterus. The lower uterine segment is formed from the isthmus of the non-pregnant uterus and appears at 32 to 34 weeks' gestation. A diagnosis of placenta praevia cannot obviously be made prior to that time and at such early gestations the placenta should be described merely as 'low lying'.

Placenta praevia is subdivided into grades I to IV, grades I and II also being described as 'minor' degrees of placenta praevia with grades III and IV as 'major' degrees of placenta praevia (Fig. 19.3). These differentiations are made dependent on the amount of placenta situated in the lower segment which is identified on ultrasound examination as the area of the uterus lying below the maternal bladder. However, caution must be taken not to overdistend the bladder which may mimic a placenta praevia by causing an increased area of the uterus to be covered by the bladder or by elongating the cervix and so cause a false impression of the proximity of the lower edge of the placenta to the internal os. Repeat examination with an empty bladder is advised. A myometrial contraction in the lower pole of the uterus may also make the diagnosis of placenta praevia difficult (Fig. 19.4). Repeat scanning after 30 minutes will allow the relaxation of a contraction.

Another helpful differentiating feature is the absence on the myometrium of the bright echo of the chorionic plate seen on the fetal surface of the placenta.

The exact relationship between the lower edge of a posterior placenta and the cervix can be difficult to ascertain because of attenuation of the ultrasound beam by the fetal head. Prior to the use of transvaginal ultrasound, a suspicion of posterior placenta praevia was raised if the distance between the presenting part and the sacral promontory was greater than 1.5 cm. The diagnosis of placenta praevia, particularly a posterior placenta praevia, can now be made with more confidence using TVS as it overcomes the problems of the overlying head and overdistension of the bladder.[13] Timor-Tritsch & Monteagudo in 1993 reviewed the use of transvaginal sonography in the diagnosis of placenta praevia. They predicted that the ease of performance and the clarity and accuracy of TVS and the additional information that could be gained about abnormalities of implantation, such as placenta accreta, would soon make TVS the gold standard imaging technique in the diagnosis of placenta praevia.[14] Their prediction is rapidly being realized. Although not yet official guidelines, it is

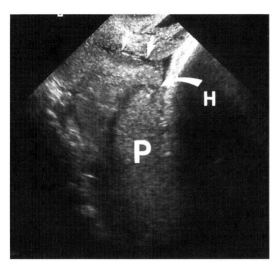

Fig. 19.5 Placenta praevia. Sagittal transvaginal scan, showing fetal head (H), cervical canal (straight arrows) and lower edge of placenta (P); curved arrow close to internal os.

prudent for all patients with potential placenta praevia to have the placental position assessed by TVS (Fig. 19.5).

Using TVS, it is more appropriate to measure the distance from the cervical os rather than to refer to 'grades' of placenta praevia. Oppenheimer et al in a prospective study suggested that the critical distance of the lower placental edge from the cervical os was 2 cm. In their study group, eight of the 21 women who had a low-lying or partial placenta praevia had a caesarean section for antepartum haemorrhage suggestive of placenta praevia. In seven of these women, the placental edge was 2 cm or less from the cervical os. 14 women with a placental edge greater than 2 cm from the cervical os had vaginal deliveries.[15] Other researchers have suggested 3 cm as the critical distance.[14] Women with a placenta nearer to the cervical os than this should be delivered by elective caesarean section at 37/38 weeks' gestation.

Should a placenta prior in early pregnancy be found to be 'low-lying', a repeat examination may be arranged at 34 weeks' gestation to exclude placenta praevia. Studies on the predictive value of a low-lying placenta at 18 weeks' gestation for placenta praevia in the final trimester, however, do not justify this practice. One study[16] gave a positive predictive value of only 1.3% and a negative predictive value of 99.8% – a result which appears better than it is because of the low incidence of placenta praevia at term. Most units advocate routine repeat scanning only if the placenta in early pregnancy is found to completely cover the os.

A succenturiate lobe is an accessory lobe of the placenta attached to the main body of the placenta by blood vessels which pass through the membranes. If noted on ultrasound examination, its presence should be reported as the succenturiate lobe may be retained following delivery resulting in postpartum haemorrhage or infection. A further potential complication is that vessels running between the succenturiate lobe and the main placenta may overly the cervical os resulting in vasa praevia. Careful ultrasound scanning, if necessary using colour Doppler studies, in the region of the internal os may make this diagnosis and prevent rupture of the vessels with subsequent fetal haemorrhage when the membranes rupture.

Retroplacental area

The most common finding in the retroplacental area is large retroplacental veins which appear as parallel hypoechoic channels between the placenta and the myometrium. They are normal but can be difficult to differentiate from a retroplacental haematoma and may be a trap for the unwary (Fig. 19.6).

A retroplacental haematoma may be found on ultrasound examination of a woman who has had a placental abruption or a threatened miscarriage. Ultrasound appearances are dependent on the age of the haemorrhage. Acute haemorrhage is hyperechoic relative to the placenta, becoming hypoechoic after about 1 week and later becoming anechoic.[17] It should be stressed, however, that the diagnosis of placental abruption is a clinical one and that the role of ultrasound in its diagnosis and management is minimal.

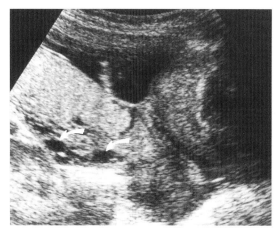

Fig. 19.6 Sagittal scan through lower uterus, showing lower edge of placenta close to internal os but also retroplacental veins (curved arrows).

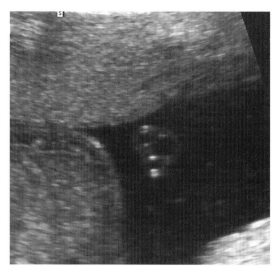

Fig. 19.7 Transverse scan through normal umbilical cord.

Umbilical cord

Examination of the umbilical cord is an important part of the examination of the pregnancy and can be seen with high-resolution ultrasound as early as 10 weeks' gestation. Details of the structure may be seen with some difficulty by 20 weeks' gestation. Details of the anatomy can be clearly seen by the third trimester. Normally, the cord consists of the central umbilical vein with the two umbilical arteries seen spiralling around it (Fig. 19.7). In 1% of pregnancies, only one umbilical artery is present (Fig. 19.8). A single umbilical artery is associated with an increased incidence of fetal anomalies, especially cardiac and central nervous system anomalies, fetal trisomies, cleft lip and palate, oesophageal atresia and ventral wall defects. The fetus should be comprehensively scanned to exclude these anomalies, when a single umbilical artery is found. In those pregnancies with a single umbilical artery, but in which no structural anomaly is detected, there is an increased incidence of intra-uterine growth retardation. Fetal growth measurements and Doppler blood flow studies should be performed.

Persistence of the right umbilical vein is a rare but serious finding and has a high risk of fetal anomaly.[18]

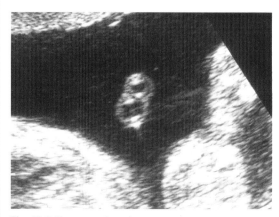

Fig. 19.8 Two-vessel cord.

Visualization of the insertion of the umbilical cord into the placenta is essential for cordocentesis and intravascular transfusion. A velamentous insertion of the cord through the membranes into the placenta may be suspected if the cord insertion site is seen distant to the placenta and confirmed by the use of colour Doppler. This is of clinical significance in the diagnosis of vasa praevia.

Cord presentation may be diagnosed by TVS, particularly if the presenting part is high. Antenatal diagnosis will prevent the emergency of cord prolapse in labour if elective caesarean section is performed prior to the onset of labour in those women in whom this finding is noted at term.

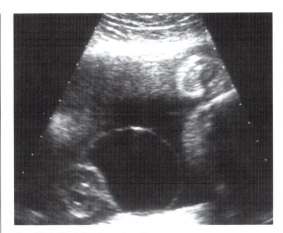

Fig. 19.9 Umbilical cord cyst.

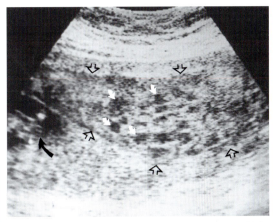

Fig. 19.10 Hydatidiform mole. Placenta contains multiple cystic areas (curved arrows). Open black arrows outline placenta.

Enlargement of the umbilical cord is commonly caused by an increased amount of Wharton's jelly and is of no clinical significance. Other causes may be umbilical cord oedema, dilatation of umbilical vessels, umbilical cord cyst (Fig. 19.9), haematoma formation and more rarely haemangioma formation. Thickening of the cord at its fetal insertion may indicate exomphalos.

Abnormalities of the placenta

The commonest placental anomaly is hydatidiform mole with an incidence which varies from 1:2000 in the UK to 1:200 in Hong Kong. The patient presents with a history of vomiting, vaginal bleeding and may have signs of pregnancy-induced hypertension. The ultrasound appearance of a mole is classic with a widespread 'snow-storm' appearance with multiple hypoechoic areas (Fig. 19.10). No fetus is present. Scanning of the ovaries is essential in these women to exclude theca lutein cysts. If a fetus is present coexistent with a hydatidiform mole, the differential diagnosis is between a partial mole (Fig. 19.11) which is commonly a triploid (69 chromosomes) pregnancy or, more rarely, a twin pregnancy with a hydatidiform mole in one sac. Careful ultrasound scanning will reveal a separate normal placenta in the latter case.

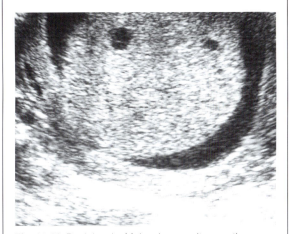

Fig. 19.11 Partial mole. Molar changes (two cystic spaces) in a large placenta. The associated fetus was triploidy.

Non-trophoblastic tumours of the placenta are less common and may be primary or secondary. Secondary deposits may be found in the placenta from a maternal malignant melanoma or from a fetal neuroblastoma.

The commonest primary tumour is a chorioangioma. Chorioangiomas appear on ultrasound as hypoechoic, occasionally echogenic, encapsulated tumours. They usually lie within the body of the placenta or close to, or protruding from, the cord insertion (Fig. 19.12). Small chorioangiomas are of no significance and may be found in approximately 1% of placentae but tumours

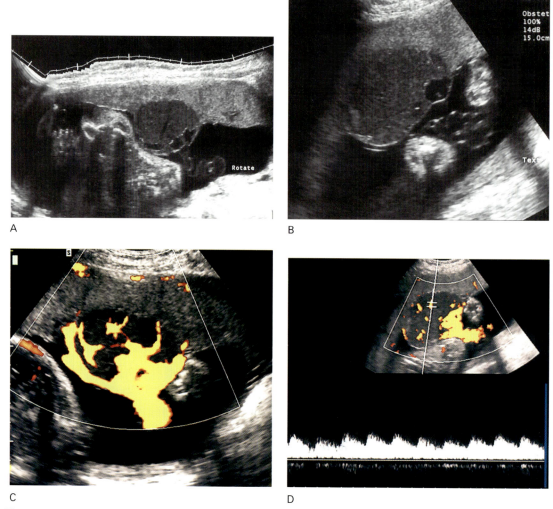

Fig. 19.12 Chorioangioma. (A) Extended field of view scan, showing chorioangioma at the cord insertion. (B) Conventional scan image. (C) Power colour flow image, showing cord vessels around the chorioangioma and vessels within tumour. (D) Doppler trace of vessels within tumour, showing high arterial flow.

over 5 cm in size require monitoring. Such tumours are associated with fetal non-immune hydrops, polyhydramnios, fetal intra-uterine growth retardation and antepartum haemorrhage. It has been suggested that there is an increased number of chorioangiomas found in the placentae of fetuses affected by fetal alcohol syndrome.[19] Large chorioangiomas at the cord insertion require careful monitoring to establish continued fetal wellbeing.

Placental teratomas may also occur but are very rare. The appearance of areas of calcification within the tumour is diagnostic.

Other features may mimic placental tumours on ultrasound. Myometrial contractions or uterine fibroids may cause a protrusion into the placenta and may be a trap for the unwary. Careful examination will identify the protrusion as being of myometrium rather than placenta. Re-examination after half an hour will help differentiate between a fibroid and contraction.

After 28 weeks' gestation, placental 'lakes' may be seen in the placenta as hypoechoic areas of varying size (Fig. 19.13). These are of no clinical significance and are caused by

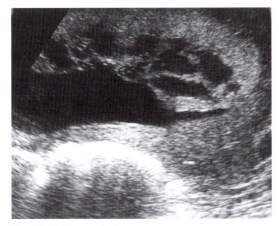

Fig. 19.13 Placental lakes.

blood-filled cavities, devoid of villi, present where venous plexus converge. Careful examination will identify blood vessels entering and leaving the 'lakes'.

Placental 'cysts' are found immediately below the chorionic plate and are also of no clinical significance, being associated with no increase in adverse pregnancy outcome. This is irrespective of the lucencies being simple or multicystic, or the size of the lucencies, even if 50% of the subchorionic placental surface is involved.[20] Haematoma may also be found beneath the chorionic plate but likewise are of no significance and in particular are not associated with an increased risk of miscarriage.[21]

A circumvallate placenta is one where the membranes are inserted some way into the fetal surface instead of the more normal insertion into the edge of the placenta and occurs in 1 to 7% of pregnancies.[22] The insertion site may cause a depression in the fetal surface which may be seen on ultrasound. The finding is of significance as such pregnancies have a high incidence of intra-uterine growth retardation and antepartum haemorrhage.

Placental infarcts are difficult to see on ultrasound examination, one series showing that 86% of infarcts were isoechoic with the placenta. The remainder of the infarcts in the series were only visible because of haemorrhage within the infarct which caused them to appear hypoechoic.[23] It

would appear, however, that in the acute phase, infarction may give a hyperechoic appearance relative to the normal placental substance. Jauniaux & Campbell reported three cases and postulated that in the acute phase congested villi and crowded intervillous spaces give rise to this appearance which then becomes isoechoic as the acute phase resolves.[24]

Abnormalities of the membranes

The appearance of a band of membranes lying within the uterine cavity may be due to chorioamniotic separation, chorioamniotic elevation or amniotic bands. A membrane may also be seen separating the sacs in multiple pregnancies. Chorioamniotic separation is a normal finding prior to the fusion of the membranes at around 16 weeks' gestation. The appearance of a separation after this time is of no clinical significance. Chorioamniotic elevation usually occurs in the presence of haemorrhage and may be seen in conjunction with retroplacental haematoma (Fig. 19.14).

The aetiology of amniotic bands is uncertain, but the most widely held theory is

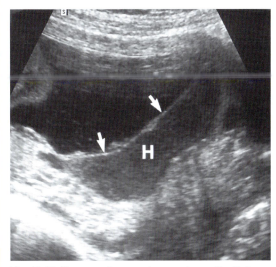

Fig. 19.14 Retromembranous haemorrhage. Sagittal scan through lower uterus, showing haemorrhage (H) lifting amniotic membrane (arrows).

that an early amnion rupture causes a band of mesoderm to be formed within the amniotic cavity which may then become attached to the developing fetus. Amniotic bands can be easily seen on ultrasound. They are of significance as they may cause a wide range of fetal anomalies which vary in severity from minor amputations or constrictions of digits to major disruption of development such as cleft lip and palate or encephalocoele. Their presence should always be looked for in pathological examination of fetuses with these anomalies as the recurrence risk is negligible, information which is essential for counselling for future pregnancies.

The finding of an amniotic band on ultrasound examination requires careful further examination to reveal whether the amniotic band is attached to the fetus.[25] If no such attachment is found, the amniotic band can be regarded as of no significance. Amniotic bands which are not attached to the fetus may be mistaken for chorioamniotic separation.

In multiple pregnancy, the thickness of the membrane separating the sacs depends on the zygosity. All dizygotic twins are dichorionic and diamniotic. They are therefore separated by a membrane which is composed of two layers of chorion and two layers of amnion. Monozygotic twins may be either dichorionic, monochorionic and diamniotic or monoamniotic depending on the time after fertilization that the separation occurred. If the twins are monochorionic, then the membrane separating them is likely to be less obvious on imaging as it comprises only two layers of amnion. In a study of 212 multiple pregnancies, of which 43 (40 twins and 3 triplets) had both pathological and ultrasound assessment, transvaginal ultrasound examination correctly predicted the chorionic and amniotic type when the scan was performed at or before 14 weeks' gestation.[26]

In conclusion, therefore, careful ultrasound study of the placenta, membranes and umbilical cord will differentiate true abnormalities of the placenta from appearances caused by normal physiological variants. Such anomalies are frequently significant in the assessment of fetal wellbeing.

References

1. Goldstein I, Zimmer EA, Tamir A, Peretz BA, Paldi E. Evaluation of normal gestational sac growth: appearance of embryonic heart beat and embryo body movements using the transvaginal technique. Obstet Gynecol 1991; 77:885–888.
2. Royal College of Radiology and Royal College of Obstetricians and Gynaecologists. Guidance on ultrasound procedures in early pregnancy. 1995.
3. Hately W, Case J, Campbell S. Establishing the death of an embryo by ultrasound: report of a public inquiry with recommendations. Ultrasound Obstet Gynecol 1995; 5:353–357.
4. Grannum PAT, Berkowitz RL, Hobbins JC. The ultrasonic changes in the maturing placenta and their relation to fetal pulmonic maturity. Am J Obstet Gynecol 1979; 133:915–922.
5. Pinette MG, Loftus-Brault K, Nardi DA, Rodis JF. Maternal smoking and accelerated placental maturation. Obstet Gynecol 1989; 73:379–382.
6. Proud J, Grant AM. Third trimester placental grading by ultrasonography as a test of fetal well-being. BMJ 1987; 294:1641–1644.
7. Neilson JP. Routine ultrasound placentography in late pregnancy. In: Enkin MW, Keirse MJNC, Renfrew MJ, Neilson JP, eds. Pregnancy and childbirth module. Cochrane Database of Systemic Reviews, Review No. 03874, 24 March 1993. Published through Cochrane Updates on disk. Oxford: Update Software; 1993: Spring.
8. Hoddick WK, Mahoney BS, Callen PW, et al. Placental thickness. J Ultrasound Med 1985; 4:479–482.
9. Jauniaux E, Ramsay B, Campbell S. Ultrasonographic investigation of placental morphologic characteristics and size during the second trimester of pregnancy. Am J Obstet Gynecol 1994; 170:130–137.
10. Hohlfeld P, Macaleese J, Capella-Pavlovski M, et al. Fetal toxoplasmosis: Ultrasonic signs. Ultrasound Obstet Gynecol 1991; 1:241–244.
11. Hoogland HJ, deHaan J, Martin CB. Placental size during early pregnancy and fetal outcome: A preliminary report of sequential ultrasound study. Am J Obstet Gynecol 1980; 138:441–443.
12. Wolf H, Oosting H, Treffers PE. Second trimester placental volume measurement by ultrasound: prediction of fetal outcome. Am J Obstet Gynecol 1989; 160:121–126.
13. Farine D, Fox HE, Jakobson S, Timor-Tritsch IE. Vaginal ultrasound for diagnosis of placenta previa. Am J Obstet Gynecol 1988; 159:566–569.
14. Timor-Tritsch IE, Monteagudo A. Diagnosis of placenta previa by transvaginal sonography. Ann Med 1993; 25(3):279–283.

15. Oppenheimer LW, Farine D, Ritchie JWK, Lewinsky RM, Telford J, Fairbanks LA. What is a low-lying placenta? Am J Obstet Gynecol 1991; 165:1026–1028.

16. McClure N, Dornan JC. Early identification of placenta praevia. Br J Obstet Gynaecol 1990; 97:959–960.

17. Nyberg DA, Cyr DR, Mack LA, Wilson DA, Shuman WP. Sonographic spectrum of placental abruption. AJR 1987; 148:161–164.

18. Jeanty P. Persistence of the right umbilical vein: an ominous prenatal finding. Radiology 1990; 177:735–738.

19. Baldwin VJ, Macleod PM, Benirschke K. Placental findings in alcohol abuse in pregnancy. Birth Defects 1982; 18(34):89.

20. Katz VL, Blanchard GF Jr, Watson WJ, Miller LC, Chescheir NC, Thorp JM Jr. The clinical implications of subchorionic lucencies. Am J Obstet Gynecol 1991; 164:99–100.

21. Pederson JF, Mantoni M. Prevalence and significance of subchorionic haemorrhage in threatened abortion: a sonographic study. AJR 1990; 154:535–537.

22. Fox J. Pathology of the placenta. Philadelphia: WB Saunders; 1978:68–72.

23. Harris RD, Simpson WA, Pet LR, Marin-Padilla M, Crow HC. Placental hypoechoic–anechoic areas and infarction: sonographic–pathologic correlation. Radiology 1990; 176:75–80.

24. Jauniaux E, Campbell S. Antenatal diagnosis of placental infarcts by ultrasonography. J Clin Ultrasound 1991; 19:58–61.

25. Mahoney BS, Filly RA, Callen PW, Golbus MS. Amniotic band syndrome: antenatal sonographic diagnosis and potential pitfalls. Am J Obstet Gynecol 1985; 152:63–68.

26. Monteagudo A, Timor-Tritsch IE, Sharma S. Early and simple determination of chorionic and amniotic type in multifetal gestations in the first fourteen weeks by high-frequency transvaginal sonography. Am J Obstet Gynecol 1994; 170:824–829.

CHAPTER 20

Fetal anomalies – the geneticist's approach

Peter A. Farndon

Introduction

The geneticist's approach to the unexpected finding of fetal structural malformations is to determine whether they constitute a recognizable abnormal pattern of morphogenesis. The pattern and nature of the anomalies can often suggest the timing and cause of an embryological insult, and together with information gleaned from family and parental medical histories, may be helpful in determining whether the insult was environmental or genetic. Even if it is not possible to reach a definitive diagnosis, this approach may generate information helpful for management and estimation of risk for future pregnancies.

This chapter outlines this approach and ends with a description and explanation of the modes of inheritance, including inherited chromosomal anomalies. Specific recurrence risks for single malformations and malformation syndromes are discussed in Chapter 21. Lists of structural malformations which may be features of rare syndromes are also given in that chapter together with a brief overview of the syndromes and their modes of inheritance.

There are several practical stages to this approach (Fig. 20.1). To:

- determine if an anomaly is isolated or associated with other abnormal findings
- determine the underlying cause from the nature and pattern of anomalies
- collect information from family, pregnancy and personal medical histories
- attempt to make a diagnosis, assess prognosis and recurrence risks using information from as many sources as possible
- discuss all the information available and possible management options with the parents.

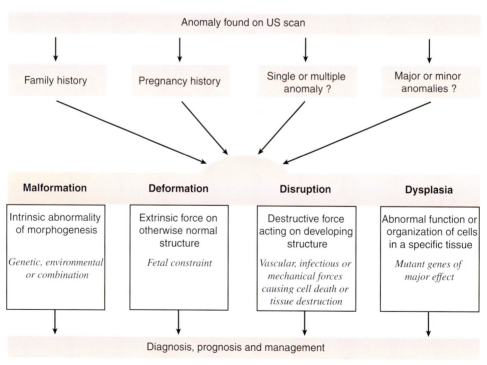

Fig. 20.1 A diagnostic approach to determine the underlying cause(s) of anomalies to aid management.

Determining if an anomaly is isolated or associated with other abnormal findings

When a detailed fetal ultrasound examination reveals an unexpected structural anomaly, the first step is to determine if the anomaly is an isolated single anomaly or whether there are other ultrasound findings.

Isolated single anomaly

Single malformations may occur as isolated anomalies, the child being otherwise completely normal. Careful detailed scanning should be performed to confirm that all other fetal structural and growth parameters are normal because single anomalies can also be markers for malformation syndromes.

The most common single primary defects[1] in liveborns are shown in Table 20.1.

Studies from Kyoto and London on induced and spontaneous abortions have been used[2] to show that congenital heart disease, cleft lip and palate and neural tube defects are at least twice as common in late embryos and early fetuses than in liveborns. The London series of spontaneous abortions at 8 to 28 weeks[3] showed single malformations in 4.7% and multiple problems in a further 4.9%.

Table 20.1

	Prevalence per 1000 births (UK)
Deformations	
Congenital hip dislocation	3.2
Talipes equinovarus	6.2
Malformations	
Cleft lip and/or cleft palate	1.2
Congenital cardiac defects	6.9
Pyloric stenosis	3–4
Defect in neural tube closure	3.6

Multiple malformations

A careful search should be made to determine if the anomaly is truly an isolated anomaly or whether there are other structural malformations, growth disturbance or unusual movements.

If several anomalies are present, they may fall into a pattern which suggests a specific diagnosis. Common recognizable patterns of major anomalies are most likely to be due to chromosomal imbalance, but certain combinations of anomalies may also suggest rare single gene or dysmorphic syndromes which can be diagnosed in utero in the absence of a previous family history. Examples are given in Chapter 21.

Determining the underlying cause from the nature and pattern of anomalies

The second step is to try to elucidate the underlying cause of the anomalies.

Reviewing the embryonic origin of the tissue or organ involved in a specific anomaly can be helpful in attempts to determine its cause or timing, particularly so with multiple abnormalities when such an approach may suggest a common embryological origin.

The nature of an anomaly is related to the stage of embryogenesis at which genetic and environmental factors acted during organogenesis or during maturation. During human development there are critical times when organ systems are susceptible and these are summarized in Figure 20.2. The embryology of each organ system is described in the relevant chapter in this book. Table 20.2 gives a summary of the timing before which insults must have occurred to result in some major anomalies.

Teratogenic influences – genetic or environmental – acting during the first 2 weeks of development are likely to result in the death of the embryo rather than cause

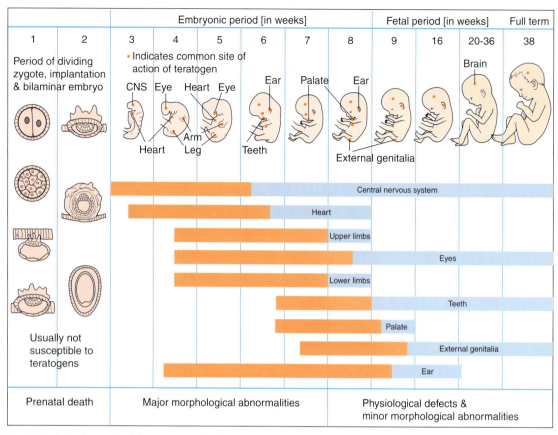

Fig. 20.2 Critical periods of development (dark shaded areas denote highly sensitive periods). (Reproduced from Moore & Persaud[13] with permission.)

Table 20.2
Embryological timing of some anomalies

Malformation	Defect in	Cause prior to
Holoprosencephaly	Prechordal mesoderm	23 days
Sirenomelia	Caudal axis	23 days
Anencephaly	Anterior neuropore	26 days
Meningomyelocoele	Posterior neuropore	28 days
Transposition of the great vessels	Direction of development of bulbous cordis septum	36 days
Radial aplasia	Development of radius	38 days
Cleft lip	Development of primary palate	6 weeks
Ventricular septal defect	Closure of ventricular septum	6 weeks
Diaphragmatic hernia	Closure of pleuropotential canal	6 weeks
Syndactyly	Programmed cell death between digits	6 weeks
Duodenal atresia	Recanalization of duodenum	7–8 weeks
Omphalocoele	Intestinal loop return to abdominal cavity	10 weeks
Bicornuate uterus	Fusion of lower portion of Mullerian ducts	10 weeks
Cleft palate	Development of secondary palate	10 weeks
Hypospadias	Fusion of urethral folds	12 weeks
Cryptorchidism	Descent of testes	7–9 months

malformations. The 3rd to the 8th week post-conception is the embryonic period during which organogenesis occurs, and so most major malformations arise during this critical period. The final stage of development is from the 3rd month to birth. As this is the period of somatic growth and maturation of tissues, few malformations may be expected to arise, but the fetus may be at risk from extrinsic factors such as fetal constraint.

Malformations initiated during early organogenesis tend to have more complex outcomes; a single malformation can result in a cascade of secondary and tertiary events resulting in what appear to be multiple anomalies (see malformation sequence below). Some defects in organs already normally developed can be clearly identified as the result of compression, constriction or immobility.

Nature of the anomalies – malformations, deformations, disruptions

Anomalies can be classified into three main types of abnormal morphogenesis – malformations, deformations and disruptions. Although it may appear academic to determine whether an anomaly is likely to be due to one of these causes, classifying anomalies in this way can help in differential diagnosis and in subsequent investigations.

Malformation

A malformation is caused by an abnormality of morphogenesis owing to an intrinsic problem within the developing structure. Underlying mechanisms include altered tissue formation, growth or differentiation caused by genetic, environmental or a combination of factors. Examples include spina bifida, cleft lip and palate, congenital heart defect and neural tube defects.

Deformation

A deformation is an abnormality of morphogenesis caused by extrinsic force on a normally developing or developed structure. Deformations usually occur in late fetal life and are caused by lack of fetal movement through mechanical, malformational or functional factors. Examples include craniofacial asymmetry, arthrogryposis and talipes. Mechanical causes include uterine anomalies and abnormal fetal positions. Malformations such as spina bifida can cause intrinsic lack of movement; renal agenesis results in a lack of amniotic fluid which constrains movement. Functional disorders include fetal neuromuscular disorders.

Disruption

A disruption is due to a destructive force acting upon an otherwise normal developing structure. Anomalies caused by disruptive forces can present a distinctive appearance because of the loss of tissue and aberrant differentiation of adjacent tissues with which adhesions may have developed. The mechanisms include cell death or tissue destruction because of vascular anomalies, anoxia, teratogens, infections or mechanical forces. Examples include some cases of facial clefts and missing digits or limbs.

Table 20.3 compares the features of malformations, deformations and disruptions.[4]

Table 20.3
Comparison of the features of malformations, deformations and disruptions

Features	Malformations	Deformations	Disruptions
Time of occurrence	Embryonic	Fetal	Embryonic/fetal
Level of disturbance	Organ	Region	Area
Perinatal mortality	+	–	+
Clinical variability of a given anomaly	Moderate	Mild	Extreme
Multiple causes of a given anomaly	Very frequent	Less common	Less common
Spontaneous correction	–	+	–
Correction by posture	–	+	–
Correction by surgery	+	±	+
Relative recurrence rate	Higher	Lower	Extremely low
Approximate frequency in newborns	2–3%	1–2%	1–2%

The pattern of anomalies – isolated anomaly, malformation syndrome/ sequence or association

An anomaly may be an isolated malformation, or may be one of several in a malformation syndrome. Some anomalies may be secondary to a primary malformation, deformation or disruption which has resulted in a malformation sequence. Even if a precise aetiological agent cannot be identified, recognizing into which group a patient's anomalies fall can result in information about genetic risks, prognosis and appropriate management for the affected individual.

When trying to elucidate if the pattern of multiple malformations is the result of a sequence or represents a true malformation syndrome, it is helpful to consider the organ systems involved and ask if all the abnormalities can be explained by a single anomaly or problem which has led to a cascade of subsequent structural defects. The converse is to consider whether the multiple structural defects present appear to be independent embryologically, and cannot be attributed to a single initiating abnormality and its consequences.

The first pattern of anomalies is described as a 'sequence', whilst the second is designated a 'malformation syndrome'.

Malformation sequence

A sequence occurs when a primary anomaly itself determines additional defects. Examples are the oligohydramnios (Potter) sequence where facial appearance, lung hypoplasia and joint contractures are all the result of constraint because of insufficient amniotic fluid. The cleft palate in the Pierre Robin sequence is caused by the normally sized tongue pressing against the palate because of micrognathia which is the primary anomaly.

The cause of the original single localized abnormality may be a malformation, deformation or disruption. Some anomalies such as anencephaly can be the result of a primary malformation or an early embryonic disruption; before the aetiology is ascribed to the latter, additional features consistent with a disruption – for instance, amniotic bands or orofacial clefting with amputations and ring constrictions – should be confirmed. Monozygotic twins have a higher frequency of disruptions[5] which are likely to have a vascular cause related to arterial-to-venous anastomoses in the placenta.

Malformation syndrome

A recognizable pattern of multiple defects is described as a 'malformation syndrome' when a common cause has resulted in a number of anatomically unrelated errors in morphogenesis. Primary developmental anomalies in two or more systems cause the structural defects. Causes include chromosomal abnormalities, teratogens and single gene defects. Examples are Down syndrome and fetal alcohol syndrome.

Association

Some recognized patterns of malformations are described by the term 'association' because the initiating cause has not been identified, and neither are the anomalies the results of a sequence.

An association is defined as a combination of anomalies which occur together more frequently than by chance alone, but which is not known to have a common cause. Examples are the VATER, VACTERL, MURCS and CHARGE associations, and are summarized in Table 20.4. When aetiology can be understood, 'associations' may well be reclassified, either within existing groups, or in new embryological groups.

Determining if any contributing information is available from family, pregnancy and personal medical histories

Family history

Documenting the family history is essential in trying to determine whether the anomalies

Table 20.4
Recognized associations. Some recognized patterns of malformations are described by the term 'association'. An association is defined as a combination of anomalies which occur together more frequently than by chance alone, but which are not known to have a common cause. Examples are the CHARGE, VATER, VACTERL and MURCS associations

CHARGE		VATER		VACTERL		MURCS	
C	coloboma	V	vertebral anomalies	V	vertebral defects	MU	Mullerian duct
H	heart defect	A	anal atresia	A	anal atresia		aplasia
A	atresia choanae	TE	tracheo-oesophageal	C	cardiovascular	R	renal aplasia
R	retarded growth		fistula		anomalies	CS	cervico-thoracic
	and/or CNS	R	radial and renal	TE	tracheo-oesophageal		somite dysplasia
	abnormalities		anomalies		fistula		
G	genital anomalies			R	radial and renal		
	and/or				anomalies		
	hypogonadism			L	limb defects		
E	ear anomalies						
	and/or deafness						

are likely to have a genetic cause, especially in groups of anomalies where recurrence would otherwise be low, e.g. congenital contractures or cleft palate. Autosomal dominant, X-linked and inherited chromosomal disorders may give a recognizable pedigree pattern, although of course an isolated case can still have a genetic cause – autosomal recessive inheritance or a new dominant mutation, for example.

Drawing a pedigree is the best way to record genetic information about a family. The agreed notation is shown in Figure 20.3. Guidelines include:

- Build up the tree from the 'bottom', starting with the affected child and siblings. 'Please give me the names of your children, and their dates of birth in order of their ages, starting with the oldest first.'
- Choose one of the parents (usually the mother) and ask about her siblings and their children, and then her parents, moving from generation to generation
- Add information on the paternal side of the family
- Use clear symbols, e.g. circles for females, squares for males. Fill in the symbol if the person is affected
- Put a sloping line through the symbol (from the bottom left-hand to the top right-hand corners) if the person has died

Symbols used in the drawing of pedigrees

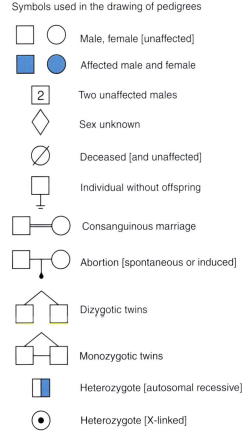

Fig. 20.3 Symbols used in the drawing of pedigrees.

- Record names, dates of birth and maiden names
- Ask for miscarriages, stillbirths or deaths in each partnership: 'How many children have you had? Have you lost any children?'

- Ask about consanguinity: 'Are you and your partner related; are there any surnames in common in the family?'
- Date and sign the pedigree.

Record at least basic details on both sides of the family, even if it appears that a disorder is segregating on one side.

Interpreting the pedigree

Table 20.5 summarizes pedigree patterns which would be suggestive of Mendelian inheritance. Other pointers include:

- a history of miscarriages, stillbirths or early neonatal deaths, especially if the causes of death are unexplained or ambiguous, suggests the possibility of a parental balanced chromosome rearrangement
- abnormal features in either parent in common with the patient raises the possibility of an autosomal dominant disorder
- the presence of consanguinity does not prove autosomal recessive inheritance, but makes it more likely

Table 20.5
Summary of pedigree patterns for single gene disorders

Autosomal dominant inheritance
1 Males and females affected in equal proportions
2 Transmitted from one generation to next ('vertical transmission')
3 All forms of transmission are observed (i.e. male to male, female to female and male to female)

Autosomal recessive inheritance
1 Males and females affected in equal proportions
2 Individuals affected in a single sibship in one generation
3 Consanguinity in the parents provides further support

X-linked recessive inheritance
1 Males affected almost exclusively
2 Transmitted through carrier females to their sons ('knight's move' pattern)
3 Affected males cannot transmit the disorder to their sons

X-linked dominant inheritance
1 Males and females are affected but affected females occur more frequently than affected males
2 Females are usually less severely affected than males
3 While affected females can transmit the disorder to male and female children, affected males transmit the disorder only to their daughters, all of whom are affected

- similarly affected male relatives of a male patient on the maternal side suggests an X-linked disorder.

Illegitimacy may explain discrepancies.

Take pregnancy and personal medical histories

Pregnancy history is of crucial importance because it may reveal a specific non-genetic cause, such as maternal illness caused by infection or drug therapy or misuse. An abnormal fetal intra-uterine position may suggest a mechanical uterine factor causing deformation or disruption. Pre-existing risk factors may be suggested from information on parental ages, occupations, past medical and drug history.

Making a diagnosis; assessing prognosis and recurrence risks

Making a definitive diagnosis of a malformation syndrome from ultrasound anomalies can be very difficult in the absence of other clues, for instance from the family history. It may not be possible to make a specific diagnosis of a syndrome prenatally; indeed, a diagnosis cannot be made in about half the patients with dysmorphic syndromes seen in tertiary referral genetic clinics even with the additional information available after birth. Diagnosis of a genetic syndrome leading to prognostic information is especially useful in planning management.

Diagnosis depends on recognizing the pattern of anomalies, but individual defects are non-specific and even rare defects may be found in several conditions. There is variable expression of features associated with a particular disorder.

Information from as many sources as possible should be used

This should include the expertise of clinical genetics units which are likely to have a clinical geneticist with specialist skills in the diagnosis of dysmorphic and multiple malformation syndromes who would be pleased to discuss cases. Clinical geneticists also have knowledge of DNA diagnosis for single gene disorders, risks associated with familial chromosome rearrangements and with organ/system anomalies, and have access to specialist literature.

Further investigations

Multiple malformations affecting several different organ systems, timed at different stages of gestation, are highly suggestive of a chromosomal disorder. Certain combinations of defects may suggest a small chromosomal deletion; close links between clinical and laboratory staff will help when determining if such additional studies are needed.

Biochemical studies currently prove helpful in only a small proportion of dysmorphic infants (e.g. peroxisomal disorders such as Zellweger syndrome).

Autopsy by an experienced paediatric pathologist is valuable in any abortion associated with malformation.

Use databases

Computerized databases are useful diagnostic tools. The London Dysmorphology Database (LDDB)[6] and POSSUM[7] are two in common use. The LDDB, for example, contains information on over 2750 non-chromosomal, multiple congenital anomaly syndromes including single gene disorders, sporadic conditions and those caused by environmental agents. A list of possible diagnoses is generated by searching on combinations of clinical features. It is often impossible to assess which are the most characteristic or constant features of a rare syndrome, and so LDDB does not rank the features in order of frequency or importance within a syndrome. Some clinical experience is therefore required to assess the likelihood of the diagnoses suggested.

Characteristics of the patient which are called 'good handles' are chosen for use in the computer search. These are anomalies which are easily recognizable as being abnormal and do not merge with normal variation. Each chosen feature should not be common in too large a number of syndromes. It is also important to consider that a feature might not be a primary phenomenon, but perhaps the end result in a sequence, e.g. a high arched palate may be the result of long-standing hypotonia and may not be an important feature in itself. Some secondary features are important, however. For instance, joint contractures as a result of fetal akinesia secondary to neuromuscular abnormalities are the most important clinical features of this group of conditions. The features of a patient selected for database searching must be the most unusual, clear-cut and unequivocal.

However, the approach must be flexible, using different combinations of features during searches as patients described in the literature may not have had all the features found in the patient awaiting diagnosis. The aim is to find a small number of possible diagnoses and then to review the features, photographs and abstracts on the database, and then the original references to see whether the overall features of the condition fit the pattern found in the patient. The features may not fit exactly with those of patients with the same syndrome in the literature as syndromes can be so variable. Equally it is important that the patient should not be forced into a diagnostic category that is not correct as this may have important management consequences. Although the computer may suggest diagnoses, clinical skill and experience in assessing variability of normal individuals and those with syndromes are required.

Assess recurrence risks

Detailed information about recurrence risks for isolated anomalies and multiple malformation syndromes are given in Chapter 21. Those risks should be read in conjunction with the background information on genetics in this chapter.

Discussing available information and diagnostic dilemmas with parents

The unexpected diagnosis of a malformation syndrome or serious genetic disorder during pregnancy may leave the family with relatively little time to understand the severity and consequences of the disorder, ascertain options open to them (including any treatments available) and discuss genetic implications. They find the support offered during this time by specially trained nurses in fetal medicine departments or clinical genetics units extremely valuable.

Discussions with families have to be honest: too often definitive answers cannot be found during gestation, even with the best information and facilities available. This uncertainty can be difficult for some families to accept in an age when medical investigations are widely expected to be able to answer all questions. In such cases, a discussion of the various possibilities and outcomes takes considerable time but it is vital that the family members fully understand the certainties or uncertainties of the collective medical opinion which has been formed. Discussions with paediatric surgeons or neonatologists about treatments available and the likelihood of success can help parents to reach decisions.

Families particularly want to know if a condition is lethal or severely disabling and if there is a high risk in a future pregnancy. Couples with a family history of abnormality who have received this information before embarking upon a pregnancy have time to decide the options which they consider correct for them. During pregnancy, difficult management decisions may have to be made extremely quickly and genetic information, including an assessment of the risk of recurrence, may play an important role when considering options.

Genetic counselling, however, is not solely the giving of a risk figure. Harper[8] has defined it as 'the process by which patients or relatives at risk of a disorder that may be hereditary are given information about the consequences of the disorder, the probability of developing and transmitting it and the ways in which it may be prevented or ameliorated'.

It is widely accepted that genetic information should be given in a non-directive manner, presenting facts, discussing options and helping couples and families to reach their own decisions. There is no 'right' or 'wrong' decision; rather a couple must make a decision which they feel is correct for their situation.

Options available to a couple may include:

- having no (more) children
- accepting the risk
- undertaking prenatal diagnosis (if available)
- seeking adoption
- gamete donation
- pre-implantation diagnosis.

A couple's choice will depend on many factors, social, economic, moral and practical.

Examining the fetus/baby after birth

Whatever the outcome of the pregnancy, all efforts must be made to achieve a diagnosis so that genetic implications can be considered. As with all aspects of genetic counselling, accuracy of diagnosis is paramount. Information obtained prenatally should be supplemented by information from neonatal examination, or from a detailed examination by a perinatal pathologist if the pregnancy is terminated or the fetus is stillborn. Photographs of the main features will be helpful when seeking the diagnostic advice of a clinical geneticist.

Diagnosis of a syndrome after birth is able to incorporate further information from the pattern of minor anomalies.

Major anomalies occur in 3 to 5% of newborns and usually require medical or surgical intervention. Minor anomalies are variants that are of no serious medical or cosmetic significance and occur in less than 4% of the population but can serve as indicators of altered morphogenesis and clues to patterns of malformation. They are found in physical features of complex and variable development and include anomalies of hair patterning, eye spacing, ear form, palmar creases and digits. As almost any minor variant may occasionally be found as a usual feature in a particular family, parents and other family members should be examined before assuming that the feature is part of the syndrome.

Three or more minor anomalies are found in only 0.5% of babies but 90% have one or more major defects as well. The finding of several minor anomalies in an individual is unusual and often indicates that a more serious problem in morphogenesis has occurred. Although minor variants are extremely helpful in the diagnosis of syndromes postnatally, most cannot be detected prenatally by ultrasound. The diagnosis of syndromes therefore relies on the patterns of major malformations, growth and fetal movement.

Identifying families at highest risk

Families with single gene disorders and parental chromosomal anomalies have the highest risks and may usually be detected by taking a family pedigree. The family may suspect that the family tree is suggestive of a genetic disorder and offer this information; in others, the high risk is appreciated only when a formal history is taken.

Confirmation of diagnosis

Accurate genetic information requires an accurate diagnosis. Confirmatory documents such as specialists' letters and results of laboratory or necropsy investigations may be required to confirm a diagnosis. Apparently unaffected individuals should be assessed to exclude mild or early disease, especially in autosomal dominant disorders such as neurofibromatosis and tuberous sclerosis.

Ultrasound examination in subsequent pregnancies

For families with a previously affected child, consulting the literature will help in determining the ultrasound marker most likely to be useful in diagnosis. Discussion and evaluation of the pattern of anomalies with a clinical geneticist with a special interest in dysmorphology may aid identification of a dysmorphic syndrome. The use of computer databases such as the LDDB and POSSUM may also be helpful. It should be noted that not all features of a syndrome may be present in an affected patient.

Syndrome recognition relies on the recognition of patterns of major and minor anomalies. Ultrasound examination during future pregnancies would be expected to detect major anomalies associated with the syndrome, but the minor anomalies, so helpful in the postnatal syndromic diagnosis, may not be diagnosable.

Variability of anomalies in malformation syndromes

The malformations in malformation syndromes can show variation in their expression. It is well recognized from syndromes of known aetiology that not every affected patient has exactly the same combination of malformations, some being more frequent than others. It is likely that single gene disorders causing malformation syndromes create their effects by altering the relative amounts of the specific gene product in a dosage-sensitive pathway; therefore differences in the appearance of the numbers and types of malformations may vary between affected individuals. This is especially true for dominant disorders. A subsequently affected fetus may show a different spectrum of anomalies from the affected child. For most syndromes of known aetiology the frequencies of given malformations are known, as is the range of variation of those malformations.

Genetic causes of malformations

Chromosomal abnormalities, specific genes or more complex genetic mechanisms may interact with environmental factors to produce an abnormal fetal phenotype.

Single congenital malformations

The genetic contribution to single birth defects has long been recognized. The observed increase in risk for first-degree relatives of people with common anomalies such as neural tube defects and cleft lip and palate was highly suggestive that a genetic component was involved. This was strengthened by the finding that there was a lesser, but still greater than background, risk for second- and third-degree relatives. Environmental factors have been identified which contribute to the occurrence of certain defects. As not all embryos subjected to a particular environmental factor develop a malformation, it is assumed that those who are affected have a genetic predisposition. The combination of genetic and environmental influences is the basis of the multifactorial model, as described below.

Isolated congenital malformations rarely have a mutation in a single gene as their cause. A few such as the autosomal dominant condition van der Woude syndrome which causes cleft lip and palate are well known, but perhaps more will be found on further examination of developmental genes such as

the *hedgehog* gene, mutations of which have been found in some cases of holoprosencephaly.

Multiple malformation syndromes

The underlying causes of multiple malformation syndromes may be known and are the result of chromosomal imbalance, single gene mutations and teratogens or they may be unknown.

Abnormalities of chromosome structure and number

Chromosomal anomalies cause developmental abnormalities by disturbing the action of multiple genes. Additional copies of genes (either by trisomy of whole chromosomes or duplication of chromosomal segments) cause abnormalities of gene dosage – in this case, increased levels of the gene products. Decreased levels of gene products are the consequence of monosomy or deletions. Specific patterns and malformations associated with aneuploidy are discussed in Chapter 14. Mosaicism and chromosomal microdeletions are other mechanisms of fetal maldevelopment and these are discussed further in a section below.

Several hypotheses have been proposed to explain the clinical effects of aneuploidy. One model proposes that the phenotype is caused by the direct effects of the specific genes located on the chromosome or segment involved.[9] If this is correct, then knowledge from the Human Genome Project will be able to be used to predict the resulting phenotype from any chromosomal imbalance. As it could be argued that there are more general similarities than differences between the aneuploid phenotypes, an alternative hypothesis suggests that the imbalance of a large number of gene products enhances the 'developmental instability' inherent in many developmental pathways.[10]

Single gene malformation syndromes

The 1997 edition of LDDB[6] lists 1812 single gene malformation syndromes: 689

autosomal dominant, 1050 autosomal recessive, 19 X-linked recessive and 54 X-linked dominant. Some of these appear to be very rare, and many are single case reports. Some of these syndromes have congenital structural malformations which would be expected to be detectable by obstetric ultrasound. A broad view would suggest that of the autosomal dominant conditions in LDDB, 74 might be detectable because of prenatal structural anomalies, 167 autosomal recessive, 19 X-linked recessive and 9 X-linked dominant conditions. Many of these are discussed further in Chapter 21.

Gene mapping and genes for major developmental pathways

The cellular pathways involved in the pathogenesis of some malformation syndromes are being delineated, often by analyzing genes identified in other species and proved to be vital for normal development. Confirming that mutations in these genes cause particular human syndromes offers the possibility of DNA diagnosis.

A review in 1994 by Wilkie et al[11] catalogued 139 genetic loci (including 65 specific genes) implicated in congenital malformations. For the majority of conditions, the affected infant has a genetic mutation, but in a few conditions the abnormality arises from maternal–fetal interaction (e.g. maternal phenylketonuria, fetal hydantoin syndrome).

Most of the specific genes cited in Wilkie's review causing malformations appear to encode enzymes or structural proteins, but it is to be expected that an increasing number which are integral parts of signalling cascades will be delineated (as in the PTCH gene which causes the Gorlin syndrome). Several genes have been implicated in congenital malformations and neoplasia later in life – the neoplasia occurring when the normal gene is inactivated by somatic mutation in a cell already containing a germ-line mutation of the other gene of the pair. They include PAX3 (Waardenburg syndrome/alveolar rhabdomyosarcoma),

RET (Hirschsprung's disease, multiple endocrine neoplasia type 2B/medullary thyroid carcinoma), WT1 (Denys–Drash syndrome/Wilms' tumour) and PTCH (polydactyly, eye anomalies and medulloblastoma and basal cell carcinomas). These examples show that similar pathways control cellular growth and differentiation in the embryo and the adult.

Types of genetic disorders

Single gene disorders

Single gene (Mendelian) disorders behave as though they are under the control of only one pair of the 70 to 100 000 genes in the human genome. As they have high risks of recurrence, it is important to recognize families where such a mode of inheritance is operating, usually by a combination of the precise clinical diagnosis and the pedigree pattern.

Table 20.5 summarizes the pedigree patterns which would be suggestive of Mendelian inheritance; more details about Mendelian inheritance are given later in this chapter.

The genes for many Mendelian disorders have been isolated and their DNA sequences read, allowing direct mutation detection in affected families. Genes for other Mendelian disorders have not yet been isolated but their positions have been localized to specific chromosomal regions. This allows the inheritance of the chromosomal region containing the disease gene to be followed through the family – 'gene tracking'. Presymptomatic diagnosis, carrier detection and prenatal diagnosis are therefore possible for many Mendelian conditions. (Box 20.1 lists common single gene conditions not usually associated with malformations.)

Genes for a small number of malformation syndromes have been identified and DNA diagnosis by mutation analysis for these is possible. Others have been localized to chromosomal regions. A list

Box 20.1
Common single gene disorders

DNA diagnosis is becoming available for some malformation syndromes caused by abnormal single genes. There are many other single gene disorders for which DNA diagnosis may be available by either direct mutation detection or by gene tracking. These include:

Dominantly inherited disorders
Achondroplasia
Adult polycystic kidney disease
Breast cancer (some families)
Familial adenomatous polyposis coli
Familial hypercholesterolaemia
Hereditary motor and sensory neuropathy
von Hippel–Lindau disease
Huntington's disease
Marfan syndrome
Multiple endocrine neoplasia
Myotonic dystrophy
Neurofibromatosis
Tuberous sclerosis

Recessively inherited disorders
Alpha-1 antitrypsin
Congenital adrenal hyperplasia
Cystic fibrosis
Friedreich's ataxia
Sickle cell disease
Spinal muscular atrophy
Tay–Sachs disease
Thalassaemia

X-linked disorders
Becker muscular dystrophy
Duchenne muscular dystrophy
Fragile-X syndrome
Haemophilia A and B

Note that for gene tracking, DNA from the affected person and family studies are required. Consult the Regional Clinical Genetics Service for availability of DNA diagnosis in other diseases: it is potentially possible for all diseases where the gene has been localized.

of some is given in Table 20.6. Although the mainstay of prenatal diagnosis for most malformation syndromes is likely to continue to be ultrasound for some time, up-to-date information should be obtained from a clinical genetics department since advances are too rapid for published literature to keep up to date and access to online databases is required. Tests useful for prenatal diagnosis may have become available or improved by the time a couple is considering another child.

Autosomal dominant inheritance

A dominant trait is one which manifests in a heterozygote (a person possessing both the abnormal and normal alleles) and is usually transmitted from one generation to the next – 'vertical transmission' (Fig. 20.4). Isolated cases within a family may arise as a new mutation. Each offspring of a parent with an autosomal dominant trait has a 1 in 2 chance of inheriting the condition (Fig. 20.5). Autosomal dominant traits can exhibit variable expressivity, reduced penetrance and sex limitation.

Indeed, some dominant traits are so variable in their expression that careful physical examination is needed to detect the minute signs that a parent has the gene, e.g. a child may inherit the gene for autosomal dominant ectrodactyly and have severe hand anomalies, but the affected parent may show signs only on radiology. Unfortunately a

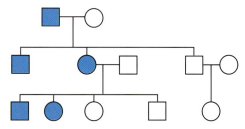

Fig. 20.4 Autosomal dominant inheritance. Three generations are affected, including male-to-male transmission.

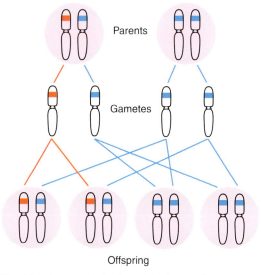

Parents

Gametes

Offspring

Fig. 20.5 Autosomal dominant inheritance. If one parent is affected by a disorder caused by a dominant trait, his/her offspring have a 50% (1 in 2) risk of also inheriting the disorder.

Table 20.6
Selected genetic disorders localized to specific chromosomal regions

Name	Chromosomes and region
van der Woude syndrome	1q32
Holoprosencephaly-2	2p21
Wardenburg syndrome, type 1	2q35
Morquio syndrome, type B (MPS IVB)	3p14.2-p21
Hurler, Hurler–Scheie, Scheie syndromes	4p16.3
Achondroplasia	4p16.3
Hypochondroplasia	4p16.3
Thanatophoric dysplasia, types 1 and 2	4p16.3
Rieger syndrome	4q25-q27
Diastrophic dysplasia	5q31-q34
Mandibulofacial dysostosis	5q32-q33.1
Saethre–Chotzen syndrome	7p21
Greig cephalopolysyndactyly	7p13
Split hand/split foot, type 1	7p11.2
Osteogenesis imperfecta, several forms	7p21.3-q22.1
Holoprosencephaly-3	7p36
Pfeiffer syndrome-1	8p11.2-p12
Branchio-oto-renal syndrome	8p13.3
Cleidocranial dysplasia	8q22
Cohen syndrome	8q22-q23
Nevoid basal cell carcinoma syndrome	9q31
Tuberous sclerosis-1	9q33-q34
Nail-patella syndrome	9q34
Apert syndrome	10q25.3-q26
Crouzon syndrome	10q25.3-q26
Pfeiffer syndrome-2	10q25.3-q26
Stickler syndrome	12q13.1-q13.3
Spondyloepiphyseal dysplasia congenita	12q13.1-q13.3
Kneist syndrome	12q13.1-q13.3
Sanfilippo syndrome (MPS IV)	12q14
Marfan syndrome	15q21.1
Rubenstein–Taybi syndrome	16p13.3
Tuberous sclerosis-2	16p13.3
Morquio syndrome, Type A (MPS IVA)	16q24.3
Neurofibromatosis, type I	17q11.2
Osteogenesis imperfecta, several forms	17q21.31-q22
Camptomelic dysplasia-1	17q24.3-q25.1
Neurofibromatosis, type 2	22q11.21-q13.1
Focal dermal hypoplasia	Xp22.31
Chondrodysplasia punctata, X-linked recessive	Xp22.3
Kallmann syndrome	Xp22.3
Coffin–Lowry syndrome	Xp22.2-p22.1
Aicardi syndrome	Xp22
Cleft palate–ankyloglossia	Xq21.1 q21.31
Simpson–Golabi–Behmel syndrome	Xq26
Borjeson–Forssman–Lehmann syndrome	Xq26-q27
Fragile X syndrome	Xq27.3
Hunter syndrome (MPS III)	Xq27.3
Oto-palato-digital syndrome, type I	Xq28
Chondrodysplasia punctata, X-linked dominant type	Xq28

parent with minor signs of a dominant trait can have a severely affected child. Very rarely, a person who must carry the gene for an autosomal dominant condition fails to show any signs of the condition. The gene is said to be 'non-penetrant' in the person without signs of the disease.

Some patients with severe autosomal dominant conditions appear to be sporadic cases. If both parents are unaffected, and there is no family history, then the child's disease is likely to be due to a new mutation. The recurrence risk for parents is small, but of course the child is at 50% risk of passing on the disease to children. There is a slight chance that a parent of a child with an apparently new dominant mutation has gonadal mosaicism – the germ line contains two populations of cells, one with the mutation, and one with the normal gene. This is likely to be the explanation for the rare cases of two children with the same autosomal dominant condition being born to unaffected parents.

Autosomal recessive conditions

An autosomal recessive trait is one in which a person who has two copies of the abnormal gene (homozygote) manifests the trait, but heterozygotes (carriers) are unaffected. A person with an autosomal recessive condition often appears to be the only person affected in a family (Fig. 20.6). Offspring of parents who are both heterozygous for the same autosomal recessive condition have a 1 in 4 chance of being affected (Fig. 20.7). An unaffected sib of an affected person has a 2 in 3 chance of being a carrier. The less common the autosomal recessive condition, the greater likelihood that the parents of a homozygote are related. If an affected person is able to reproduce, children will be at risk only if the partner is a carrier.

X-linked recessive inheritance

Sex-linked recessive traits are determined by genes on the X chromosome and so are usually manifest only in males who have a single copy of the gene (Fig. 20.8). Although females have two X chromosomes, only one is active in most cells at most times (in accordance with the Lyon hypothesis). A

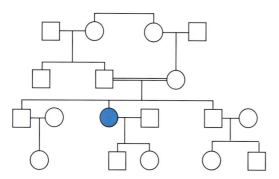

Fig. 20.6 Autosomal recessive inheritance. Siblings in only one generation are affected. In this family, their parents are first cousins.

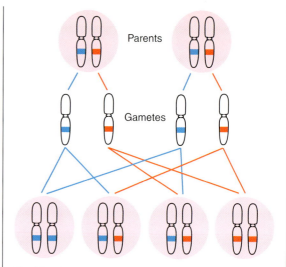

Fig. 20.7 Autosomal recessive inheritance. If both parents carry the same abnormal gene for a recessive condition, their offspring have a 25% (1 in 4) risk of inheriting the abnormal gene from both parents and being affected.

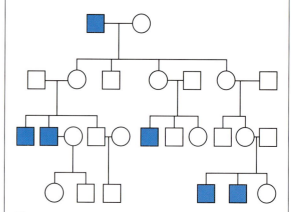

Fig. 20.8 X-linked inheritance. This family shows that the grandfather had a non-lethal X-linked disorder (e.g. haemophilia). Males affected in several generations are linked through unaffected females. Daughters of affected men are obligatory carriers.

female heterozygous for an X-linked condition is therefore a mosaic of normal and affected cells. This chance pattern of X inactivation can make carrier detection in X-linked recessive disorders very difficult. For example, about 30% of known carriers of haemophilia A or Duchenne muscular dystrophy have biochemical carrier tests within the normal range. Many cases of the more serious diseases are caused by new mutations which also makes it difficult to counsel parents unless reliable carrier detection is available. However, DNA techniques may be able to answer these questions with certainty.

Offspring, boys or girls, of females heterozygous for an X-linked recessive allele have a 1 in 2 chance of inheriting the allele from their mother (Fig. 20.9).

Daughters of affected males are obligate heterozygotes. If male-to-male transmission can be demonstrated, then X-linkage is ruled out. Rarely, females show signs of an X-linked recessive disease because they are homozygous for the allele (e.g. colour blindness), have a single X chromosome (Turner's syndrome), have a structural rearrangement of an X chromosome, or are heterozygous but show skewed or non-random X-inactivation.

Unusual patterns of inheritance

Unusual patterns of inheritance may be explained by phenomena such as genetic

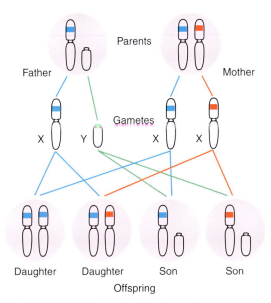

Fig. 20.9 X-linked recessive inheritance. If a woman carries an abnormal recessive gene on one of her X chromosomes, she has a 25% (1 in 4) risk at each conception of an affected male.

heterogeneity, mosaicism, anticipation, imprinting, uniparental disomy and mitochondrial mutations.

Genetic heterogeneity

Genetic heterogeneity occurs when a single clinical disorder can be caused by several genes. Examples include tuberous sclerosis, which is caused by mutations in a gene on either chromosome 9 or chromosome 16, and retinitis pigmentosa which has autosomal dominant and recessive and X-linked recessive forms. When considering diagnosis by gene tracking for a family it is obviously important that genetic heterogeneity has been excluded.

Mosaicism

Mosaicism occurs when an individual's tissues or organs contain more than one genetic line of cells – the mutant line of cells may contain a chromosome anomaly or sometimes a mutant single gene. This can be a very difficult prenatal diagnostic counselling problem because the phenotype will lie somewhere between the full disorder and normal, and further tests are usually indicated. Even so, the proportion of abnormal cells in one tissue cannot be taken as the proportions elsewhere. Similarly, it is not possible to give exact figures for the risk to offspring of individuals with chromosome or single gene mosaicism because of the very nature of mosaicism which depends on the numbers and disposition of mutant cells in the gonads.

Placental mosaicism with a chromosomally normal fetus is a well-recognized phenomenon.

Mosaicism for chromosomes 18 and 21 frequently predicts fetal abnormality. Trisomy 13 mosaicism predicts abnormality in about 50% of cases. There is a high incidence of fetal abnormality associated with mosaic trisomy 9 and mosaic trisomy 22. Mosaicism for a structurally abnormal additional chromosome appears to carry a greater risk than autosomal trisomy mosaicism.

However, another concern when autosomal trisomy mosaicism is found at prenatal diagnosis is that a trisomic fetus may have 'lost' one of the three copies of the chromosome in some cells to 'correct' the imbalance. If both remaining copies of the chromosome originated from the same parent (uniparental disomy), this too could give an abnormal phenotype.

Uniparental disomy

Uniparental disomy (UPD) implies that two copies of a given chromosome or chromosome segment have been inherited from one parent, no contribution at these loci coming from the other parent. UPD for chromosome 15q11-13 is one of the mechanisms leading to Angelman syndrome and Prader–Willi syndrome. In triploidy, a hydatidiform mole is produced if there are two paternal contributions; two maternal contributions result in a growth-retarded embryo and underdeveloped placenta.

Genomic imprinting

Imprinting results in differential expression of parental alleles during development from the embryo to the adult. Alteration of imprinted loci can result in neuro-developmental disorders, abnormalities of growth and malformations. Angelman and Prader–Willi syndromes show different parental imprints at chromosome 15q11-13 as does the Beckwith-Wiedemann syndrome (characterized by overgrowth, exomphalos and facial dysmorphism) at 11p15.

Chromosomal anomalies

The karyotype report: nomenclature

Karyotyping is labour intensive as high resolution (or extended) chromosome preparations reveal over 850 bands. Occasionally, only a limited analysis may be possible because of poor elongation of the chromosomes.

The karyotype of a cell is reported in an internationally agreed format giving a precise description of an abnormality. It has three parts separated by a comma:

- the total number of chromosomes (e.g. 46, 45, 47)
- the sex chromosome constitution (e.g. XX, XY, X, XXY)
- abnormalities or variants of whole chromosomes or their arms ('p' and 'q' refer to the short ('petit') and long arms respectively).

Breakpoints involved in structural rearrangements are described according to the arm involved, the region of that arm, and then by band and sub-band(s) within that region. For example, band Xq27.3 is found on the long arm of the X chromosome, in region 2, band 7 and sub-band 3.

Examples:

- Normal: 46,XY normal male
- Sex chromosome aneuploidy: 47,XXY Klinefelter syndrome
- Autosomal aneuploidy: 47,XX,+21 Female with trisomy 21 (Down syndrome)
- Deletion: 46,XY,del(18)(q21) deletion of part of long arm of one chromosome 18 from band q21 to the end of the long arm
- Translocation: 46,XX,t(3;11)(p14;p13) Female with balanced reciprocal translocation between chromosomes 3 and 11, with breakpoints on the short arms – at p14 on chromosome 3 and p13 on chromosome 11.

Cytogenetics laboratories are always pleased to discuss reports of abnormalities.

Aneuploidies

Chromosomal aneuploidies cause malformations by disturbing the actions of multiple genes by increasing the amounts of gene products in trisomies or duplications, and by reducing gene products in monosomies or deletions.

Chromosomal microdeletions/ contiguous gene syndromes

Contiguous gene syndromes, also known as microdeletion syndromes, have extremely variable clinical manifestations depending on the amount of genetic material involved. Molecular techniques (usually fluorescence in situ hybridization) must be employed for the diagnosis of those where the gain or loss of material is beyond the limit of light microscopy. Table 20.7 lists the common conditions. The ones likely to present with structural anomalies during ultrasound scanning are:

Miller–Dieker syndrome del(17)(p13):
  Lissencephaly
Shprintzen syndrome del(22)(q11):
  Heart lesions.

Some recurrent pattern malformation syndromes suspected to have a chromosomal basis but with no abnormality on conventional microscopy (such as Cornelia de Lange syndrome) may eventually be found to have microdeletions.

Chromosomal translocations

A translocation is formed when there has been transfer of material between chromosomes, requiring breakage of both chromosomes, with repair in an abnormal arrangement. If the exchange results in no loss or gain of DNA, the individual is clinically normal and is said to have a balanced translocation. Such a translocation carrier is, however, at risk of producing chromosomally unbalanced gametes which may result in a chromosomally abnormal baby, miscarriage, stillbirth or infertility depending on the origin and amount of chromosomal material involved. Generally,

---

Table 20.7
Chromosomal microdeletion syndromes

Alagille (20p12)
Alpha-thalassaemia with mental handicap (16p13)
Angelman syndrome (15q11–q13)
Beckwith–Wiedemann (11p15)
DiGeorge/velocardiofacial (usually 22q11; rarely 10p13)
Langer–Giedion (8q24)
Miller–Dieker lissencephaly (17p13.3)
Prader–Willi (15q11–q13)
Rubenstein–Taybi (16p13.3)
Smith-Magenis (17p11.2)
Williams (7q11)
Wilms' tumour–aniridia and WAGR (11p13)

---

the smaller the segment involved, the greater the chance of viable offspring. The cytogenetic literature may reveal whether a viable child with the potentially unbalanced products of the particular translocation has been reported. It may be possible to calculate a theoretical risk figure, so the clinical genetics or cytogenetics services should be consulted. For most couples, however, the precise risk figure is not the vital consideration, rather it is the possibility of prenatal diagnosis in future pregnancies.

There are two types of translocations:

a. Reciprocal translocation

In reciprocal translocations, chromosomal material distal to (i.e. beyond) the breaks in two chromosomes is exchanged. Either the long or short arms of any pair of chromosomes may be involved.

When a fetus has inherited a parental, apparently balanced, reciprocal translocation, there appears to be no increased incidence of phenotypic abnormality in the child, especially if the translocation is present without effect in several family members.

b. Robertsonian (centric fusion)

A Robertsonian translocation is one in which effectively all of one chromosome is joined end to end with another. This translocation is one of the most common, balanced structural rearrangements in the general population with a frequency in newborn surveys of about 1 in 900.

Deletions/duplications of chromosomal material

A child can inherit either the normal homologue or the chromosome with the deletion or duplication from a parent with partial autosomal monosomy or trisomy. The risk of the child inheriting the parental chromosomal abnormality is therefore theoretically 50%.

Multifactorial inheritance

By far the major contribution of genetic

factors to morbidity and mortality is through the many common diseases and malformations which show a familial tendency but do not follow simple Mendelian patterns – multifactorial conditions. Together they are more common than single gene and chromosomal abnormalities. Examples in the newborn are cleft lip and palate, club-foot, pyloric stenosis, congenital heart disease and neural tube defects; in adults, examples are diabetes, schizophrenia and peptic ulcer. Multifactorial conditions are considered to be determined by the summation of the effects of multiple genes at different loci, together with environmental factors.

The additive effects of these multiple genes cause the population to demonstrate a susceptibility based on a Gaussian distribution. It is postulated that there is a liability threshold; people whose genetic predisposition is above this will manifest the disease.

It is usual to use empiric risk figures in genetic counselling. These are the observed recurrence risks for different relatives of an affected individual. These are obtained through population studies, and strictly apply only to the population from which they were collected.

After two children have been born with a multifactorial condition, the recurrence risk rises because a couple must have either a particularly high genetic susceptibility or suffer chronic environmental insult, or both.

Thus genetic counselling for multifactorial conditions depends on a detailed pedigree and good, relevant and up-to-date empirical data.

Human malformations associated with environmental factors

Environmental factors may be wholly or partly responsible for some malformations. The main categories are given in Table 20.8.

Many single congenital malformations are not solely genetically determined but are the result of the interplay between genetic and environmental factors. Neural tube defects are an excellent example of how the environmental component can be modified by maternal treatment with folic acid which has been shown to reduce the rate of recurrence in susceptible individuals by one-half.[12]

Teratogens

A teratogen is an environmental agent that can cause abnormalities of form or function in a fetus exposed to the agent. Susceptibility to teratogenesis depends on the genotype of the conceptus, timing of exposure, dosage and interaction with other environmental factors and maternal genetic factors.

Table 20.8
Environmental factors contributing to human structural anomalies

Agent	Example	Structural anomaly
Drugs	Alcohol	Microcephaly, dysmorphism, heart defect
	Androgens	Masculinization of females
	Cocaine	Vascular disruptions
	Phenytoin	Cleft lip and palate, heart defect
	Sodium valproate	Mandibular/ear abnormalities
	Vitamin A	Spina bifida
Infection	Rubella	Microcephaly, cataracts, heart defect
	Toxoplasma	Hydrocephalus
	Varicella	Limb defects, scarring
Maternal factors	Diabetes	Neural tube defect, heart defect,
	Phenylketonuria	Microcephaly, heart defect
Physical agents	Hyperthermia	Neural tube defect, central nervous system anomalies
	X-rays	Microcephaly

Timing of exposure

If exposure to the teratogen occurs before the differentiation of the three germ layers, either embryonic death results or no abnormalities are apparent. A high degree of sensitivity then occurs during organogenesis from about days 18 to 60, with a peak susceptibility at approximately 30 days. The type of malformation is dependent on which organ is susceptible at exposure, an organ being most susceptible early in its differentiation. Because the fetal period (2nd to 9th months) is characterized by histogenesis (refined cellular and tissue changes) and functional maturation, teratogenic insults during this time will result mainly in mental and growth retardation.

Dose and interaction with other environmental and genetic factors

For some, but not all, teratogens there is a dose-related effect, higher doses resulting in more malformations. The potency of some teratogens can be increased in the presence of other environmental factors: the teratogenicity of some anti-convulsants is increased, for example, if used in combination with another drug. There also appears to be a difference in susceptibility between individuals: the same dose of sodium valproate is associated with a neural tube defect in the fetus of one mother but not another.

Mechanisms of teratogens in the causation of malformations

Teratogens affect morphogenesis, development and differentiation through cell death, failed cell interactions or alterations in the movement of cells. As these affect the basic processes of cells, a teratogen may have a general effect on several tissues. Likewise, different teratogens may produce common effects. Some teratogens do, however, produce a characteristic pattern of anomaly: these are included in the tables in Chapter 21.

References

1. Leck I. The contribution of epidemiologic studies to understanding human malformations. In: Stevenson R E, Hall J G, Goodman R M (eds) Human malformations and related anomalies, vol 1. New York: Oxford University Press; 1993:70.
2. Leck I. Fetal malformations. In: Barron S L, Thomason A M, eds. Obstetrical epidemiology. London: Academic Press; 1983:263.
3. Creasy M R, Crolla J A, Alberman E D. A cytogenetic study of spontaneous abortions using banding techniques. Hum Genet 1976;31:177.
4. Cohen M M. The child with multiple birth defects. 2nd ed. New York: Oxford University Press; 1997:41.
5. Van Allen M I. Structural anomalies resulting from vascular disruption. Pediatr Clin North Am 1992;39:255–277.
6. London Dysmorphology Database (1997 version). Published on CDROM. Oxford: Oxford University Press; 1997.
7. POSSUM (Pictures of standard syndromes and undiagnosed malformations). Australia: Murdoch Institute.
8. Harper P S. Practical genetic counselling. 4th ed. Oxford: Butterworth-Heinemann; 1993.
9. Shapiro B L. Down syndrome – a disruption of homeostasis. Am J Med Genet 1983;14:241–269.
10. Epstein C J. Mechanisms of the effects of aneuploidy in mammals. Ann Rev Genet 1988;22:5–75.
11. Wilkie A O M, Amberger J S, McKusick V A. A gene map of congenital malformations. J Med Genet 1994;31:507–517.
12. MRC Vitamin Study research group. Prevention of neural tube defects: results of the Medical Research Council Vitamin Study. Lancet 1991;338:131.
13. Moore K L, Persaud T V N. The developing human – clinically oriented embryology. 6th ed. Philadelphia: WB Saunders; 1993.

Further reading

Baraitser M, Winter R M. Multiple congenital anomalies: a diagnostic compendium. London: Chapman and Hall; 1991.

Buyse M L. Birth defect encyclopedia. Center for Birth Defects Information Services Inc, Cambridge, MA: Blackwell Scientific;1990.

Donnai D, Winter R M. Congenital malformation syndromes. London: Chapman and Hall Medical;1995.

Gardner R J M, Sutherland G R. Chromosome abnormalities and genetic counselling. 2nd ed. Oxford: Oxford University Press;1996.

Gorlin R J, Cohen M M Jr, Levin L S. Syndromes of the head and neck. 3rd ed. New York: Oxford University Press;1990.

Graham J M Jr. Smith's recognisable patterns of human deformation. 3rd ed. Philadelphia: WB Saunders; 1996.

Harper P S. Practical genetic counselling. 4th ed. Oxford: Butterworth-Heinemann;1993.

Jones K L. Smith's recognizable patterns of human malformation. 5th ed. Philadelphia: WB Saunders; 1997.

Graham J M Jr. Smith's recognizable patterns of human deformation. 2nd ed. Philadelphia: WB Saunders; 1988.

McKusick V A. Mendelian inheritance in man. 11th ed. Baltimore: Johns Hopkins University Press;1994.

Rimoin D L, Connor J M, Pyeritz R E. Emery and Rimoin's principles and practice of medical genetics. 3rd ed. London: Churchill Livingstone; 1996.

Scriver C R, Beaudet A L, Sly W S, Valle D. The metabolic and molecular basis of inherited disease. 7th ed. New York: McGraw-Hill; 1995.

Shepard T H. Catalog of teratogenic agents. 8th ed. Baltimore: Johns Hopkins University Press; 1995.

Taybi H, Lachman R S. Radiology of syndromes, metabolic disorders and skeletal dysplasias. 4th ed. Chicago: Year Book;1996.

Databases

On-line Mendelian Inheritance in Man – URL: http://www.ncbi.nlm.nih.gov/omim/

London Dysmorphology Database (1997 version) contains information on over 2750 non-chromosomal multiple anomaly syndromes. Published on CDROM. Oxford: Oxford University Press.

Schinzel A. Human chromosome abnormality database. Oxford: Oxford University Press.

POSSUM (Pictures of standard syndromes and undiagnosed malformations). Australia: Murdoch Institute.

CHAPTER 21

Isolated malformations and multiple anomaly syndromes: features and recurrence risks

Peter A. Farndon

Introduction

The previous chapter outlined a geneticist's approach to diagnosis when a fetus is found to have one or more anomalies at ultrasound examination. This chapter:

- discusses factors to be considered in assessing recurrence risks for isolated anomalies and syndromes
- briefly explores the components of a risk – the burden of the disorder and the probability of its occurrence
- presents tables of syndromes associated with particular anomalies
- lists details of important syndromes.

Once a precise diagnosis has been made – or in the absence of a diagnosis a view formed as to the most likely aetiology – an assessment of the recurrence risk can be made. Points to consider are shown in Box 21.1. However, couples respond to the same mathematical figure differently (as discussed below), taking into account the 'burden' of the disease as well as the mathematical probability. Even where the burden is considered to be severe and the risk is high a couple may still wish to proceed with future pregnancies because there is the reassurance that the major structural malformation or syndrome could be diagnosable prenatally by ultrasound.

The timing and giving of genetic information

Timing

Some couples wish to have information about recurrence risks when discussing management options for an affected pregnancy, but thoughts about the future and the probability of having an unaffected child may form only a small part in the immediate reactions of most couples. The optimal timing for giving genetic information may therefore vary from couple to couple – an appointment for more detailed 'genetic counselling' being given some time later. If the couple decide to end the affected pregnancy, invaluable information will be available from photographs, X-rays (if appropriate) and autopsy, which may alter the diagnosis. A liveborn child can be examined and appropriate investigations undertaken to determine the likely diagnosis, as outlined in Chapter 20.

Box 21.1
Points to consider when assessing recurrence risks

1. Look for clues in the family tree suggestive of a single gene disorder or inherited chromosomal anomaly (see Chapter 20, Table 20.5).
   If a single gene disorder is recognized, risks for other family members can be calculated from knowledge of inheritance.
   If an inherited chromosome anomaly is discovered (for instance a translocation) the risk may be high. Refer to a clinical geneticist for family studies.

2. Try to determine if the pattern and timing of anomalies suggests a malformation, deformation or disruption (see Chapter 20).
   Deformations and disruptions most usually have low recurrence risks, depending on their causes.

3. Are the anomalies isolated or multiple?
   If isolated malformation, look in the text below (some have low risk, e.g. isolated gastrointestinal atresia). Many have multifactorial risk of 2 to 5%.
   If multiple anomalies, try to determine whether a specific syndrome can be recognized from the pattern of anomalies. (See Tables 21.1–21.20 which lists syndromes associated with particular anomalies. Consult literature and computer databases as outlined in Chapter 20).
   If the pattern is caused by a de novo chromosome anomaly, there is a low risk to future pregnancies.
   If a known syndrome can be recognized, the literature may suggest a specific risk if sufficient cases have been reported.
   If the pattern of anomalies remains unknown, the overall empiric risk of 3% is often used (but beware of previously unreported recessive conditions).

The diagnosis of a serious genetic disorder or malformation syndrome during pregnancy may require difficult management decisions to be taken urgently. The family may have relatively little time to understand the severity and consequences of the disorder, ascertain the options open to them (including any treatments available) and discuss genetic implications. Families particularly want to know whether a condition is lethal or severely disabling, whether there is a high risk for a future pregnancy and whether specific prenatal diagnosis would be available.

Giving genetic information

It is widely accepted that genetic information should be given in a non-directive manner, presenting facts, discussing options and helping couples and families to reach their own decisions. Wherever possible, both partners should be seen together to discuss abnormalities found at prenatal diagnosis and the genetic implications.

The genetic consultation and genetic counselling

Genetic counselling is more than the giving of a risk figure. Harper (1998) has defined it as 'the process by which patients or relatives at risk of a disorder that may be hereditary are given information about the consequences of the disorder, the probability of developing and transmitting it and the ways in which it may be prevented or ameliorated'. There are three steps in genetic counselling.

Making an accurate diagnosis

Steps to consider in making the diagnosis are outlined in Chapter 20. Risks can be assessed in accordance with the guidelines below.

Explaining the features and genetics of the condition in language easily understood

Although some people perceive risks only as 'high' or 'low', most wish to understand how a risk figure has been reached, which may need a discussion about modes of inheritance

and mechanisms of genetic disease. Giving a risk figure in the form of a fraction (e.g. 1 in 2; ½) or odds (50:50) or a percentage (50%) has the advantage that it is less likely to lead to confusion – the perception of what constitutes 'high' or 'low' risk varies with the individual. Some families find it easier to understand risk figures presented as odds, others as percentages. Most clinical geneticists use both during a consultation, concentrating on the one which the patients find easiest to understand.

The decision as to what constitutes an 'acceptable' risk will vary with the disorder and the individual, and how they view the two components of the risk figure – the probability of the condition occurring and the burden of the disease.

Families may view the same mathematical figure entirely differently. For example, if one considers autosomal dominant conditions (with a '1 in 2 risk'), the family may view the effect of the disease as mild (e.g. brachydactyly) or very severe (e.g. Huntingdon's disease). Their view may also take into account whether screening and treatment are available (as in bilateral retinoblastoma or in adenomatous polyposis coli): such issues may need to be discussed during the genetic consultation.

Supporting the family whilst they come to terms with often very difficult decisions

Most units would feel that ongoing support should be provided to families during this time, usually by specially trained nurses or other health care professionals.

Calculating risks

The probability of another child being affected with a similar condition can be calculated accurately if Mendelian inheritance is the cause, but for many isolated malformations or syndromes the underlying causes are unknown, and so an empiric figure, based on a population study, may have to be used. The characteristics of Mendelian inheritance and other genetic mechanisms are outlined in Chapter 20.

Isolated anomalies

Many disorders affecting only one organ system appear to have a genetic component but do not follow a clear pattern of Mendelian inheritance nor have an identifiable chromosomal abnormality. They are said to have 'polygenic' or 'multifactorial' causation, as discussed in Chapter 20.

Recurrence risk data for isolated malformations therefore have to be derived empirically – from observation of recurrences in population studies. Figures are available for many of these conditions, but theoretically should be used only in the population from which they were obtained. It is important to take a family history and examine the affected person to ensure no other associated malformations are present which may raise the possibility of a syndromic diagnosis which could be monogenic. Some isolated malformations (such as tracheo-oesophageal atresia and most intestinal atresias) appear to be largely sporadic.

Recurrence figures for isolated anomalies are given system by system in the text which follows. Experience has shown, however, that most single primary defects do behave as multifactorial traits, with an observed recurrence risk for first degree relatives of between 2 and 5%.

The multifactorial theory predicts that the genetic component is caused by the summation of the effects of several genes. However, DNA and clinical studies are beginning to suggest that for some malformations the disorder is not a single entity but a heterogeneous group of disorders – some inherited in a Mendelian fashion, others where an inherited component interacts with environmental factors and others which are due largely to environmental factors. Indeed, mutations in single genes have been identified which are responsible in some cases for cleft lip and for Hirschsprung's disease.

Anomalies caused by chromosomal imbalance

If the multiple malformation syndrome is caused by chromosomal imbalance, the recurrence risk is low (< 1%) if the parents' chromosomes are normal. In this case, it might be expected that the chromosomal anomaly was the result of a de novo event at meiosis; the recurrence risk is not zero, however, because of the risk of undetectable parental gonadal mosaicism for the chromosomal anomaly.

For autosomal trisomies the empiric risk of a liveborn child with aneuploidy is about 1% until age 30 years from when the recurrence risk is that associated with maternal age.[1] If the malformation syndrome is the result of an unbalanced rearrangement associated with a parental translocation or inversion the recurrence risk could be extremely high; referral to a clinical genetics unit is recommended for family studies.

Anomalies and syndromes caused by mutations in single genes

Hundreds of multiple malformation syndromes are inherited as single gene traits: 1812 are listed in the 1997 edition of the London Dysmorphology Database. Chromosomal locations for many have been identified (see Table 20.6). Many multiple malformation syndromes caused by single genes have been carefully delineated and the range of phenotypic features well documented. Others, especially where only a few cases have been reported, await further delineation. Diagnosis is usually by pattern recognition and pedigree analysis; for others diagnosis may be possible by genetic mutation analysis, or by radiological, biochemical or haematological investigations.

Detailed explanations of the single gene modes of inheritance (dominant, recessive and X-linked) are given in Chapter 20. Diagrams there explain how the disease genes are expected to segregate in offspring, allowing a precise probability of recurrence to be calculated.

Unknown syndromes

Specific risks are available for some named multiple malformation syndromes, but more usually the general empiric risk of 3% has to be used in the absence of a specific diagnosis.

It is difficult to obtain recurrence risks for many syndromes because of their rarity, and although the overall observed recurrence risk is 3%, there always remains the concern that a new syndrome could have an autosomal recessive mode of inheritance.

Environmental factors

It is unusual to be able to identify a specific environmental factor as the cause of a malformation, but when this is the case it gives important information for genetic counselling. As most exposures are sporadic, there is a low risk of recurrence in future pregnancies.

Recurrence risks for isolated anomalies, associations and malformation syndromes

Anomalies are listed system by system. Recurrence risks and practice points for isolated anomalies are given in the main text with associated tables giving lists of syndromes associated with the particular anomaly. Details of most of the syndromes can be found in the list at the end of the chapter.

Table 21.1
Syndromes with short limbs at birth

Achondrogenesis types 1 and 2 (lethal)	Autosomal recessive/new dominant mutation
Beemer lethal short rib syndrome	Probably autosomal recessive
de Lange	Mostly sporadic uncertain
Camptomelic dysplasia	Autosomal dominant (new mutation likely)
Chondrodysplasia punctata (severe rhizomelic form)	Autosomal recessive
Diastrophic dysplasia	Autosomal recessive
Dyssegmental dysplasia	Most sporadic; some may be autosomal recessive
Ellis–van Creveld	Autosomal recessive
Femoral hypoplasia – unusual facies	Autosomal dominant, sporadic, diabetic mother
Fibrochondrogenesis	Autosomal recessive
Grebe	Autosomal recessive
Hypochondrogenesis	Sporadic, (?AD new mutation)
Hypophosphatasia (severe autosomal recessive form)	Autosomal recessive
I-cell mucolipidosis type 2	Autosomal recessive
Jeune (asphyxiating thoracic dystrophy)	Autosomal recessive
Kniest – severe neonatal form	Possibly autosomal recessive
Kyphomelic dysplasia	Possibly autosomal recessive
Lethal multiple pterygium syndrome – type Chen	Autosomal recessive
Metatropic dysplasia	Both autosomal dominant and autosomal recessive forms
Osteogenesis imperfecta (type II)	See text; some new dominant mutations
Rhizomelic chondrodysplasia punctata (autosomal recessive)	Autosomal recessive
Roberts (pseudothalidomide)	Autosomal recessive
Robinow (fetal face)	Both autosomal dominant and autosomal recessive pedigrees reported
Rudiger	Autosomal recessive
Schneckenbecken dysplasia	Autosomal recessive
Seckel	Autosomal recessive
Short-rib-polydactyly type 1 (Saldino–Noonan)	Autosomal recessive
Short-rib-polydactyly type 2 (Majewski)	Autosomal recessive
Spondyloepiphyseal dysplasia congenita	Most autosomal dominant, some autosomal recessive lethal cases reported
Spondylohumerofemoral dysplasia	Unknown; cases appear sporadic
Many chromosomal anomalies	Sporadic, or due to familial rearrangement

LIMBS

Heart defects are commonly associated with limb anomalies – some of these syndromes are listed in the table in the cardiovascular section below.

Symmetrical bone dysplasias

Most of the severe dysplasias are autosomal recessive; a few are autosomal dominant, often caused by new mutation (Table 21.1). Ultrasound is extremely helpful in future pregnancies as short limbs can be identified by 20 weeks' gestation. A minority of skeletal anomalies have low recurrence risks – such as isolated butterfly or hemi-vertebrae, or absent sacrum.

Limb defects

A high proportion of bilateral limb anomalies follow Mendelian inheritance (Table 21.2). As many of the dominant conditions can be very variable, detailed physical examination of the parents' limbs together with radiographs should be undertaken before assuming a child has a new dominant mutation. Families find ultrasound in subsequent pregnancies extremely helpful as the degree of severity can be predicted. Developmental genes (including SHOX and TBOX) causing limb defects are being studied.

Isolated unilateral anomalies are usually considered to be non-genetic.

Table 21.2
Syndromes involving polydactyly, syndactyly or limb reduction defects

Polydactyly	
Acrocallosal syndrome	Autosomal recessive
Apert syndrome	Autosomal dominant
Bardet–Biedel	Autosomal recessive
Ellis–van Creveld	Autosomal recessive
Fetal valproate	Environmental
Goltz	XLD
Gorlin syndrome	Autosomal dominant
Juberg–Hayward	Autosomal recessive
Jeune thoracic dystrophy	Autosomal recessive
Maternal diabetes (pre-axial polydactyly)	Environmental
Meckel–Gruber syndrome	Autosomal recessive
Mohr–Majewski OFD IV (postaxial polydactyly)	Autosomal recessive
Trisomy 13	Usually sporadic
Syndactyly	
Apert syndrome	New autosomal dominant mutation
Goltz	XLD
Other craniosynostosis syndromes	Usually autosomal dominant
Oro-facial-digital (type 1)	XLD (male lethal) most commonly
Poland anomaly	Usually sporadic
Limb reduction defects	
Adams–Oliver	Autosomal dominant
Amniotic bands	Usually sporadic
de Lange syndrome	Usually sporadic
Fanconi pancytopenia	Autosomal recessive
Fetal cocaine	Environmental
Fetal thalidomide	Non-genetic
Fetal valproate	Environmental
Goltz	XLD
Holt–Oram syndrome	Autosomal dominant
Roberts syndrome	Autosomal recessive
Thrombocytopenia-absent radius	Autosomal recessive
VATER association	Usually sporadic

Polydactyly

Postaxial polydactyly in the absence of other anomalies can be a relatively common autosomal dominant condition with variation in expression and lack of penetrance. It is especially common in African populations. It is a primary feature of many severe autosomal recessive conditions, especially the short-rib syndromes. Table 21.2 lists syndromes with polydactyly. Pre-axial polydactyly is more unusual, and should institute a search for other syndromic features.

Ectrodactyly (split hands/feet)

Most isolated cases of bilateral ectrodactyly follow autosomal dominant inheritance. It may be necessary to X-ray the hands of both parents to exclude variation in expression. If the X-rays are normal there remains a small risk of recurrence due to gonadal mosaicism. The combination of ectrodactyly and cleft lip and palate (with ectodermal dysplasia) is found in the autosomal dominant EEC syndrome. Table 21.3 lists syndromes associated with ectrodactyly.

Limb reduction defects

It can be very difficult to be certain about the aetiology of limb reduction defects, but asymmetry is usually considered to indicate that the cause was likely to be non-genetic – for instance in the amnion disruption sequence where asymmetrical amputation defects occur. Cocaine can cause reduction defects; thalidomide was a major cause in the past.

The VATER association combines asymmetrical limb defects with vertebral, anal, tracheo-oesophageal, renal and cardiac defects. The recurrence risk is low. (See the syndrome list at the end of the chapter.)

Sirenomelia

Cases appear to be sporadic.

Osteogenesis imperfecta

The non-lethal autosomal dominant type is the commonest form, which can show great variation in severity both within and between families. Occasionally an affected child can present in utero with fractures.

Type II OI includes severe forms of OI which cause stillbirth or are lethal in the neonatal period (see the syndrome list at the end of the chapter for references). Radiological examination should be performed to determine the subtype to allow accurate genetic information. Where radiology is not available and there is no family history, an overall recurrence risk of 7% is given.

Type IIa is lethal, causing limb shortening and intra-uterine fractures. Most cases appear to be due to new dominant mutations, and so the recurrence risk is very low (perhaps 1% due to gonadal mosaicism).

Types IIb and IIc have higher empiric recurrence risks: about 7%, increasing to 25% if consanguinity is present.

Type III is also severe, but is not lethal in the perinatal period. The empiric recurrence risk is about 7%.

Table 21.3 Syndromes with split hands or feet	
Acro-renal-mandibular syndrome	Possibly autosomal recessive
de Lange	Mostly sporadic
Ectrodactyly cleft palate	Autosomal dominant
Ectrodactyly syndrome	Autosomal dominant
Ectrodactyly – ectodermal dysplasia – clefting (EEC)	Autosomal dominant with variable expression
Goltz (focal dermal hypoplasia)	XLD with assumed intra-uterine lethality in males
Juberg–Hayward	Autosomal recessive

Table 21.4
Syndromes with fractures

Antley–Bixler	Autosomal recessive
Camptomelic variant	Uncertain
Kozlowski	Uncertain
Osteogenesis imperfecta	(See text)

Fractures

Syndromes are listed in Table 21.4 and their details given in the syndrome list at the end of the chapter.

Congenital contractures

Any condition which prevents or reduces fetal movement may result in contractures. Causes include myopathies, neuropathies, brain dysfunction due to chromosomal imbalance, and lack of amniotic fluid.[2] Congenital contractures may therefore result from non-genetic or genetic causes and achieving a precise diagnosis requires careful investigation of the affected patient and detailed pregnancy and family histories.

There are some autosomal dominant distal arthrogryposis syndromes where the effects can be variable between family members, but occasionally an apparently severely affected child is born. Prognosis is excellent with physiotherapy.

Talipes

A neurological or constraint cause must be excluded. The empiric risk for sibs for talipes equinovarus is 3% overall.[3]

VERTEBRAL COLUMN AND CRANIUM

Neural tube defects

Recurrence risk is 1/20, but this can be reduced by up to one-tenth if preconceptional folic acid is taken by the mother.[4] It is important to exclude the autosomal recessive Meckel–Gruber syndrome which is associated with polycystic kidneys, as well as the other syndromes shown in Table 21.6.

Hydrocephalus

Hydrocephalus in the absence of neural tube defects usually has a low recurrence risk (1–2%). Hydrocephalus caused by aqueduct stenosis is a special case, as it can be X-linked, so a detailed maternal family history should be taken. Affected boys may have a

Table 21.5
Syndromes with vertebral defects

Acro-renal-mandibular syndrome	Possibly autosomal recessive
Dyssegmental dysplasia	?Autosomal recessive, most sporadic
Exstrophy of cloaca	Usually sporadic
Goldenhar (facio-auriculo-vertebral)/hemifacial microsomia	Mostly sporadic/autosomal dominant
Incontinentia pigmenti	XLD with presumed intra-uterine lethality in males
Jarcho–Levin spondylothoracic dysplasia	Autosomal recessive
Klippel–Feil	Usually sporadic
Larsen (lethal variant)	Autosomal recessive
Maternal diabetes	Environmental
Multiple pterygium (lethal)	Autosomal recessive
MURCS association	
Robinow	Autosomal dominant and autosomal recessive pedigrees reported
Schisis association	Mostly sporadic
Spondylocostal dysplasia	Autosomal dominant and autosomal recessive families reported
VATER association	Sporadic
3q-	
4p-	
dup(7q)	
Tri 8	
13q-	

Table 21.6
Syndromes with neural tube defects

Cranial defects	
Amniotic bands	Mostly sporadic
Fetal valproate	Environmental
HARD (±E) Walker–Warburg syndrome	Autosomal recessive
Joubert – cerebellar vermis aplasia plus other anomalies	Autosomal recessive
Meckel–Gruber (dysencephalia splanchnocystica)	Autosomal recessive
Roberts (pseudothalidomide)	Autosomal recessive
Schisis association	Mostly sporadic
Spinal dysraphism	
Fetal valproate	Environmental
Klippel–Feil	Usually sporadic
Maternal diabetes	Environmental
Radial aplasia – thrombocytopenia (TAR)	Autosomal recessive
Schisis association	Mostly sporadic
Spondylocostal dysplasia	Autosomal dominant and autosomal recessive families reported
Tri 18	
Wildervanck-cervico-oculoacoustic syndrome	Uncertain; ?? X-LD

characteristic thumb position. It may be best to discuss such cases with a genetic unit as mutation analysis of the L1CAM gene may be a possibility. The autosomal recessive HARD±E (Walker–Warburg) syndrome has lissencephaly and retinal changes as well as hydrocephalus.

Dandy–Walker syndrome

As an isolated anomaly Dandy–Walker syndrome has a risk similar to that of isolated hydrocephalus.

Hydrancephaly

This is most likely to be due to an environmental cause as the risk of recurrence appears to be negligible.

Microcephaly

Genetic microcephaly may not become apparent until the third trimester or after birth. When infections, metabolic disorders and syndromes have been excluded, the remaining cases have an empiric recurrence risk of 1/6,[5] suggesting a high likelihood that they have genetic causes.

Encephalocoele

Isolated encephalocoele is usually taken to be part of the neural tube defect complex.

Table 21.7
Syndromes with webbing of the neck or nuchal cystic hygroma

Klippel–Feil	Usually sporadic
Lethal multiple pterygium syndrome	Autosomal recessive
Noonan	Autosomal dominant
Roberts (pseudothalidomide)	Autosomal recessive
6q-	
9p-	
Turner syndrome	

Encephalocoele is also part of the autosomal recessive conditions HARD±E (Walker–Warburg) and Meckel–Gruber syndromes (see syndrome list).

Neck webbing/cystic hygroma

Table 21.7 lists syndromes

THE FACE

Cleft lip and palate

Cleft lip and/or palate can be isolated anomalies, occur in syndromes, or be associated with maternal drug treatment (especially anti-convulsants). A particularly important syndrome to recognize is the Shprintzen syndrome (interstitial deletion of chromosome 22q11) as 9% of patients have cleft palate.[6]

Isolated cleft palate appears genetically different from cleft lip, with or without cleft palate. It is unusual in a family with isolated cleft palate to have family members affected by clefting of the lip. The exception is where cleft palate is a manifestation of the dominantly inherited Van der Woude syndrome (see the syndrome list later).

When recurrences occur in families where there is clefting of the lip, with or without cleft palate, all combinations of cleft lip and palate can occur, which can vary in severity, degree and involvement. Recurrence risks increase with severity of cleft lip and the number of affected sibs, and if the proband is female.

A sib of someone with cleft lip, with or without cleft palate, has an overall risk of facial clefting of about 4%. The risk to a sib of someone with an isolated cleft palate is 1.8% – also chiefly of cleft palate. When it is known for certain that there are no other affected family members, the risk to a sib of someone with cleft lip with or without cleft palate is about 2.2%. Risks to offspring are now becoming available: 4.3% if the parent has cleft lip and palate, 3% if the parent has an isolated cleft palate.[7] Although the observed recurrence risks of non-syndromic facial clefting generally concur with the

multifactorial form of inheritance, it is likely that major genes will be shown to be implicated, such as transforming growth factor-α. Studies to identify such genes are in progress.

Syndromes associated with lateral facial clefting are given in Table 21.8.

Median cleft lip

This has a different embryological basis from lateral cleft lip, and has its own syndromic associations, some of which are shown in Table 21.9. It is common in trisomy 13, and a minor degree of upper lip clefting may be a sign of autosomal dominant holoprosencephaly.

Pierre Robin sequence

This sequence is the combination of micrognathia, cleft palate and glossoptosis. It is causally heterogeneous but held to be the result of a small jaw causing failure of the tongue to descend, so interfering with the closure of the palatal shelves, resulting in a U-shaped cleft palate. There can be many

Table 21.8
Syndromes with non-midline cleft lip

Amniotic bands	Mostly sporadic
Ectrodactyly cleft palate	Autosomal dominant
Fraser (cryptophthalmos) syndrome	Autosomal recessive
Ectrodactyly-ectodermal dysplasia-clefting	Autosomal dominant with variable expression
Fetal hydantoin	Environmental
Fetal trimethadione	Environmental
Fryns – acral defects – cloudy corneae – diaphragmatic defects	Autosomal recessive
Hypertelorism – clefting – microtia	Autosomal recessive
Hydrolethalus	Autosomal recessive
Juberg–Hayward	Autosomal recessive
Meckel–Gruber (dysencephalia splanchnocystica)	Autosomal recessive
Neu–Laxova	Autosomal recessive
Lethal multiple pterygium syndrome	Autosomal recessive
Popliteal pterygium: severe autosomal recessive form	Autosomal recessive
Rapp–Hodgkin ectodermal dysplasia	Autosomal dominant
Roberts (pseudothalidomide)	Autosomal recessive
Schisis association	Mostly sporadic
Van der Woude	Autosomal dominant
Varadi–Papp oro-facio-digital-like syndrome (OFD type VI)	Autosomal recessive
4p-	
4q-	
7q-	
dup(10p)	
dup(11p)	
Tri 13	

Table 21.9
Syndromes with midline cleft upper lip

Beemer (lethal short-rib syndrome)	Probably autosomal recessive; uncertain
Clefting – premaxilla agenesis	Autosomal dominant
Cleft lip and palate with pituitary deficiency	Mostly sporadic
Holoprosencephaly	Autosomal dominant, autosomal recessive, sporadic, chromosomal
Oral-facial-digital type 2 – Mohr	Autosomal recessive
Oral-facial-digital (type 1)	X LD
Short-rib – polydactyly type 2 (Majewski)	Autosomal recessive
Trisomy 13	
18p-	

Table 21.10
Syndromes with a significantly small mandible

Acro-renal-mandibular syndrome	Possibly autosomal recessive
Fetal amniopterin/methotrexate syndrome	
Cerebro-costo-mandibular	Autosomal recessive; AD
Fetal trimethadione	
Femoral hypoplasia – unusual facies	Sporadic; autosomal dominant; diabetic mother
Goldenhar (facio-auriculo-vertebral)/hemifacial microsomia	Mostly sporadic; AD
Hydrolethalus	Autosomal recessive
Hypoglossia-hypodactyly	Mostly sporadic
Stickler (hereditary arthro-ophthalmopathy)	Autosomal dominant
Treacher Collins (mandibulofacial dysostosis)	Autosomal dominant in most cases
Plus many chromosomal anomalies	

causes of micrognathia, including single gene inheritance, chromosome anomaly, bone dysplasia, and teratogens. Robin sequence should therefore institute a search for a possible cause, and not be regarded as a diagnosis in its own right. Stickler syndrome is an autosomal dominant condition which can present with Pierre Robin sequence. Table 21.10 lists syndromes causing a significantly small mandible.

EYES

Cyclopia

This is aetiologically heterogeneous and can be a feature of holoprosencephaly (qv). It is associated with chromosomal anomalies (especially chromosomes 18 and 13) but otherwise appears to be a sporadic condition (with an extremely low risk of recurrence).

Microphthalmia and anophthalmia

Unilateral cases of microphthalmia and anophthalmia are usually considered to be non-genetic, but cannot be distinguished absolutely from genetic forms.

Microphthalmia is a feature of many chromosomal anomalies as well as single gene disorders. Complete bilateral anophthalmia is usually autosomal recessive.

Cryptophthalmos

This may have autosomal recessive inheritance, associated with relatively

Table 21.11
Recurrence risks to sibs (for any congenital heart defect) where the isolated cardiac defect in the first sib is shown below.[8] Single gene and chromosomal causes have been excluded

Defect	Risk %
Ventricular septal defect	3.2
Hypoplastic left heart	3.2
Patent ductus	3.1
Atrial septal defect	2.7
Endocardial cushion defect	2.5
Tetralogy of Fallot	2.4
Pulmonary stenosis	2.2
Coarctation of aorta	2.1
Aortic stenosis	2.0
Transposition	1.4
Truncus	4.1
Pulmonary atresia	1.2
Tricuspid atresia	1.0
Ebstein anomaly	0.9
Interrupted aortic arch	2.0

normal eye development but with absence or fusion of the upper or lower lids.

Crytophthalmos is a frequent feature of the autosomal recessive Fraser syndrome (qv), which also has congenital malformations of the genitalia, kidneys, larynx and digits.

CARDIOVASCULAR SYSTEM

Congenital heart disease[8]

About 3 to 5% of congenital heart disease is caused by single mutant genes, 8 to 10% by chromosome imbalance and 85% by multifactorial inheritance which includes

environmental factors. It is observed that following the birth of a child with a congenital cardiac anomaly, a subsequently affected child may have a different cardiac defect. A possible explanation is the timing of environmental triggers on a genetic predisposition, resulting in different defects at different stages of cardiac embryogenesis. If the parent has a congenital heart defect, or there is a family history, referral should be made to a clinical genetics unit.

Recurrence risks for isolated cardiac anomalies are given in Table 21.11; Table 21.12 lists syndromes associated with some

Table 21.12
Syndromes associated with congenital heart disease

Atrioventricular defect

CHARGE association	Uncertain
Chromosome 16 maternal disomy	Disomy
Dandy–Walker malformation	Uncertain
Ellis–van Creveld syndrome	Autosomal recessive
Hydrolethalus syndrome	Autosomal recessive
Hypochondrogenesis	Sporadic; (? new AD mutation)
Ivemark – asplenia or polysplenia	Uncertain
Jarcho–Levin (spondylothoracic dysplasia)	Autosomal recessive
Mohr–Majewski syndrome	Autosomal recessive
Oral-facial-digital syndrome type II	Autosomal recessive
Pallister–Hall (ano-cerebro-digital) syndrome	Autosomal dominant
Short-rib – polydactyly syndrome type 2 (Majewski)	Autosomal recessive
Smith–Magenis syndrome	Microdeletion

Tetralogy of fallot

Adams–Oliver – scalp defects; terminal transverse defects	Autosomal dominant
Arterio-hepatic dysplasia (Alagille)	Autosomal dominant/microdeletion
Baller–Gerold – craniostenosis; radial aplasia	Autosomal recessive
Carpenter – acrocephalopolysyndactyly type II	Autosomal recessive
CHARGE association	Uncertain
DiGeorge syndrome	Autosomal dominant/microdeletion
Fetal alcohol syndrome	Environmental
Fetal primidone	Environmental
Fetal thalidomide	Environmental
Fetal vitamin A syndrome	Environmental
Frontonasal dysplasia	Uncertain
Goldenhar (facio-auriculo-vertebral) syndrome/hemifacial microsomia	Mostly sporadic; autosomal dominant
Ivemark – asplenia or polysplenia	Uncertain
Mohr–Majewski syndrome	Autosomal recessive
Nager acrofacial dysostosis	Autosomal dominant
Robinow (fetal face) syndrome	Autosomal recessive/autosomal dominant
Thrombocytopenia – absent radius (TAR) syndrome	Autosomal recessive
Velo-cardio-facial syndrome	Autosomal dominant/microdeletion

Transposition of the great arteries

Carpenter – acrocephalopolysyndactyly type II	Autosomal recessive
Ivemark – asplenia or polysplenia	Uncertain
Johanson–Blizzard syndrome	Autosomal recessive
Maternal diabetes syndrome	Environmental
Short-rib syndrome, Beemer–Langer type	Autosomal recessive
Short-rib – polydactyly syndrome type I (Saldino–Noonan)	Autosomal recessive
Situs inversus (familial)	Autosomal recessive

Table 21.13
Syndromes featuring heart defects with upper or lower limb anomalies

Aase–Smith – hydrocephalus-CP-joint contractures	Autosomal dominant
Acrofacial – dysostosis with postaxial defects	Possibly autosomal recessive
Carpenter (acrocephalopolysyndactyly)	Autosomal recessive
de Lange	Sporadic
Ellis–van Creveld	Autosomal recessive
Fanconi pancytopenia	Autosomal recessive
Fetal alcohol syndrome	Environmental
Fetal hydantoin	Environmental
Fetal trimethadione	Environmental
Goltz (focal dermal hypoplasia)	XLD with assumed intra-uterine lethality in males
Holt–Oram	Autosomal dominant
Hydrolethalus	Autosomal recessive
Lethal multiple pterygium syndrome	Autosomal recessive
Meckel–Gruber (dysencephalia splanchnocystica)	Autosomal recessive
Noonan	Autosomal dominant
Radial aplasia-thrombocytopenia (TAR)	Autosomal recessive
Roberts (pseudothalidomide)	Autosomal recessive
Rubinstein–Taybi	Mostly sporadic; microdeletion 16p
Short-rib – polydactyly type 1 (Saldino–Noonan)	Autosomal recessive
Smith–Lemli–Opitz (RSH)	Autosomal recessive
VATER association	Sporadic
Velo-cardio-facial	Occasionally autosomal dominant/microdeletion

congenital heart defects. Cardiac anomalies are often associated with limb defects; syndromes are shown in Table 21.13.

Submicroscopic deletion of the long arm of chromosome 22 (Shprintzen syndrome, 22q minus; velo-cardio-facial syndrome) is being increasingly recognized as a cause of CHD.[6] Fluorescence in situ hybridization (FISH) studies are necessary for diagnosis. Several congenital cardiac anomalies are associated with this syndrome – see Table 21.14. If the parents have normal FISH studies, the recurrence risk is low. For further details see the syndrome list later.

Table 21.14
Heart defects in 22q-syndrome in 545 patients[6]

	%
Normal	20
Other clinically non-significant	5
Tetralogy of Fallot	17
Ventricular septal defect	14
Interrupted aortic arch	14
Pulmonary atresia/ventricular septal defect	10
Truncus arteriosus	9
Pulmonary valve stenosis	2
Atrial septal defect	1
Atrioventricular septal defect	<1
Transposition of great arteries	<1
Complex heart disease	<1
Other significant abnormalities	5

GASTROINTESTINAL TRACT

There are relatively few single gene disorders which result in congenital malformations of the gastrointestinal tract. Recurrence figures are usually obtained from empiric studies and are generally low.

Oesophageal atresia

Oesophageal atresia (usually together with tracheo-oesophageal fistula) is found with other malformations (congenital heart disease, genitourinary anomalies, imperforate anus, skeletal anomalies) in about 50% of patients. The VATER association is a recognized pattern (qv). The recurrence risk obtained from empiric studies[9] is < 1%.

Diaphragmatic hernia (Table 21.15)

Recurrences of isolated diaphragmatic hernia are extremely rare. The empiric recurrence risk is low,[10] about 1%.

Omphalocoele (Table 21.16) and gastroschisis

The sib recurrence risk for isolated omphalocoele[11] is low (< 1%). Anomalies of

Table 21.15
Syndromes with diaphragmatic defects

Fryns – acral defects – cloudy corneae – diaphragmatic defects	Autosomal recessive
Lethal multiple pterygium syndrome	Autosomal recessive
Neural tube defects	
Rudiger	Autosomal recessive
Schisis association	Mostly sporadic
4p-	

Table 21.16
Syndromes with omphalocoele

Amniotic bands	Mostly sporadic
Beckwith–Wiedemann	Duplication, deletion, disomy 11p
CHARGE association	Unknown. Most cases sporadic
Meckel–Gruber syndrome	Autosomal recessive
OEIS	Usually sporadic
Schisis association	Mostly sporadic
Trisomy 13	
Trisomy 18	
Triploidy	

the cardiovascular, genitourinary and central nervous systems occur in 67% of patients with an omphalocoele. It is important to consider the Beckwith–Wiedemann syndrome (omphalocoele, macroglossia, somatic overgrowth) because of the intractable neonatal hypoglycaemia, and autosomal dominant inheritance in some cases. Gastroschisis has a very low sib recurrence risk.

Bowel atresias and malrotations

Most gastrointestinal atresias are sporadic, commonly believed to be due to intra-uterine vascular anomalies. Multiple intestinal atresias and apple-peel syndrome are two autosomal recessive conditions (qv).

Hirschsprung's disease

Hirschsprung's disease was long considered to be multifactorial in its inheritance, with empiric risks of 7.2% for sibs of an affected female, 2.6% for sibs of an affected male.[12] It is now known that this phenotype can result from one of several genes operating either alone or in combination. Dominant mutations in the RET gene account for approximately 50% cases, a recessive mutation in endothelin receptor type B (EDNRB) gene accounting for about 5%. Short segment disease occurs in about 25% of RET cases, and in more than 95% of EDNRB-related cases.[13] Genes for endothelin-3 and glial cell line-derived neurotrophic factor have also been implicated. Mutations of these genes give dominant, recessive or polygenic patterns.[14]

RENAL TRACT

Renal cystic disorders

Differentiation must be made between polycystic kidney disease and multicystic renal dysplasia.

Multicystic renal dysplasia can have multiple causes – including syndromes, teratogens, chromosomal imbalance or secondary to obstruction. Renal dysplasia is often associated with structural malformations of other organ systems. As renal dysplasia can be part of the spectrum of an autosomal dominant disorder also resulting in renal agenesis (unilateral or bilateral), renal ultrasound of both parents may be warranted. When all other causes have been eliminated, empiric risk figures are 3.6% for sibs of a perinatal lethal case.[15]

Polycystic kidney disease has Mendelian inheritance, autosomal recessive for the neonatal and infantile types. Although it was considered that autosomal recessive polycystic kidney disease presented early, it is now known that it may not present until later in childhood. Hepatic fibrosis is also a feature in the autosomal recessive disorder. It is rare for autosomal dominant (adult) polycystic kidney disease to present prenatally or neonatally, but the diagnosis in a parent has been known to follow ultrasound finding of fetal cysts. The histology is different from the autosomal recessive condition, in which the renal cysts are due to collecting duct ectasia. The adult dominant disorder (chromosome 16) and the recessive disorder are not allelic. Prenatal diagnosis using DNA markers on chromosome 6 is being assessed.[16] Table 21.17 lists syndromes which can have multiple renal cysts.

Renal tubular dysgenesis

An autosomal recessive condition of renal tubular dysgenesis has recently been described.[17] The proximal convoluted tubules are short and poorly developed, leading to oligohydramnios, Potter sequence and neonatal respiratory failure. Demonstration of oligohydramnios in the absence of genitourinary abnormalities should suggest this diagnosis, and if confirmed by pathological examination warrants genetic counselling. Amniotic fluid volumes may be normal prior to the 22nd week of gestation.

Renal agenesis

It is important that renal ultrasound examination for unilateral renal agenesis be performed on both parents who have had a child with renal agenesis because bilateral or unilateral renal agenesis can be caused by a single autosomal dominant gene with variable expressivity and reduced penetrance. Normal renal ultrasound examination of parents should not preclude ultrasound in subsequent pregnancies, however, as parents with apparently normal renal tracts have had recurrences. The empiric risk for a sib is around 4% for renal anomalies[15] rising to 9% for a related urogenital anomaly.

Syndromes are listed in Table 21.18.

Prune belly syndrome

This has a congenital deficiency of the abdominal musculature, usually associated with urinary tract abnormalities such as a grossly dilated bladder, hydronephrosis and hydro-ureter. Many causes of abdominal distension can result in the phenotype: urethral obstruction, tumours, ascites. Most cases are sporadic. The megacystis-microcolon-intestinal hypoperistalsis syndrome is an important differential diagnosis.

Bladder exstrophy

The recurrence risk for bladder exstrophy[18] is

Table 21.17
Syndromes with multiple renal cysts (renal dysplasia or polycystic kidneys)

Acro-renal-mandibular syndrome	Possibly autosomal recessive
Congenital urogenital adysplasia	Autosomal dominant in some cases
Ellis–van Creveld	Autosomal recessive
Fryns – acral defects – cloudy corneae – diaphragmatic defects	Autosomal recessive
Ivemark – asplenia or polysplenia	Mostly sporadic, but occasional affected sibs reported
Jeune	Autosomal recessive
Meckel–Gruber (dysencephalia splanchnocystica)	Autosomal recessive
Oral-facial-digital (type 1)	XLD
Prune belly	Mostly sporadic
Roberts (pseudothalidomide)	Autosomal recessive
Short-rib – polydactyly type 1 (Saldino–Noonan)	Autosomal recessive
Short-rib – polydactyly type 2 (Majewski)	Autosomal recessive
Tuberous sclerosis	Autosomal dominant
Zellweger (cerebro-hepato-renal) syndrome	Autosomal recessive
Partial dup(9)	
Trisomy 13 and 18; triploidy	

Table 21.18
Syndromes with renal agenesis

Acro-renal-mandibular syndrome	Autosomal recessive
Antley–Bixler synostosis; bent femurs; multiple fractures	Autosomal recessive
Branchio-oto-renal (BOR) syndrome	Autosomal dominant
Caudal regression	Autosomal recessive/sporadic/environmental
Chromosome 16 maternal disomy	Disomy
DiGeorge syndrome	Autosomal dominant/microdeletion
Ectrodactyly – ectodermal dysplasia – clefting (EEC)	Autosomal dominant
Fanconi pancytopenia	Autosomal recessive
Fetal cocaine	Environmental
Fetal thalidomide	Environmental
Fetal warfarin	Environmental
Fraser – cryptophthalmos syndrome	Autosomal recessive
Fryns – acral defects – cloudy corneae – diaphragmatic defects	Autosomal recessive
Goldenhar (facio-auriculo-vertebral) syndrome/hemifacial microsomia	Mostly sporadic; autosomal dominant
Maternal diabetes syndrome	Environmental
Mohr–Majewski syndrome	Autosomal recessive
MURCS association	Uncertain
Nager acrofacial dysostosis	Autosomal dominant
Pallister–Hall (ano-cerebro-digital) syndrome	Autosomal dominant
Popliteal pterygium (Bartsocas–Papas) syndrome – severe autosomal recessive form	Autosomal recessive
Renal dysplasia (familial)	Autosomal recessive/autosomal dominant
Rokitansky – vaginal atresia; rudimentary uterus	Uncertain
Sirenomelia	Uncertain
Smith–Lemli–Opitz syndrome type II (severe lethal form)	Autosomal recessive
Smith–Magenis syndrome	Microdeletion 17
Tetraploid/diploid mosaicism	Mosaic
Townes – imperforate anus; triphalangeal thumbs; ear anomalies	Autosomal dominant
VATER association	Sporadic
Velo-cardio-facial syndrome	Autosomal dominant/microdeletion

low (< 1%). It is a cardinal feature of the OEIS syndrome.

Hydronephrosis

Bilateral hydronephrosis most commonly is the result of obstruction; the recurrence risk being that of the underlying cause. Syndromes are listed in Table 21.19.

GENITAL ANOMALIES

Genital ambiguity occurs in some single gene multiple malformation syndromes (shown in Table 21.20), but these are generally rare. Simple hypospadias or cryptorchidism are common features of a large number of syndromes.

Table 21.19
Syndromes with hydronephrosis

Cryptophthalmos (Fraser)	Autosomal recessive
Megacystis-microcolon-intestinal hypoperistalsis syndrome	Autosomal recessive in severe neonatal cases
Prune belly	Mostly sporadic
Rudiger	Autosomal recessive
Schinzel–Giedion – hypertrichosis – mid-face retraction	Autosomal recessive

Multiple malformation syndromes: inheritance, features and references

- In the following descriptions of syndromes, the emphasis is on associated structural malformations which are likely to be detected by obstetric ultrasound.
- No attempt has been made to indicate the frequency of the structural malformations within the syndrome.
- 'Soft' dysmorphic features (such as minor digital anomalies, anomalies of eye

Table 21.20
Syndromes with 46XY chromosome complement and Mullerian structures

Camptomelic dysplasia	Autosomal dominant; new mutation likely
Double vagina with cardiac, pulmonary and genital malformations	Uncertain
Drash syndrome (nephritis, pseudohermaphroditism, Wilms' tumour)	Mostly sporadic
Nivelon syndrome (chondrodysplasia, pseudohermaphrodism)	Autosomal recessive
Persistent Mullerian duct syndrome	Autosomal recessive
Robinow syndrome	Autosomal recessive/autosomal dominant
Smith–Lemi–Opitz syndrome type II	Autosomal recessive
Verloes syndrome (male pseudohermaphroditism, Mullerian structure; mental retardation)	Autosomal recessive

spacing, ear anomalies) so helpful in postnatal diagnosis have, in general, not been given.

- The original papers should be consulted to aid in diagnosis of the newborn.
- Published reports of prenatal diagnosis are given in the references, but note that techniques available for prenatal diagnosis may change: for instance DNA diagnosis for single gene disorders may become possible when the gene is localized or cloned.

Aarskog syndrome (Facio-digito-genital syndrome, Aarskog–Scott syndrome)

Autosomal dominant/X-linked dominant.

Features

Short stature, proportionate (3–10 centile in males); rhizomelia; hypertelorism; pulmonary stenosis and ventricular septal defect (rare); brachydactyly.

This syndrome (with hypertelorism and a distinctive appearance of the fingers) is unlikely to present at obstetric ultrasound but is in the differential diagnosis of short stature. Mental retardation, seldom severe, is present in only a minority. Most cases have been males and transmission can occur through unaffected females but male to male transmission has been reported occasionally. The Aarskog gene (FGD1) at Xp11.2 is a Rho/Rac guanine nucleotide exchange factor.

References
Aarskog D. A familial syndrome of short stature associated with facial dysplasia and genital anomalies. J Pediatr 1970;77:856–861.

Pasteris N G, Cadle A, Logie L J, et al. Isolation and characterization of the faciogenital dysplasia (Aarskog–Scott syndrome) gene: a putative Rho-Rac guanine nucleotide exchange factor. Cell 1994;79:669–678.

Porteous M E M, Goudie D R. Syndrome of the month. Aarskog syndrome. J Med Genet 1991;28:44–47.

Achondrogenesis types 1 and 2

Type 1: Autosomal recessive.
Type 2: New autosomal dominant mutation.

Features

Macrocephaly; flat nose; short long bones with wide metaphyses; brachydactyly; short ribs; unossified vertebrae with platyspondyly; small pelvis.

Achondrogenesis type 1 (Parenti–Fraccaro type) and type 2 (Langer–Saldino type) cannot be distinguished clinically. Both show severe micromelia, relatively large head, short neck, short trunk and protuberant abdomen, and result in perinatal death. Radiologically, ossification of the skull, spine and pelvis is more deficient in type 1 than in type 2. The long bones are more severely micromelic in type 1 and there are spiky metaphyseal spurs in both, but more so in type 1. Type 1 has two subclasses: in type 1A there are multiple rib fractures and almost complete lack of spinal ossification. Differential diagnosis includes hypochondrogenesis and lethal spondylo-epiphyseal dysplasia congenita. Mutations demonstrated in the diastrophic dysplasia sulphate transporter gene in achondrogenesis type 1B (Superti-Furga et al., 1996). Type 2 is caused by new dominant mutations of COL2A1.

References
Balakumar K. Antenatal diagnosis of Parenti–Fraccaro type achondrogenesis. Indian Pediatr 1990;27:496–499.

Borochowitz Z, Lachman R, et al. Achondrogenesis type I: delineation of further heterogeneity and identification of two distinct subgroups. J Pediatr 1988;112:23–31.

Superti-Furga A, Hastbacka J, Wilcox W R, et al. Achondrogenesis type 1B is caused by mutations in the diastrophic dysplasia sulphate transporter gene. Nature Genetics 1996;12:100–102.

Whitley C B, Gorlin R J. Achondrogenesis: new nosology with evidence of genetic heterogeneity. Radiology 1983;148:693–698.

References for achondrogenesis type 2 (Langer–Saldino type achondrogenesis)
Chen H, Liu C T, Yang S S. Achondrogenesis: a review with special consideration of achondrogenesis type II (Langer–Saldino). Am J Med Genet 1981;10:379–394.

Soothill P W, Vuthiwong C, Rees H. Achondrogenesis type 2 diagnosed by transvaginal ultrasound at 12 weeks' gestation. Prenat Diagn 1993;13:523–528.

Tongsong T, Srisomboon J, Sudasna J. Prenatal diagnosis of Langer–Saldino achondrogenesis. J Clin Ultrasound 1995;23:56–58.

Acrocallosal syndrome

Autosomal recessive.

Features

High birthweight (> 90th centile); macrocephaly with prominent forehead; anencephaly; agenesis of corpus callosum; interhemispheric cyst; hypertelorism; cleft palate; pulmonary stenosis; VSD and ASD; eventration of diaphragm; hypospadias; pre- or postaxial polydactyly of hands and/or feet.

The main characteristics (which may be variable between sibs) are severe mental retardation, agenesis of the corpus callosum and pre-axial polydactyly involving both feet. One case had a large interhemispheric cyst. The forehead is prominent and broad with moderate hypertelorism. Anencephaly appears to be part of the spectrum.

References
Gelman-Kohan Z, Antonelli J, Ankori-Cohen H, et al. Further delineation of the acrocallosal syndrome. Eur J Pediatr 1991;150:797–799.

Hendriks H J E, Brunner H G, Haagen T A M, Hamel B C J. Acrocallosal syndrome. Am J Med Genet 1990;35:443–446.

Lurie I W, Naumchik I V, Wulfsberg E A. The acrocallosal syndrome: expansion of the phenotypic spectrum. Clin Dysmorphol 1994;3:31–34.

Schinzel A. Four patients including two sisters with the acrocallosal syndrome (agenesis of the corpus callosum in combination with preaxial hexadactyly). Hum Genet 1982;62:382.

Schinzel A. The acrocallosal syndrome in first cousins: widening of the spectrum of clinical features and further support for autosomal recessive inheritance. J Med Genet 1988;25:332–336.

Acro-renal-mandibular syndrome

Autosomal recessive.

Features

Strikingly small mandible; split hands and/or feet; absent fingers/toes; hemivertebrae; renal agenesis/cystic dysplasia; malformed uterus.

This syndrome, reported in sibs, has striking mandibular hypoplasia, asymmetrical upper limb defects (split hands or radial ray defects) and either splitting or monodactyly in the feet, with small tarsal bones. One sib had bilateral renal agenesis and the other cystic dysplasia; both had abnormalities of the uterine cavity.

Reference
Halal F, Desgranges M-F, Leduc B, et al. Acro-renal-mandibular syndrome. Am J Med Genet 1980;5:277–284.

Adams–Oliver syndrome

Autosomal dominant.

Features

Scalp defects; terminal transverse defects of limbs – from absent digits to more severe reduction deformities; tetralogy of Fallot; pulmonary stenosis; ventricular septal defect.

The limb defects usually consist of relatively minor terminal reductions of the fingers and toes but occasionally severe limb defects (such as below knee hemimelia) can be present because of the extreme variability. The limb defects can give the appearance of amniotic band disruptions. As well as the scalp defects, small defects of the underlying skull bones are occasionally found; acrania has been reported. Congenital heart defects may be part of the condition.

References
Bamforth J S, Kaurah P, Byrne J, Ferreira P. Adams–Oliver syndrome: a family with extreme variability in clinical expression. Am J Med Genet 1994;49:393–396.
Fryns J P. Syndrome of the month: congenital scalp defects with distal limb reduction anomalies. J Med Genet 1987;24:493–496.
Kuster W, Lenz W, et al. Congenital scalp defects with distal limb anomalies (Adams–Oliver syndrome): report of ten cases and review of the literature. Am J Med Genet 1988;31:99–116.
Zapata H H, Sletten L J, Pierpont M E M. Congenital cardiac malformations in Adams–Oliver syndrome. Clin Genet 1995;47:80–84.

Amniotic bands/early amnion rupture

Sporadic.

Features

Anterior encephalocoele; anencephaly; craniosynostosis; anophthalmia; facial clefting; cleft upper lip; cleft palate; ectopia cordis; exomphalos; reduction deformity of arms and legs, with missing digits; constriction rings of digits and limbs; syndactyly.

Amniotic bands can cause a bizarre combination of craniofacial and limb defects. Facial clefts can have unusual extensions, e.g. the lip and the eyelids may be involved as part of an oblique facial cleft, and severe cranial abnormalities can occur resembling anencephaly or holoprosencephaly. Amputation defects are common, sometimes associated with constriction rings of the digits or limbs. Although usually sporadic, some single gene disorders can mimic this condition (e.g. Adams–Oliver syndrome). Early rupture of the amnion results in additional body wall defects and a shortened cord. Postnatally the presence of constriction rings can be helpful in making the diagnosis, as are unusual forms of syndactyly and configurations of digits suggesting that they have been held together.

References
Burton D J, Filly R A. Sonographic diagnosis of the amniotic band syndrome – pictorial essay (Editorial). Am J Roentgenol 1991;156:555–558.
Goldstein I, Winn H N, Hobbins J C. Prenatal diagnostic criteria for body stalk anomaly. Am J Perinatol 1989;6:84–85.
Goldstein R B, Filly R A. Prenatal diagnosis of anencephaly: spectrum of sonographic appearances and distinction from the amniotic band syndrome. Am J Roentgenol 1988;151:547–550.
Jauniaux E, Vyas S, Finlayson C. Early sonographic diagnosis of body stalk anomaly. Prenat Diagn 1990;10:127–132.
Patten R M, Van Allen M, Mack L A, et al. Limb-body wall complex: in utero sonographic diagnosis of a complicated fetal malformation. Am J Roentgenol 1986;146:1019–1024.

Antley–Bixler syndrome (Trapezoidocephaly-multiple synostotic osteodysgenesis syndrome)

Autosomal recessive.

Features

Brachycephaly; craniosynostosis; clover-leaf skull; frontal bossing; proptosis; choanal atresia/stenosis; depressed nasal bridge; thin ribs; ambiguous genitalia; vaginal atresia; renal agenesis; horseshoe kidneys; radiohumeral synostosis; bowed femur; joint contractures; multiple fractures; thin bones.

The main features are premature closure of the coronal and lambdoidal sutures, proptosis, severe depression of the nasal bridge (± choanal stenosis or atresia). There is brachycephaly with frontal bossing, radiohumeral synostosis, medial bowing of the ulnae, bowing of the femora, slender hands and feet, fractures. Some patients have congenital heart disease, renal anomalies and abnormalities of the female genitalia.

References
Antley R M, Bixler D. Invited editorial comment: developments in the trapezoidocephaly-multiple synostosis syndromes. Am J Med Genet 1983;14:149–150.
Hassell S, Butler M G. Antley–Bixler syndrome: report of a patient and review of literature. Clin Genet 1994;46:372–376.
Jacobson R L, Dignan P S, Miodovnik M, Siddiqi T A. Antley–Bixler syndrome. J Ultrasound Med 1992;11:161–164.
Savoldelli G, Schinzel A. Prenatal ultrasound detection of

humero-radial synostosis in a case of Antley–Bixler syndrome. Prenat Diagn 1982;2:219–223.

Schinzel A, Savoldelli G, Briner J, et al. Antley–Bixler syndrome in sisters: a term newborn and a prenatally diagnosed fetus. Am J Med Genet 1983;14:139–147.

Apert syndrome (acrocephalosyndactyly type I)

Autosomal dominant; most cases new mutations.

Features

Craniosynostosis; proptosis; cleft palate; fusion of vertebrae; hydronephrosis; radio-humeral synostosis; brachydactyly; osseous and skin syndactyly of fingers and toes; postaxial polydactyly of toes.

This is one of the most serious of the craniosynostosis syndromes and is usually caused by new mutations in the FGFR2 gene. At birth all the cranial sutures are abnormal, apart from the lambdoidal, and the head is tower-shaped, flat from front to back with a prominent forehead. The eyes are prominent, the nose beaked and the palate high or cleft. The hands and feet show fusion of digits 2–5, sometimes including the thumb. Pre-axial polydactyly of the feet is occasionally seen. Cardiovascular and genitourinary anomalies each occur in about 10% of cases.

References

Cohen M M Jr, Kreiborg S. An updated pediatric perspective on the Apert syndrome. Am J Dis Child 1993;147:989–993.

Narayan H, Scott I V. Prenatal ultrasound diagnosis of Apert's syndrome. Prenat Diagn 1991;11:187–192.

Parent P, Le Guern H, Munck M R, Thoma M. Apert syndrome, an antenatal ultrasound detected case. Genetic Counseling 1994;5:297–301.

Wilkie A O M, Slaney S F, Oldridge M, et al. Apert syndrome results from localized mutations of FGFR2 and is allelic with Crouzon syndrome. Nature Genetics 1995;9:165–172.

Apple peel congenital intestinal atresia

Autosomal recessive.

Features

Hydrocephaly; microphthalmia; spina bifida; atrial septum defect; small bowel atresia; intestinal duplication; intestinal malrotation; common mesentery; anal atresia; biliary atresia; ureteropelvic junction obstruction.

A duodenal or high jejunal atresia associated with an absence of the small bowel mesentery and occlusion of the superior mesenteric artery, results in the appearance of a twisted loop of small bowel arising from the caecum and twisted around the marginal artery. This syndrome accounts for less than 5% of all intestinal atresias. The syndrome usually presents in the neonatal period with an intestinal obstruction. Fifteen percent of cases have non-intestinal malformations including imperforate anus, biliary atresia, spina bifida, hydrocephalus, microphthalmia, atrial septal defects and ureteropelvic junction obstruction.

References

Blyth H, Dickson J A S. Apple peel syndrome (congenital intestinal atresia): a family study of seven index patients. J Med Genet 1969;6:275–277.

Manning C, Strauss A, Gyepes M T. Jejunal atresia with 'apple peel' deformity. A report of eight survivors. J Perinatol 1989;9:281–286.

Seashore J H, et al. Familial apple peel jejunal atresia. Pediatrics 1987;80:540–544.

Bardet–Biedl (Laurence–Moon–Bardet–Biedl) syndrome

Autosomal recessive.

Prenatal features

Proportionate short stature; tricuspid incompetence; malformed uterus; brachydactyly; postaxial polydactyly of fingers and toes.

Seventy percent of cases of Bardet–Biedl syndrome have polydactyly which can be unilateral. Syndactyly and brachydactyly are very common. (Patients with Laurence–Moon syndrome have spasticity, are thin and do not have polydactyly.) Postnatally both conditions present with retinal dystrophy, mental handicap and hypogenitalism, and 90% have renal problems which can lead to renal failure. Female urogenital abnormalities are common, including vaginal atresia, septate vagina, ectopic urethra, and hypoplasia or duplication of the uterus and fallopian tubes. Linkage studies show at least two loci (on chromosome 16 and possibly 11q and 15q).

References

Carmi R, Elbedour K, Stone E M, Sheffield V C. Phenotypic differences among patients with Bardet–Biedl syndrome linked to three different chromosome loci. Am J Med Genet 1995;59:199–203.

Green J S, Parfrey P S, Harnett J D, et al. The cardinal manifestations of Bardet–Biedl syndrome, a form of Laurence–Moon–Biedl syndrome. N Engl J Med 1989;321:1002–1009.

Ritchie G, Jequier S, Lussier-Lazaroff J. Prenatal renal ultrasound of Laurence–Moon–Biedl syndrome. Pediatr Radiol 1988;19:65–66.

Camptomelic dysplasia

Autosomal dominant: new mutation likely.

Features

Macrocephaly; craniosynostosis; small mandible; cleft palate; platyspondyly; narrow thorax; laryngomalacia; 11 pairs of ribs; small scapulae; pubic ossification defect; ambiguous genitalia; male pseudo-hermaphroditism; hydronephrosis; bowed femur and tibia; talipes equinovarus.

Bowing of the femur and tibia are hallmarks of this often neonatally lethal condition which has characteristic X-ray changes. The majority of patients with an XY karyotype have ambiguous genitalia. There is a large head, small jaw, cleft palate and flat nasal bridge. The narrow chest results in respiratory distress. Congenital dislocation of the hip and bilateral talipes equinovarus occur in the majority. A third of patients have cardiac defects (VSD, ASD, Fallot tetralogy) and a third have hydronephrosis, mostly unilateral. Other frequent malformations include laryngomalacia or tracheomalacia, hydrocephalus and arrhinencephaly. There may be 11 pairs of ribs. The sib recurrence risk is only about 5%, suggesting that many cases may be caused by new autosomal dominant mutations. Mutations have indeed been demonstrated in the SOX9 gene, an SRY-related gene at 7q23-qter, in some patients.

References

Cordone M, Lituania M, Zampatti C, et al. In utero

ultrasonographic features of campomelic dysplasia. Prenat Diagn 1989;9:745–750.

Houston C S, Opitz J M, Spranger J W, et al. The campomelic syndrome: review, report of 17 cases, and follow-up on the currently 17-year-old boy first reported by Maroteaux et al in 1971. Am J Med Genet 1983;15:3–28.

Mansour S, Hall C M, Pembrey M E, Young I D. A clinical and genetic study of campomelic dysplasia. J Med Genet 1995;32:415–420.

Wagner T, Wirth J, Meyer J, et al. Autosomal sex reversal and campomelic dysplasia are caused by mutations in and around the SRY-related gene SOX9. Cell 1994;79:1111–1120.

Winter R, Rosenkranz W, Hofmann H, et al. Prenatal diagnosis of campomelic dysplasia by ultrasonography. Prenat Diagn 1985;5:1–8.

Chondrodysplasia punctata, rhizomelic type (RCD)

Autosomal recessive.

Features

Proportional short stature; flat nasal bridge and flat face; cleft palate; coronal clefts of vertebrae; platyspondyly; rhizomelia of upper and lower limbs; club-foot; joint contractures; stippled epiphyses; metaphyseal dysplasia.

This form of chondrodysplasia punctata is characterized by symmetrical rhizomelic shortening of the limbs with enlarged joints and contractures and is lethal. There may be ichthyosiform skin changes and cataracts. Epiphyseal stippling and flared metaphyses at birth are helpful diagnostically, together with coronal clefts of the vertebrae. About two-thirds of patients die in the first year of life with others dying in late infancy; survival beyond 5 years is rare. Survivors develop microcephaly and mental retardation. There are two types. Mutations in the PEX7 gene which encodes the peroxisomal type 2 targeting signal receptor located on 6q22–q24 have been found in RCD type 1. Type 2 shows deficiency of the enzyme acyl-CoA dihydroxyacetone phosphate acyltransferase (DHAPAT) caused by mutations in that gene. These infants show the clinical features of rhizomelic CP but lack the biochemical anomalies of impairment of plasmalogen biosynthesis, elevated phytanic acid and deficiency of dihydroxyaceto-nephosphate acyltransferase.

References

Gendall P W, Baird C E, Becroft D M. Rhizomelic chondrodysplasia punctata: early recognition with antenatal ultrasonography. J Clin Ultrasound 1994;22:271–274.

Gray R G, Green A, Schutgens R B H, et al. Antenatal diagnosis of rhizomelic chondrodysplasia punctata in the second trimester. J Inherit Metab Dis 1990;13:380–382.

Heymans H S A, Oorthuys J W E, Nelck G, et al. Peroxisomal abnormalities in rhizomelic chondrodysplasia punctata. J Inherit Metab Dis 1986;9(Suppl 2):329–331.

Hoefler G, Hoefler S, Watkins P A, et al. Biochemical abnormalities in rhizomelic chondrodysplasia punctata. J Pediatr 1988;112:726–733.

Hoefler S, Hoefler G, Moser A B, et al. Prenatal diagnosis of rhizomelic chondrodysplasia punctata. Prenat Diagn 1988;8:571–576.

Moser A B, Rasmussen M, Naldu S, et al. Phenotype of patients with peroxisomal disorders subdivided into sixteen complementation groups. J Pediatr 1995;127:13–22.

Sastrowijoto S H, Vandenberghe K, Moerman P, et al. Prenatal ultrasound diagnosis of rhizomelic chondrodysplasia punctata in a primigravida. Prenatal Diagn 1994;14:770–776.

de Lange syndrome (Cornelia de Lange syndrome, Brachmann–de Lange syndrome)

Aetiology uncertain.

Features

Short stature; microcephaly; microphthalmia; micrognathia; cleft palate; diaphragmatic hernia; intestinal malrotation; reduction deformity of arms and digits; split hand.

Upper limb defects in this mental retardation syndrome vary from proximally placed thumbs to absence deformities and ectrodactyly. The majority have low birth-weight, short stature and microcephaly. There is a characteristic facial appearance, and generalized hirsutism. Kliewer gives fetal growth data. Diaphragmatic hernia appears to be relatively common. Children with duplication of 3q also show some features of de Lange syndrome.

References

Bruner J P, Hsia Y E. Prenatal findings in Brachmann–de Lange syndrome. Obstet Gynecol 1990;76:966–968.

Hawley P P, Jackson L G, Kurnit D M. Sixty-four patients with Brachmann–de Lange syndrome: a survey. Am J Med Genet 1985;20:453–459.

Jackson L, Kline A D, Barr M A, Koch S. de Lange syndrome: a clinical review of 310 individuals. Am J Med Genet 1993;47:940–946.

Jelsema R D, Isada N B, Kazzi N J, et al. Prenatal diagnosis of congenital diaphragmatic hernia not amenable to prenatal or neonatal repair: Brachmann–de Lange syndrome. Am J Med Genet 1993;47:1022–1023.

Kliewer M A, Kahler S G, Hertzberg B S, Bowie J D. Fetal biometry in the Brachmann–de Lange syndrome. Am J Med Genet 1993;47:1035–1041.

Double vagina with cardiac, pulmonary and genital malformations

Aetiology uncertain.

Features

Diaphragmatic hernia; anomalous venous return (Scimitar sequence); tetralogy of Fallot; dextrocardia; ventricular septal defect; lung hypoplasia; accessory spleen; ambiguous genitalia; male pseudo-hermaphroditism; vaginal duplication; horseshoe kidneys.

This syndrome was originally reported in two unrelated males (46,XY) with ambiguous external genitalia, undescended small testes, double vagina, complex congenital heart disease (tetralogy of Fallot, dextrocardia, ASD, single atrium, anomalous pulmonary venous return), right lung hypoplasia and diaphragmatic eventration or mal-insertion. Rhabdomyomatous dysplasia of the lung and Scimitar sequence (pulmonary venous return of the right lower lobe of the lung to the liver) have been recorded.

References

Maaswinkel-Mooij P D, Stokvis-Brantsma W H. Phenotypically normal girl with male pseudohermaphroditism, hypoplastic left ventricle, lung aplasia, horseshoe kidney, and diaphragmatic hernia. Am J Med Genet 1992;42:647–648.

Meacham L R, Winn K J, Culler F L, Parks J S. Double vagina, cardiac, pulmonary, and other genital malformations with 46,XY karyotype. Am J Med Genet 1991;41:478–481.

Toriello H V, Higgins J V. Report of another child with sex reversal and cardiac, pulmonary, and diaphragm defects (Letter). Am J Med Genet 1992;44:252.

Drash syndrome (Denys–Drash syndrome)

Most cases sporadic.

Features

Congenital hernia of diaphragm (one case); female pseudo-hermaphroditism; male pseudo-hermaphroditism; true hermaphroditism

The cardinal feature is an XY genotype with either normal female or ambiguous genitalia, usually presenting with early onset hypertension and proteinuria leading to renal failure, and an association with relatively early onset Wilms' tumour and gonadoblastomas developing in streak gonads. Most cases are sporadic; germline mutations have been demonstrated in the zinc-finger domains of the WT1 (Wilms' tumour) gene. Ultrasound examination may be requested in subsequent pregnancies, rather than the diagnosis being made prenatally in the proband.

References

Clarkson P A, Davies H R, Williams D M, et al. Mutational screening of the Wilms's tumour gene, WT1, in males with genital abnormalities. J Med Genet 1993;30:767–772.

Mueller R F. Syndrome of the month. The Denys–Drash syndrome. J Med Genet 1994;31:471–477.

Ectrodactyly syndrome (Cleft hand/foot; split hand/foot)

Autosomal dominant.

Features

Split hand; split foot; polydactyly.

Autosomal dominant inheritance is the commonest mode of transmission. Expression is very variable – occasionally individuals have polydactyly and some gene carriers show no signs at all. Cases have been described with chromosomal anomalies of chromosomes 2q, 6q, 7q and 10q.

Reference

Buss P W. Syndrome of the month. Cleft hand/foot: clinical and developmental aspects. J Med Genet 1994;31:726–730.

Ectrodactyly-cleft palate syndrome

Autosomal dominant.

Features

Cleft palate; split hand; split foot.

This condition may be the same as EEC (qv). A large family was reported where cleft palate and ectrodactyly were segregating – singly or together – but in the absence of skin changes.

Reference

Opitz J M, Frias J L, Cohen M M. The ECP syndrome, another autosomal dominant cause of monodactylous ectrodactyly. Eur J Pediatr 1980;133:217–220.

Ectrodactyly-ectodermal dysplasia-clefting syndrome (EEC syndrome)

Autosomal dominant.

Features

Sparse hair; cleft lip and palate; renal agenesis; renal cysts; hydronephrosis; split hand and foot.

Variable ectrodactyly may occur in this syndrome with ectodermal features (sparse fine dry hair, small and/or missing teeth, and thin ridged nails) and cleft lip and palate. Facial clefting is common but not an essential part of the syndrome. Urogenital anomalies (megaureter, vesicoureteric reflux, hydronephrosis and hypospadias) are present in about 50% of cases. Mental development is usually normal. All the features are very variable and extreme care must be taken in examining and counselling parents of an apparently isolated case. Linkage studies suggest loci on 7q and 19.

References

Bronshtein M, Gershoni-Baruch R. Prenatal transvaginal diagnosis of the ectrodactyly, ectodermal dysplasia, cleft palate (EEC) syndrome. Prenat Diagn 1993;13:519–522.

Buss P W, Hughes H E, Clarke A. Twenty-four cases of the EEC syndrome: clinical presentation and management. J Med Genet 1995;32:716–723.

Buss P W. Syndrome of the month. Cleft hand/foot: clinical and developmental aspects. J Med Genet 1994;31:726–730.

Kohler R, Sousa P, Jorge C S. Prenatal diagnosis of the ectrodactyly, ectodermal dysplasia, cleft palate (EEC)

syndrome. J Ultrasound Med 1989;8:337–339.

Rodini E S O, Richieri-Costa A. EEC syndrome: report on 20 new patients, clinical and genetic considerations. Am J Med Genet 1990;37:42–53.

Ellis–van Creveld syndrome (EVC syndrome; chondroectodermal dysplasia)

Autosomal recessive.

Features

Short limbs prenatal onset; Dandy–Walker malformation; midline cleft upper lip; narrow thorax; pre- or postaxial polydactyly of fingers, less usually of toes.

Postaxial polydactyly, mostly involving the hands but occasionally the feet, meso/acromelic shortening of the limbs, multiple oral frenulae and congenital heart defect (usually ASD) are major features. Neonatal teeth may be present. The chest is narrow and the radiological changes are indistinguishable from Jeune's syndrome, as the iliac bones are small with a downwardly directed spike in the region of the triradiate cartilage. Ribs and long bones are short, thorax long and narrow, and the femora and humeri thick and bowed. The gene has been mapped to 4p16.

References

Brueton L A, Dillon M J, Winter R M. Ellis–van Creveld syndrome, Jeune syndrome, and renal-hepatic-pancreatic dysplasia: separate entities or disease spectrum? J Med Genet 1990;27:252–255.

Mahoney M J, Hobbins J C. Prenatal diagnosis of chondroectodermal dysplasia (Ellis–van Creveld syndrome) with fetoscopy and ultrasound. N Engl J Med 1977;297:258–260.

Zangwill K M, Boal D K B, Ladda R L. Dandy–Walker malformation in Ellis–van Creveld syndrome. Am J Med Genet 1988;31:123–129.

Fetal akinesia/hypokinesia sequence (Pena–Shokeir syndrome)

Causally heterogenous (see below).

Features

Short stature, prenatal onset; hydrocephaly; cleft palate; short webbed neck; kyphosis; lung hypoplasia; limited movement of large joints leading to joint contractures; club-foot, varus; multiple fractures; slender bones.

The 'Pena–Shokeir syndrome' phenotype results from lack of fetal movement, causing multiple ankyloses, pulmonary hypoplasia, facial anomalies and polyhydramnios. Presentation can be with multiple prenatal fractures. Causes include congenital myopathy, degeneration of the anterior horn cells, or abnormalities of the cerebral cortex and cerebellum, including ischaemia and anoxic damage. A recurrence risk of 10 to 15% is generally given because some, but not all, cases are autosomal recessive. If a reliable pathological opinion demonstrates long-standing ischaemic/anoxic damage of the central nervous system at autopsy, it may be possible to reduce this risk.

References

Ajayi R A, Keen C E, Knott P D. Ultrasound diagnosis of the Pena–Shokeir phenotype at 14 weeks of pregnancy. Prenat Diagn 1995;15:762–764.

Hall J G. Analysis of Pena–Skokeir phenotype (Invited editorial comment). Am J Med Genet 1986;25:99–117.

Kirkinen P, Herva R, Leisti J. Early prenatal diagnosis of a lethal syndrome of multiple congenital contractures. Prenat Diagn 1987;7:189–196.

Muller L M, De Jong G. Prenatal ultrasonographic features of the Pena–Shokeir I syndrome and the trisomy 18 syndrome. Am J Med Genet 1986;25:119–129.

Pena S D J, Shokeir M H K. Syndrome of camptodactyly, multiple ankyloses, facial anomalies and pulmonary hypoplasia – further delineation and evidence for autosomal recessive inheritance. BDOAS 1976;12(5):201–208.

Persutte W H, Lenke R R, et al. Antenatal diagnosis of Pena–Shokeir syndrome (type I) with ultrasonography and magnetic resonance imaging. Obstet Gynecol 1988;72:472–475.

Sherer D M, Sanko S R, Metlay L A, Woods J R. Absent fetal movement response with a blunted cardioacceleratory fetal response to external vibratory acoustic stimulation in a fetus with the Pena–Shokeir syndrome (fetal akinesia and hypokinesia sequence). Am J Perinatol 1992;9:1–4.

Fetal cocaine syndrome

Environmental.

Features

Short stature; microcephaly; cerebral atrophy; cerebellar abnormalities; agenesis of corpus callosum; posterior encephalocoele; holoprosencephaly; porencephaly; schizencephaly; meningocoele; hemivertebrae; pulmonary stenosis; ventricular septal defect; absent ribs; anterior abdominal wall defects; intestinal atresias; renal agenesis; hydronephrosis; reduction deformity of arms; split hand.

Maternal cocaine exposure may cause fetal vascular disruption or placental vasoconstriction. Common abnormalities are limb reduction defects, genitourinary defects, and microcephaly with nervous system defects such as porencephaly, agenesis of the corpus callosum, septo-optic dysplasia, schizencephaly, and midline cerebral cysts. Intra-uterine growth retardation and developmental delay are also associated. There is a characteristic facial appearance with puffy eyelids, grooves above hypoplastic supraorbital ridges, short nose, large fontanelles, and excess skin at the glabella.

References

Dominguez R, Vilacoro A A, Slopis J M, Bohan T P. Brain and ocular abnormalities in infants with in utero exposure to cocaine and other street drugs. Am J Dis Child 1991;145:688–695.

Gieron-Korthals M A, Helal A, Martinez C R. Expanding spectrum of cocaine induced central nervous system malformations (Case report). Brain Dev 1994;16:253–256.

Hume R F Jr, Gingras J L, Martin L S, et al. Ultrasound diagnosis of fetal anomalies associated with in utero cocaine exposure: further support for cocaine-induced vascular disruption teratogenesis. Fetal Diagn Ther 1994;9:239–245.

van den Anker J N, Cohen-Overbeek T E, Wladimiroff J W, Sauer P J J. Prenatal diagnosis of limb-reduction defects due to maternal cocaine use (Letter). Lancet 1991;2:1332.

Fetal thalidomide syndrome (thalidomide embryopathy)

Environmental.

Features

Short trunk; anophthalmia; microphthalmia; cleft lip and palate; meningo-myelocoele; absent sacrum; hemivertebrae; Fallot tetralogy; pulmonary stenosis; truncus arteriosus; ventricular septal defect;

pulmonary segmentation defects; bowel atresias; renal agenesis; horseshoe kidneys; hydronephrosis; absent upper and lower limbs; reduction deformity of arms and legs; club-foot, varus; polydactyly.

As well as severe limb defects there were associated craniofacial, cardiac, abdominal and urogenital abnormalities in many cases reported following maternal ingestion in the years 1959–61.

References

Kajii T, Kida M, Takahashi K. The effect of thalidomide intake during 113 human pregnancies. Teratology 1973;8:163–166.

Newman C G H. Teratogen update: clinical aspects of thalidomide embryopathy – a continuing preoccupation. Teratology 1985;32:133–144.

Smithells R W, Newman C G H. Recognition of thalidomide defects. J Med Genet 1992;29:716–723.

Fetal valproate syndrome

Environmental.

Features

Low birthweight; microcephaly; neural tube defect; craniosynostosis (metopic suture); reduction deformity of arms; postaxial polydactyly of fingers; absent or hypoplastic thumbs; club-foot, varus.

Diagnosis by ultrasound is likely to be in those fetuses where neural tube defects or limb anomalies (pre- and postaxial polydactyly and radial defects) have occurred. Some affected infants have distinctive dysmorphic features with brachycephaly, high forehead, shallow orbits and prominent eyes. The proportion of infants affected when the mother is on monotherapy is said to be between 2.5 and 10%; risk figures at the lower end of the range are usually given where there has not been a previously affected child. In one prospective series a major malformation occurred in 4/14 cases.

References

Clayton-Smith J, Donnai D. Syndrome of the month. Fetal valproate syndrome. J Med Genet 1995;32:724–727.

Omtzigt J G C, Los F J, Hagenaars A M, et al. Prenatal diagnosis of spina bifida aperta after first-trimester valproate exposure. Prenat Diagn 1992;12:893–897.

Sharony R, Garber A, Viskochil D, et al. Preaxial ray reduction defects as part of valproic acid embryofetopathy. Prenat Diagn 1993;13:909–918.

Fetal varicella syndrome

Environmental.

Features

Short stature; hypoplasia of arms and legs.

On the rare occasions when the fetus is infected transplacentally, extensive skin scarring can occur, associated with hypoplasia of affected limbs. Low birth-weight, mild mental retardation, lax abdominal wall, eye defects and neuropathic bladder are other features.

References

Alkalay A L, Pomerance J J, Rimoin D L. Fetal varicella syndrome. J Pediatr 1987;111:320–323.

Enders G, Miller E, Craddock-Watson J, et al. Consequences of varicella and herpes zoster in pregnancy: prospective study of 1739 cases. Lancet 1994;1:1547–1550.

Jones K L, Johnson K A, Chambers C D. Offspring of women infected with varicella during pregnancy: a prospective study. Teratology 1994;49:29–32.

Pastuszak A L, Levy M, Schick B, et al. Outcome after maternal varicella infection in the first 20 weeks of pregnancy. N Engl J Med 1994;330:901–905.

Fibrochondrogenesis

Autosomal recessive.

Features

Rhizomelic shortening of upper and lower limbs; brachycephaly; prominent eyes; cleft palate; short neck; coronal clefts of vertebrae; platyspondyly; narrow thorax; short ribs; small pelvis.

This rare, lethal, rhizomelic chondrodysplasia causes a short neck, narrow chest, flat face, prominent eyes and occasionally cleft palate. Radiological features are short broad tubular bones with slightly irregular metaphyses and peripheral spur formation. The iliac bones are small and inferiorly broad with spurs on the lower margins. The vertebral bodies are flat with sagittal midline clefting in most. The ribs are short and cupped at their anterior ends.

References

Bankier A, Fortune D, Duke J, Sillence D O. Fibrochondrogenesis in male twins at 24 weeks gestation. Am J Med Genet 1991;38:95–98.

Eteson D J, Adomian G E, Ornoy A, et al. Fibrochondrogenesis: radiologic and histologic studies: distinctive cartilage histology. Am J Med Genet 1984;19:277–290.

Whitley C B, Langer L O Jr, Ophoven J, et al. Fibrochondrogenesis: lethal, autosomal recessive chondrodysplasia with distinctive cartilage histopathology. Am J Med Genet 1984;19:265–275.

Fraser syndrome (Cryptophthalmos syndrome)

Autosomal recessive.

Features

Anophthalmia; cryptophthalmos; microphthalmia; cleft lip and palate; malformed uterus; renal agenesis.

The main features of this variable condition are a 'hidden eye', syndactyly and abnormal genitalia. Cryptophthalmos can be bilateral, unilateral or asymmetrical, sometimes with a covering of skin which can extend from the forehead to the cheeks. Usually the globe is present under the fused eyelids. Laryngeal stenosis, renal agenesis, and genital abnormalities (hypospadias, clitoromegaly) are common. Mental retardation occurs in 80% of survivors. Cryptophthalmos may also occur without other malformations.

References

Boyd P A, Keeling J W, Lindenbaum R H. Fraser syndrome (cryptophthalmos-syndactyly syndrome): a review of eleven cases with postmortem findings. Am J Med Genet 1988;31:159–168.

Gattuso J, Patton M A, Baraitser M. The clinical spectrum of the Fraser syndrome: report of three new cases and review. J Med Genet 1987;24:549–555.

Schauer G M, Dunn L K, Godmilow L, et al. Prenatal diagnosis of Fraser syndrome at 18.5 weeks gestation, with autopsy findings at 19 weeks. Am J Med Genet 1990;37:583–591.

Fryns syndrome

Autosomal recessive.

Features

Agenesis of corpus callosum; arhinencephaly; heterotopia; cleft lip and palate; short neck; anomalous venous return; ventricular septal defect; lung hypoplasia secondary to diaphragm defect; pulmonary segmentation defects; intestinal malrotation and atresia; bicornuate uterus; renal agenesis; absent phalanges; club-foot, varus.

Hydramnios in the presence of normal fetal growth is suggestive of this syndrome, as is a diaphragmatic defect (with secondary lung hypoplasia) together with renal abnormalities. There is a characteristic face: coarse features, broad flat nasal bridge, cloudy cornea, small jaw, cleft lip and palate and abnormal ears. There are absent or hypoplastic finger nails and distal phalanges. Intestinal malrotation or atresias and a bicornuate uterus are also found. Central nervous system malformations are common, as are cardiovascular lesions including ASD, VSD and persistent left superior vena cava. Growth may be above the 75th centile and there may be true macrocephaly. Several chromosome aberrations show similar features: duplication of 1q24-31, terminal 6q deletion, partial trisomy 22, mosaic trisomy 9 and trisomy 22.

References

Ayme S, Julian C, Gambarelli D, et al. Fryns syndrome: report on 8 new cases. Clin Genet 1989;35:191–201.

Fryns J-P. Prenatal diagnosis and long survival of Fryns syndrome. Prenat Diagn 1995;15:97–98.

Gadow E C, Lippold S, Serafin E, et al. Prenatal diagnosis and long survival of Fryns' syndrome. Prenat Diagn 1994;14:673–676.

Moerman P, Fryns J-P, et al. The syndrome of diaphragmatic hernia, abnormal face and distal limb anomalies (Fryns syndrome): report of two sibs with further delineation of this multiple congenital anomaly (MCA) syndrome. Am J Med Genet 1988;31:805–814.

Pellissier M C, Philip N, Potier A, et al. Prenatal diagnosis of Fryns' syndrome. Prenat Diagn 1992;12:299–304.

Goldenhar syndrome (Facio-auriculo-vertebral syndrome; hemifacial microsomia; oculoauriculovertebral syndrome)

Possibly autosomal dominant/sporadic.

Features

Encephalocoele; hydrocephaly; microphthalmia; cleft lip and palate; fusion of vertebrae; hemivertebrae; segmentation defects of spine; anomalous venous return; Fallot tetralogy; pulmonary stenosis; ventricular septal defect.

This condition principally affects the face (bilaterally but asymmetrically) – small ear, acrostomia, failure of formation of the mandibular ramus and condyle. An epibulbar dermoid is considered a necessary diagnostic feature. Cervical vertebral anomalies are common. It can be associated with other structural malformations such as cardiac defects (5–58% of cases). Severe central nervous system involvement is rare but hydrocephalus, microcephaly, encephalocoele and severe retardation have been reported. Inheritance is uncertain – irregular dominant families have been described.

References

Benacerraf B R, Frigoletto F D. Prenatal ultrasonographic recognition of Goldenhar's syndrome. Am J Obstet Gynecol 1988;159:950–952.

Jeanty P, Zaleski W, Fleischer A C. Prenatal sonographic diagnosis of lipoma of the corpus callosum in a fetus with Goldenhar syndrome. Am J Perinatol 1991;8:89–90.

Kumar A, Friedman J M, Taylor G P, Patterson M W H. Pattern of cardiac malformation in oculoauriculovertebral spectrum. Am J Med Genet 1993;46:423–426.

Rollnick B R, Kaye C I, Nagatoshi K, et al. Oculoauriculovertebral dysplasia and variants: phenotypic characteristics of 294 patients. Am J Med Genet 1987;26:361–376.

Goltz syndrome (focal dermal hypoplasia)

X-linked dominant.

Features

Microcephaly; anophthalmia; microphthalmia; cleft lip and palate; split hand; polydactyly; osseous syndactyly of fingers.

The limb defects are variable – syndactyly of fingers 3 and 4, polydactyly, missing fingers, missing part of a limb. The variable skin lesions include congenital skin hypoplasia through which fat may herniate, linear pigmented streaks and telangiectasia.

Papillomas develop around the lips, gums or the side of the nose. Scalp hair may be sparse or brittle and the nails dysplastic. The eyes are frequently affected, mostly asymmetrically, with chorioretinal or iris colobomata, but unilateral anophthalmos has been reported. Most cases are female and inheritance is thought to be X-linked dominant with early intra-uterine lethality in males. A locus has been mapped to Xp22.31.

References

Goltz R W. Focal dermal hypoplasia syndrome. An update (Editorial comment). Arch Dermatol 1992;128:1108–1111.

Temple I K, MacDowall P, Baraitser M, Atherton D J. Syndrome of the month. Focal dermal hypoplasia (Goltz syndrome). J Med Genet 1990;27:180–187.

Greig syndrome (frontodigital syndrome; cephalopolysyndactyly syndrome)

Autosomal dominant/microdeletion.

Features

Macrocephaly; asymmetrical skull; agenesis of corpus callosum; communicating hydrocephalus; frontal bossing; postaxial polydactyly of fingers more common than pre-axial; skin syndactyly of fingers; broad thumbs and hallux; syndactyly and pre- and postaxial polydactyly of toes.

In the hands postaxial polydactyly is more common than pre-axial polydactyly, but both occur. The thumbs are often broad; the thumb nail or terminal phalanx may be bifid. In the feet the hallux is often duplicated with syndactyly of toes 1, 2 and 3, and postaxial polydactyly is less common. The face has a high forehead with frontal bossing, macrocephaly, hypertelorism and a broad nasal base. Agenesis of the corpus callosum and mild cerebral ventricular dilatation are occasionally seen. The gene maps to 7p13; the GLI3 zinc-finger gene has been reported to be interrupted by translocations in some Greig syndrome families.

References

Baraitser M, Winter R M, Brett E M. Greig cephalopolysyndactyly: report of 13 affected individuals in three families. Clin Genet 1983;24:257–265.

Greig D M. Oxycephaly. Edinburgh Med J 1926;33:189–218.

HARD ± E syndrome (Warburg syndrome; Walker–Warburg syndrome)

Autosomal recessive.

Features

Cerebellar abnormalities; agyria; lissencephaly; Dandy–Walker malformation; posterior encephalocoele; hydrocephaly; anterior chamber abnormalities; Rieger anomaly; buphthalmos; microphthalmia.

This neurodevelopmental syndrome has severe mental retardation, anterior chamber eye defects, retinal dysplasia and hydrocephalus. The brain pathology is a form of lissencephaly (type 2) with agyria, absent cortical layer, absent or small corpus callosum and septum pellucidum, and a small, dysplastic cerebellum and brain stem with absence of the posterior vermis. A small encephalocoele can be present at the vertex.

References

Chitayat D, Toi A, Babul R, et al. Prenatal diagnosis of retinal nonattachment in the Walker–Warburg syndrome. Am J Med Genet 1995;56:351–358.

Crowe C, Jassani M, Dickerman L. The prenatal diagnosis of the Walker–Warburg syndrome. Prenat Diagn 1986;6:177–186.

Donnai D, Farndon P A. Syndrome of the month: Walker–Warburg syndrome (Warburg syndrome, HARD ± E syndrome). J Med Genet 1986;23:200–203.

Farrell S A, Toi A, Leadman M L, et al. Prenatal diagnosis of retinal detachment in Walker–Warburg syndrome. Am J Med Genet 1987;28:619–624.

Maynor C H, Hertzberg B S, Ellington K S. Antenatal sonographic features of Walker–Warburg syndrome. Value of endovaginal sonography. J Ultrasound Med 1992;11:301–303.

Vohra N, Ghidini A, Alvarez M, Lockwood C. Walker–Warburg syndrome: prenatal ultrasound findings. Prenat Diagn 1993;13:575–580.

Hay–Wells syndrome (AEC syndrome; ankyloblepharon-ectodermal dysplasia-clefting syndrome)

Autosomal dominant.

Features

Buphthalmos, hypoplastic maxilla, cleft upper lip, cleft palate.

This is a rare cause of facial clefting. The ankyloblepharon is caused by strands consisting of a central core of vascular connective tissue surrounded by epithelium. Eroded skin at birth and recurrent scalp infections, or chronic scalp erosions, are common features of the condition. The hair can be totally absent, or sparse and wiry, and the nails absent or dystrophic. Teeth can be pointed and widely spaced.

References

Greene S L, Michels V V, Doyle J A. Variable expression in ankyloblepharon-ectodermal defects-cleft lip and palate syndrome. Am J Med Genet 1987;27:207–212.

Hay R J, Wells R S. The syndrome of ankyloblepharon, ectodermal defects, and cleft lip and palate. Br J Dermatol 1976;94:277–289.

Shwayder T A, Lane A T, Miller M E. Hay–Wells syndrome. Pediatr Dermatol 1986;3:399–402.

Spiegel J, Colton A. AEC syndrome: ankyloblepharon, ectodermal defects, and cleft lip and palate. Report of two cases. J Am Acad Dermatol 1985;12:810–815.

Holoprosencephaly

Autosomal recessive, autosomal dominant, sporadic, chromosomal.

Features

Microcephaly; holoprosencephaly; arhinencephaly; hypotelorism; cleft upper lip (non-midline); midline cleft upper lip; cleft palate.

A form of holoprosencephaly caused by chromosome abnormality on 7q is now known to be due to haploinsufficiency of the human sonic hedgehog gene and is designated holoprosencephaly type 3. Mutations in this gene have been found in some dominant families. Dominant families can show incomplete penetrance and variable expression – a parent may have a single central maxillary incisor as the only sign, or mild hypotelorism or anosmia. The risk of an obligate carrier having a severely affected infant is 16 to 21%; the risk of milder manifestations is 13 to 14%. Recurrence risks after an isolated case of holoprosencephaly with normal chromosomes are 5 to 6%.

About a third of cases have a cytogenetic abnormality, including del(18p) del(7q36), dup(3p24-pter), del(21q22.3) and trisomy 13.

References

Berry S M, Gosden C, Snijders R J M, Nicolaides K H. Fetal holoprosencephaly: associated malformations and chromosomal defects. Fetal Diagn Ther 1990;5:92–99.

Bronshtein M, Wiener Z. Early transvaginal sonographic diagnosis of alobar holoprosencephaly. Prenat Diagn 1991;11:459–462.

Collins A L, Lunt P W, Garrett C, Dennis N R. Holoprosencephaly: a family showing dominant inheritance and variable expression. J Med Genet 1993;30:36–40.

McGahan J P, Nyberg D A, Mack L A. Sonography of facial features of alobar and semilobar holoprosencephaly. Am J Roentgenol 1990;154:143–148.

Nelson L H, King M. Early diagnosis of holoprosencephaly. J Ultrasound Med 1992;11:57–59.

Siebert J R, Cohen M M Jr, Sulik K K, Shaw C-M, Lemire R J. Holoprosencephaly: An overview and atlas of cases. New York: John Wiley & Sons Ltd; 1990.

Toma P, Costa A, Magnano G M, et al. Holoprosencephaly: prenatal diagnosis by sonography and magnetic resonance imaging. Prenat Diagn 1990;10:429–436.

Holt–Oram syndrome

Autosomal dominant.

Features

Hypoplastic clavicles; atrial septum defect; conduction defects; ventricular septal defect; reduction deformity of arms and digits; hypoplastic humerus, radius or ulna; radio-humeral and radio-ulnar synostosis; absent or hypoplastic thumbs.

The limb abnormalities are very variable. Bilateral upper limb defects can range from thumb hypoplasia and radial aplasia to severe phocomelia. Heart lesions (the other component of the syndrome) are predominantly ASD, or more rarely VSD and other lesions, including ECG anomalies where no structural cardiac defects are present. Wrist X-rays and careful assessment of the heart should detect mildly affected family members as penetrance is probably close to 100%. This syndrome can be caused by mutations in the TBX5 gene on 12q24.1, but there is heterogeneity as some families do not show linkage to this locus.

References

Brons J T J, Van Geijn H P, et al. Prenatal ultrasound diagnosis of the Holt–Oram syndrome. Prenat Diagn 1988;8:175–182.

Hurst J A, Hall C M, Baraitser M. Syndrome of the month: the Holt–Oram syndrome. J Med Genet 1991;28:406–410.

Newbury-Ecob R, Leanage R, Raeburn J A, Young I D. Holt–Oram syndrome: a clinical genetic study. J Med Genet 1996;33:300–307.

Hypertelorism-microtia-clefting (HMC syndrome)

Autosomal recessive.

Features

Small ears; hypertelorism; bifid nasal tip; cleft lip and palate.

This is another single gene cause of facial clefting. As all cases of cleft lip and palate have some degree of hypertelorism, in considering this diagnosis the hypertelorism should be more severe than would otherwise be expected in isolated cleft lip and palate.

Reference

Baraitser M. The hypertelorism microtia clefting syndrome. J Med Genet 1982;19:387–388.

Hypoglossia-hypodactyly (Hanhart syndrome; adactylia-aglossia; oromandibular-limb hypogenesis syndrome)

Uncertain.

Features

Cleft palate; hypoplastic tongue; reduction deformity of arms or legs; absent fingers.

This condition is variable with limb abnormalities varying from absence of digits to absence of the distal part of a whole limb. The jaw is small. Intelligence is usually normal. There is a definite association with the Möbius syndrome. Firth reported four possible cases where chorionic villus sampling was carried out at 8 to 9 weeks and later reported an inverse correlation between severity of limb defect following CVS and gestation, suggesting that CVS might be the cause in some cases.

References

Firth H V, Boyd P A, Chamberlain P, et al. Severe limb abnormalities after chorion villus sampling at 56–66 days' gestation. Lancet 1991;1:762–763.

Firth H V, Boyd P A, Chamberlain P F, et al. Analysis of limb reduction defects in babies exposed to chorionic villus sampling. Lancet 1994;1:1069–1071.

Gorlin R J, Cohen M M, Levin L S. Syndromes of the head and neck. 3rd ed. Oxford: Oxford University Press; 1990: 666–673.

Herrmann J, Pallister P D, Gilbert E F, et al. Studies of malformation syndromes of man XXXXIB. Nosologic studies in the Hanhart and the Möbius syndrome. Eur J Pediatr 1976;122:19–55.

Shechter S A, Sherer D M, Geilfuss C J, et al. Prenatal sonographic appearance and subsequent management of a fetus with oromandibular limb hypogenesis syndrome associated with pulmonary hypoplasia. J Clin Ultrasound 1990;18:661–665.

Sheu B-C, Shyu M-K, Tseng L-H, Lin C-J, Hsieh F-J. Prenatal detection of limb defects after chorionic villus sampling. Prenat Diagn 1995;15:1075–1077.

Hypophosphatasia

Autosomal recessive (severe type).
Autosomal dominant (childhood/adult type).

Features

Short stature; narrow thorax; beaded short ribs; bowing of femur and tibia; multiple fractures; wide metaphysis.

One form of this condition can present in utero, the other in childhood or in adulthood. The 'infantile' form can result in stillbirth or early death from respiratory insufficiency. The limb bones are deformed and sometimes fractured, and may suggest lethal osteogenesis imperfecta. The ends of the long bones have a rachitic appearance, and the skull is poorly ossified and assumes a globular shape. The severe type is autosomal recessive and has been mapped to 1p36.1-34. The two distinct clinical forms of the disorder usually run true in families, however they have occasionally been observed together. Mis-sense mutations have been demonstrated in the tissue-non-specific alkaline phosphatase gene (ALPL) in both severe and mild cases.

References

Benzie R, Doran T A, Escoffery W, et al. Prenatal diagnosis of hypophosphatasia. BDOAS 1976;12(6):271–282.

Blau K, Rattenbury J M, Pryse-David J, et al. Prenatal detection of hypophosphatasia: cytological and genetic considerations. J Inherit Metab Dis 1978;1:37–39.

Brock D J H, Barron L. First-trimester prenatal diagnosis of hypophosphatasia: experience with 16 cases. Prenat Diagn 1991;11:387–391.

Henthorn P S, Whyte M P. Infantile hypophosphatasia: successful prenatal assessment by testing for tissue-non-specific alkaline phosphatase isoenzyme gene mutations. Prenat Diagn 1995;15:1001–1006.

Kishi F, Matsuura S, Murano I, et al. Prenatal diagnosis of infantile hypophosphatasia. Prenat Diagn 1991;11:305–310.

Mulivar R A, Memuti M, Zackai E H, Harris H. Prenatal diagnosis of hypophosphatasia: genetic, biochemical, and clinical studies. Am J Hum Genet 1978;30:271–282.

Orimo H, Nakajima E, Hayashi Z, Kijima K, Watanabe A, Tenjin H, Araki T, Shimada T. First-trimester prenatal molecular diagnosis of infantile hypophosphatasia in a Japanese family. Prenat Diagn 1996;16:559–563.

Rathbun J C. Hypophosphatasia: a new developmental anomaly. Am J Dis Child 1948;75:822–826.

Warren R C, Mckenzie C, Rodeck C H, et al. First trimester diagnosis of hypophosphatasia with a monoclonal antibody to the liver/bone/kidney isoenzyme of alkaline phosphatase. Lancet 1985;2:856–858.

Wladimiroff J W, Niermeijer M F, et al. Early prenatal diagnosis of congenital hypophosphatasia: case report. Prenat Diagn 1985;5:47–52.

Jarcho–Levin (spondylothoracic dysplasia; occipito-facio-cervico-thoracic-abdomino-digital syndrome)

Autosomal recessive.

Features

Short trunk; cleft palate; short neck; fusion of vertebrae; hemivertebrae; platyspondyly; segmentation defects of spine; short thorax; atrioventricular septal defect; pulmonary stenosis; ventricular septal defect; pulmonary segmentation defects; fused thin ribs; hydronephrosis.

The majority of cases with this severe spondylocostal dysplasia do not survive the first year because of the severe respiratory problems. There is a short trunk, prominent anterior rib margin, and a short immobile neck. Occasionally there are urogenital abnormalities such as undescended/absent testes, unilateral hydronephrosis and imperforate anus. The ribs appear fan-like or crab-like on X-ray, sometimes with hemivertebrae. Congenital heart disease (AV septal defect, pulmonary artery atresia, aorta arising anteriorly from the morphological right ventricle) and lung segmentation defects have been reported.

References

Apuzzio J J, Diamond N, Ganesh V, et al. Difficulties in the prenatal diagnosis of Jarcho–Levin syndrome. Am J Obstet Gynecol 1987;156:916–918.

Karnes P S, Day D, Berry S A, Pierpont M E M. Jarcho–Levin syndrome; four new cases and classification of subtypes. Am J Med Genet 1991;40:264–270.

Lenoir S, Rolland M, Sarramon M F. Prenatal ultrasound diagnosis of the Jarcho–Levin syndrome. J Genet Hum 1989;37:425–430.

Marks F, Hernanz-Schulman M, Horii S, et al. Spondylothoracic dysplasia. Clinical and sonographic diagnosis. J Ultrasound Med 1989;8:1–5.

Romero R, Ghidini A, Eswara M S, et al. Prenatal findings in a case of spondylocostal dysplasia type I (Jarcho–Levin syndrome). Obstet Gynecol 1988;71:988–990.

Tolmie J L, Whittle M J, McNay M B, et al. Second trimester prenatal diagnosis of the Jarcho–Levin syndrome. Prenat Diagn 1987;7:129–134.

Juberg–Hayward syndrome

Autosomal recessive.

Features

Low birthweight; short stature; microcephaly; small mandible; cleft lip and palate; short neck; scoliosis; absent ribs; extra ribs; horseshoe kidneys; small kidneys; dislocated elbow; hypoplastic radii and ulnae; cleft hand; polydactyly; hypoplastic thumbs, proximally placed.

The minimal criteria are microcephaly, cleft lip/palate and hypoplastic distally displaced thumbs. The forearm bones can be short with limited elbow extension. The alae nasi and columella can be hypoplastic, with a broad nasal root. Boys in the original sibship were more severely affected than girls.

Reference

Juberg R C, Hayward J R. A new familial syndrome of oral, cranial, and digital anomalies. J Pediatr 1969;74:755–762.

Kozlowski syndrome (osteocraniostenosis)

Uncertain.

Features

Undermineralization of skull; craniosynostosis; microphthalmia; platyspondyly; thin ribs; multiple fractures; wide metaphysis; thin bones but with osteosclerosis.

All reported cases have had intra-uterine dwarfism, thin ribs and long bones, and multiple fractures. One case had metaphyseal widening. One infant died at 20 minutes and had hydrops, frontal bossing, short tapering fingers with poorly developed nails and poor skull ossification.

References

Kozlowski K, Kan A. Intrauterine dwarfism, peculiar facies and thin bones with multiple fractures – a new syndrome. Pediatr Radiol 1988;18:394–398.

Sharma B K, Kapoor R, Ramji S, et al. Thin ribs, thin tubular bones, abnormal facies and intrauterine growth retardation: a lethal syndrome. Br J Radiol 1990;63:654–656.

Verloes A, Narcy F, Grattagliano B, et al. Osteocraniostenosis. J Med Genet 1994;31:772–778.

Larsen syndrome, lethal variant

Autosomal recessive.

Features

Hypertelorism; micrognathia; cleft lip and palate; segmentation defects of spine; laryngotracheomalacia; flared ribs/anterior splaying; shoulder dislocation; broad thumbs; club-foot; multiple joint dislocations; wide metaphysis.

There may be a lethal variant of Larsen syndrome. Apart from neonatal death due to pulmonary hypoplasia and laryngotracheomalacia, the main distinguishing features appear to be abnormal palmar creases and a form of metaphyseal dysplasia.

References

Chen H, Chang C-H, Perrin E, et al. A lethal, Larsen-like multiple joint dislocation syndrome. Am J Med Genet 1982;13:149–161.

Clayton-Smith J, Donnai D. A further patient with the lethal type of Larsen syndrome. J Med Genet 1988;25:499–500.

Mostello D, Hoechstetter L, Bendon R W, et al. Prenatal diagnosis of recurrent Larsen syndrome: further definition of a lethal variant. Prenat Diagn 1991;11:215–225.

Maternal diabetes syndrome

Environmental.

Features

Large size; microcephaly; neural tube defects; absent sacrum; ventricular septal defect; transposition of the great vessels; situs inversus; intestinal atresias; polysplenia; renal agenesis; hydronephrosis; bowed long bones; hypoplastic long bones; hypoplastic thumbs; polydactyly.

Infants of diabetic mothers have a 2 to 3 times increased incidence of congenital anomalies. These include pre-axial polydactyly of the feet, neural tube defects, cardiac defects (transposition of the great vessels, coarctation of the aorta, VSD, ASD, cardiomyopathy), situs inversus, renal anomalies (hydronephrosis, renal agenesis, duplication of the renal tracts), intestinal atresias, radius and ulna hypoplasia, and forms of caudal regression including sacral agenesis.

References

Brown Z A, Mills J L, Metzger B E, et al. Early sonographic evaluation for fetal growth delay and congenital malformations in pregnancies complicated by insulin-requiring diabetes. National Institute of Child Health. Diabetes Care 1992;15:613–619.

Gomez K J, Dowdy K, Allen G, et al. Evaluation of ultrasound diagnosis of fetal anomalies in women with pregestational diabetes: University of Florida experience. Am J Obstet Gynecol 1988;159:584–586.

Kalter H. Case reports of malformations associated with maternal diabetes: history and critique. Clin Genet 1993;43:174–179.

Landon M B, Mintz M C, Gabbe S G. Sonographic evaluation of fetal abdominal growth: predictor of the large-for-gestational-age infant in pregnancies complicated by diabetes mellitus. Am J Obstet Gynecol 1989;160:115–120.

Martinez-Frias M L. Epidemiological analysis of outcomes of pregnancy in diabetic mothers: identification of the most characteristic and most frequent congenital anomalies. Am J Med Genet 1994;51:108–113.

Pachi A, Maggi E, Giancotti A, et al. Prenatal sonographic diagnosis of diastematomyelia in a diabetic woman. Prenat Diagn 1992;12:535–539.

Meckel–Gruber syndrome (dysencephalia splanchnocystica)

Autosomal recessive.

Features

Microcephaly; hydrocephaly; posterior encephalocoele; microphthalmia; cleft lip and palate; polysplenia; multiple renal cysts; polydactyly.

The main features are occipital encephalocoele associated with microcephaly, hydrocephaly or anencephaly, anophthalmia or microphthalmia, polymicrogyria, cleft lip and palate, polycystic kidneys, hepatic fibrosis and cysts, ambiguous genitalia, congenital heart defect and postaxial polydactyly. Expression can be variable between sibs: the most consistent features are the hepatic and renal lesions. Pre-axial polydactyly and bowing of the long bones can also occur. The syndrome has been mapped to 17q21-q24 but there may be clinical and genetic heterogeneity.

References

Braithwaite J M, Economides D L. First-trimester diagnosis of Meckel–Gruber syndrome by transabdominal sonography in a low-risk case. Prenat Diagn 1995;15:1168–1170.
Nyberg D A, Hallesy D, Mahony B S, et al. Meckel–Gruber syndrome: importance of prenatal diagnosis. J Ultrasound Med 1990;9:691–696.
Pachi A, Giancotti A, Torcia F, et al. Meckel–Gruber syndrome: ultrasonographic diagnosis at 13 weeks gestational age in an at-risk case. Prenat Diagn 1989;9:187–190.
Ramadani H M, Nasrat H A. Prenatal diagnosis of recurrent Meckel syndrome. Int J Gynaecol Obstet 1992;39:327–332.
Salonen R. The Meckel syndrome: clinicopathological findings in 67 patients. Am J Med Genet 1984;18:671–689.
Saw P D, Rouse G A, DeLange M. Meckel syndrome – sonographic findings. J Diagn Med Sonogr 1991;7:8–11.
Wininger S J, Donnenfeld A E. Syndromes identified in fetuses with prenatally diagnosed cephaloceles. Prenat Diagn 1994;14:839–843.

Mohr–Majewski syndrome (oral-facial-digital syndrome type IV)

Autosomal recessive.

Features

Cerebral atrophy/Dandy–Walker malformation; polymicrogyria; micrognathia; midline cleft upper lip; cleft palate; cleft tongue; lobulated tongue; atrial septum defect; anomalous venous return; Fallot tetralogy; ventricular septal defect; renal agenesis; multiple renal cysts; hydronephrosis; severely hypoplastic tibia; club-foot, varus.

This syndrome has clinical features intermediate between Mohr (OFD II) and Majewski syndromes (short-rib – polydactyly II), with a midline cleft or notch of the upper lip, multiple oral frenulae, fleshy nodules or hamartomas of the tongue, and a high or cleft palate. Postaxial polydactyly is common. The tibia is severely hypoplastic. The ribs are short, or relatively normal allowing survival. Congenital heart defects include single atrium, VSD, anomalous pulmonary venous drainage, and tetralogy of Fallot. Some cases have cerebral abnormalities including Dandy–Walker malformation or cerebral atrophy and micropolygyria. Anal atresia has been reported.

References

Nevin N C, Thomas P S. Orofaciodigital syndrome type IV: report of a patient. Am J Med Genet 1989;32:151–154.
Silengo M C, Bell G L, Biagioli M, et al. Oro-facial-digital syndrome II. Transitional type between the Mohr and the Majewski syndromes: report of two new cases. Clin Genet 1987;31:331–336.
Toriello H V. Review. Oral-facial-digital syndromes, 1992. Clin Dysmorphol 1993;2:95–105.

Multiple gastrointestinal atresias

Autosomal recessive; uncertain.

Features

Multiple atresias of small and large bowel.

Familial occurrence of small bowel atresia is rare, but a few families (one consanguinous) have been reported where sibs had multiple atresias of the small and large bowel. This condition is separate from apple peel syndrome.

References

Boyd P A, Chamberlain P, Gould S, et al. Hereditary multiple intestinal atresia – ultrasound findings and outcome of pregnancy in an affected case. Prenat Diagn 1994;14:61–64.
Chiba T, Ohi R, Kamiyama T, Yoshida S. Ileal atresia with perforation in siblings. Eur J Ped Surg 1991;1:51–53.
Gungor N, Balci S, Tanyel F C, Gogus S. Familial

intestinal polyatresia syndrome. Clin Genet 1995;47:245–247.

Skoll M A, Marquette G P, Hamilton E F. Prenatal ultrasonic diagnosis of multiple bowel atresias. Am J Obstet Gynecol 1987;156:472–473.

Young I D, Kennedy R, Ein S H. Familial small bowel atresia and stenosis. J Pediatr Surg 1986;21:792–793.

Multiple pterygium syndrome (lethal)

Autosomal recessive.

Features

Low birthweight; short limbs; microcephaly; cerebellar abnormalities; hydranencephaly; hypertelorism; cleft lip and palate; cystic hygroma; fusion of vertebrae; lung hypoplasia; multiple joint webbing; radio-ulnar synostosis; synostosis of fingers.

Multiple joint contractures with skin webs, hypoplastic lungs, a history of polyhydramnios, oedema of the skin, cystic hygromas of the neck, hypertelorism with downward slanting palpebral fissures, and cleft palate are the main features but may be dependent on the age of onset in utero of growth retardation, the degree of neck swelling and the presence or absence of bony fusions of the vertebrae and long bones. A few cases have had central nervous system abnormalities – hydranencephaly, holoprosencephaly, and intracerebral cysts with dilated ventricles.

References

Chen H, Immken L, Lachman R, et al. Syndrome of multiple pterygia, camptodactyly, facial anomalies, hypoplastic lungs and heart, cystic hygroma, and skeletal anomalies: delineation of a new entity and review of lethal forms of multiple pterygium syndrome. Am J Med Genet 1984;17:809–826.

Grubben C, Gyselaers W, Moerman P, et al. The echographic diagnosis of fetal akinesia. A challenge towards etiological diagnosis and management. Genetic Counseling 1990;1:35–40.

Hall J G. Editorial comment: the lethal multiple pterygium syndromes. Am J Med Genet 1984;17:803–807.

Isaacson G, Gargus J J, Mahoney M J. Lethal multiple pterygium syndrome in an 18-week fetus with hydrops. Am J Med Genet 1984;17:835–839.

Kirkinen P, Herva R, Leisti J. Early prenatal diagnosis of a lethal syndrome of multiple congenital contractures. Prenat Diagn 1987;7:189–196.

Lockwood C, Irons M, Troiani J, et al. The prenatal sonographic diagnosis of lethal multiple pterygium syndrome: a heritable cause of recurrent abortion. Am J Obstet Gynecol 1988;159:474–476.

Martin N J, Hill J B, Cooper D H, et al. Lethal multiple pterygium syndrome: three consecutive cases in one family. Am J Med Genet 1986;24:295–304.

Zeitune M, Fejgin M D, et al. Prenatal diagnosis of the pterygium syndrome. Prenat Diagn 1988;8:145–150.

Nail-patella syndrome (osteo-onychodysplasia)

Autosomal dominant.

Features

Cleft lip and palate; dislocated elbow; Madelung deformity; absent or hypoplastic patella.

Occasionally this condition causes facial clefting. It principally affects the nails, skeleton and kidney. The small nails are abnormal from birth. Skeletal abnormalities include talipes equinovarus and other joint contractures, posterior iliac horns, a malformed capitellum of the radius, Madelung deformity and absent or hypoplastic patellae. Nephropathy may manifest with proteinuria or intermittent nephrotic syndrome and 8 to 10% will progress to renal failure. It has been suggested that prenatal diagnosis might be possible by renal biopsy, but nephropathy does not occur in all families. The gene has now been cloned and the condition shown to be caused by mutations in the LIM-homeodomain protein LMX1B on 9q34.1.

References

Beals R K, Eckhardt A L. Hereditary onycho-osteodysplasia (nail-patella syndrome). A report of nine kindreds. J Bone Joint Surg A 1969;51:505–516.

Gubler M-C, Levy M. Prenatal diagnosis of nail-patella syndrome by intrauterine kidney biopsy (Letter). Am J Med Genet 1993;47:122–123.

Guidera K J, Satter-White Y, Ogden J A, et al. Nail patella syndrome: a review of 44 orthopaedic patients. J Pediatr Orthop 1991;11:737–742.

Neu–Laxova syndrome

Autosomal recessive.

Features

Severe microcephaly; agenesis of corpus callosum; lissencephaly; prominent eyes;

cataract; absent eyelids; flat nose; cleft lip and palate; short neck; vertical talus; joint contractures; oedema.

This syndrome is characterized by severe microcephaly, intra-uterine growth retardation, absent eyelids (in some), microphthalmia, cataracts, a hypoplastic nose, multiple joint contractures, skin syndactyly of the fingers, collodion skin and subcutaneous oedema. Central nervous system abnormalities include lissencephaly, agenesis of the corpus callosum and a hypoplastic cerebellum. Some infants are severely affected with staring eyes, limb contractures and grossly swollen hands and feet. In others the phenotype may be less striking. The limb defects are probably caused by fetal akinesia.

References

Kainer R, Pretchtl H F R, Dudenhausen J W, Unger M. Qualitative analysis of fetal movement patterns in the Neu–Laxova syndrome. Prenat Diag 1996;16:667–669.

Muller L M, De Jong G, Mouton S C E, et al. A case of the Neu–Laxova syndrome: prenatal ultrasonographic monitoring in the third trimester and the histopathological findings. Am J Med Genet 1987;26:421–430.

Neu R L, Kajii T, Gardner L I, et al. A lethal syndrome of microcephaly with multiple congenital anomalies in three siblings. Pediatrics 1971;47:610–612.

Russo R, D'Armiento M, et al. Neu–Laxova syndrome: pathological, radiological, and prenatal findings in a stillborn female. Am J Med Genet 1989;32:136–139.

Shapiro I, Borochowitz Z, Degani S, et al. Neu–Laxova syndrome: prenatal ultrasonographic diagnosis, clinical and pathological studies and new manifestations. Am J Med Genet 1992;43:602–605.

Tolmie J L, Mortimer G, Doyle D, et al. The Neu–Laxova syndrome in female sibs: clinical and pathological features with prenatal diagnosis in the second sib. Am J Med Genet 1987;27:175–182.

Nevoid basal cell carcinoma syndrome (Gorlin syndrome; basal cell nevus syndrome)

Autosomal dominant.

Features

Macrocephaly; hydrocephaly; microphthalmia; cleft lip; cardiac fibromas; bifid/fused ribs; polydactyly.

Fetal ultrasound can be used to detect macrocephaly, ventriculomegaly, cardiac fibromas or polydactyly before birth. Bifid, fused, partially missing, or anteriorly splayed ribs occur in about 60% of cases. The facial features can be characteristic with macrocephaly, frontal and temporo-parietal bossing and hypertelorism. The multiple nevoid basal cell carcinomas usually appear after puberty. Caused by mutations in the patched gene: the congenital malformations may be the result of haploinsufficiency, tumours occurring later in life when the wild-type gene is inactivated in individual cells.

References

Bialer M G, Gailani M R, McLaughlin J A, et al. Prenatal diagnosis of Gorlin syndrome (Letter). Lancet 1994;2:477.

Coffin C M. Congenital cardiac fibroma associated with Gorlin syndrome. Pediatr Pathol 1992;12:255–262.

Evans D G R, Ladusans E J, Rimmer S, et al. Complications of the naevoid basal cell carcinoma syndrome: results of a population based study. J Med Genet 1993;30:460–464.

Evans D G R, Sims D G, Donnai D. Family implications of neonatal Gorlin's syndrome. Arch Dis Child 1991;66:1162–1163.

Gorlin R J. Nevoid basal-cell carcinoma syndrome. Medicine 1987;66:98–113.

Hogge W A, Blank C, Roochvarg L B, et al. Gorlin syndrome (naevoid basal cell carcinoma syndrome): prenatal detection in a fetus with macrocephaly and ventriculomegaly. Prenat Diagn 1994;14:725–727.

Nivelon syndrome

Autosomal recessive.

Features

Severe intra-uterine growth retardation, short limbs, hypoplastic scapulae, dense clavicles, short first metacarpals, short fibulae, hypoplasia of the cerebellar vermis, narrow thorax, absent or short thin ribs, ambiguous genitalia, 46,XY with Mullerian structures.

Reported in female sibs. The first had 46,XY karyotype, female internal genitalia, an unusual face, severe intrauterine growth retardation with short limbs and a narrow thorax. Radiographs revealed short, thin ribs, trapezoid vertebral bodies, hypoplastic scapulae, dense clavicles and short first metacarpals. The fibulae were short and the pelvis was wide with short ilia. Hypoplasia of the cerebellar vermis was demonstrated but neurological examination was reported as normal. The palpebral fissures were short and upslanting and the ears large. The irides were hypoplastic and there was an irreducible myosis and a coloboma of the optic disc. A second sib was terminated at 28 weeks – she had similar features but a 46,XX karyotype.

Reference

Nivelon A, Nivelon J-L, Mabille J-P, et al. New autosomal recessive chondrodysplasia-pseudohermaphrodism syndrome. Clin Dysmorphol 1992;1:221–227.

OEIS syndrome (omphalocele-exstrophy of bladder-imperforate anus-spinal defects syndrome)

Usually sporadic.

Features

Spinal dysraphism; hemivertebrae; congenital heart anomaly; lung hypoplasia; small/large bowel atresia; intestinal malrotation; omphalocoele; imperforate anus; ambiguous/absent genitalia; bladder exstrophy; exstrophy of the cloaca; renal dysplasia; dilated ureters.

Below an apparent omphalocoele in the lower part of the abdomen is an everted bladder, into which shortened small bowel and a blind colonic remnant may open. There is associated imperforate anus and abnormal or absent genitalia, and frequently hemivertebrae or segmentation defects of the lumbar spine and sacrum. Most cases are sporadic, and may be caused by early amnion rupture.

References

Carey J C, Greenbaum B, Hall B D. The OEIS Complex (omphalocele, exstrophy, imperforate anus, spinal defects). BDOAS 1978;14(6B):253–263.
Gosden C, Brock D J H. Prenatal diagnosis of exstrophy of the cloaca. Am J Med Genet 1981;8:95–109.
Hendren W H. Cloacal malformations: experience with 105 cases. J Pediatr Surg 1992;27:890–901.
Kutzner D K, Wilson W G, Hogge W A. OEIS complex (cloacal exstrophy): prenatal diagnosis in the second trimester. Prenat Diagn 1988;8:247–254.
Lande I M, Hamilton E F. Antenatal sonographic visualization of cloacal dysgenesis. J Ultrasound Med 1986;5:275.
Meizner I, Bar-Ziv J. Prenatal ultrasonic diagnosis of cloacal exstrophy. Am J Obstet Gynecol 1985;153:802–803.
Smith N M, Chambers H M, Furness M E, Haan E A. The OEIS complex (omphalocele-exstrophy-imperforate anus-spinal defects): recurrence in sibs. J Med Genet 1992;29:730–732.

Oral-facial-digital syndrome type I

X-linked dominant.

Features

Agenesis/hypoplasia of corpus callosum; hydrocephaly; porencephaly; midline cleft lip; cleft alveolar ridges; cleft palate; cleft tongue; lobulated tongue; renal cysts; hydronephrosis; postaxial polydactyly of fingers; skin syndactyly of fingers; bifid hallux; pre- and postaxial polydactyly of toes.

The main features include midline cleft lip, multiple oral frenulae, asymmetrical cleft palate, clefting of the maxillary alveolar ridge, lobulated tongue with hamartomata, facial milia in infancy and hypoplasia of the alae nasi. Brachydactyly of hands and feet, asymmetrical syndactyly of the hands and polydactyly of the hallux occur. Other abnormalities include polycystic kidneys, partial alopecia and central nervous system abnormalities leading to mental retardation (hydrocephaly, porencephaly, Dandy–Walker cysts, neuronal migration defects and agenesis of the corpus callosum). The gene (at Xp22.3-p22.2) is lethal in males, the majority dying in utero.

References

Baraitser M. Syndrome of the month: the orofaciodigital (OFD) syndromes. J Med Genet 1986;23:116–119.
Toriello H V. Review. Oral-facial-digital syndromes, 1992. Clin Dysmorphol 1993;2:95–105.

Oral-facial-digital syndrome type II (Mohr syndrome)

Autosomal recessive.

Features

Short stature; microcephaly; Dandy–Walker malformation; hydrocephaly; porencephaly; bifid nasal tip; micrognathia; midline cleft lip; oral frenulae; cleft palate; midline cleft tongue; lobulated tongue; polydactyly of fingers and toes; bifid thumb and/or hallux; pseudoarthrosis of tibia.

This syndrome is similar to OFD–1 but affects males and females, and can usually be differentiated from it postnatally – the hair is normal, the tip of the nose may be bifid and milia are not pronounced in infancy. Otherwise the facial and oral features are similar to OFD–1. Conductive hearing loss occurs in OFD–2. Although there may be postaxial polydactyly, bilateral duplication of the hallux is characteristic. Pseudarthrosis of the tibia can be a feature. Mental retardation may be less frequent than in OFD–1.

References

Iaccarino M, Lonardo F, Giugliano M, et al. Prenatal diagnosis of Mohr syndrome by ultrasonography. Prenat Diagn 1985;5:415–418.

Reardon W, Harbord M G, Hall-Craggs M A, et al. Central nervous system malformations in Mohr's syndrome. J Med Genet 1989;26:659–663.

Suresh S, Rajesh K, Suresh I, Raja V, Gopish D, Gnanasoundari S. Prenatal diagnosis of orofaciodigital syndrome: Mohr type. J Ultrasound Med 1995;14:863–866.

Toriello H V. Heterogeneity and variability in the oral-facial-digital syndromes. Am J Med Genet 1988;Suppl 4:149–159.

Toriello H V. Review. Oral-facial-digital syndromes, 1992. Clin Dysmorphol 1993;2:95–105.

Osteogenesis imperfecta type II

Autosomal dominant (usually new mutation)/autosomal recessive.

Features

Short limbs; ossification defects of skull; Wormian bones; narrow thorax; bowing of long bones; multiple fractures.

This severe, usually lethal form of osteogenesis imperfecta is subdivided into sub-groups on radiological features. All infants have short, deformed limbs with clinical evidence of bowing and abnormal angulation of the long bones. The chest is narrow. The subtypes have different recurrence risks from extremely low to perhaps 25% but the overall observed risk is about 7% (probably as a result of germline

mosaicism for a new dominant mutation). OI type II can be caused by mutations in either the COL1A1 or COL1A2 genes. Referral to a genetics unit is recommended.

References

Brons J T J, Van Der Harten H J, Wladimiroff J W, et al. Prenatal ultrasonographic diagnosis of osteogenesis imperfecta. Am J Obstet Gynecol 1988;159:176–181.

Cole W G, Dalgleish R. Syndrome of the month. Perinatal lethal osteogenesis imperfecta. J Med Genet 1995;32:284–289.

Elejalde B R, Elejalde M M. Prenatal diagnosis of perinatally lethal osteogenesis imperfecta. Am J Med Genet 1983;14:353–359.

Ghosh A, Woo J S K, Wan C W, Wong V C W. Simple ultrasonic diagnosis of osteogenesis imperfecta type II in early second trimester. Prenat Diagn 1984;4:235–240.

Munoz C, Filly R A, Golbus M S. Osteogenesis imperfecta type II: prenatal sonographic diagnosis. Radiology 1990;174:181–185.

Patel Z M, Shah H L, Madon P F. Prenatal diagnosis of lethal osteogenesis imperfecta (OI) by ultrasonography. Prenat Diagn 1983;3:261–263.

Stephens J D, Filly R A, Callen P W, et al. Prenatal diagnosis of osteogenesis imperfecta type II by real-time ultrasound. Hum Genet 1983;64:191–193.

Thompson E M, Young I D, Hall C M, Pembrey M E. Recurrence risks and prognosis in severe sporadic osteogenesis imperfecta. J Med Genet 1987;24:390–405.

Thompson E M. Non-invasive prenatal diagnosis of osteogenesis imperfecta. Am J Med Genet 1993;45:201–206.

Young I D, Thompson E M, Hall C M, Pembrey M E. Osteogenesis imperfecta type IIA: evidence for dominant inheritance. J Med Genet 1987;24:386–389.

Pena–Shokeir syndrome

See fetal akinesia sequence.

Persistent Mullerian duct syndrome

Autosomal recessive.

Features

Hirschsprung syndrome; male pseudo-hermaphroditism; 46,XY with Mullerian structures.

This phenotype can be produced by a mutation in either the gene encoding anti-Mullerian hormone or in the gene coding for the AMH receptor. Males have persistent Mullerian structures including fallopian tubes and uterine remnants. External genitalia may be ambiguous or normal and the presenting abnormality may be an inguinal hernia containing Mullerian structures. Affected sibs and parental consanguinity have been described.

References

Brook C G D, Wagner H, Zachmann M, et al. Familial occurrence of persistent Mullerian structures in otherwise normal males. BMJ 1973;1:771–773.

Fuqua J S, Sher E S, Perlman E J, et al. Abnormal gonadal differentiation in two subjects with ambiguous genitalia, Mullerian structures, and normally developed testes: evidence for a defect in gonadal ridge development. Hum Genet 1996;97:506–511.

Rangnekar G V, Loya B M, Goswami L K, Sengupta L K. Premature centromeric divisions and prominent telomeres in a patient with persistent Mullerian duct syndrome. Clin Genet 1990;37:69–73.

Rosenthal I M. Molecular basis for persistent Mullerian duct syndrome. Int Pediatr 1992;7:53–56.

Polydactyly-cleft lip (Thurston syndrome; oral-facial-digital syndrome type V)

Autosomal recessive.

Features

Midline cleft lip; oral frenulae; postaxial polydactyly of fingers and toes.

The combination of postaxial polydactyly with a midline cleft of the upper lip appears to be a condition distinct from the oral-facial-digital syndromes, and to have autosomal recessive inheritance.

References

Chowdhury J. A study of five siblings with median cleft lips and polydactyly. Paris, Trans 6th Int Congr Plast Reconstr Surg 1975;208–211.

Toriello H V. Heterogeneity and variability in the oral-facial-digital syndromes. Am J Med Genet 1988;Suppl 4:149–159.

Popliteal pterygium syndrome

Autosomal dominant.

Features

Cleft lip and palate; absent digits; webbing of knee; club-foot, varus; broad hallux; syndactyly.

The main features are cleft lip/palate, lower lip pits (similar to those seen in Van der Woude syndrome), popliteal webs (pterygia), syndactyly or absence of fingers or toes, hypoplastic toenails with a characteristic pyramid of skin overlying the nail of the great toe, and genital anomalies consisting of a small penis and hypoplastic scrotum in males, and hypoplastic labia majora and clitoromegaly in females. Occasionally pterygia are seen elsewhere, for example in the groin. The syndrome is very variable.

References

Froster-Iskenius U G. Syndrome of the month. Popliteal pterygium syndrome. J Med Genet 1990;27:320–326.

Hunter A. The popliteal pterygium syndrome: report of a new family and review of the literature. Am J Med Genet 1990;36:196–208.

Popliteal pterygium syndrome, severe autosomal recessive form (Bartsocas–Papas syndrome)

Autosomal recessive.

Features

Microcephaly; hypertelorism; eyelid synechiae; cleft lip and palate; short neck; hypoplastic diaphragm; oesophageal atresia; renal agenesis; reduction deformity of arms and legs; limited movement of elbow with webbing; absent digits; osseous syndactyly of fingers; flexion deformities of large joints; limited movement of knee; webbing of knee; club-foot, varus; absent toes.

Severe webbing at the knee limiting leg extension and cleft lip and palate are the main clinical features. Ankyloblepharon has been reported in 50% of cases, filiform strands connecting upper and lower lids. The nose is hypoplastic, and the jaw small. Limb abnormalities include absent thumbs with syndactyly of the fingers, talipes equinovarus and syndactyly of the toes. Hypoplasia of the penis and an abnormal scrotum are the main genital abnormalities. Some cases have other features such as renal agenesis, oesophageal atresia, hypoplastic diaphragm and anal atresia.

References

Bartsocas C S, Papas C V. Popliteal pterygium syndrome – evidence for a severe autosomal recessive form. J Med Genet 1972;9:222–226.

Hennekam R C M, Huber J, Variend D. Bartsocas-Papas syndrome with internal anomalies: evidence for a more generalized epithelial defect or new syndrome? Am J Med Genet 1994;53:102–107.

Rapp–Hodgkin ectodermal dysplasia syndrome

Autosomal dominant.

Features

Cleft lip and palate.

The main features are hypohidrosis, absent or sparse eyelashes and eyebrows, absent secondary sexual hair, oligodontia, dystrophic nails and cleft palate/lip. This may be the same condition as AEC syndrome.

References

Breslau-Siderius E J, Lavrijsen A P M, Otten F W A, et al. The Rapp–Hodgkin syndrome. Am J Med Genet 1991;38:107–110.
Rapp R S, Hodgkin W E. Anhidrotic ectodermal dysplasia, autosomal dominant inheritance with palate and lip anomalies. J Med Genet 1968;5:269–272.

Roberts (pseudothalidomide) syndrome (SC-phocomelia syndrome)

Autosomal recessive.

Features

Microcephaly; hydrocephaly; craniosynostosis; hypertelorism; prominent eyes; cleft lip and cleft palate; nuchal bleb; absent gall bladder; polysplenia; malformed uterus; large penis; renal cysts; radio-humeral synostosis; hypoplastic or absent radii/ulnae and fibulae/tibiae; syndactyly of fingers; absent or hypoplastic thumbs.

The severe shortening of the limbs, with radial defects and oligodactyly or syndactyly are likely to be the features detected on prenatal ultrasound. Facial features include hypertelorism, severe cleft lip and a prominent premaxilla. Other defects include large genitalia, congenital heart defects and cystic kidneys. Many affected infants die in the newborn period, and survivors may have mental retardation. The chromosomes show characteristic 'puffing' around the centromere and this has been used for prenatal diagnosis.

References

Allingham-Hawkins D J, Tomkins D J. Heterogeneity in Roberts syndrome. Am J Med Genet 1995;55:188–194.
Gruber A, Rabinerson D, Kaplan B, Ovadia Y. Prenatal diagnosis of Roberts syndrome (Letter). Prenat Diagn 1994;14:511–512.
Robins D B, Ladda R L, Thieme G A, et al. Prenatal detection of Roberts–SC phocomelia syndrome: report of 2 sibs with characteristic manifestations. Am J Med Genet 1989;32:390–394.
Sherer D M, Shah Y G, Klionsky N, Woods J R Jr. Prenatal sonographic features and management of a fetus with Roberts–SC phocomelia syndrome (pseudothalidomide syndrome) and pulmonary hypoplasia. Am J Perinatol 1991;8:259–262.
Stioui S, Privitera O, Brambati B, et al. First-trimester prenatal diagnosis of Roberts syndrome. Prenat Diagn 1992;12:145–149.
Tomkins D J. Premature centromere separation and the prenatal diagnosis of Roberts syndrome. Prenat Diagn 1989;9:451–452.
Van Den Berg D J, Francke U. Roberts syndrome: a review of 100 cases and a new rating system for severity. Am J Med Genet 1993;47:1104–1123.

Robinow syndrome

Autosomal dominant/autosomal recessive.

Features

Short limbs; macrocephaly; prominent forehead; hypertelorism; prominent eyes; cleft lip and palate; hemivertebrae; coarctation; Fallot tetralogy; patent ductus arteriosus; pulmonary stenosis; tricuspid stenosis; ventricular septal defect; micropenis; mesomelia of upper limbs.

Mesomelic limb shortening is usually (but not always) apparent. Other features include a prominent forehead, hypertelorism, wide mouth, small nose with anteverted nostrils, micropenis, hydronephrosis or urinary tract infections, cleft lip and palate, and hemivertebrae. Autosomal dominant and recessive families have been reported. Congenital heart defects include ASD, Fallot tetralogy, coarctation of the aorta, valvular and peripheral pulmonary stenosis, VSD and PDA.

References

Loverro G, Guanti G, Caruso G, Selvaggi L. Robinow's

syndrome: prenatal diagnosis. Prenat Diagn 1990;10:121–126.

Robinow M, Silverman F N, Smith H D. A newly recognized dwarfing syndrome. Am J Dis Child 1969;117:645–651.

Robinow M. The Robinow (fetal face) syndrome: a continuing puzzle. Clin Dysmorphol 1993;2:189–198.

Short-rib-polydactyly syndrome type 1 (Saldino–Noonan syndrome)

Autosomal recessive.

Features

Short limbs; coronal clefts of vertebrae; narrow thorax due to short ribs; atrial septum defect; coarctation; ventricular septal defect; transposition of the great vessels; hydrops; renal cysts; postaxial polydactyly of fingers and toes.

This condition is lethal in the neonatal period. As well as short ribs and polydactyly, urogenital and anorectal abnormalities are common including imperforate anus, vaginal atresia, urethrovaginal fistula, persistent cloaca and ureteral atresia. Many cases have a congenital heart defect. Radiographs are helpful in making the diagnosis – the base of the ilium is hypoplastic and the vertebrae rounded, sometimes with coronal clefts. The ends of the long bones are either pointed or have a convex central area of ossification with lateral metaphyseal spikes.

References

Grote W, et al. Prenatal diagnosis of a short-rib-polydactylia syndrome type Saldino–Noonan at 17 weeks' gestation. Eur J Pediatr 1983;140:63–66.

Richardson M M, Beaudet A L, Wagner M L, et al. Prenatal diagnosis of recurrence of Saldino–Noonan dwarfism. J Pediatr 1977;91:467–471.

Saldino R M, Noonan C D. Severe thoracic dystrophy with striking micromelia, abnormal osseous development, including the spine, and multiple visceral anomalies. Am J Roentgenol 1972; 114:257–263.

Sillence D O. Invited editorial comment: Non-Majewski short rib-polydactyly syndrome. Am J Med Genet 1980;7:223–229.

Short-rib-polydactyly syndrome type 2 (Majewski syndrome)

Autosomal recessive.

Features

Short limbs; macrocephaly; cleft upper lip (midline and non-midline), lip and palate; narrow thorax; coarctation; ventricular septal defect; ambiguous genitalia; renal cysts; pre- and postaxial polydactyly of fingers; postaxial polydactyly of toes; hydrops.

This lethal form of short-rib-polydactyly has a midline cleft of the upper lip and relatively normal pelvic and long bones, apart from the tibiae, which have a characteristic oval shape, and ambiguous genitalia. The differential diagnosis includes Ellis–van Creveld syndrome and Mohr–Majewski compound. Central nervous system anomalies include cerebellar vermis hypoplasia, arachnoid cysts in the posterior cranial fossa, agenesis or hypoplasia of the corpus callosum, and pachygyria or neuronal heterotopia.

References

Gembruch U, Hansmann M, Fodisch H J. Early prenatal diagnosis of short rib-polydactyly (SRP) syndrome type 2 (Majewski) by ultrasound in a case at risk. Prenat Diagn 1985;5:375.

Montemarano H, Bulas D I, Chandra R K, Tifft C. Prenatal diagnosis of glomerulocystic kidney disease in short-rib polydactyly syndrome type II, Majewski type. Pediatr Radiol 1995;25:469–471.

Spranger J, Grimm B, Weller M, et al. Short rib-polydactyly (SRP) syndrome, types Majewski and Saldino–Noonan. Z Kinderheilkd 1974;116:73–94.

Thomson G S M, Reynolds C P, Cruikshaw K J. Antenatal detection of recurrence of Majewski dwarf (short rib-polydactyly syndrome type II Majewski). Clin Radiol 1982;33:509–517.

Toftager-Larsen K, Benzie R J. Fetoscopy in prenatal diagnosis of the Majewski and the Saldino-Noonan type of short rib-polydactyly syndromes. Clin Genet 1984;26:56–60.

Sirenomelia (sacrococcygeal dysgenesis association; Duhamel anomaly)

Uncertain.

Features

Absent sacrum; fusion of vertebrae; hemivertebrae; situs inversus; intestinal atresia; bladder exstrophy; absent bladder; renal agenesis; hydronephrosis; sirenomelia.

The lower limbs are fused together,

sometimes with a single femur, with two tibiae and fibulae rotated by 180 degrees. Associated malformations include absent external genitalia, imperforate anus, lumbosacral vertebral and pelvic abnormalities and renal agenesis. Some cases have situs inversus. The condition has been thought to be part of the caudal regression spectrum.

References

Sirtori M, Ghidini A, et al. Prenatal diagnosis of sirenomelia. J Ultrasound Med 1989;8:83–88.

Twickler D, Budorick N, Pretorius D, et al. Caudal regression versus sirenomelia: sonographic clues. J Ultrasound Med 1993;12:323–330.

Van Zalen-Sprock M M, Van Vugt J M G, Van der Harten J J, Van Geijn H P. Early second-trimester diagnosis of sirenomelia. Prenat Diagn 1995;15:171–177.

Smith–Lemli–Opitz syndrome type I and type II (severe lethal form)

Autosomal recessive.

Features of type 2 SLO

Microcephaly; cleft lip and palate; hypoplastic anterior tongue; pulmonary segmentation defects; thin ribs; absent gall bladder; ambiguous genitalia; renal agenesis; renal cysts; postaxial polydactyly of fingers and toes.

There are two types, one of which is lethal in the neonatal period. Type 1 can be difficult to diagnose clinically relying on facial features, significant 2–3 syndactyly of the toes and hypospadias. Type 2 is the type likely to be diagnosed at ultrasound because of the maformations.

In the severe lethal form the male external genitalia can be ambiguous or female. Postaxial polydactyly in the hands, and a valgus deformity of the feet with syndactyly of several toes, are characteristic. A cleft palate and hypoplasia of the anterior portion of the tongue are common, unilobar lungs, hypoplastic kidneys, agenesis of the gall bladder, cerebellar hypoplasia, cardiac defects and enlarged pancreatic islets with giant cells. The Rutledge syndrome of multiple anomalies is probably the same as the lethal form of SLO syndrome.

Both phentoypes are caused by deficiency of 7-dehydrocholesterol reductase (11q12-q13). Prenatal diagnosis has been performed by measuring 7-dehydro-cholesterol levels in amniotic fluid, but may well be superseded by linkage analysis or direct mutation analysis.

References

Abuelo D N, Tint G S, Kelley R, et al. Prenatal detection of the cholesterol biosynthetic defect in the Smith–Lemli–Opitz syndrome by the analysis of amniotic fluid sterols. Am J Med Genet 1995;56:281–285.

Curry C J R, Carey J C, Holland J S, et al. Smith–Lemli–Opitz syndrome – type II: multiple congenital anomalies with male pseudohermaphroditism and frequent early lethality. Am J Med Genet 1987;26:45–57.

Dallaire L, Mitchell G, Giguere R, et al. Prenatal diagnosis of Smith–Lemli–Opitz syndrome is possible by measurement of 7-dehydrocholesterol in amniotic fluid. Prenat Diagn 1995;15:855–858.

Greene C, Pitts W, Rosenfeld R, et al. Smith–Lemli–Opitz syndrome in two 46,XY infants with female external genitalia. Clin Genet 1984;25:366–372.

Hyett J A, Clayton P T, Moscoso G, Nicolaides K H. Increased first trimester nuchal translucency as a prenatal manifestation of Smith–Lemli–Opitz syndrome. Am J Med Genet 1995;58:374–376.

Johnson J A, Aughton D J, Comstock C H, et al. Prenatal diagnosis of Smith–Lemli–Opitz syndrome, type II. Am J Med Genet 1994;49:240–243.

McGaughran J M, Clayton P T, Mills K A, et al. Prenatal diagnosis of Smith–Lemli–Opitz syndrome. Am J Med Genet 1995;56:269–271.

Mills K, Mandel H, Montemagno R, Soothill P W, Gershoni-Baruch R, Clayton P T. First trimester prenatal diagnosis of Smith–Lemli–Opitz syndrome (7-dehydrocholesterol reductase deficiency). Pediatr Res 1996;39:816–819.

Wassif C A, Maslen C, Kachilele-Linjewile S et al. Mutations in the human sterol delta-7-reductase gene at 11q12–13 cause Smith–Lemli–Opitz syndrome. Am J Hum Genet 1998,63.55 62.

Split hand/foot-tibial defects

Autosomal recessive/autosomal dominant.

Features

Dysplastic ears; hypoplastic or absent radii, ulna, femur, patella, tibia, fibula, digits; split hand/foot; pre- or postaxial polydactyly of fingers or toes.

Limb anomalies can range from hypoplastic great toes to transverse hemimelia of all four limbs. Some cases have other limb anomalies such as hypoplastic ulnae, bifurcation of the femurs, absent patellae or postaxial polydactyly. Cup-shaped ears appear to be a manifestation. Penetrance in families with associated limb abnormalities is 66%, resulting in skipped generations.

References

Majewski F, Kuster W, ter Haar B, et al. Aplasia of tibia with split-hand/split-foot deformity. Report of six families with 35 cases and considerations about variability and penetrance. Hum Genet 1985;70:136–147.

Richieri-Costa A, Ferrareto I, et al. Tibial hemimelia: report on 37 new cases, clinical and genetic considerations. Am J Med Genet 1987;27:867–884.

Zlotogora J. On the inheritance of the split hand/split foot malformation. Am J Med Genet 1994;53:29–32.

Stickler syndrome (hereditary arthro-ophthalmopathy, Marshall–Stickler syndrome, Wagner syndrome)

Autosomal dominant.

Features

Deafness; proptosis; small nose; flat nasal bridge; flat face; mid-face hypoplasia; micrognathia; cleft palate; coronal clefts of vertebrae; platyspondyly; spondylo-epiphyseal dysplasia; wide metaphysis.

This autosomal dominant syndrome can be extremely variable, presenting at birth with Pierre Robin sequence (cleft palate, micrognathia and glossoptosis) when radiological examination may show vertebral coronal clefts, mild platyspondyly and flaring of the metaphyses of the long bones (described as the Weissenbacher–Zweymuller syndrome). These features later become normal, although a mild epiphyseal dysplasia may develop. As the severe myopia may lead to retinal detachment, ophthalmic follow-up is recommended. The face may be very distinctive early in life with mid-face hypoplasia and a very depressed nasal root.

Mutations of COL2A1 cause the syndrome in some families, but there is genetic heterogeneity. A few families have mutations of the COL11A1 or COL11A2 genes which appear not to be associated with eye abnormalities.

References

Temple I K. Syndrome of the month. Stickler's syndrome. J Med Genet 1989;26:119–126.

Zlotogora J, Granat M, Knowlton R G. Prenatal exclusion of Stickler syndrome. Prenat Diagn 1994;14:145–148.

Thanatophoric dysplasia

Probably new dominant mutation.

Features

Short limbs; macrocephaly; platybasia; clover-leaf skull; prominent forehead; flat nasal bridge; platyspondyly; narrow thorax; small scapulae; hypoplastic ilia; bowed femur ('telephone receiver' appearance); metaphyseal flaring.

This is the most common lethal bone dysplasia, probably caused by sporadic mutations in the FGFR3 gene. The limbs are extremely short, the fingers short with a trident configuration, and the chest very narrow resulting in death from respiratory failure. The head is large with a prominent forehead. The femurs are characteristically curved ('telephone receiver'), the long bones are short with metaphyseal flaring and cupping, the iliac wings are hypoplastic and the vertebral bodies show severe flattening. Some cases have a clover-leaf skull, which can be discordant in affected sibs.

References

Brandon P S, Rouse G A, DeLange M. Sonography of thanatophoric dwarfism: a review. J Diagn Med Sonogr 1990;6:24–28.

Kassanos D, Botsis D, Katassos T, et al. Prenatal sonographic diagnosis of thanatophoric dwarfism. Int J Gynaecol Obstet 1991;34:373–376.

MacDonald I M, Hunter A G W, et al. Growth and development in thanatophoric dysplasia. Am J Med Genet 1989;33:508–512.

Tavormina P L, Shiang R, Thompson L M, et al. Thanatophoric dysplasia (types I and II) caused by distinct mutations in fibroblast growth factor receptor 3. Nature Genetics 1995;9:321–328.

Tuberous sclerosis (TS, epiloia)

Autosomal dominant.

Prenatal features

Brain tumour; tumours of the heart.

TS rarely presents prenatally but may do so with cardiac rhabdomyomata which may regress. At least 51% of infants with a cardiac rhabdomyoma are said to have TS. Giant cell astrocytomas of the brain occur in about 5% of individuals which can obstruct the exit of the third ventricle. Recurrence risks to normal parents of an isolated case are less than 5%, but not negligible. Mutations either in a gene on chromosome 9 or on chromosome 16 are responsible – in families with an appropriate structure prenatal diagnosis may be possible by linkage analysis. The spectrum of mutations is currently being delineated. The gene for adult polycystic kidney disease is contiguous with the TS gene on chromosome 16, and if this gene is also disrupted renal cysts can result.

References

Blethyn J, Jones A, Sullivan B. Prenatal diagnosis of unilateral renal disease in tuberous sclerosis. Br J Radiol 1991;64:161–164.

Chitayat D, McGillivray B C, et al. Role of prenatal detection of cardiac tumours in the diagnosis of tuberous sclerosis. Prenat Diagn 1988;8:577–584.

Gava G, Buoso G, Beltrame G L, et al. Cardiac rhabdomyoma as a marker for the prenatal detection of tuberous sclerosis. Case report. Br J Obstet Gynaecol 1990;97:1154–1157.

Groves A M M, Fagg N L K, Cook A C, Allan L D. Cardiac tumours in intrauterine life. Arch Dis Child 1992;67:1189–1192.

Journel H, Roussey M, Plais M H, et al. Prenatal diagnosis of familial tuberous sclerosis following detection of cardiac rhabdomyoma by ultrasound. Prenat Diagn 1986;6:283–289.

Platt L D, Devore G R, Horenstein J, et al. Prenatal diagnosis of tuberous sclerosis: the use of fetal echocardiography. Prenat Diagn 1987;7:407–411.

van Oppen A C C, Breslau-Siderius E J, Stoutenbeek P, et al. A fetal cystic neck mass associated with maternal tuberous sclerosis. Case report and literature review. Prenat Diagn 1991;11:915–920.

Webb D W, Thomas R D, Osborne J P. Cardiac rhabdomyomas and their association with tuberous sclerosis. Arch Dis Child 1993;68:367–370.

Webb D W, Thomas R D, Osborne J P. Echocardiography and genetic counselling in tuberous sclerosis. J Med Genet 1992;29:487–489.

Werner H Jr, Mirlesse V, Jacquemard F, et al. Prenatal diagnosis of tuberous sclerosis. Use of magnetic resonance imaging and its implications for prognosis. Prenat Diagn 1994;14:1151–1154.

Ulnar-mammary (Pallister) syndrome

Autosomal dominant.

Features

Anal atresia; malformed uterus; vaginal septum; small penis; dislocated elbow; bowed radius; hypoplastic or absent ulna; ectrodactyly; postaxial polydactyly of fingers.

The main features of this condition (which shows incomplete penetrance) are ulnar ray defects with missing digits or postaxial polydactyly, anal atresia, small penis, absent kidneys, uterine malformations and hypoplasia of the apocrine glands and breasts.

References

Gonzalez C A, et al. Studies of malformation syndromes of man XXXXIIB. Mother and son affected with the ulnar-mammary syndrome type Pallister. Eur J Pediatr 1976;123:225–235.

Pallister P D, Herrmann J, Opitz J M. Studies of malformation syndromes in man XXXXII. A pleiotropic dominant mutation affecting skeletal, sexual and apocrine-mammary development. BDOAS 1976;12(5):247–254.

Schinzel A, Illig R, Prader A. The ulnar-mammary syndrome: an autosomal dominant pleiotropic gene. Clin Genet 1987;32:160–168.

Schinzel A. Ulnar-mammary syndrome. J Med Genet 1987;24:778–781.

Van der Woude syndrome (lip pits syndrome)

Autosomal dominant.

Features

Cleft lip and palate; lower lip pits.

This condition is important to diagnose because of the high recurrence risk. About 2% of cases of cleft lip/palate are thought to be associated with lower lip pits. Eighty percent of gene carriers have symmetrical pits or eminences of the lower lip, usually situated at the vermilion border on either side of the midline. A parent may have verrucous eminences of the lower lip as the only sign. About 50% of gene carriers have clefts (one-third cleft palate alone; two-thirds cleft lip with or without cleft palate). This condition is genetically heterogenous with at least two loci (on chromosome 2q and 1q).

References

Dommergues M, Le Merrer M, Couly G, et al. Prenatal diagnosis of cleft lip at 11 menstrual weeks using embryoscopy in the van der Woude syndrome. Prenat Diagn 1995;15:378–381.

Schinzel A, Klausler M. Syndrome of the month: the van der Woude syndrome (dominantly inherited lip pits and clefts). J Med Genet 1986;23:291–294.

Varadi–Papp syndrome (oral-facial-digital syndrome type VI)

Autosomal recessive.

Features

Dandy–Walker malformation; hamartoma of brain; holoprosencephaly; craniosynostosis; small mandible; cleft upper lip (non-midline or lateral); cleft palate; lobulated tongue; congenital cardiac anomaly; small penis; small kidneys; polydactyly of fingers and toes; club-foot, varus; absent pituitary.

This type of oral-facial-digital syndrome has short stature, mental retardation, cleft lip and palate, lingual nodules, and duplication of the halluces with an extra finger with a bifid 3rd metacarpal. Additional features include absence of the olfactory bulbs and tracts, congenital heart disease and cryptorchidism, renal agenesis, sagittal and metopic craniosynostosis.

References

Munke M, McDonald D M, Cronister A, et al. Oral-facial-digital syndrome type VI (Varadi syndrome): further clinical delineation. Am J Med Genet 1990;35:360–369.

Stephan M J, Brooks K L, Moore D C, et al. Hypothalamic hamartoma in oral-facial-digital syndrome type VI (Varadi syndrome). Am J Med Genet 1994;51:131–136.

Varadi V, Szabo L, Papp Z. Syndrome of polydactyly, cleft lip/palate or lingual lump, and psychomotor retardation in endogamic gypsies. J Med Genet 1980;17:119–122.

VATER association (VACTERL association)

Sporadic.

Features

Wide cranial sutures; cleft palate; fusion or segmentation defects of vertebrae; congenital cardiac anomaly; anal atresia/stenosis; tracheo-oesophageal fistula; exstrophy of the cloaca; renal agenesis, multiple renal cysts, horseshoe kidney; hypoplastic or absent radii; pre-axial polydactyly of fingers; skin syndactyly of fingers; absent or hypoplastic thumbs.

VATER is the association of Vertebral defects, Anal atresia or stenosis, Tracheo-oesophageal fistula, Radial defects and Renal anomalies. The acronym has been expanded to VACTERL to include Cardiac defects and non-radial Limb defects. Most cases are sporadic.

Hassink reviewed 264 patients with anorectal malformations and noted that additional congenital defects were present in 67%. The majority of these were urogenital tract abnormalities. Forty-four percent of cases were felt to have features compatible with the VACTERL association. Five percent of patients had trisomy – mainly trisomy 21 without associated fistulae. McMullen studied cases ascertained because of tracheo-oesophageal fistula. Of 140 index cases they found that 29% had one other feature of VATER association and 17% at least two features; 1.4% of sibs had a feature of VATER association including one sib with oesophageal atresia. One out of 41 children of affected individuals (2.4%) had a tracheo-oesophageal fistula in addition to a congenital heart defect and a radial ray anomaly.

References

Brons J T J, Van Der Harten H J, Van Geijn H P, et al. Prenatal ultrasonographic diagnosis of radial-ray reduction malformations. Prenat Diagn 1990;10:279–288.

Czeizel A, Ludanyi I. An aetiological study of the VACTERL-association. Eur J Pediatr 1985;144:331–337.

Hassink E A M, Rieu P N M A, Hamel B C J, Severijnen R S V M, vd Staak F H J, Festen C. Additional congenital defects in anorectal malformations. Eur J Pediatr 1996;155:477–482.

Hearn-Stebbins B, Sherer D M, Abramowicz J S, et al. Prenatal sonographic features associated with an imperforate anus and rectourethral fistula. J Clin Ultrasound 1991;19:508–512.

Kawana T, Ikeda K, Nakagawara A, et al. A case of VACTERL syndrome with antenatally diagnosed duodenal atresia. J Pediatr Surg 1989;24:1158–1160.

McMullen K P, Karnes P S, Moir C R, Michels V V. Familial recurrence of tracheoesophageal fistula and associated malformations. Am J Med Genet 1996;63:525–528.

Quan L, Smith D W. The VATER association: vertebral defects, anal atresia, tracheoesophageal fistula with esophageal atresia, radial dysplasia. BDOAS 1972;8(2):75–78.

Rittler M, Paz J E, Castilla E E. VACTERL association, epidemiologic definition and delineation. Am J Med Genet 1996;63:529–536.

Weaver D D, Mapstone C L, Yu P-L. The VATER association: analysis of 46 patients. Am J Dis Child 1986;140:225–229.

Velo-cardio-facial syndrome (VCFS, Shprintzen syndrome)

Autosomal dominant/microdeletion.

Features

Short stature; microcephaly; micrognathia; facial clefting – upper lip, cleft palate, submucous cleft palate; meningomyelocoele; coarctation of aorta; Fallot tetralogy; pulmonary stenosis; tricuspid stenosis; ventricular septal defect.

Facial clefting and heart defects are the features which could present prenatally. It has been recommended that FISH analysis for the 22q11 microdeletion causing this syndrome be performed when a conotruncal anomaly is detected. The main features are cardiac anomalies with an unusual facial appearance, cleft palate (often submucous), short stature, and micrognathia, as well as a host of other features. It is variable in severity – both between and within families – presumably depending on the number of genes involved in a particular microdeletion. Indeed the phenotype spans DiGeorge syndrome, velo-cardio-facial (Shprintzen) syndrome, isolated conotruncal cardiac defects and truncus arteriosus. In some families the VCFS segregates as an autosomal dominant condition, in the absence of a demonstrable microdeletion of chromosome 22.

References

Driscoll D A, Salvin J, Sellinger B, et al. Prevalence of 22q11 microdeletions in DiGeorge and velocardiofacial syndromes: implications for genetic counselling and prenatal diagnosis. J Med Genet 1993;30:813–817.

Goldberg R, Motzkin B, Marion R, et al. Velo-cardio-facial syndrome: a review of 120 patients. Am J Med Genet 1993;45:313–319.

Raymond F L, Simpson J M, Mackie C M, Sharland G K. Prenatal diagnosis of 22q11 deletions: a series of five cases with congenital heart defects. J Med Genet 1997;34:679–682.

Ryan A, Goodship J, Wilson D I, et al. Spectrum of clinical features associated with interstitial chromosome 22q11 deletions: a European collaborative study. J Med Genet 1997;34:798–804.

Verloes syndrome

Autosomal recessive.

Features

Microcephaly; microphthalmia; anal atresia; 46,XY with Mullerian structures; hypospadias; small penis.

Two 46,XY sibs were reported by Verloes with genital ambiguity, persistent Mullerian structures, obesity, short stature and mental retardation. The facies were coarse with deep-set, microphthalmic eyes and thick lips. One sib had an anal atresia and a sacral spina bifida.

References

de Die-Smulders C, Van Schrojenstein L-de Valk H, Fryns J P. Confirmation of a new MR/male pseudohermaphroditism syndrome, Verloes type. Genetic Counseling 1994;5:73–75.

Schipper J A, Delemarre-v d Waal H A, Jansen M, Sprangers M A J. Case report: testicular dysgenesis and mental retardation in two incompletely masculinized XY-siblings. Acta Paediatr Scand 1991;80:125–128.

Verloes A, Gillerot Y, Delfortrie J, et al. Male pseudohermaphroditism with persistent Mullerian structures, mental retardation and Borjeson–Forssman–Lehmann-like features: a new syndrome? Genetic Counseling 1990;1:219–225.

References

1. Gardner R J M, Sutherland G R. Down syndrome, other full aneuploidies and polyploidy. In: Chromosome abnormalities and genetic counseling. 2nd ed. Oxford: Oxford University Press;1996:256.

2. Hall J G. Arthrogryposes (multiple congenital contractures). In: Emery A E H, Rimoin D L, eds. Principles and practice of medical genetics. 3rd ed. Edinburgh: Churchill Livingstone; 1996:1869–2915.

3. Wynne-Davies R. Family studies and aetiology of clubfoot. J Med Genet, 1965;2:227–232.

4. MRC Vitamin study research group. Prevention of neural tube defects: results of the Medical Research Council Vitamin Study. Lancet 1991;238:131–137.

5. Tolmie J L, McNay M, Stephenson J B P, et al. Microcephaly: genetic counselling and antenatal diagnosis after the birth of an affected child. Am J Med Genet 1987;27:583–594.

6. Ryan A K, Goodship J A, Wilson D I, et al. Spectrum

of clinical features associated with interstitial chromosome 22q11 deletions: a European collaborative study. J Med Genet, 1997;34:798–804.

7. Harper P S. In: Practical Genetic Counselling. 5th ed. Oxford: Butterworth-Heinemann; 1998:211–212.

8. Nora J J, Berg K, Nora A H. Cardiovascular diseases: genetics, epidemiology and prevention. Oxford: Oxford University Press; 1991.

9. David T J, O'Callaghan E. Oesophageal atresia in the South-West of England. J Med Genet 1975;12:1–11.

10. David T J, lllingworth C A. Diaphragmatic hernia in the South-West of England. J Med Genet 1976;13:253–262.

11. Czeizel A. Recurrence risk of omphalocoele (letter to editor). Lancet 1979;ii:470.

12. Passarge E. The genetics of Hirschprung's disease: evidence for heterogeneous etiology and a study of sixty-three families. N Engl J Med 1967;276:138–143.

13. Chakravati A. Endothelin receptor-mediated signalling in Hirschsprung's disease. Hum Molec Genet 1996;5:303–307.

14. Hofstra R M W, Osinga J, Buys C H C M. Mutations in Hirschsprung's disease: when does a mutation contribute to the phenotype? Eur J Hum Genet 1997;5:180–185.

15. Roodhooft A M, Birnholz J C, Holmes L B. Familial nature of congenital absence and severe dysgenesis of both kidneys. N Engl J Med 1984;310:1341–1345.

16. Zerres K, Mucher G, Becker J, et al. Prenatal diagnosis of autosomal recessive polycystic kidney disease (ARPKD): molecular genetics, clinical experience, and fetal morphology. Am J Med Genet 1998;76:137–144.

17. Allanson J E, Hunter A G W, Mettler G S, Jimenenz C. Renal tubular dysgenesis: a not uncommon autosomal recessive syndrome: a review. Am J Med Genet 1992;43:811–814.

18. Ives E, Coffey R, Carter C O. A family study of bladder exstrophy. J Med Genet 1980; 17:139–141.

Further reading

Baraitser M, Winter R M. Multiple congenital anomalies: a diagnostic compendium. London: Chapman and Hall;1991.

Buyse M L. Birth defect encyclopedia. Center for Birth Defects Information Services Inc, Cambridge, MA: Blackwell Scientific;1990.

Donnai D, Winter R M. Congenital malformation syndromes, London: Chapman and Hall Medical;1995.

Gardner R J M, Sutherland G R. Chromosome abnormalities and genetic counseling. 2nd ed. Oxford: Oxford University Press;1996.

Gorlin R J, Cohen M M Jr, Levin L S. Syndromes of the head and neck. 3rd ed. New York: Oxford University Press; 1990.

Graham J M Jr. Smith's recognisable patterns of human deformation. 3rd ed. Philadelphia: WB Saunders; 1996.

Graham J M Jr. Smith's recognizable patterns of human deformation. 2nd ed. Philadelphia: WB Saunders; 1988.

Harper P S. Practical genetic counselling. 5th ed. Oxford: Butterworth-Heinemann;1998.

Jones K L. Smith's recognisable patterns of human malformation. 5th ed. Philadelphia: WB Saunders; 1997.

McKusick V A. Mendelian inheritance in man, 12th ed. Baltimore: Johns Hopkins University Press;1998.

Rimoin D L, Connor J M, Pyeritz R E. Emery and Rimoin's principles and practice of medical genetics. 3rd ed. London: Churchill Livingstone;1996.

Scriver C R, Beaudet A L, Sly W S, Valle D. The metabolic and molecular basis of inherited disease. 7th ed. New York: McGraw-Hill;1995.

Shepard T H. Catalog of teratogenic agents. 8th ed. Baltimore: Johns Hopkins University Press;1995.

Taybi H, Lachman R S. Radiology of syndromes, metabolic disorders and skeletal dysplasias. 4th ed. Chicago: Year Book Publishers;1996.

Databases

On-line Mendelian Inheritance in Man – URL: http://www.ncbi.nlm.nih.gov/omim/

London Dysmorphology Database (1997 version) contains information on over 2750 non-chromosomal multiple anomaly syndromes. Published on CDROM. Oxford: Oxford University Press.

Schinzel A, Human chromosome abnormality database. Oxford: Oxford University Press.

POSSUM (Pictures of standard syndromes and undiagnosed malformations). Australia: Murdoch Institute.

CHAPTER 22

Counselling patients undergoing prenatal tests and following the diagnosis of fetal abnormality

Lenore Abramsky

Introduction

In this chapter of this book about how to screen for and diagnose fetal anomalies, I invite the reader to examine the context in which prenatal screening and diagnostic tests are offered. Counselling, testing, and any subsequent action all happen within an ethical and legal framework. The consequences of decisions taken in the light of test results will be profound and will include a large psychosocial element. This chapter will look first at the ethical, legal and emotional aspects of antenatal testing and then examine the very important role of counselling in the whole process. I will argue that the counselling must start *before* rather than after the abnormality is detected.

A test with a difference

Medical tests in most branches of medicine are done in order to obtain information enabling the doctor to make a diagnosis, to initiate appropriate treatment when necessary, and to give a prognosis. By the act of presenting themselves as patients, people having these tests have signified their acceptance of the goal of maintaining or improving their health. Prenatal diagnostic tests are, for the most part, fundamentally different in their aim. In the majority of cases, the identification of an abnormality in the fetus is the first step towards the parents being offered the option of terminating the pregnancy.[1,2] While there are effective prenatal and perinatal treatments for some conditions which can be diagnosed in utero, for the majority, the question is one of whether or not the parents wish to continue with the pregnancy given the problems that the baby is likely to have. Some parents will welcome the added control such information can give them over their own and their future offspring's destiny, while others will consider such tinkering with nature to be totally unacceptable.

Ethical issues

An individual's, a group's, or society's acceptance or rejection of prenatal diagnosis and selective termination of handicapped fetuses will be largely determined by their answers to the following questions:[3–6]

- At what point does the conceptus become a person with rights?
- What is the relative importance of the rights of the fetus compared to those of the mother?
- Is any life (whatever the quality) better than no life?

There is, of course, no guarantee that both members of the couple will answer the above questions in the same way. In addition, it is entirely possible that the parents and the carers will answer these questions differently.

An important ethical issue which needs addressing is that of minor variations from the norm which are sometimes identified when investigations are done to detect serious pathology. Since the only information the parents know about their baby is its imperfection, this can on rare occasions lead to a request being made to interrupt a pregnancy for a minor and/or correctable condition. Such requests need to be considered on a case-by-case basis, but in deciding how to respond, health care professionals need to consider the ethical implications for society if selective termination of pregnancy becomes available because a baby does not have all the traits desired by the parents.

Ethical issues in fetal medicine are more complex than those in other areas of medicine, because:

- there are always at least two patients to be considered (mother and fetus) and there may be a conflict of interests – what is good for one may be harmful for the other. In a twin or higher order pregnancy, one course of action may be best for one baby (such as early delivery), and a different course of action best for the other baby.
- The child-to-be cannot express his or her wishes.

Legal issues

Prenatal diagnostic investigations

An individual doctor generally will not be liable to prosecution for offering or not offering an investigation if the doctor is acting in accordance with the practice in his or her unit. However, if a doctor does not offer an amniocentesis to a 40-year-old pregnant woman in his or her care at a unit in which all women over the age of 35 are routinely offered an amniocentesis, this is a different matter. The doctor could well be in difficulties if the woman later delivers a liveborn baby with Down's syndrome and says that she would have had the amniocentesis and terminated an affected fetus if the offer had been made.

If the offer of a test is accepted and there is a pregnancy loss or an inaccurate result, there would be no legal consequences provided the offer of the test was appropriate (consistent with accepted medical practice), the test was carried out with an acceptable level of expertise and care, and the woman was intellectually competent and had been adequately counselled about the risks so that she was able to give informed consent.[7]

Pregnancy termination

The legal framework in which fetal medicine functions will to some extent reflect the ethical backdrop on which the laws were formulated. For example, in the Republic of Ireland, where the developing fetus enjoys the same ethical status as an adult, termination of pregnancy for any reason is prohibited by law. In the UK, on the other hand, termination of pregnancy for a number of possible reasons is allowed until the time of viability, currently set at 24 weeks. However, after 24 weeks, termination of pregnancy is allowed only for a few specific reasons, one being that if the baby were born, there would be 'a substantial risk that it would suffer from serious handicap'.[8] The more restrictive legislation for terminations done after viability reflects the increased ethical status which is enjoyed by the viable fetus. It is a source of concern to some practitioners that the words 'substantial' and 'serious' have not been further defined. It is anticipated that at some stage they will be tested in the courts.

When counselling couples regarding fetal abnormality and the options for further action which would be both medically and legally acceptable, the practitioner must be up to date or seek expert advice on both areas. From the legal point of view, a doctor may be subject to criminal prosecution if he or she performs a pregnancy termination without satisfying the terms of the Abortion Act.[9] On the other hand, if a doctor does not mention the possibility of termination of pregnancy in a case which most obstetricians would think met the criteria, there is a possibility that this could result in legal action.[10] However, although a doctor may be obliged to inform a patient of the possibility of having a termination of pregnancy for fetal abnormality, the doctor is not obliged to do the procedure him or herself if he or she feels it is unethical.[11]

At the birth of an abnormal baby

If a child is born with a serious abnormality, there are five possibilities:

- The condition was not amenable to antenatal detection.
- The mother was not offered the investigations which might have detected the condition.
- She was offered the investigations but declined to have them.
- She had the investigations but the condition was not diagnosed.
- The condition was diagnosed but the couple elected to go on with the pregnancy.

The parents need to be clear about which of the possibilities occurred. It is very important from the medicolegal point of view to be able to distinguish these five different scenarios by reading the case notes.

Emotional issues

The burden of choice

When screening tests are offered to women who thought themselves to be at low risk (such as those of low maternal age with no family history of congenital anomalies), anxiety is generated. They are forced to consider the possibility that their baby may not be 'perfect'. The offer poses dilemmas for couples. Do they want the information? Are they prepared to take any risks involved in obtaining the information? What would they do if an abnormality was detected? In attempting to make these decisions, many people experience intrapersonal conflict such as: (a) conflict between long-standing ethical beliefs and what they feel they could cope with or (b) the fear of having a handicapped baby and the fear of miscarrying a normal baby because of invasive tests. In addition, some people experience interpersonal conflict (such as the two members of a couple disagreeing). Making important decisions can be very stressful, and a decision about whether or not to have antenatal tests is now inevitable if a pregnant woman is to be involved in her own care in an informed manner.

For 'high-risk' couples, such as known carriers of genetic or chromosomal abnormalities, the offer of prenatal diagnostic tests can bring great relief from the fear of giving birth to a severely handicapped child. Of course, along with the relief comes the enormous anxiety attached to deciding upon and having (or not having) tests, awaiting results and acting upon them. Having said that, it is the existence of such tests which gives many 'high-risk' couples the courage to try again for a healthy baby.

If the offer of tests is accepted or if tests are done without informed consent (as often happens with anomaly scanning), the results are usually reassuring (sometimes falsely), but this is not always the case. Some couples are faced with further decisions such as whether or not to have more tests (and if so, which ones?) or whether or not to terminate the pregnancy (and if so, how?). Again, all

the intrapersonal and interpersonal conflicts may arise.

If a serious abnormality is diagnosed antenatally, the parents must make the terribly difficult decision of whether to continue the pregnancy or to have a termination. Whatever course of action they choose, it will have far-reaching consequences for them as individuals and as a couple.

Throughout the last decade, I have counselled many hundreds of couples who have had to make this difficult choice. For some the decision was clear-cut, while for others it was much less clear, but I do not remember ever meeting a couple who were not profoundly upset by the experience. They have many different ways of expressing their despair, but one common theme recurs – the terrible burden of the choice.[12] Many couples who have experienced a previous miscarriage say that although it was very sad, at least they did not have to make a decision and live with the extra feelings of doubt or guilt that that involves.

For those couples who have a baby with a severe abnormality whether or not it was diagnosed antenatally, the existence of prenatal diagnostic tests has altered the way in which society and individuals will view the birth of that baby. On the one hand, parents may blame carers for not detecting the handicap and giving them a chance to decide whether or not to carry on with the pregnancy. On the other hand, friends and relatives of the couple may look askance at them and ask hurtful questions such as 'Why didn't you have a test?'. Many people are under the erroneous impression that all abnormalities can and should be detected antenatally and that all couples would wish to terminate an affected fetus.

Living with the decision

If parents decide to terminate a pregnancy, they are likely to have even more complicated and ambivalent feelings than those which normally accompany a bereavement, and the grieving process can be a particularly complex one. They are mourning both their dream, normal baby whom they could not have and the abnormal baby that they decided not to have. They will feel relieved that they will not have to look after a handicapped child, but guilty that they decided to end the life of their own child. They are feeling extremely unlucky that the baby had an abnormality but grateful that it was discovered antenatally. They feel sad about the loss but guilty about feeling sad since they chose to terminate the pregnancy. If they have a religious faith, they are likely to feel a great need for their God while at the same time feeling angry at God for letting this happen to an innocent baby. They may be feeling both love for their baby and disgust and anger at what they imagine is a monster.[13–16]

When the abnormality in question would be lethal before or soon after birth, the trauma of terminating the pregnancy replaces what would otherwise be the trauma of a stillbirth or neonatal death. I am not aware of any published evidence which demonstrates that one is less emotionally damaging than the other, although a large study looking at this issue is currently underway.* There is, however, some evidence that couples who terminate a pregnancy cope better if they create memories about the baby by seeing, holding and naming it, taking photographs and having a funeral.[17] That, and the many times I have heard couples express feelings of intense guilt about terminations – 'I must have done something wrong or I would not still feel so terrible about it 10 years later ... if only I could turn the clock back.' or 'I didn't give birth to my baby, I only gave death.' has led me to believe that it is possible that in some cases we do more harm than good by identifying lethal abnormalities during pregnancy and terminating the pregnancy.[18]

When, however, the abnormality is not lethal before or soon after birth but is seriously handicapping, the alternative to prenatal diagnosis and termination of an affected pregnancy may be a lifetime of looking after a very handicapped child or of watching a much-loved child slowly deteriorate and die, and that child may (depending upon the condition) suffer a great deal of pain and/or have a poor quality of life. Many people, but not all, may feel that the very sad choice of ending the life of a wanted baby is preferable.

Whether people decide to carry on with a pregnancy or to terminate it, the two halves of the couple may have very complicated feelings towards each other. They will usually feel protective of each other but some may feel angry at their partner. They may both feel that they have failed or may blame each other or both of these. One may feel that the other is blaming him or her, particularly if the abnormality has definitely come from one partner (such as a dominantly inherited or X-linked inherited condition). They may also feel that they have let down their other children or the would-be grandparents, and sometimes feel unable to tell them what has happened.

Clearly, the reaction of each individual to an unhappy pregnancy outcome will be different, but some groups appear to be more vulnerable than others to the stresses induced by termination of pregnancy for fetal abnormality. Vulnerable groups include young and immature couples, couples whose pre-pregnancy relationship was in difficulties, isolated couples or individuals, women who have had infertility or a very poor obstetric history prior to the pregnancy in question, women with secondary post-termination infertility, people who already had emotional problems prior to the pregnancy in question, and people who have not resolved their feelings about a previous, significant bereavement.[19]

Fathers report two particular problems which make it difficult for them to grieve: they feel that they must be strong in order to support their partners both emotionally and at a practical level, and they suffer from our culturally induced male reluctance to show their feelings.[20,21]

---

*Detection of fetal abnormality at different gestations: impact on parents and service implications (Statham H, Solomou W, Green J. Centre for Family Research, Cambridge).

Counselling

Sensitive, accurate and thorough counselling is required at all stages in the prenatal screening/diagnosis chain if we hope to avoid unnecessary emotional damage to the parents. This counselling can be loosely divided into four stages:

- pre-test counselling which enables parents to make an informed choice about whether or not to have particular tests
- post-test counselling during which:
  — the results of investigations and options for future action are explained to parents
  — the couple are supported in their attempts to make decisions
- post-decision counselling during which:
  — parents are given information which has been gained from subsequent investigations
  — parents are given help to deal with their feelings about continuing or terminating the pregnancy
  — implications for the future are explained
- counselling for the next pregnancy during which parents are helped:
  — to cope with the enormous burden of anxiety which accompanies the next pregnancy even if all goes well
  — to make decisions about prenatal diagnostic tests.

The different types of counselling require different skills, and this usually means that a variety of people will be involved. It is important that there is still a sense of continuity, and the parents should always feel that there is one familiar and easy-to-contact person to whom they can turn when they have questions or need to talk.

While the purpose and type of counselling will vary with the situation, certain minimum conditions will always be necessary. Time, privacy and a comfortable setting are essential. The counsellor must herself or himself understand anything which is being explained and must be able to explain it in language which is understood by the parents. The counsellor must respect the parents and be able to convey a feeling of respect and caring. The counsellor must encourage the parents to express and explore their own feelings. Such a person may come from any one of a number of backgrounds – medical, nursing, midwifery, counselling, sonography or religious.

Pre-test counselling

The very existence of prenatal screening and diagnostic tests creates a major dilemma in counselling. If we offer tests to women, some will interpret the offer as a recommendation and will feel obliged to have them. If we do not offer tests and leave only the articulate, well-informed women to request them, we are not distributing care equitably. People may have a right to know important information about themselves which can be known, but they also have a right not to know it if they would prefer this.[22]

By offering a woman screening or diagnostic tests, we are implying that her baby could have an abnormality and that we think it might be better for her to terminate the pregnancy if the baby were affected. It is hard for women to refuse such tests because (a) they think society in general and the doctor or midwife in particular think it is irresponsible to refuse tests and (b) they think they will never forgive themselves if they have a child with an abnormality that could have been detected.[23]

Some would say that the above-mentioned problems make the ideal of non-directive, pre-test counselling unattainable.[24] This may be true, but we should not let that discourage us from trying to come as close as possible to achieving that goal.

Counselling before prenatal screening or diagnostic tests is necessary if a woman is to be offered the most appropriate tests and if she is to give informed consent to having or not having a test. This counselling may begin as early as her first contact with a health professional when she discovers she is pregnant, or before conception in the case of high-risk couples.

Prior to tests being offered, the health care

professional must give the woman a chance to express her worries, desires and opinions. A careful history should be taken (including her own and her partner's medical problems, previous obstetric history, in-/sub-fertility, problems with the current pregnancy, ethnic group, age, whether or not she and her partner are consanguinous, and family history). This will usually involve the pregnant woman talking a great deal more than the midwife/doctor/ counsellor. If this is not the case, the health care professional should give thought as to why. It will also involve the person who is counselling listening carefully and being sensitive to what is being said and to what is *not* being said.

The health care professional must give the woman an opportunity to say what she does and does not wish to know and, by implication, which tests she would like to know more about, and must also give information about the tests. Let us consider the question of what information needs to be given about any test being offered if the woman is to make a truly informed choice.[25–29]

Box 21.1
Basic information

The basic information needed is:

- what condition or conditions does the test screen for/diagnose?
- what are the effects of this/those condition/s?
- what is the chance that this/those condition/s are present in the fetus?
- how, when and where will the test be done?
- what will it feel like?
- what (if any) risks will it pose to the pregnancy?
- what (if any) pre-test care and/or aftercare will be needed?
- how, when, and where will the results be given?
- is the test being offered a screening test or a diagnostic test?
- what conditions will not be screened for/diagnosed on this test?
- how often does the test fail to work, and why?
- what does a positive result mean, and what are the chances of her having a positive result?
- what does a negative result mean, and what are the chances of her having such a result?
- what other methods are available to screen for/diagnose the condition in question?
- what options will be available to the parents in the event of a positive result and what will these options involve?

The above information needs to be given to parents in a form which is understandable and should ideally be given both verbally and in writing in a language in which they are fluent.

Those counselling must remember at all times the distinction between giving information about the possible consequences of different courses of action and giving advice as to which course of action should be taken. It is irrelevant what the counsellor thinks the woman should do or what he or she would do in a similar situation.

The issue of whether or not pre-test counselling such as that outlined above is appropriate before a woman has an anomaly scan is an important one. Many doctors and midwives feel that it is not necessary to counsel women before they have an ultrasound scan, since the scan itself is not thought to pose a physical threat to the pregnancy. However, this reasoning does not take into account the damage which can be done by giving someone information which that person would rather not have. While one can ask a woman before she has had a scan if she would want to know if her baby had a structural abnormality, it is not possible to ask that question after the scan has been done and an abnormality has been detected. It is my opinion that scans should be presented to women as prenatal diagnostic tests and that if they are not, the woman has not given informed consent for the procedure. Ultrasound is, after all, our most powerful tool in prenatal diagnosis.[30–32]

Post-test counselling

After a woman has had a test, the results need to be communicated. If the results of the test are negative, the couple should be informed immediately so that they do not spend more anxious moments than necessary. If the results are positive, the various possibilities for further investigations or action must be carefully explained and their optional nature made clear.

When a woman is having a test, she should know from the outset when, where and how she will obtain the results. Of course, the time-lag between doing the test and having the results will vary with the type of test, and this will play a part in how the results are given. For example, the findings of an ultrasound scan will be available as it is being done. The woman should be told at the beginning of the scan whether the person scanning will be silent for a time or will talk her through it. A couple may become extremely anxious if the sonographer/doctor silently looks and does measurements and says nothing but has not warned them that this will happen. If all looks well, this should be communicated as soon as possible, while ensuring that the woman knows the limitations of the scan. If a possible problem is identified, this needs to be discussed with the parents before they leave the unit. They need to know what the worries are, what further investigations (if any) will be offered, and what courses of action are open to them. Attempts to arrange further investigations without telling the parents about a potential problem usually result in a great deal of anxiety, because the parents have picked up that there is a problem through the non-verbal communication of the sonographer/doctor. If they do not pick this up, the woman may go off to a specialist centre for a further scan completely unaware that there may be a problem and may arrive there on her own or with young children in tow and no-one to help.[33]

Following a test, if a definitive diagnosis has been made and the prognosis is known with a high degree of certainty, this information needs to be given, and the various options open to the parents must be presented. They may need many sessions and much discussion about the various options before they can reach a decision about what to do. Sometimes, although the diagnosis is clear, the prognosis is less so, and it may be necessary to arrange for consultations with various specialists who can give an informed opinion although an element of uncertainty may remain. If the fetus has been diagnosed as having a condition which will require surgery after birth, the parents may benefit from talking

with the appropriate surgeon who can explain what will happen.

Sometimes it is not possible to make an antenatal diagnosis and parents are left with the agonizing choice of whether to 'chance it' and hope the baby is not affected or to terminate the pregnancy knowing that the baby might well be entirely normal. Examples of such conditions are de novo apparently balanced translocations, maternal exposure to a teratogen, ventriculomegaly, or a male fetus in a woman who carries (or might carry) an X-linked recessive condition for which antenatal diagnosis is not currently possible.[34] In such a situation, parents are usually given a risk figure for the child being affected. While this may be of some help (a 90% chance of being affected is much greater than a 5% chance), it still means the parents must make a decision in the face of uncertainty.

Many conditions are variable in the amount of problems they cause in the affected individual. Parents trying to decide whether or not to carry on with such a pregnancy may ask to meet other parents who have affected children. This can be helpful, but there are many potential problems associated with this. They may make their decision based on how well or badly the affected child/children they meet are doing and how well the family is coping. This means that their decision might be primarily a function of whom they happen to meet. If the meeting is arranged by a support group, there are many possible biases. For example, parents who are members of a Klinefelter support group may be the parents of the most affected boys who have been karyotyped postnatally because of problems.

When a couple is deciding whether or not to continue with a pregnancy complicated by fetal abnormality, they will need to know not only what the prognosis for the baby would be if they continued the pregnancy, but also what the emotional consequences to themselves might be if they terminated the pregnancy. They need to be aware that although they may decide that termination is the better option for them, it is never an easy option. Most people who terminate a pregnancy for fetal abnormality suffer a profound and complicated grief reaction.[35–37]

Unrecognized weaknesses in the relationship between the couple may surface under the strain. In addition, tensions may develop between them and friends or relatives, particularly if any of the friends or relatives are pregnant or have new babies. Parents may find themselves unable to cope with their living children or may become terribly anxious about and overprotective of them and of each other.

Parents also need to know how a termination would be done, and if there is a choice of methods, such as a choice between prostaglandin induction or dilatation and evacuation (D&E) under general anaesthetic, and they need to know the pros and cons of the two methods. Women should be aware that having a D&E may be physically and emotionally easier at the time, but that it means they will not be able to see and hold their baby which many people find a very important part of the healing process. They also need to know that having a D&E means that a post-mortem examination will not be possible; this may not be important in the face of a known chromosomal or gene abnormality, but it may be very important if the termination is for a structural abnormality of unknown aetiology.

Post-decision counselling

When a serious abnormality has been diagnosed antenatally, the parents will have had to decide whether they wish it to be treated aggressively (in the case of a severe but potentially treatable structural malformation), to 'let nature take its course' or to terminate the pregnancy. Whatever they have decided, there will be emotional consequences, and sensitive counselling will be required. For some, this may involve just a chance to have a full explanation and the answers to their questions. For others, counselling may be required over an extended period.[38]

For parents continuing the pregnancy

If parents decide to continue with the pregnancy in the face of severe fetal abnormality, they will need a good deal of support. They will probably want a lot of information from professionals and from other couples who have been through a similar experience, but they will also need the opportunity to talk about their feelings. Some people prefer to do this outside the medical setting, but others find they get the most helpful support from members of the hospital or primary health care team. Counselling of some sort may continue to be of value after the birth of the baby.

For parents terminating the pregnancy

Couples who elect to have a termination of pregnancy for fetal abnormality should always be offered post-termination counselling. This offer should include both genetic counselling and an opportunity to discuss psychosocial problems caused, highlighted or exacerbated by the termination.

Support during the next pregnancy

In the pregnancy immediately following an unsuccessful one, parents are likely to suffer from a great deal of anxiety.[42] I attribute this to the fact that they have 'lost their innocence'. They now know that bad things can happen to them and not just to other people. As such, in addition to the reasonable fear that the same thing could happen again, they may have the fear that even if that does not happen, something else is bound to go wrong.

They will benefit from knowing that they have an advocate on the staff: someone who knows them well, is aware of their anxieties, will go over all the issues again, will help to ensure that they have any investigations which are appropriate, and will offer support while they wait for results. Parents who have had a miscarriage following an amniocentesis or chorionic villus sampling of a fetus found to be unaffected will need special help with the very difficult decision as to whether or not to test a subsequent pregnancy.

Box 21.2
Principles of good counselling

Genetic counselling

A couple having a pregnancy affected by fetal abnormality should be offered genetic counselling whether or not they decide to terminate the pregnancy. As a minimum, they need to know:[39]

- the name of the condition
- how it will affect a child
- what causes it (in so far as this is known)
- what the recurrence risk is
- what steps (if any) can be taken to prevent its recurrence
- what prenatal diagnostic tests will be available to them in a future pregnancy
- how (if at all) the presence of the abnormality in their fetus affects the risk of such an abnormality occurring in the babies of other family members.

The couple should be encouraged to ask questions, and these should be answered in a clear and honest way with the counsellor admitting ignorance where appropriate and offering to obtain the answer if one is known.

The results of investigations done (such as post-mortems, karyotypes, DNA tests, and virology) should be carefully explained. It may be that further investigations are appropriate for themselves or their relatives, and these should be offered, in writing where appropriate, and should be carried out if the offer is accepted.

For most people, the above information will involve many words and concepts with which they are not familiar; but even if this is not the case, it should be remembered that people who are very upset are unlikely to remember clearly all that they are told. Ideally, the counselling should be backed up with a letter outlining all they have been told. Couples need to be given the phone number and address of someone whom they know and can contact in the event of further questions on their part.

Bereavement counselling

Why?

Many people may think that as death and pregnancy loss are natural phenomena, it is being a bit precious to suggest that people having a termination for fetal abnormality should routinely be offered counselling. They may say that for thousands of years people have been handling death and pregnancy loss without the benefit of bereavement counselling; not to mention the fact that in the case of termination for abnormality, the parents have 'chosen' to have a pregnancy loss.

I would counter this argument with a few observations. Until very recently, most people lived near extended family and friends whom they had known since childhood. Thus they had a stronger support network than is now the case for many people. Just a couple of generations back, many more people were actively religious which gave them the comfort of their faith and the support of their religious leader and other members of the congregation. Not long ago, death was a fact of life; it happened at home, and it happened fairly regularly to people of all ages. Now death has been removed to hospital, and its very mention is taboo. Its inevitability is denied in ordinary speech. It is common for people to say 'if something happens to him' rather than to say 'when he dies'. Thus, it may be that counselling is needed much more now for 'ordinary' bereavement than it might have been in the past.

Finally, I would argue, termination of pregnancy for fetal abnormality is not a natural phenomenon. Miscarriages, stillbirths, and the birth of handicapped babies are all tragedies – but they are natural. Termination of pregnancy in a particular situation may be the best alternative, but it is not natural; it is medical intervention. In all areas of medicine, there is the danger of introducing iatrogenic problems. Termination of pregnancy for fetal abnormality is no exception; and many of the problems it causes are psychosocial. We owe parents our help in their attempts to deal with problems that we have played a part in creating.

Termination of pregnancy for fetal abnormality is a special sort of loss. As outlined above, it brings with it many strong and confusing emotions and parents may benefit from sessions devoted to discussing these feelings. It is important for the counsellor in these sessions to have an understanding of the fetal abnormality; and if this person is not doing the genetic counselling, he or she should attend the session. This presents an excellent opportunity to offer bereavement counselling if that has not already begun.

When?

Ideally, a couple will get to know the counsellor before the decision to terminate the pregnancy is made and will discuss it with her or him. They will then see the counsellor when they are in hospital for the termination and will have a chance to discuss how they will deal with the event itself and the immediate aftermath and some of the problems they are likely to face later.

An offer should be made of a visit from a chaplain; the question of whether or not the couple want a funeral should be explored. The fact that many people find it helpful to see, hold, name and photograph the baby should be discussed in most cases; but of course couples must not be made to feel that they should do anything which does not feel right for them. They should be given the name, address and phone number of a relevant support group.

At some time before they go home, it is helpful to talk with parents about some of the feelings they may experience, so that they are less shocked by them. Parents may benefit from being warned that in addition to being sad, they are likely to feel angry and may be resentful and jealous of friends and relatives who are pregnant. They may fear that they are going mad because of the way they are feeling or acting. Other people may not know what to say to them and so may act as if nothing has happened, avoid them, or say such hurtful things as 'Never mind, you can always have another one'. Finally, they need to know that the road to emotional recovery can be a long and bumpy one. It may take them much longer to recover than they or others would imagine, and during the recovery there will be times when they think they have gone back to the beginning. They may also find that they grieve in different ways from each other which can create problems. Many people say that the knowledge that all of the above is 'normal' in the circumstances has been an enormous help to them.

Before parents leave the hospital, a follow-up appointment with the counsellor should be offered. If they do not want this, they should be asked if they would prefer the counsellor to contact them or if they would rather make contact themselves if and when they feel the need. The drawback with leaving the initiative with them is that people who are having difficulty coping or who are very depressed

Box 21.2 (contd)

usually are unable to summon up the emotional energy to seek help – especially from someone they barely know.

What does bereavement counselling involve?

The process is, of course, different with every person, but there are some general similarities which can be summarized as follows:[40,41]

- The counsellor acknowledges the parents' loss. This is done implicitly by talking about 'the baby' instead of 'the fetus' and by enquiring if they have named the baby and, if so, using the name. If appropriate, the counsellor may ask to see photos of the baby. Recognition of the loss should also be done explicitly.
- Recognition of the loss and the fact that the counsellor is comfortable with the parents expressing strong feelings and has time for them will give the parents 'permission to grieve.'
- Sharing of feelings will offer some relief from the sense of isolation which parents often feel and will allow them to

acknowledge and cope with such feelings as sadness, anger and guilt.
- The counsellor may help them to open up communication between themselves if this has become blocked, or between the couple and their friends, relatives or colleagues.
- Finally, when the time comes, the counsellor can 'give them permission to stop grieving'. Many people feel very guilty when the grief becomes less intense; the acknowledgement of these feelings by the counsellor can reduce their impact.

If a parent is having particular difficulties coming to terms with the loss, there may be one or more underlying problems that need to be discussed. In my experience, the most common one is that there is unresolved grief for an earlier loss (not necessarily of a child). The person is usually very relieved to have a chance to spend time talking about that, and at some sessions this may be done to the exclusion of talking about the recent termination.

Communication problems

Giving information

There are many possible reasons for failure to communicate information effectively. One reason may be that the person doing the explaining does not fully understand that which he or she is explaining. There is much evidence to show that GPs, doctors and midwives are sometimes expected to explain concepts without being offered sufficient training.[43–45] How can someone explain a screening test, for example, if the person does not clearly understand the difference between a screening test and a diagnostic test? How can one explain the recurrence risk for cystic fibrosis without understanding both the mechanism of autosomal recessive inheritance and the concept of probability? I have met people who were counselling mothers about serum screening results who not only did not understand the concept of a multiple of the median (MoM) but did not even know how to find the median. If the person explaining does not understand and is at best only repeating explanations learned by rote, communication will be inadequate, inaccurate and probably confusing.

While understanding something oneself is

a necessary condition for being able to explain it well, it is not sufficient. Some people have a talent for making complicated concepts easy to understand, while others have a talent for making simple concepts difficult to understand. The latter people need to practise the art of explaining.

Another reason for failure to communicate information might be that although the explainer understands it, he or she has not correctly assessed the patient's level of understanding or medical sophistication and is pitching the explanation at the wrong level – either assuming that people know vocabulary or concepts that they do not understand, or, conversely, explaining in a simplistic way to a person who wants to have and is able to understand an in-depth explanation. I learned this lesson in the early years of my counselling when I was explaining chromosomes in a very simplistic way to someone whom I then learned had a PhD in molecular biology!

Explanations involve using a common language. If the carer and the patient do not share a common language, the gulf has to be bridged by an interpreter. The best solution is to find a medical or paramedical person who fully understands the situation and can explain it. If this is not possible, another interpreter must be found. It is very important that the person translating understands his or her role. In fetal medicine, it is not unusual to find that the interpreter is digesting the information and passing it on in such a way that it is inaccurate and that any decisions made reflect the interpreter's beliefs and wishes rather than the patient's. One must make it very clear to an interpreter that this is not appropriate and that the translation should be verbatim. The counsellor should be wary if after he or she says one sentence, the interpreter speaks for about 5 minutes when giving the translation!

Other barriers to effective communication of facts are lack of sufficient time to explain carefully or lack of a private quiet place in which to do it.

Finally, if the couple are extremely distressed either because of what they are being told or for some other reason, they will have difficulty taking in information. They may find the information so unacceptable that they will deny it. It is not uncommon to have to go over and over the same information, not because the parents are intellectually unable to understand it, but because they are emotionally unable to accept it.

Making assumptions

The issue of making false assumptions is a more elusive one. Many of us have a tendency to think that deep down, if only they realized it, other people think just like we do. If we would want a certain piece of information, then so would they; if we would want to take a particular course of action, then so would they. This, of course, is not true. At the same time, and in contradiction to this, we also sometimes assume that we know, because of someone's professed beliefs and/or ethnic group or social class, what they will want to do. Yet, in practice, we are often surprised. I have known devout Catholics who have had their fetus tested for abnormalities and who have terminated an affected pregnancy. I have met declared atheists who declined (on ethical grounds) to have any tests or who chose (on ethical grounds) to continue a pregnancy with a severely handicapped fetus. We must all

guard against making assumptions and thereby making decisions for people. This can only be done by questioning ourselves as to why we have or have not offered a particular course of action or have explained something in one way rather than another.

Allowing the patient to communicate to us

It can be uncomfortable, even frightening, to let someone express intense emotional pain. Some people are better at dealing with this than others. Some doctors and nurses send out a very clear non-verbal message which says 'Please hold yourself together and don't show me your pain.' while others tend to comfort people with reassurance, hugs, or cups of tea, instead of (rather than in addition to) letting them express their sorrow.

One important idea we must all remember is that just as it is sometimes necessary to cause a patient physical pain in order to treat a physical problem, it can be necessary to cause emotional pain in order to help people come to terms with a loss. Most people find it distressing to talk about a loss, but they may need to do it.

The other issue – that of confronting our own fears of loss – is a far more difficult one. Loss of loved ones through death is one of the few near certainties in life; it can only be avoided by having no loved ones or by dying before all of them. Our own eventual death is perhaps the only absolute certainty. Both of the above are frightening to most of us, and supporting someone else through a loss can be an unwelcome reminder of our own and our loved ones' mortality.

Finally, we all feel inadequate in the face of other people's grief at bereavement. This is because we are, in a sense, inadequate. We cannot give them what they want – the return of the loved one. We must not demand the impossible of ourselves. All we can hope to do is to make the totally unacceptable just a little less awful by allowing people to express their sorrow and being there to share it with them.

Staff issues

Ethics and personal choice

Many people specialize in obstetrics because of an interest in assisting in the process of bringing forth life. While it is true that doctors choosing this specialty today may do so because of an interest in fetal medicine – the detection and possible treatment or termination of the abnormal – the majority probably still are those who are attracted by the idea of being involved in a happy event, the birth of a live, healthy baby. This is even more true of people going into midwifery.[46]

Among medical and midwifery staff, there will be those who find termination of pregnancy under any circumstance to be unethical. Of those who do not hold this view, there will be an enormous variation in the conditions which need to be met before they feel that a termination is justified. It is never right to ask a member of staff to take any part in an activity which he or she feels is unethical. However, this can create practical problems since, for example, all staff working in an antenatal clinic in which any form of prenatal screening tests is offered will be involved to some extent. Suffice it to say that this problem does not go away if it is ignored. It must be recognized and dealt with.

Training

Doctors and midwives cannot be expected to counsel couples appropriately if they do not (a) understand thoroughly what they are explaining and (b) know the principles of good counselling for prenatal diagnosis as outlined above. It is unfair to both professionals and patients if a prenatal screening or diagnostic programme is operated by inadequately trained staff. When such a programme is to be introduced, it is imperative that resources are allocated to staff training and that ongoing staff education is built into the programme.

Support and supervision

Counselling couples who are deciding whether or not to have prenatal diagnostic tests and those who are found to have a pregnancy affected with serious fetal abnormality is extremely stressful. If staff are to continue to do it well and to avoid damaging their own emotional health, they need to have an opportunity to talk about their worries, uncertainties and sadness with colleagues and with a supervisory counsellor. Time should be built into their schedule for this to be done formally, and the working day should allow for moments of informal discussion. Some units find it useful to have group discussion sessions on a regular basis or when a number of tragedies occur within a short space of time.[47,48]

Conclusions

I hope that the message of this chapter is a clear and simple one – that good counselling for prenatal diagnosis can only occur if the staff are well-informed, honest and kind, if they respect the thoughts and feelings of the parents, and if they have time and space in which to do the counselling. The onus falls upon senior staff to ensure that these conditions are met.

References

1. Crawfurd M. Ethical and legal aspects of early prenatal diagnosis. Br Med Bull 1983; 39(4):310–314.
2. Weatherall DJ. Foreword. In: Brock DJ, Rodeck CH, Ferguson Smith MA, eds. Prenatal diagnosis and screening. Edinburgh: Churchill Livingstone; 1992.
3. Cohen M, Nagel T, Scanlon T, eds. The rights and wrongs of abortion. Princeton, NJ: Princeton University Press; 1974.
4. Bewley S. Ethical issues in prenatal diagnosis. In: Abramsky L, Chapple J, eds. Prenatal diagnosis: the human side. London: Chapman and Hall; 1994.
5. Dunstan GR. Screening for fetal and genetic abnormality: social and ethical issues, J Med Genet 1988; 25:290–293.
6. Cranley MS. Roots of attachment: the relationship of parents with their unborn. In: Lederman RP, Raff BS, Caroll P, eds. Perinatal parental behaviour: Nursing research and implications for the newborn health. New York: Alan R. Liss; 1981.
7. Montgomery J. Legal issues in prenatal diagnosis. In: Abramsky L, Chapple J, eds. Prenatal diagnosis:

the human side. London: Chapman and Hall: 1994.

8. Morgan D, Lee R, Blackstone's guide to the Human Fertilisation and Embryology Act 1990. London: Blackstone Press; 1991.

9. Powers MJ. The duties of the obstetrician. In: Clements RV, ed. Safe practice in obstetrics and gynaecology: A medico-legal handbook. Edinburgh: Churchill Livingstone: 1994.

10. Paintin DB. Induced abortion. In: Clements RV, ed. Safe practice in obstetrics and gynaecology: A medico-legal handbook. Edinburgh: Churchill Livingstone; 1994.

11. The Abortion Act 1967. Section 4: Conscientious objection to participation in treatment. London: HMSO.

12. Brown J. The choice: A piece of my mind. JAMA 1989; 262(19):2735.

13. White-van Mourik MCA. Looking in from the outside. In: Abramsky L, Chapple J, eds. Prenatal diagnosis: the human side. London: Chapman and Hall; 1994.

14. White-van Mourik MCA. Termination of a second-trimester pregnancy for fetal abnormality: psychosocial aspects. In: Clarke A, ed. Genetic counselling: practice and principles. London: Routledge; 1994.

15. Statham H. The parents' reactions to termination of pregnancy for fetal abnormality: from a mother's point of view. In: Abramsky L, Chapple J, eds. Prenatal diagnosis: the human side. London: Chapman and Hall; 1994.

16. Lloyd J, Lawrence KM. Sequelae and support after termination of pregnancy for fetal malformation. BMJ 1985; 290:907–909.

17. SATFA. A handbook for parents when an abnormality is diagnosed in their baby, Essex: Good News Press; 1990.

18. Palmer K. Peace and pain. BMJ 1994; 309:279.

19. White-van Mourik MCA, Connor JM, Ferguson-Smith MA. The psychosocial sequelae of a second-trimester termination of pregnancy for fetal abnormality. Prenat Diagn 1992; 12:189–204.

20. Hall R. The parents' reactions to termination of pregnancy for fetal abnormality: from a father's point of view. In: Abramsky L, Chapple J, eds. Prenatal diagnosis: the human side. London: Chapman and Hall; 1994.

21. O'Dowd T. The needs of fathers. BMJ 1992; 306:1484–1485.

22. Abramsky L. Counselling prior to prenatal testing. In: Abramsky L, Chapple J, eds. Prenatal diagnosis: the human side. London: Chapman and Hall; 1994.

23. Sjogren B, Uddenberg N. Decision making during the prenatal diagnostic procedure. A questionnaire and interview study of 211 women participating in prenatal diagnosis. Prenat Diagn 1988; 8:263–273.

24. Clarke A. Is non-directive genetic counselling possible? Lancet 1991; 338:998–1001.

25. Green JM. Calming or harming? A critical review of psychological effects of fetal diagnosis on pregnant women. Galton Institute Occasional Papers, Second Series, No. 2; 1990.

26. Boppart I, et al. Special report. Maternal serum alpha-fetoprotein screening for neural tube defects. Results of a consensus meeting. Prenat Diagn 1985; 5:77–83.

27. King's Fund Forum. Screening for fetal and genetic abnormality. BMJ 1987; 295:1551–1553.

28. Davis AJ. Informed consent: how much information is enough? Nursing Outlook 1985; 33:40–42.

29. Donnai D. The management of the patient having fetal diagnosis. Baillière's Clin Obstet Gynaecol 1987; 1:737–745.

30. Chitty LS, Hunt GH, Moore J, Lobb MO. Effectiveness of routine ulltrasonography in detecting fetal structural abnormalities in a low risk population. BMJ 1991; 303:1165–1169.

31. Levi S, Hyjazi Y, Schaaps JP, Defoort P, Coulon R, Buekens P. Sensitivity and specificity of routine antenatal screening for congenital anomalies by ultrasound: the Belgian Multicentric Study. Ultrasound Obstet Gynecol 1991; 1:102–110.

32. Shirley IM, Bottomley F, Robinson VP. Routine radiographer screening for fetal abnormalities by ultrasound in an unselected low risk population. Br J Radiol 1992; 65(775):564–569.

33. Hollingsworth J. The sonographer's dilemma. In: Abramsky L, Chapple J, eds. Prenatal diagnosis: the human side. London: Chapman and Hall; 1994.

34. Garrett C, Carlton L. Difficult decisions in prenatal diagnosis. In: Abramsky L, Chapple J, eds. Prenatal diagnosis: the human side. London: Chapman and Hall; 1994.

35. Seller M, Barnes C, Ross S, Barby T, Cowmeadow P. Grief and mid-trimester fetal loss. Prenat Diagn 1993; 13:341–348.

36. Blumberg BD. The emotional implications of prenatal diagnosis. In: Emery AEH, Pullen IM, eds. Psychological aspects of genetic counselling. London: Academic Press; 1984:202–217.

37. Becker J, Glinski L, Laxova R. Long-term emotional impact of 2nd trimester pregnancy termination after detection of fetal abnormality. Am J Hum Genet 1984; 36:122s.

38. White-van Mourik MCA, Connor JM, Ferguson-Smith MA. Patient care before and after termination of pregnancy for neural tube defects. Prenat Diagn 1990; 10:497–505.

39. Harper PS. Practical genetic counselling. Bristol: John Wright; 1981.

40. Worden JW. Grief counselling and grief therapy. London: Tavistock; 1983.

41. Murray Parkes C. Bereavement: studies of grief in adult life. London: Penguin; 1986.

42. Statham H, Green JM. The effects of miscarriage and other 'unsuccessful' pregnancies on feelings early in a subsequent pregnancy. J Reprod Infant Psychol 1994; 12:45–54.

43. Smith DK, Slack J, Shaw RW, Marteau TM. Lack of knowledge in health professionals: a barrier to providing information to patients? Qual Health Care 1994; 3:75–78.

44. Smith DK, Shaw RW, Slack J, Marteau TM. Training

obstetricians and midwives to present screening tests: evaluation of two brief interventions. Prenat Diagn 1995; 15:317–324.

45. Boulton M, Griffiths J, Hall D, McIntyre M, Oliver B, Woodward J. Improving communication: a practical programme for teaching trainees about communication issues in the general practice consultation. Med Educ 1984; 18:269–274.

46. Friedrich E. Caring for the carers. In: Abramsky L, Chapple J, eds. Prenatal diagnosis: the human side. London: Chapman and Hall; 1994.

47. National Association for Staff Support. A charter for staff support. Woking, Surrey: National Association for Staff Support; 1992.

48. Jenkins R. Prevalence of mental illness in the workplace. In: Jenkins R, Coney N, eds. Prevention of mental ill health at work: a conference. London: HMSO; 1992.

CHAPTER 23

Neuro-behavioural studies in fetuses with abnormality

David James and Srini Vindla

Introduction and background

The identification and assessment of fetuses with structural abnormality have been possible for many years, with X-rays preceding the use of ultrasound (US). However, recognition of structural abnormalities has limitations, especially in the area of predicting outcome. In principle, as in all areas of medicine, the ideal approach is for complementary methods of assessment to be used with evaluation of structure and function producing the clearest view of diagnosis and prognosis. But the evaluation of function in the fetus with abnormality is a relatively new concept and a clinical science that is in its infancy.[1]

As with the developments in the evaluation of structural abnormality of the fetus, advances in US have been an essential prerequisite to developments in the area of assessment of function. However, to date, most of this work has been conducted in a research setting which suffers from the limitations of being impractical, labour intensive, inconvenient and subjective.[2] Typically, all such research methods use direct real-time observation by one or two observers with one or two US transducers, simultaneous recording on video and fetal heart rate (FHR) recording with Doppler US and all the signals integrated onto a polygraph. Analysis of all this data requires laborious playback and comparison of polygraph and video recordings.[1-3] More recent developments are overcoming these inherent problems of traditional fetal behavioural analysis.[1]

Behaviour is defined as the interaction of an organism with its environment.

Fetal behaviour can be studied in three ways:

1. By passive observation of fetal activity[4]
2. By recording the reaction of a fetus to a stimulus[5]
3. By documenting fetal habituation, i.e. the cessation of a response to a repeated stimulus.[6]

This last response represents a simple form of learned behaviour and potentially is the most sophisticated method of assessment of the three.

Passive behaviour

Movements

Fetal movements in early pregnancy have been studied by several groups. Van Dongen and Goudie[7] described four patterns of behaviour in fetuses between 10 and 12 weeks – periods of absence of movements (not lasting longer than 5 min), periods of rolling, flexion, extension and head rotation involving all parts of the body, periods of isolated limb movements and periods of strong pulsed movements of the thorax similar to hiccups. The most detailed analysis of fetal movements in early pregnancy has been performed by De Vries and colleagues.[8,9] They reported that the first movements seen in the fetus were extensions and flexions of the fetal spine visible from 7 weeks. This was followed by the onset of a wide variety of distinct types of movement over the next 6 to 8 weeks. Indeed, all the movements observed in term fetuses were already present by 15 weeks, provided a sufficiently long observation time was used to compensate for the low incidence of many movements (such as breathing) in early pregnancy (see Table 23.1). The only difference in these early movements and those seen at term is in their greater sophistication, co-ordination and integration later in pregnancy.

As pregnancy advances a cyclicity of fetal behaviour develops. The first to be recognized is a diurnal pattern which has been reported from as early as 20 to 22 weeks[10] through to the end of pregnancy.[11,12] All these studies found peaks of fetal activity occurring in the late evening and appear to be related to maternal corticosteroid levels.[13]

For the end of the second trimester shorter cycles of fetal behavioural variation can be recognized. Initially, the fetus shows alternating rest-activity cycles (also called

Table 23.1
The appearance of fetal movements in early pregnancy (adapted from Reference[8])

Movement	Gestation of first appearance
Any movement	7
Startle	8
Generalized movements	8
Hiccups	8
Isolated arm movements	9
Head retroflexion	9
Hand-face contact	10
Breathing	10
Jaw opening	10
Stretching	10
Head anteflexion	10
Yawn	11
Suck and swallow	12

Table 23.3
Characteristics of behavioural states in full-term normal human fetuses (from Reference[16])

State	% Time observed	Mean duration (min)	Range (min)
1F	30.1	21.8	3–38
2F	57.5	31.6	3–94
4F	9.5	37.8	4–137

No 3F was observed in this study. State was not defined for 2.9% of the observational period.

active-quiet and ultradian rhythms).[14] Thus, for example, prior to 24 weeks the longest period of inactivity or quiescence in the human fetus is 6 minutes; whereas after 32 weeks most quiet intervals are between 10 and 40 minutes.[15] Using this arbitrary 6-minute rule, rest-activity cycles are rarely seen prior to 24 weeks, but by 29 weeks they are seen in over 80% of recordings from normal fetuses.[15]

This continuing development of the fetal neurological system can be seen in the manifestation of behavioural states by the end of pregnancy.

Behavioural states are fixed and recurring associations between body movements, eye movements and heart rate in the fetus which change within 3 minutes.[4] They are defined in Table 23.2 and their characteristics are described in Table 23.3. The existence of State 3F is disputed. Pillai and James[16] found no evidence of its existence in over 138 hours of observation of normal fetuses and furthermore, even in the original

descriptions, the state was only present for short periods.[4] Behavioural states are present in over 80% of recordings from normal fetuses at 36 weeks.[16]

Tone

There is a progressive increase in the tone of the fetus as pregnancy advances. This reflects maturation of both the central nervous system (especially the cerebellum) and the musculoskeletal system. This may be useful as a general neurological screening tool in the future. If features of this aspect of development could be quantified and documented, then it may play a role in the diagnosis and/or evaluation of fetal neuromuscular disorders in pregnancies of women with a family history of such conditions or even in general population screening.

Fetal heart rate (FHR)

The development of FHR characteristics during normal pregnancy represents a combination of the effects of both local and central factors.[17]

During normal pregnancy the mean baseline FHR declines significantly as gestation advances, with the mean value

Table 23.2
Behavioural states in full-term normal human fetuses (from Reference[4])

State description	Somatic movements	Eye movements	Baseline FHR pattern
1F	Absent except for occasional startle	Absent	Low variation
2F	Present in bursts	Present	High variation
3F*	Absent	Present	High variation
4F	Present	Present	Sustained tachycardia

The existence of State 3F is disputed (see text and Reference[16]).

being approximately 155 bpm at 16 weeks and falling by approximately one bpm per week to reach a mean value of 130 bpm at 40 weeks.[17] Thus the normal range of the FHR at the start of the third trimester is 120–160 bpm, whereas at term it is 110–150 bpm. Most of the other features of the FHR are positively correlated with advancing gestation. Thus, as pregnancy progresses there are significant rises in the proportion of fetal movements associated with FHR accelerations, the rate of rise of the accelerations and the maximum height of the accelerations.[17] There is also an initial increase in the variability of the baseline FHR over the first two trimesters. However, over the last trimester this continues to rise in periods of activity but falls again in periods of quiescence.[17]

Mouthing

A sinusoidal FHR pattern may reflect an underlying pathology (see below); however, it can also be a normal feature often found in association with fetal mouthing movements.[18]

Respiratory activity

Human fetal breathing movements have been recognized for over a century and have been defined as downward movement of the diaphragm with outward movement of the abdominal contents and inward displacement of the thorax.[19] It is now well established that breathing is a normal feature of fetal life and is episodic in nature with circadian and ultradian biological rhythms.[20] These are stimulated by glucose[21] and carbon dioxide[22] and inhibited by hypoxia.[23]

The onset of both hiccups and breathing has been described at 8 to 10 weeks,[8] corresponding to the time of development of the diaphragm. However, their developmental trends are very different with fetal hiccups being the predominant type of diaphragmatic movement up to 26 weeks and fetal breathing being more common thereafter.[24] This suggests that the centres controlling fetal breathing are not only different but also are more complex than those that control hiccups. The early

appearance of both types of activity suggests their ontogeny may depend on relatively simple mechanisms. However, the subsequent developmental course of fetal breathing suggests a profound influence from higher centres. Data on the developmental trends in hiccups is lacking; however, the observation that they declined in incidence with advancing pregnancy suggests that any subsequent brain influence is likely to be inhibitory.[1]

Stimulated behaviour

The response of normal fetus to a single stimulus has been extensively studied, though the nature of the stimulus has varied. The most commonly studied stimulus is the 'acoustic larynx'[5] which emits a broad band of frequencies resulting in both vibratory and acoustic components to the stimulus. A normal healthy human fetus responds to such a vibro-acoustic stimulus (VAS) by moving and increasing its heart rate.[25] The earliest response has been noted at 22 weeks, but by 28 weeks all females and by 30 weeks all male fetuses appear to respond in some degree.[26] However, the appearance of fetal movement and FHR responses appear to be developmentally distinct processes.

After stimulation a mean increase in the FHR is noted consistently from 26 weeks. After 30 weeks there is also a significant rise in the basal FHR. From about 33 weeks, in addition to the early increase in FHR, a delayed response occurs whereby there is an increase in the number of FHR accelerations and incidence of gross body movements, commencing between 10 and 30 minutes after exposure to the stimulus and remaining for up to 1 hour after exposure.[5] Prior to 32 weeks there is no alteration in the gross fetal body movements.[27] This suggests that the initial FHR response to stimulation develops neurologically distinctly from the body movement component. By 36 weeks another developmental trend is a significant decrease in the percentage of time that breathing occurs after the stimulus.[5]

Habituation

Habituation is a decrease and eventual cessation of a behavioural response that occurs after an initially novel stimulus is repeatedly presented. It is widely accepted as a basic form of learning and a normal pattern reflects an intact and fully functioning central nervous system.[28] A number of different stimuli have been used. Peiper[29] was the first to report the cessation of the fright response (i.e. habituation) in the human fetus to repetitive sound stimuli using a car horn. Leader and colleagues[6,30] examined habituation of the fetal movement response to repeated vibro-acoustic stimulation using the acoustic larynx. They demonstrated that 93% of fetuses from very low-risk pregnancies habituated their movement response after 10 to 50 stimuli. Madison et al[31] using two different vibro-acoustic stimuli in randomized methods confirmed that this decrement in observed response is genuine habituation and not response fatigue by demonstrating dishabituation. More recently habituation of the FHR response to repeated stimulation has been demonstrated.[28]

A gestational effect has also been reported for fetal habituation with the rate of habituation becoming significantly faster as gestational age increases. This phenomenon is thought to reflect the maturation of the neural circuitry responsible for this form of learning.[32]

Finally, fetal habituation has been used to study cognition and language development. Term fetuses are able to discriminate between different sounding vowels,[33] to recognize their mother's voice and to differentiate between male and female voices.[34]

Computerized evaluation of fetal behaviour

In an attempt to overcome the limitations of fetal behavioural analysis in the research setting described above (impractical, labour intensive, inconvenient and subjective) work has been undertaken to make the assessment more relevant and applicable to clinical practice. The two approaches used for this purpose are:[1]

1. The identification and recording of fetal behaviour (principally FHR and fetal movement) using Doppler ultrasound.
2. The analysis by computer of the signals thus generated.

These methods have been applied to the study of passive fetal behaviour using FHR alone,[35] fetal movements alone[36] and FHR and fetal movements in combination;[1,37] stimulated behaviour[38] and habituation.[39]

Biological influences on fetal behaviour

A number of biological or physiological factors influence fetal behaviour. They are summarized in Table 23.4. Arguably, the two most important factors are gestational age and behavioural state. There is no agreement about the influence of uterine contractions and labour on fetal behaviour.[40,44,45] Similarly, there are conflicting reports in the literature about the effects of heat and maternal exercise,[46–49] although this is perhaps not surprising given the varied nature of the thermal stress and exercise used in the different studies.

Fetal behaviour in abnormal pregnancies but no congenital abnormality

A number of pathologies in pregnancy are known to influence behaviour in structurally normal fetuses.

Intra-uterine growth retardation (IUGR)

The alteration of fetal behaviour in growth

Table 23.4
Biological/physiological factors which influence fetal behaviour (from Reference[40])

Behavioural characteristic	Biological variable and effect	Reference
Heart rate	Advancing gestation produces: fall in baseline, increased correlation of accelerations and movements, faster rate of rise of accelerations, greater height of accelerations, differentiation of baseline variability with state development	17
	Ethnic differences exist	42
Movement	Diurnal variation in fetal activity from about 20–22 weeks	41
	Advancing gestation produces organization into rest/activity cycles and eventually behavioural states	15
Respiratory	Advancing gestation produces: proportion of time spent exhibiting: a) breathing movements are increased and b) hiccups is reduced	24
	More breathing movements seen in active states	24
	Maternal glucose consumption increases fetal breathing activity	41
	Maternal caffeine consumption increases fetal breathing activity	43

retardation has been studied by several groups. The definitions of IUGR have varied in the different reports. The causes of growth restriction are many and include congenital abnormality and infection. The most common identifiable cause is uteroplacental insufficiency and is the commonest cause in most of the studies of fetal behaviour in association with IUGR, although many of the reports have failed to document the cause.

The results of long term outcome studies are inconsistent. Several studies have shown that fetuses with IUGR are at risk of neurodevelopmental disability in infancy.[50,51] Furthermore, the degree of fetal academia associated with chronic hypoxia is correlated to the degree of intellectual impairment seen in childhood.[52] In contrast, other studies have reported accelerated neurological development in infants that were chronically malnourished in utero.[53,54]

As a generalization the studies of fetal behaviour in IUGR have shown a reduction in both the quantity and quality of fetal movements. Bekedam and Visser[23] reported that there was a reduction in movements in IUGR fetuses but that there was an overlap with normally grown fetuses. They also noted a reduction in the fast component

movements in IUGR fetuses. Sival and colleagues, however, found no difference in the quality and quantity of fetal movements in IUGR except in the presence of oligohydramnios.[55,56] This would suggest that the effect of pathological undergrowth on fetal movements occurs relatively late in the disease process.[23,57]

There are a number of groups who have studied the ways in which IUGR can influence FHR patterns. We have reported a significant delay in the maturation of FHR patterns with IUGR.[58] Visser and colleagues[59] demonstrated a progressive degeneration of FHR variability in fetuses with IUGR.

Several workers have reported a lower incidence and shorter duration of fetal breathing in IUGR.[58,60,61] This is in keeping with the findings in chronically hypoxic fetal lambs.[62]

When the different features of fetal behaviour are considered in combination, IUGR has been consistently shown to result in a delay in appearance of behavioural states.[58,63] Furthermore, in the pathologically growing fetus it appears that this effect on fetal behaviour predates any FHR changes such as loss of acceleration and appearance of decelerations by several weeks.[58]

The response of human fetuses with IUGR to VAS has been studied.[64,65] Two groups of intra-uterine growth restricted fetuses were exposed to VAS. First, a group of IUGR fetuses in pregnant women between 33 and 40 weeks' gestation were studied. Prior to stimulation the fetuses moved less often and also had a decrease in long term FHR variation compared to a group of normally grown controls. Following stimulation the two groups behaved in a similar fashion.[64] However, when the response of fetuses developing IUGR prior to 32 weeks' gestation was studied no significant changes in FHR and fetal activity patterns was found in response to stimulation.[65] The authors speculated that in this subgroup of growth restricted fetuses a delay in the functional maturation of fetal sensory receptors may have occurred due to chronic nutritional deprivation.

Fetuses with IUGR have also been shown to manifest abnormalities in habituation. For example, 93% of fetuses from totally normal uncomplicated pregnancies will habituate their movement response to VAS after exposure to 10–50 stimuli. In contrast only 34% of IUGR fetuses will habituate their movement response after 10 to 50 stimuli.

Maternal diabetes

This maternal metabolic disorder has many implications for the fetus including congenital abnormality and excessive growth. Behaviour has been shown to be altered in infants of diabetic mothers.[66]

Behaviour in the fetuses of diabetic mothers has also been studied. Studies in early pregnancy have shown that there is a delay in the onset of motor development (except breathing which occurs at an earlier gestation) when compared to a group of normal control fetuses.[67] The quantity of movements is also less than in control fetuses. After the 12th week of gestation there is increased activity in the fetuses of diabetic mothers mainly due to an increase in the incidence of fetal breathing movements.[68]

Maternal drug administration

The effects on the fetus of drugs administered to the mother have been widely studied. The main reported effects are summarized in Table 23.5. There are conflicting reports in the literature of the effects of maternally administered steroids on fetal behaviour. Some groups have found that steroids decrease heart rate variation and fetal activity,[78,79] while another group has found that the administration of steroids, in fact, has no effect on the fetal activity but caused a rise in fetal heart rate variation.[80] Some of these differences may be due to differences in gestational age in the fetuses studied and also the underlying pathology and its severity leading to the need for steroid therapy.

Other pathological conditions

Fetal infection has been reported to be associated with reduced FHR variability,

Table 23.5
The effects of drugs on fetal behaviour

Drug	Effects	Reference
Tranquillizers, narcotics, methadone, atropine, barbiturates, pancuronium, anticonvulsants	General depression — reduced FHR variability — reduced movements — reduced breathing	40,69, 70,71, 72
Amphetamines	Increased PHR variability and movements	40
Magnesium sulphate	Reduced FHR variability, reduced movements and FHR response to VAS	73,74
Ethanol	Reduced FHR variability, movement and breathing	75
Indomethacin, terbutaline	Increased fetal movements and breathing	76
Prostaglandin E$_2$	Reduced fetal movements and breathing	77

fetal movements and breathing.[81] Yet there have been other reports disputing this view.[82] The phenomenon of fetal brain death is now well documented.[83] Such fetuses characteristically have less fetal activity and an FHR with reduced variability. The majority of such cases arise from transient though severe hypoxic episodes which do not result in fetal death.

More subtle forms of fetal neurodevelopmental compromise, of an uncertain aetiology, may be identified using fetal behavioural examination. Such cases may not necessarily result in gross abnormalities of fetal activity or FHR pattern, but may present with a failure to develop integrated behavioural states, with complete dissociation of fetal eye and somatic movements and FHR pattern.[84]

Severe fetal anaemia or a massive fetal blood loss can result in a characteristic sinusoidal FHR pattern.[85,86]

It is not surprising that fetal cardiac problems are associated with abnormalities of the FHR. The influence of structural abnormalities is discussed below. However, other conditions include maternal systemic lupus erythematosus (producing a fetal bradycardia by transplacental passage of Ro antibodies),[87] maternal auto-immune thyrotoxicosis (producing a fetal tachycardia due to transplacental passage of thyroid stimulating antibodies),[88] and cardiac failure from a variety of causes (producing initially a loss of variability and decelerations).[40]

Finally, fetal mouthing in an otherwise quiescent fetus may indicate neurological integrity. We have reported absence of this feature in quiescent fetuses who were acidotic from a variety of causes.[18]

Behaviour in fetuses with abnormality

Passive behaviour and fetal abnormality

Anencephaly was one of the first conditions to be studied. Visser and colleagues reported an observational study in eight anencephalic fetuses between 16 and 35 weeks.[89] All fetuses had a poorly differentiated range of movements with only half the normal 14 different patterns being observed at most. For example, retro- and anteflexion of the fetal head, jaw opening, sucking, swallowing, stretching and yawning were never seen. Generalized movements were present in all fetuses, isolated arm movements in all but one, and startles and isolated leg movements in all but two fetuses. Breathing was observed on three occasions. Hiccups, which occur relatively frequently during the first half of pregnancy in normal fetuses (see above), were observed in only one of six fetuses studied before 20 weeks. The clearest abnormality concerned the quality of the individual movements and especially that of the general movements. In all fetuses these movements were forceful, jerky in character and of large amplitude and caused large positional shifts in the uterus. They started abruptly, and during the movement the same force and amplitude continued until the movement suddenly stopped. This is in contrast to the fluent appearance and the waxing and waning of these movements in normal fetuses. Although there were large interfetal differences, the execution of these movements was highly consistent within the individual fetus. The authors tried to relate the pathological behaviour to the anatomical defect in the seven cases where post-mortems were performed. They concluded that the presence or absence of the hindbrain was critical to certain types of behaviour. Thus when the hindbrain was absent there was a 'burst-pause' pattern to the generalized movements and also those movements were in excess of that normally seen at any given gestation.[89] From this work it has been suggested that the high rate of fetal activity at younger gestations giving way to a lower rate with advancing fetal maturity supports the hypothesis that such maturation is associated with the development of inhibitory neural pathways. The fact that anencephalic fetuses maintain this high level of activity throughout pregnancy, suggests that such inhibitory pathways derive from the cerebral cortex.[1] Anencephalic fetuses also exhibit persistent abnormalities of the FHR, namely a pattern of poor variability with short-lived shallow decelerations.[90] It is of note that this FHR pattern is very similar to that seen in the normal immature fetus at about 18 weeks.[17]

Fetuses with trisomy 18 have been reported as manifesting abnormal movement patterns in a study by Hepper & Shahidulla.[91] In addition, they reported such fetuses have abnormal eye movements.

Bizarre fetal behaviour has also been reported in a fetus with the lethal multiple abnormality syndrome of Smith–Lemli–Opitz Type II (autosomal recessive).[92] The fetal behaviour was studied in detail at 36 weeks. Analysis revealed absence of any behavioural state patterns (1F to 4F) previously described in healthy fetuses of 36 weeks' gestation and absence of any cyclicity of behaviour which is usually observable in fetuses throughout the last trimester. Fetal eye movements briefly accompanied somatic movements but otherwise were absent. Somatic movements were isolated rather than occurring in bursts, and were much less frequent than normally observed during state 2F, but were more frequent than in state 1F. Mouthing movements were absent. Shallow fetal breathing movements were observed intermittently during 10 minutes of the recording, the longest sustained interval being 96 seconds. Fetal heart-rate acceleration accompanied every somatic movement. In summary, the behaviour was bizarre, not confirming to any of the recognized behavioural state patterns normally present in fetuses of 36 weeks' gestation.

Normal fetal growth and development during pregnancy is highly dependent upon adequate fetal movement. Limitation of movement, regardless of the underlying cause, can result in a particular pattern of abnormal fetal morphogenesis. This phenotype is termed the fetal akinesia deformation sequence (FADS). The aetiology of fetal akinesia may be generally classified into one of five categories: neuropathy,

Table 23.6
Syndromes associated with the fetal akinesia deformation sequence (FADS)

Pena–Shokeir syndrome
Neu–Laxova syndrome
Neu–Laxova variant
Restrictive dermopathy
Lethal multiple pterygium syndrome
Cerebro-oculofacioskeletal syndrome
Oligohydramnios sequence
Trisomy 18
Alpers progressive infantile neuronal poliodystrophy
Arthrogryposis multiplex congenita
Gaucher's disease type II
Congenital myotonic dystrophy
Teratogens
Congenital infection

myopathy, restrictive dermopathy, teratogen exposure, or restricted movement due to intra-uterine constraint. It has been well reviewed by Hammond & Donnenfeld.[93] Syndromes/conditions associated with FADS are listed in Table 23.6. Although there is significant genetic heterogeneity for the aetiology of decreased fetal movement, the resulting phenotypic findings are often similar. These include intra-uterine growth retardation (IUGR), congenital contractures, underdevelopment of the limbs, pulmonary hypoplasia, abnormal amniotic fluid volume, craniofacial changes (hypertelorism, micrognathia, short neck, low-set ears, cleft palate), and a short umbilical cord. In most cases of FADS there is restricted limb movement; however, where there is associated hydramnios (due to defective swallowing), it is possible that overall body movement may be increased (presumably due to a lack of physical constraints). Clearly many of the cases of FADS have abnormalities of fetal tone which is easily identifiable on ultrasound (e.g. Pena–Shokeir syndrome,[93] congenital myotonic dystrophy,[94] lethal multiple pterygium syndrome[95] and various forms of arthrogryposis). Some cases of FADS are associated with fetal hydrops which in itself has been shown to be associated with fetal hypomobility irrespective of the cause.[96] In cases of hydrops, in addition to reduced fetal activity there is often reduced fetal heart rate variability. In addition, in a few cases, a fetal tachyarrhythmia will be recognized which is the cause of the hydrops. Maxwell and colleagues[97] reported their experience of 23 pregnancies between 22 and 38 weeks with fetal tachycardia. Twelve were cases of supraventricular tachycardia, eight of atrial flutter, and three cases in which the rhythm varied between supraventricular tachycardia and atrial flutter. In 11 cases the fetus had developed non-immune fetal hydrops before referral; 12 cases were non-hydropic at referral but one of this group of fetuses became hydropic during treatment. No relation was found between the rate or type of arrhythmia and the presence or absence of intra-uterine heart failure.

Fetuses with central nervous system (CNS) malformations of varied aetiology produce abnormal behaviour. Horimoto and colleagues[98] undertook a labour intensive study screening 1426 singleton pregnancies at term for fetal brain impairment in utero. Ultrasound examination of the CNS looking for structural abnormalities was coupled with behavioural assessment using fetal activity and FHR analysis. Ten fetuses were identified from the study population with structural abnormalities of the CNS and/or behaviour and they were subjected to more detailed behavioural assessment observing movement of the fetal extremities, fetal breathing, eye and mouth movements as well as distribution of quiescent versus active FHR patterns. Two fetuses had temporary abnormal behaviour in utero which reverted to normal before delivery and in whom no neurological abnormality was found in the newborn period. The remaining eight fetuses were found to have brain impairment after birth. The findings in all 10 fetuses are summarized in Table 23.7. In summary, the eight fetuses could be divided into three groups:

- Those with lesions at, or caudal to, the pons-medulla that were specifically identified by fetal behavioural analysis (Cases 1 and 2)
- Diffuse lesions on the brain which, although resulting in abnormal behaviour, could not be localized by this behaviour (Cases 3, 4 and 5)

- Lesions localized on the cerebral hemisphere but with no abnormal behaviour (Cases 6, 7 and 8)

Horimoto and colleagues in their report[98] proposed that their screening system should be introduced into routine clinical practice. However, that view is arguably unrealistic given the labour intensive and time consuming nature of the behavioural evaluation. We have taken a different approach using a computer based method which we believe would be more practical for both screening and diagnosis.

Over a 12-month period, Doppler ultrasound recordings were obtained from 43 fetuses ranging from 28 to 36 weeks' gestation with a conventional 1.5 MHz transducer and a Sonicaid TEAM Fetal Monitor (Oxford Instruments, Abingdon). Two groups of fetuses were studied. There were 27 normal fetuses in the first group; they were studied longitudinally. The second group consisted of 16 fetuses with congenital malformations of which 10 had structural CNS abnormalities, 1 had Down's syndrome and 5 had other congenital abnormalities (2 fetuses had congenital heart disease, 1 had a congenital diaphragmatic hernia, 1 had arthrogryposis and 1 had cystic fibrosis with meconium peritonitis). The latter two cases were further complicated by hydramnios. A clinical summary of the 16 abnormal cases is given in Tables 23.8A and 23.8B.

All fetuses were recorded for a minimum duration of 60 minutes. We were unable to obtain a full 60 minutes recording on one occasion in Case 3 (42 minutes), Case 11 and Case 16 (51 minutes) due to maternal non-compliance. The recordings took place in a quiet room with the patients in a semi-recumbent position. The patients were requested not to smoke for the duration of and from 2 hours prior to the study. The study was undertaken approximately 2 hours after a meal. The transducer was strapped to the maternal abdomen at the site corresponding to the back of the fetus, overlying the fetal heart. Real-time ultrasound was used to optimize the position.

Table 23.7
Correlation between fetal behavioural patterns and postnatal findings (from Reference[98])

Case no.	Movement of extremities	Breathing movement	EM/NEM period alternation	Eye movement pattern[†]	Regular mouthing	Active/ resting FHR pattern	Postnatal diagnosis	Lesion location and distribution	Age	Neurological signs
1*	Absent	Present	Normal	Present	Present	Present	Spinal cord haemorrhage	Spinal cord (C_{5-6})	20 months	Quadriplegia, sensory disturbance
2*	Present	Absent	Absent	Present	‡	Absent	Möbius' syndrome with central hypoventilation	Pons-medulla	3 years	No spontaneous respirations, mental retardation
3*	Present	Present	Normal	Present	Absent	Present	Undetermined	Cerebral white matter, diffuse	3 years	Mental retardation, cerebral palsy
4	Present	Present	Disproportional	Present	Present	Present	Neuronal migration abnormality, hydrocephalus, cerebellar hypoplasia	Cerebral hemisphere diffuse, brain stem, cerebellum	27 months	Mental retardation, cerebral palsy, epilepsy
5	Present	Present	Absent	Absent	‡	Absent	Holoprosencephaly (alobar)	Diffuse	Died shortly after birth	–
6	Present	Present	Normal	Present	Present	Present	Arachnoid cyst	Right frontal lobe	8 months	Not noted
7	Present	Present	Normal	Present	Present	Present	Arachnoid cyst	Right quadrigeminal cistern to intrahemispheric fissure	7 months	Not noted
8	Present	Present	Normal	Present	Present	Present	Hydrocephalus, encephalocoele	Occipital lobe	11 months	Not noted
9	Present	Present	Absent– normal	Present	Present	Present	Normal	None	7 months	Not noted
10	Present	Present	Normal	Absent– present	Present	Present	Normal	None	1 month	Not noted

EM/NEM = eye movement/no eye movement.
*Previously reported.
[†]Rapid eye movement and slow eye movement.
[‡]Undeterminable because of lack of EM/NEM alternation.

Of the 43 fetuses, 26 were monitored longitudinally until delivery on a fortnightly (4 fetuses) or monthly (22 fetuses) basis. The remaining 17 cases were monitored once.

A 'C' based computer programme analyzes the recorded digitized FHR and fetal activity count (FAC) data obtained from the TEAM monitor. The FHR baseline rate and variation were derived by analyzing a sliding 3-minute window of data every 0.275 seconds. Three minutes were chosen as the time interval to conform with conventional behavioural analysis methods.[99] For each 3-minute window of data the mean heart rate was calculated together with the standard deviation. The standard deviation was used to differentiate between low and high variation.[100] If the standard deviation for the 3-minute period was less than or equal to 3 bpm then the sliding window was said to exhibit low variation. If the standard deviation exceeded 3 bpm then the sliding window was said to exhibit high variation. In this way an update of variation could be made every 0.275 seconds.

The baseline rate was only determined after periods of low variation, as defined above, had been identified. It was defined as being equal to the mean FHR for the 3-minute window of low variation. It was then projected through periods of high variation to allow detection of accelerations. The baseline rate could therefore be updated every 0.275 seconds if consecutive sliding windows were identified as having low variation allowing changes in baseline rate to

Table 23.8A
Fetuses with CNS abnormality studied by computerized analysis of fetal behaviour (Reference[99])

Case number	Maternal age (years)	Gravida	Abnormality	Gestational age at birth (weeks)	Mode of delivery	Sex	Weight (g)	Outcome and comments
1	30	5	Walker–Warburg syndrome	36	NSD	F	2140	Baby died aged 14 days
2	38	2	Acrofacial dysostosis*	29	EmCS	M	1600	Baby died aged 12 hours
3	34	5	Agenesis corpus callosum, mild ventriculomegaly	32	NSD	M	2260	Alive, poorly controlled fits, remains in hospital at 4 months
4	28	2	Porencephaly (alloimmune fetal thrombocytopenia)	37	AVD	M	2760	Alive, hypotonic and cortical blindness at six weeks, failure to thrive
5	28	1	Marked ventriculomegaly, hypoplastic cerebellum, agenesis of corpus callosum	31	EmCS	M	1820	Baby died aged 72 hours
6	23	1	Hydrocephalus, Arnold–Chiari malformation	37	EmCS	F	3600	Shunt inserted, no major neurological deficit at 5 months of age
7	30	1	Mild ventriculomegaly	39	EmCS	M	4000	Mild ventriculomegaly, normal neurological assessment at 7 days of age
8	35	2	Mild ventriculomegaly	37	EICS	M	2680	Normal neurological assessment at 7 days
9	32	5	Open neural tube defect, Arnold–Chiari malformation, hydrocephalus	37	EICS	M	3700	Paralysis below level T10, surgical closure of NTD performed day 2
10	37	5	Alobar holoprosencephaly, ASD	37	NSD	M	2980	Baby died aged 60 minutes

*Hydrocephalus, cerebellar hypoplasia, right inner ear hypoplasia, radial hypoplasia, vertebral anomalies, absent left kidney and ureter.

Table 23.8B
Fetuses with non-CNS abnormality studied by computerized analysis of fetal behaviour (Reference[99])

Case number	Maternal age (years)	Gravida	Abnormality	Gestational age at birth (weeks)	Mode of delivery	Sex	Weight (g)	Outcome and comments
11	38	1	Congenital diaphragmatic hernia	37	EICS	F	3120	Alive, CDH corrected, normal neurological status at 6 months of age
12	30	1	Tricuspid atresia, fetal hydrops	33	EmCS	F	1790	Baby died aged 12 hours
13	25	2	Fallot tetralogy, meconium peritonitis	33	EmCS	M	2040	Alive, ileostomy, normal neurological status
14	31	1	Down's syndrome	37	NSD	F	2350	Alive, VSD and characteristic features of Down's syndrome
15	34	1	Cystic fibrosis, meconium peritonitis	33	EmCS	M	2160	Ileostomy, failure to thrive, normal neurological status at 5 months of age
16	22	2	Arthrogryposis, hydramnios, pulmonary hypoplasia	35	EmCS	F	2200	Baby died aged 6 hours

NSD – normal spontaneous delivery; EmCS – emergency caesarean section; ASD – atrial septal defect; EICS – elective caesarean section; VSD – ventricular septal defect; CDH – congenital diaphragmatic hernia; AVD – assisted vaginal delivery; NTD – neural tube defect.

be followed. When a second period of low variation occurred after an episode of high variation the baseline rate was recalculated.

Individual FAC markers indicated by the TEAM monitor were used to analyze fetal activity during the recording. The markers were used to represent both the occurrence and the duration (number of 0.25 second markers) of fetal movements. A single movement of a fetal part could result in the generation of more than one FAC. The occurrence of an FAC in a 0.25 second epoch indicated that fetal movement was detected during that time period and that it was not necessarily a separate movement from preceding or succeeding epoch recordings.

Each heart rate and movement data file was analyzed by the above described programme and results summarized as follows:

- Percentage of time in low variation FHR
- Percentage of time in high variation FHR
- The FAC rate in low variation FHR
- The FAC rate in high variation FHR.

The 27 normal fetuses had no evidence of perinatal asphyxia or neurological abnormality in the early neonatal period. The median gestation at birth was 40 weeks (range 36–42) and median birthweight was 3.46 kg (range 2.52–4.96). Twenty-four had normal vaginal deliveries, two an assisted vaginal delivery and one had a caesarean section for cephalo-pelvic disproportion.

The percentage of time that the fetuses exhibited low and high variation heart rate patterns are shown in Figures 23.1 and 23.2 respectively. There was no significant change of FHR variation with gestation. However, there was a significant fall in FAC between 28 weeks' gestation and 36 weeks' gestation in both low ($P = 0.02$) and high ($P = 0.04$) FHR variation (Figs 23.3, 23.4).

Figures 23.1 and 23.2 also show the percentage of time spent in low and high variation FHR pattern by the abnormal fetuses. Half of the cases (Cases 2, 3, 5, 6, 7, 10, 11 and 16) had FHR variation within the 10th to 90th centiles of the normal range. Seven of the abnormal fetuses (Cases 4, 8, 9, 12, 13, 14 and 15) exhibited low variation FHR pattern for a period greater than the

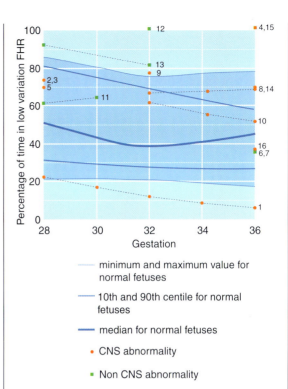

Fig. 23.1 Computerized analysis of fetal behaviour in normal and abnormal fetuses – percentage of time in low variation FHR pattern (from Reference[99]).

90th centile. Only one abnormal fetus (Case 1) exhibited high variation FHR pattern for an excessive percentage of time.

Figures 23.3 and 23.4 also show the FAC data for the abnormal fetuses. Six of the abnormal fetuses (Cases 5, 7, 8, 10, 11 and 16) consistently exhibited an FAC above the 90th centile in both low and high variation FHR patterns. A seventh fetus (Case 4) exhibited high FAC in low variation FHR pattern but no periods of high variation FHR pattern were noted. In contrast, three abnormal fetuses (Cases 2, 3 and 15) exhibited FAC below the 10th centile in both low and high variation FHR patterns (Fig. 23.4). Of the remainder of abnormal fetuses, Cases 13 and 14 exhibited predominantly normal FAC in both low and high variation FHR patterns, each having only one point outside the 10th to 90th centiles. Cases 1 and 9 showed normal FAC in low variation FHR pattern but exhibited predominantly low FAC in high variation FHR pattern. Case 6 had

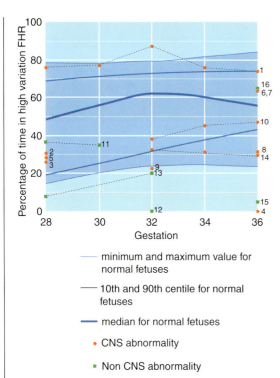

Fig. 23.2 Computerized analysis of fetal behaviour in normal and abnormal fetuses – percentage of time in high variation FHR pattern (from Reference[99]).

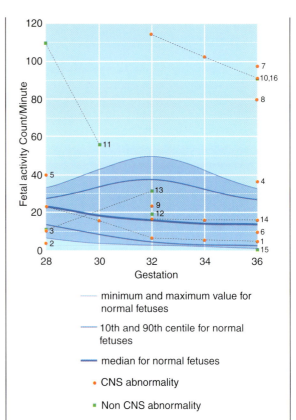

Fig. 23.3 Computerized analysis of fetal behaviour in normal and abnormal fetuses – fetal activity count in low variation FHR (from Reference[99]).

normal FAC in low variation FHR pattern and borderline low FAC in high variation FHR pattern. In Case 12 although a normal FAC in low variation FHR pattern was recorded, no high variation FHR pattern was observed (Fig. 23.2).

These observations are summarized in Table 23.9. In fetuses with abnormality the FAC was abnormal in the majority of recordings. One case (Case 14, Down's syndrome) had normal FAC values in both low and high FHR variation in all but one recording (however, in contrast, that case had consistently abnormal FHR values). In contrast, 8 of the 16 abnormal fetuses had normal FHR values (Cases 2, 3, 5, 6, 7, 10, 11 and 16). At 28 weeks' gestation, five of the six fetuses had abnormal FAC recordings whilst only two of the six had an abnormal FHR pattern. At 36 weeks' gestation seven out of the nine fetuses had an abnormal FAC and five out of nine fetuses had an abnormal FHR pattern duration.

Of the 16 fetuses with abnormality 10

survived and 6 died. In the group of fetuses with CNS anomalies, the four fetuses that died (Cases 1, 2, 5 and 10) and the four fetuses that had major morbidity (Cases 3, 4, 6, 9) all had abnormal FAC values (Table 23.9). No such relationship was seen in the other cases.

Fetuses with different abnormalities showed different profiles of abnormal behaviour (Table 23.9). Furthermore, abnormal behaviour was not confined to those fetuses with structural abnormalities of the CNS. Fetuses with similar abnormalities tended to have similar profiles of behaviour.

It is interesting to speculate why the fetuses are behaving so differently from the normal population. Case 1 (Walker–Warburg syndrome) is a complex condition characterized by agyria, hydrocephalus, cerebellar hypoplasia, brain stem gliosis and retinal dysplasia.[100] The absence of supramedullary fibres which act in an

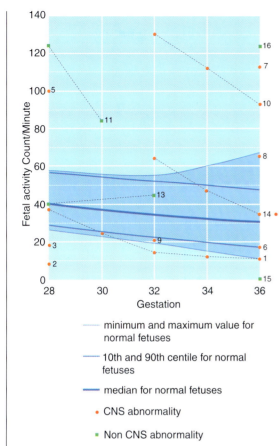

Fig. 23.4 Computerized analysis of fetal behaviour in normal and abnormal fetuses – fetal activity count in high variation FHR (from Reference[99]).

inhibitory fashion on the vagus in particular might be expected to increase the variation of the fetal heart as we observed.[101] Figure 23.4 shows that the fetus had an FAC which fell below the 10th centile as gestation increased. This could be due to the cerebellar hypoplasia which would result in hypotonia.[102]

Case 2 (acrofacial dysotosis) represents a non-random association of vertebral defects, radial hypoplasia, hydrocephalus, cerebellar hypoplasia and renal anomalies.[103] The presence of vertebral column defects leading to spinal nerve compression and cerebellar hypoplasia may result in a decreased FAC as we observed (Figs 23.3, 23.4).

Case 3 (agenesis of the corpus callosum) behaved normally in utero with respect to percentage time spent in low and high

variation FHR (Figs 23.1, 23.2). The FAC rate was below the 10th centile in both low and high FHR variation (Figs 23.3, 23.4). The corpus callosum functions as the connector of all identical points in the cortex of both hemispheres. It plays an important part in co-ordination and learned behaviour thus an abnormal movement pattern would be a consistent finding.

Cases 5, 7 and 8 (ventriculomegaly) and Case 10 (holoprosencephaly) moved at a greater rate than the normal subjects in both low and high variation FHR patterns (Figs 23.3, 23.4). These pathologies can be associated with a disruption of the corticospinal tracts and the normal inhibitory action of these neurones on the peripheral tracts may be absent, leading to excessive movements.

Case 4 (porencephaly) also shows an increased FAC in low variation FHR pattern only (Fig. 23.3) as it did not exhibit any high variation FHR pattern (Fig. 23.2). The major haemorrhagic lesions and subsequent loss of neural tissue in this fetus could disrupt the normal brain function.

Case 11 (congenital diaphragmatic hernia and hydramnios) exhibited unusually high movement patterns (Figs 23.2, 23.3). Postnatally, successful corrective surgery was performed. This baby had no neurological sequelae up to the age of 12 months. The presence of hydramnios with the resultant larger intra-uterine space and less constraint could account for the high FAC rate.

Cases 12 (tricuspid atresia and fetal hydrops) and 13 (Fallot tetralogy and meconium peritonitis) are cardiac anomalies and both exhibited a high percentage of low variation FHR pattern (Fig. 23.1). Our observations might be a reflection of systemic illness in both fetuses (hydrops and peritonitis respectively) rather than the cardiac anomalies per se (see above).

Case 10 (Down's syndrome) spent an unusual amount of time in low variation FHR pattern. A previous report has described an unusually low baseline fetal heart rate in a Down's syndrome case in early pregnancy.[104] To our knowledge, this is

NEUROBEHAVIOURAL STUDIES IN FETUSES WITH ABNORMALITY

Table 23.9
Summary of computerized fetal behaviour characteristics in 16 fetuses with abnormalities (from Reference[99])

Gestation (weeks)	Case number	Low variation FHR pattern	High variation FHR pattern	FAC low variation FHR pattern	FAC high variation FHR pattern
28	1	<10	>90	N	N
	2	N	N	<Min	<Min
	3	N	N	<10	<Min
	5	N	N	>Max	>Max
	11	N	N	>Max	>Max
	13	>Max	<Min	<10	N
30	1	<Min	<90	N	<10
	11	N	N	>Max	>Max
32	1	<Min	<Max	N	<Min
	9	>Max	<Min	N	<10
	10	N	N	>Max	>Max
	12	>Max	<Min	N	Not applicable
	13	>Max	<Min	N	N
	14	N	N	N	>Max
34	1	<Min	>90	N	<Min
	10	N	N	>Max	>Max
	14	>90	<10	N	N
36	1	<Min	=90	N	=Min
	4	>Max	<Min	>Max	Not applicable
	6	N	N	N	<10
	7	N	N	>Max	>Max
	8	>90	<10	>Max	>90
	10	N	N	>Max	>Max
	14	>90	<10	N	N
	15	>Max	<Min	<Min	<Min
	16	N	N	>Max	>Max

<10: Value less than 10th centile of normal population;
>90: Value greater than 90th centile of normal population;
N: Value within normal range;
=: Value equal to the centile;
>Max: Value greater than maximum value of normal population;
<Min: Value less than minimum value of normal population.

the first report of such an unusual fetal heart rate pattern in a case of Down's syndrome in late pregnancy. It is known that functional CNS abnormalities are associated with Down's syndrome; for example, there is a preponderance to develop Alzheimer's disease.[105] After birth, such babies spend a greater than normal proportion of time asleep and low heart rate variation has been thought to be indicative of a physiological state similar to sleep in the fetus.[106] These observations may reflect aberrant autonomic nervous system function as previously reported.[107]

Case 15 (cystic fibrosis) was a chronically ill fetus with meconium peritonitis. The abnormal behavioural profile is arguably a reflection of this.

Case 16 had a diagnosis of arthrogryposis with hydramnios which is the prenatal onset of joint contractures. Reports have suggested such cases can present with reduced fetal movements.[108] In our case the FAC was well above the 90th centiles (Figs 23.3, 23.4). This may be accounted for by the fact that in our case only the distal part of the limbs were affected in this case and that hydramnios was present, resulting in less intra-uterine constraint (as in Case 11).

Our method is able to demonstrate and also measure abnormal fetal behaviour. It appears to hold out hope as a functional adjunct to the evaluation of a fetus with abnormality. Given its advantage over conventional behavioural studies in being applicable in a routine clinical setting it lends itself for evaluation as a screening test. However, at present fetal monitor technology allows us to only assess fetuses from 24 weeks' gestation onwards, so potential problems are not identified until a relatively late stage in pregnancy. This issue is further compounded by the possibility that neurobehavioural handicap might only become apparent in the latter stages of pregnancy when a failure in expected maturation is noted. In addition the anxiety, false-positive and false-negative rates associated with any screening test are potential problems that would have to be carefully documented.

There was no overall relationship between FHR and FAC abnormality and neonatal outcome. However, in the group of fetuses with CNS abnormalities, those with abnormalities leading to neonatal death (Cases 1, 2, 5 and 10) and major morbidity (Cases 3, 4, 6 and 9) tended to have an abnormal FAC. The figures are, however, too small to analyze statistically. The trend that emerges needs further investigation. Eventually this could lead to prenatal identification of 'severe' and 'less severe' cases.

It is difficult to draw any firm conclusions about the relationship between fetal behavioural patterns and neurological status in the survivors with congenital abnormality because of the small numbers, the largely short term follow-up data and the differing pathologies monitored. Further evaluation of the computerized fetal behavioural programme is necessary. However, this method holds out the possibility of easier study of the relationship between neurodevelopmental compromise acquired during pregnancy, before labour and delivery, and subsequent disability manifest in childhood.

Stimulated behaviour and fetal abnormality

Apart from exhibiting abnormalities in passive behaviour, anencephalic fetuses do not show a response to VAS[26] nor do they habituate.[66]

There has been a case report of a partial response to VAS in a fetus with the Pena-Shokeir syndrome.[109] In that case, VAS failed to elicit any fetal movements; however, a blunted, brief acceleration of the FHR was noted. At autopsy the fetus had skeletal

neurogenic atrophy yet an anatomically normal auditory system. The authors suggest the normal prolonged increase in the FHR after VAS stimulation is sustained by active fetal movements, absent in the index case because of joint contractures.

Habituation and fetal abnormality

Habituation in the presence of fetal abnormality has been studied and reported in two conditions – anencephaly and trisomy 21.

Anencephalic fetuses fail to respond to VAS, thus it is impossible to demonstrate habituation.[26,66]

In an elegant study reported by Hepper & Shahidullah[110] fetuses with trisomy 21 were either slower to habituate or failed to habituate altogether. Furthermore, the Down's syndrome fetuses showed a longer latency of response to the initial stimulus.

Continuum of fetal and infant behaviour

At present there is limited data about the continuity between the behaviour observed in utero and that seen in childhood. However, those reports that do exist support the case for there being clear continuity.

In normal babies there is a clear similarity between the behaviour they exhibit prior to birth and that which they manifest in the early newborn period.[106] Habituation characteristics in normal fetuses in late pregnancy have been shown to correlate significantly with developmental scores at 1 year of age.[66] In addition, there have been anecdotal reports of fetuses with behavioural abnormality detected in utero, considered neurologically normal, who subsequently were found to have serious neurodevelopmental abnormality identified in infancy.[111]

Conclusions

It is clear that in the near future fetuses with abnormality will be evaluated by ultrasound not only to clarify anatomical detail as at present but also to document function.

Computerized methods of fetal behavioural analysis represent a significant advance. They offer great advantages in terms of speed, convenience and objectivity which will be essential for both screening and diagnosis.

Finally, there is a need for such methods to be applied at an earlier stage in pregnancy, in particular before 24 weeks. However, it is possible that some abnormalities of fetal neurodevelopment may only be detected at a late stage in pregnancy.

Acknowledgement

We are grateful to Mrs Lynda Straw for secretarial assistance in the preparation of the manuscript.

References

1. James D, Pillai M, Smolenic J. Neurobehavioural development in the human fetus. In: Lecanuet J P, Fifer W P, Krasnegor N A, Smotherman W P, eds. Fetal development – a psychobiological perspective. New Jersey: Lawrence Erlbaum Assoc; 1995: 107–128.
2. Vindla S, James D. Fetal behaviour as a test of fetal wellbeing (Commentary). Br J Obstet Gynaecol 1995;102:597–600.
3. Pillai M, James D. Development of human fetal behaviour. A review. Fetal Diagn Ther 1990;5:15–32.
4. Nijhuis J, Prechtl H F R, Martin C B, Bots R S G M. Are there behavioural states in the human fetus? Early Hum Dev 1982;6:177–195.
5. Gagnon R, Hunse C, Fellows F, Carmichael L, Patrick J. Human fetal responses to vibratory acoustic stimulation from twenty-six weeks to term. Am J Obstet Gynecol 1987;157:1375–1381.
6. Leader L R, Baillie P, Martin B, Vermeulen E. The assessment and significance of habituation to a repeated stimulus by the human fetus. Early Hum Dev 1982;7:211–219.
7. Van Dongen L G R, Goudie E G. Fetal movement patterns in the first trimester of pregnancy. Br J Obstet Gynaecol 1980;87:191–193.
8. De Vries J I P, Visser G H A, Prechtl H F R. The emergence of fetal behaviour: I. Qualitative aspects. Early Hum Dev 1982;15:301–322.
9. De Vries J I P, Visser G H A, Prechtl H F R. The emergency of fetal behaviour: III. Individual differences and consistences. Early Hum Dev 1988;16:85–104.
10. De Vries J I P, Visser G H A, Mulder E J H, Prechtl H F R. Diurnal and other variations in fetal movement and heart rate patterns at 20 to 22 weeks. Early Hum Dev 1987;15:333–348.
11. Nasello-Paterson C, Natale R, Connors G. Ultrasonic evaluation of fetal body movements over twenty-four hours in the human fetus at twenty-four to twenty-eight weeks gestation. Am J Obstet Gynecol 1988;158:312–316.
12. Patrick J, Campbell K, Carmichael L, Natale R, Richardson B. Patterns of gross fetal body movements over 24 hours observation interval in the last 10 weeks of pregnancy. Am J Obstet Gynecol 1982;136:471–477.
13. Arduini D, Rizzo G, Parlati E, et al. Modifications of ultradian and circadian rhythms of fetal heart rate after fetal-maternal adrenal gland suppression: A double blind study. Prenat Diagn 1986;6:409–417.
14. Sorohin Y, Bottoms S F, Dierker L J, Rosen M G. The clustering of fetal heart rate changes and fetal movements between 20 and 30 weeks of gestation. Am J Obstet Gynecol 1982;143:952–957.
15. Pillai M, James D. The importance of the behavioural states in biophysical assessment of the term human fetus. Br J Obstet Gynaecol 1990;97:1130–1134.
16. Pillai M, James D K. Behavioural states in normal mature human fetuses. Arch Dis Child 1990;65:39–43.
17. Pillai M, James D K. The development of fetal heart rate patterns during pregnancy. Obstet Gynecol 1990;76:812–816.
18. Pillai M, James D K. Sinusoidal fetal heart rate associated with fetal mouthing. Eur J Obstet Gynecol Reprod Biol 1990;38:151–156.
19. Marsal K. Ultrasonic assessment of fetal activity. Clin Obstet Gynecol 1983;10:541–563.
20. Van Woerden E E, van Geijn H P, Caron F J M, Mantel R, Swartjes J M, Arts N F T. Fetal hiccups. Characteristics and relation to fetal heart rate. Eur J Obstet Gynecol Reprod Biol 1989;30:209–216.
21. Natale R, Patrick J, Richardson B. Effects of human maternal venous plasma glucose concentrations on fetal breathing movements. Am J Obstet Gynecol 1978;132:36–41.
22. Connors G, Hunse C, Carmichael L, Natale R, Richardson B. The role of carbon dioxide in the generation of human fetal breathing movements. Am J Obstet Gynecol 1988;158:322–327.
23. Bekedam B J, Visser G H A. Effects of hypoxemic events on breathing, body movements and heart rate variations: A study in growth-retarded human fetuses. Am J Obstet Gynecol 1985;153:52–57.
24. Pillai M, James D K. Hiccups and breathing in the human fetus. Arch Dis Child 1990;65:1072–1075.
25. Leader L R, Baillie P, Martin B, Molteno C. Fetal responses to vibrotactile stimuli: a possible predictor of fetal and neonatal outcome. Aust NZ J Obstet Gynaecol 1984;24:251–256.
26. Groome L J, Gotleib S J, Neely C L, Waters M D. Development trends in fetal habituation to vibroacoustic stimulation. Am J Perinatol 1993;10:46–49.

27. Gagnon R. Stimulation of fetuses with sound and vibration. Semin Perinatol 1989;13:393–402.

28. Leader L R, Bennett M J. Fetal habituation and its clinical application. In: Leven M I, Lilford R J, eds. Fetal and Neonatal Neurology and Neurosurgery. Edinburgh: Churchill Livingstone: 45–60.

29. Peiper A. Sinnesemphfindungen des Kindes vor seiner Gerbert. Monat Kinderheilkunde 1925;29:237–241.

30. Leader L R, Baillie P, Martin B, Vermenlen E. Fetal habituation in high risk pregnancies. Br J Obstet Gynaecol 1982;89:441–446.

31. Madison L S, Adubato S A, Madison J K, et al. Foetal response decrement: True habituation. Development and Behavioural Pediatrics 1986;7:14–29.

32. Groome L J, Watson J E, Dykman R A. Heart rate changes following habituation testing of the motor response in normal human fetuses. Early Hum Dev 1994;36:69–77.

33. Hepper P, Scott D, Shahidullah S. Newborn and fetal response to maternal voice. Journal of Reproductive Infant Psychology 1992;11:147–153.

34. Lecanuet J P, Granier-Deferre C, Jacquet A Y, Capponi I, Ledru I. Prenatal discriminating of a male and female voice uttering the same sentence. Early Development Parent 1993;2:217–228.

35. Dawes G S, Redman C W G, Smith J H. Improvements in the registration and analysis of fetal heart rate records at the bedside. Br J Obstet Gynaecol 1985;92:317–325.

36. Melendez T D, Rayburn W P, Smith C V. Characterisation of fetal body movement recorded by the Hewlett-Packard M-1350-A fetal monitor. Am J Obstet Gynecol 1992;167:700–702.

37. James D, Parker M, Smoleniec J. Comprehensive fetal assessment using three ultrasound characteristics. Am J Obstet Gynecol 1992;166:1486–1495.

38. Ling N P. Auditory evoked response of the human fetus: simplified methodology. J Perinat Med 1991;19:177–183.

39. Groome L J, Mooney M M, Dykman R A. Motor and cardiac response during habituation testing: Demonstration of exaggerated cardiac reactivity in a subgroup of normal human fetuses. Am J Perinatol 1994;11:73–79.

40. James D. Limitations of fetal biophysical assessment. Contemp Rev Obstet Gynaecol 1991;3:69–73.

41. Patrick J, Campbell K, Carmichael L, Natale R, Richardson B. A definition of human fetal apnoea and the distribution of fetal apnoeic intervals during the last ten weeks of pregnancy. Am J Obstet Gynecol 1980;136:471–477.

42. Johnson M J, Paine L L, Mulder H H, Cezar C, Gegor C, Johnson T R. Population differences of fetal biophysical and behavioural characteristics. Am J Obstet Gynecol 1992;166:138–142.

43. Salvador H S, Koos B J. Effects of regular and decaffeinated coffee on fetal breathing and heart rate. Am J Obstet Gynecol 1989;160:1043–1047.

44. Petrikovsky B M, Ventzileos A M, Nochimson D J. Heart rate cyclicity during labor in healthy term fetuses. Am J Perinatol 1989;6:289–291.

45. Reddy U M, Paine L L, Gegor C L, Johnson M J, Johnson T R. Fetal movement during labour. Am J Obstet Gynecol 1991;165:1073–1076.

46. Wim H N, Hess O, Goldstein I, Wackers F, Robbins J C. Fetal responses to maternal exercise: effect on fetal breathing and baby movement. Am J Obstet Gynecol 1994;11:263–266.

47. Clapp J F, Little K D, Capeless E L. Fetal heart rate response to sustained recreational exercise. Am J Obstet Gynecol 1993;168:198–206.

48. Vaha-Eskeli K, Erkkola R. The effect of short-term heat stress on uterine contractility, fetal heart rate and fetal movements at late pregnancy. Eur J Obstet Gynecol Reprod Biol 1991;38:9–14.

49. Watson W J, Katz V L, Hackney A C, Gall M M, McMurray R G. Fetal responses to maximal swimming and cycling exercise during pregnancy. Obstet Gynecol 1991;77:382–386.

50. Coomy J O, Fitzhardings P M. Handicap in the preterm small-for-gestational-age infant. J Pediat 1979;94:779–786.

51. Ounsted M, Moar V, Scott A. Growth in the first four years: II Diversity within groups of small-for-dates and large-for-dates babies. Early Hum Dev 1982;7:29–39.

52. Soothill P W, Ajuyi R A, Campbell S, Ross E M, Nicolaides K H. Fetal oxygenation at cordocentesis, maternal smoking and childhood neuro-development. Eur J Obstet Gynecol Reprod Biol 1995;59:21–24.

53. Gould J B, Gluck L, Kulovich M V. The relationship between accelerated pulmonary maturity and accelerated neurological maturity in certain chronically stressed pregnancies. Am J Obstet Gynecol 1977;127:181–186.

54. Bekedam D J, Visser G H A, de Vries J J, Prechtl H F R. Motor behaviour in the growth retarded fetus. Early Hum Dev 1985;12:155–165.

55. Sival D A, Visser G H A, Prechtl H F R. The effect of intrauterine growth retardation on the quality of general movements in the human fetus. Early Hum Dev 1992;28:119–132.

56. Sival D A, Visser G H A, Prechtl H F R. The relationship between quantity and quality of prenatal movements in pregnancies complicated by growth retardation and premature rupture of membranes. Early Hum Dev 1992;30:193–209.

57. Sadovsky E, Yaffe H. Daily fetal movement recording and fetal prognosis. Obstet Gynecol 1973;41:845–849.

58. James D, Pillai M. Behavioural development and intrauterine growth retardation. Current Obstetrics and Gynaecology 1993;3:196–199.

59. Visser G H A, Bekedam D J, Ribbert L S M. Changes in antepartum heart rate patterns with progressive deterioration of the fetal condition. Int J Biomed Comput 1990;25:239–246.

60. Rizzo G, Arduini D, Romanini C, Mancuso S. Fetal behaviour in growth retardation: its relationship to fetal blood flow. Prenat Diagn 1987;7:229–238.

61. Vleit M A T, Martin C B, Nijhuis J G, Prechtl H F R.

The relationship between fetal activity and behavioural states and fetal breathing movements in normal and growth retarded fetuses. Am J Obstet Gynecol 1985;153:582–588.

62. Natale R, Clelow F, Dawes G S. Measurements of fetal forelimb movements in lambs in utero. Am J Obstet Gynecol 1981;140:545–551.

63. Arduini D, Rizzo G, Caforio L, Boccolini M R, Romanini C, Mancuso S. Longitudinal assessment of behavioural transitions in healthy human fetuses during the last trimester of pregnancy. J Perinat Med 1991;1:67–72.

64. Gagnon R, Hunse C, Carmichael L, Fellows F, Patrick J. Fetal heart rate and activity patterns in growth-retarded fetuses: changes after vibratory acoustic stimulation. Am J Obstet Gynecol 1988;158:265–271.

65. Gagnon R, Foreman J, Hunse C, Patrick J. Effects of low frequency vibration on human term fetuses. Am J Obstet Gynecol 1989;161:1479–1489.

66. Yogman M W, Cole P, Als J, Lester B M. Behaviour of newborns of diabetic mothers. Infant Behavior and Development 1982;5:331–340.

67. Mulder E J H, Visser G H A. Growth and motor developments in fetuses of women with type-1 diabetes. I. Early growth patterns. Early Hum Dev 1991;25:91–106.

68. Mulder E J H, Visser G H A. Growth and motor developments in fetuses of women with type-1 diabetes. II. Emergence of specific movement patterns. Early Hum Dev 1991;25:107–115.

69. Chajotte C, Forman L, Gandhi J. Heart rate patterns in fetuses exposed to cocaine. Obstet Gynecol 1991;78:323–325.

70. Wittmann B K, Segal S. A comparison of the effects of single- and split-dose methadone administration on the fetus: ultrasound evaluation. Int J Addict 1991;26:213–218.

71. Tabor B L, Soffici A R, Smith-Wallace T, Yonekura M L. The effect of maternal cocaine use on the fetus: changes in antepartum fetal heart rate tracings. Am J Obstet Gynecol 1991;165:1278–1281.

72. Swartjes J M, van Geijn H P, Meinardi H, van Woerden E E, Mantel R. Fetal motility and chronic exposure to antiepileptic drugs. Eur J Obstet Gynecol Reprod Biol 1992;45:37–45.

73. Atkinson M W, Belfort M A, Saade G P, Moise K J. The relation between magnesium sulfate therapy and fetal heart rate. Obstet Gynecol 1994;83:967–970.

74. Shere D M. Blunted fetal response to vibroacoustic stimulation associated with maternal intravenous magnesium sulfate therapy. Am J Perinatol 1994;11:401–403.

75. Katz V L, Seeds J W. Fetal and neonatal cardiovascular complications from beta-sympathomimetic therapy for tocolysis. Am J Obstet Gynecol 1989;161:1–4.

76. Haltak M, Moise K, Hira N, Dorman K F, Smith E O, Cotton D B. The effect of tocolytic agents (indomethacin and terbutaline) on fetal breathing and body movements: a prospective randomised

double-blind, placebo-controlled clinical trial. Am J Obstet Gynecol 1992;167:1059–1063.

77. Sorokin Y, Hallak M, Klein O, Kalderon I, Abramovici H. Effects of induction of labor with prostaglandin E, on fetal breathing and body movements: controlled, randomised, double-blind study. Obstet Gynecol 1992;80:788–791.

78. Mulder E J, Derks J B, Zouneveld M F, Bruinse H W, Visser G H. Transient reduction in fetal activity and heart rate variation after maternal betamethasone administration. Early Hum Dev 1994; 36:49–60.

79. Derks J B, Mulder E J, Visser G H. The effects of maternal betamethasone administration on the fetus. Br J Obstet Gynaecol 1995;102:40–46.

80. Dawes G S, Serra-Serra V, Moulden M, Redman C W. Dexamethasone and fetal heart rate variation. Br J Obstet Gynaecol 1994;101:675–679.

81. Ventzileos A M, Campbell W A, Ingardia C J, et al. Fetal biophysical profile and its predictive value. Obstet Gynecol 1983;91:271–278.

82. Del Valle G O, Joffe G M, Izquierdo L A, Smith J F, Gilson G J, Current L B. The biophysical profile and the nonstress test: poor predictors of chorionamnionitis and fetal infection inprolonger premature rupture of membranes. Obstet Gynecol 1992;80:106–110.

83. Nijhuis J G, Kruyt N, Van Wijck J A M. Fetal brain death: two case reports. Br J Obstet Gynaecol 1987;95:197–200.

84. Brar H S, Platt K D. Fetal biophysical score and fetal well-being. In: Hill A, Volpe J J, eds. Fetal Neurology. New York: Raven Press; 95–115.

85. Boylan P. Sinusoidal like tracing in a fetus with rhesus-hemolytic anemia. Am J Obstet Gynecol 1983;145:892–893.

86. Rosenn B, Ben Chetrit A, Palti Z, Hurwitz A. Sinusoidal fetal heart rate pattern due to massive fetomaternal transfusion. Int J Gynaecol Obstet 1990;31:271–273.

87. Lubbe W F, Butler W S, Palmer S J, Liggins G C. Lupus anticoagulant in pregnancy. Br J Obstet Gynaecol 1984;91:357–363.

88. Ramsay I. Thyroid disease. In: de Swiet M, ed. Medical disorders in Obstetric Practice. Oxford: Blackwell Scientific; 385–404.

89. Visser G H A, Laurini R N, De Vries J I P, Bekedam D J, Prechtl J F R. Abnormal motor behaviour in anencephalic fetuses. Early Hum Dev 1985;12:173–182.

90. De Hann J, van Bemmell J H, Stolte L A M, et al. Quantitative evaluation of fetal heart rate patterns. II. The significance of the fixed heart rate during pregnancy and labour. Eur J Obstet Gynecol Reprod Biol 1971;3:103–110.

91. Hepper P G, Shahidullah S. Trisomy 18: behavioural and structural abnormalities. An ultrasonographic case study. Ultrasound Obstet Gynecol 1992;2:48–50.

92. Pillai M, Garrett C, James D. Bizarre fetal behaviour associated with lethal congenital abnormalities: A case report. Eur J Obstet Gynecol Reprod Biol 1991;39:215–218.

93. Hammond E, Donnenfeld A E. Fetal akinesia. Obstet Gynecol Surv 1995;50:240–249.

94. Hsu C-D, Feng T I, Crawford T O, Johnson T R B. Unusual fetal movement in congenital myotonic dystrophy. Fetal Diagn Ther 1993;8:200–202.

95. Anthony J, Mascarenhas L, O'Brien J, Battachargee A K, Gould S. Lethal multiple pterygium syndrome. The importance of fetal posture in mid-trimester diagnosis by ultrasound: discussion and case report. Ultrasound Obstet Gynecol 1993;3:212–216.

96. Robin N H, Curtis M T, Mulla W, et al. Non-immune hydrops fetalis associated with impaired fetal movement: a case report and review. Am J Med Genet 1994;53:251–254.

97. Maxwell D J, Crawford D C, Curry P V M, Tynan M J, Allan L D. Obstetric importance, diagnosis and management of fetal tachycardias. BMJ 1988;297:107–110.

98. Horimoto N, Koyanagi T, Maeda H, et al. Can brain impairment be detected by in utero behavioural patterns? Arch Dis Child 1993;69:3–8.

99. Vindla S, Sahota D S, Coppens M, James D K. Computerised analysis of behaviour in fetuses with congenital abnormalities. Ultrasound Obstet Gynecol 1997;9:302–309.

100. Larroche J C, Encha-Razavi F. Abnormalities of the fetal central nervous system. In: Wigglesworth J S, Singer D B, eds. Textbook of Fetal and Perinatal Pathology. Cambridge, Massachusetts: Blackwell Scientific Publications: 1991;798–800.

101. Schifferli P Y, Caldeyro-Barcia R. Effects of atropine and beta-adrenergic drugs on the heart rate of the human fetus. In: Boreus L O, ed. Fetal Pharmacology. New York: Raven Press: 1973:259–279.

102. Walton J, ed. Brain's Textbook of Neurology. Oxford: Oxford University Press; 1993:39.

103. Rodriguez J I, Palacios J, Urioste M. New acrofacialdysostosis syndrome in three sibs. Am J Med Genet 1990;35:484–489.

104. Schats R, Jansen C A M, Wladimiroff J W. Abnormal fetal heart rate pattern in early pregnancy associated with Down's Syndrome. Hum Reprod 1990;5:877–879.

105. Cole G, Neal J W, Fraser W I, Cowie V A. Autopsy findings in patients with mental handicap. Journal of Intellectual Disability Research 1994;38:9–26.

106. Pillai M, James D. Are the behavioural states of the newborn comparable to those of the fetus? Early Hum Dev 1990;22:39–49.

107. Kakigi R, Kuroda Y. Brain stem auditory evoked potentials in adults with Down's syndrome. Electroencephalogr Clin Neurophysiol 1992;84:293–295.

108. Jones K L. Smith's Recognizable Patterns of Human Malformation. 4th ed. London: WB Saunders 1988:140–141.

109. Shever D M, Sanko S R, Meltaj L A, Woods J R. Absent fetal movement response with a blunted cardioacceleratory fetal response to external vibratory acoustic stimulation in a fetus with the Pena–Shokeir syndrome (fetal akinesia and hypokinesia). Am J Perinatol 1992;9:1–4.

110. Hepper P G, Shahidullah S. Habituation in normal and Down's syndrome fetuses. Q J Exp Psychol 1992;44B:305–317.

111. Pillai M, James D. Absence of fetal breathing and abnormal fetal behaviour in prolonged preterm ruptured membranes: case report. Ultrasound Obstet Gynecol 1992;2:44–47.

Index